Handbook of
Cancer Chemotherapy

Handbook of Cancer Chemotherapy

Third Edition

Edited by
Roland T. Skeel, M.D.

Professor of Medicine and Chief of Hematology and Oncology, Medical College of Ohio; Attending Physician, Medical College of Ohio Hospital, Toledo

Little, Brown and Company
Boston/Toronto/London

Contents

Contributing Authors

Jane B. Alavi, M.D.
Associate Professor of Medicine, University of
Pennsylvania School of Medicine,
Philadelphia

Robert S. Benjamin, M.D.
Professor of Medicine and Chief of Melanoma Sarcoma
Section, Department of Medical Oncology, The University
of Texas M.D. Anderson Cancer Center, Houston

Ronald C. DeConti, M.D.
Professor of Medicine, Albany Medical College; Chief of
Oncology, Albany Veterans Administration Medical
Center, Albany, New York

William D. DeWys, M.D.
Medical Oncologist, Capital Area Permanente Medical
Group, Washington, D.C.

Ralph R. Dobelbower, M.D., Ph.D.
Professor and Chairman of Radiation Therapy, Medical
College of Ohio; Attending Physician, Medical College of
Ohio Hospital, Toledo; Medical Director, Marion Regional
Cancer Center, Marion, Ohio

Kathy S. N. Franco, M.D.
Associate Professor of Psychiatry, University of Vermont
College of Medicine; Director of Consultation-Liaison
Psychiatry, Medical Center Hospital of Vermont,
Burlington

Roberto Franco-Saenz, M.D.
Professor of Medicine and Chief of Endocrinology and
Metabolism, Medical College of Ohio; Attending
Physician, Medical College of Ohio Hospital,
Toledo

Samir N. Khleif, M.D.
Medical Oncology Staff Fellow, National Cancer
Institute, Bethesda, Maryland

Neil A. Lachant, M.D.
Associate Professor of Medicine, Medical College of Ohio;
Attending Physician, Medical College of Ohio Hospital,
Toledo

Robert B. Livingston, M.D.
Professor of Medicine and Head of Oncology, University
of Washington School of Medicine; Staff Physician,
University Hospital, Seattle

Rodger D. MacArthur, M.D.
Assistant Professor of Medicine, Medical College of Ohio;
Attending Physician, Medical College of Ohio Hospital,
Toledo

Gerald W. Marsa, M.D.
Clinical Associate Professor of Radiation Therapy,
Medical College of Ohio, Toledo; Radiation Oncologist,
Flower Memorial Hospital, Sylvania, Ohio

John C. Marsh, M.D.
Professor of Medicine and Lecturer in Pharmacology,
Yale University School of Medicine; Attending Physician
(Internal Medicine), Yale-New Haven Hospital,
New Haven, Connecticut

Hollis W. Merrick, M.D.
Associate Professor of Surgery, Medical College of Ohio;
Attending Physician, Medical College of Ohio Hospital,
Toledo

Larry Nathanson, M.D.
Professor of Medicine, State University of New York at
Stony Brook Health Sciences Center, Stony Brook;
Director of Oncology, Hematology Division, Winthrop-
University Hospital, Mineola, New York

Martin M. Oken, M.D.
Professor of Medicine, University of Minnesota Medical
School—Minneapolis; Director, Virginia Piper Cancer
Institute, Abbott Northwestern Hospital, Minneapolis

Robert F. Ozols, M.D., Ph.D.
Chairman of Medical Oncology, Fox Chase Cancer
Center, Philadelphia

David R. Parkinson, M.D.
Head of Biologics Evaluation Section, Investigational
Drug Branch, Cancer Therapy Evaluation Program,
Division of Cancer Treatment, National Cancer Institute,
Bethesda, Maryland

Walter D. Y. Quan, M.D.
Medical Oncology Fellow, Department of Medicine,
Medical College of Ohio, Toledo

Jane W. Ringlein, R.N., M.S.N.
Adjunct Clinical Faculty, Medical College of Ohio School
of Nursing; Instructor, School of Nursing, St. Vincent
Hospital and Medical Center, Toledo

Ana Rubio, M.D., Ph.D.
Senior Instructor, Community and Preventive Medicine,
University of Rochester School of Medicine and
Dentistry, Rochester, New York

David J. Schifeling, M.D.
Assistant Professor of Medicine, University of Tennessee,
Memphis, College of Medicine, Memphis

Bahu S. Shaikh, M.D.
Clinical Associate Professor of Medicine, Medical College
of Ohio, Toledo; Attending Physician, Flower Hospital,
Sylvania, Ohio

Joy D. Skeel, M.Div.
Associate Professor and Director of Medical Humanities,
Department of Psychiatry, Medical College of Ohio,
Toledo

Roland T. Skeel, M.D.
Professor of Medicine and Chief of Hematology and
Oncology, Medical College of Ohio; Attending Physician,
Medical College of Ohio Hospital, Toledo

Mary R. Smith, M.D.
Associate Professor of Medicine and Pathology, Medical
College of Ohio; Attending Physician, Medical College of
Ohio Hospital, Toledo

Richard S. Stein, M.D.
Associate Professor of Medicine, Vanderbilt University
School of Medicine, Nashville, Tennessee

Michael Weintraub, M.D.
Associate Professor of Community and Preventive
Medicine, Pharmacology, and Medicine, University of
Rochester School of Medicine and Dentistry, Rochester,
New York

Peter White, M.D.
Professor of Medicine and Associate Dean, Medical
College of Ohio; Attending Physician, Medical College of
Ohio Hospital, Toledo

Preface

A long-term goal of cancer chemotherapy is to cure cancers that are not amenable to surgical eradication. This is possible for a small percentage of some common tumors, particularly when there is only micrometastasis, and for a larger fraction of some less common tumors. But for most patients, chemotherapy remains palliative, at best. The hope for radically improved, more specific medical treatment for cancer has been stimulated by the tremendous recent growth of information on the molecular basis of cancer development. While this new knowledge offers the potential for more specific and effective therapy of cancer by interference with oncogenes and oncogene products, or manipulating "anti-oncogenes" or their products, its practical value in the treatment of patients remains unrealized. In contrast, continuing research into ways to enhance inherent biologic responses of the host to cancer has resulted in improved therapy in several cancers, and current trials that combine the biologic therapies with each other and with chemotherapy offer a realistic expectation of continued progress during the 1990s. The past several years has also witnessed the introduction of new chemotherapeutic agents, more effective combinations, and better ways of using older agents that have resulted in cures of selected cancers and better palliation in many others.

The recent introduction of biologic response modifiers into clinical practice and major changes in the chemotherapy of some cancers have led to large modifications of several sections of the *Handbook of Cancer Chemotherapy*. A chapter on the principles of biologic therapy has been added, and the indications, dose schedules, and toxicities of these agents are added to the chapter on antineoplastic drugs. The uses of biologic agents alone and with chemotherapy are discussed in the chapters on individual cancers. Several chapters have undergone major revision or expansion necessitating two separate chapters. Thus, there are now individual chapters on acute and chronic leukemias as well as a new chapter on myeloproliferative and myelodysplastic syndromes. The management of infections, one of the most complex and critical of all complications of intensive cancer chemotherapy, has been greatly expanded and given a separate chapter. Acute chemotherapy symptom management has been expanded and separated from the principles of nursing management. The chapter discussing the acquired immunodeficiency syndrome (AIDS) has been narrowed to emphasize the malignancies associated with AIDS, for which experience in treating this disease has grown in the past five years. The increasingly important area of ethical considerations in cancer therapy is expanded to give the reader a better understanding of basic concepts and their application to patients undergoing cancer treatment.

The *Handbook* continues to be a practical pocket reference with a wealth of information for oncology specialists, nononcology physicians, house officers, oncology nurses, and medical students. Unlike any other book, it combines in one place the rationale and the specific details necessary to safely administer chemotherapy for most human cancers. We believe that with the additions and revisions in this edition the *Handbook* will continue to be a valuable resource to all kinds of physicians, nurses, and students.

R.T.S.

Basic Principles and Considerations of Rational Chemotherapy

Biologic and Pharmacologic Basis of Cancer Chemotherapy

Roland T. Skeel

I. **General mechanisms by which chemotherapeutic agents control cancer.** The purpose of treating cancer with chemotherapeutic agents is to prevent cancer cells from multiplying, invading, metastasizing, and ultimately killing the host (patient). Most agents currently in use appear to exert their effect primarily on cell multiplication and tumor growth. Because cell multiplication is a characteristic of many normal cells as well as cancer cells, most cancer chemotherapeutic agents also have toxic effects on normal cells, particularly those with a rapid rate of turnover, such as bone marrow and mucous membrane cells. The goal in selecting an effective drug, therefore, is to find an agent that has marked growth inhibitory or controlling effect on the cancer cell with minimal toxic effect on the host. In the most effective chemotherapeutic regimens, the drugs are capable not only of inhibiting but of completely eradicating all neoplastic cells while sufficiently preserving normal marrow and other target organs to allow a return to normal, or at least satisfactory, function.

Ideally, the pharmacologist or medicinal chemist would like to look at the cancer cell, discover how it differs from the normal host cell, and then design a chemotherapeutic agent to capitalize on that difference. In practice, often less rational means are used. The effectiveness of agents is discovered by treating either animal or human neoplasms, after which the pharmacologist attempts to discover why the agent works as well as it does. With few exceptions, the reasons chemotherapeutic agents are more effective against cancer cells than normal cells are poorly understood.

Inhibition of cell multiplication and tumor growth can take place at several levels within the cell.

1. Macromolecular synthesis and function
2. Cytoplasmic organization
3. Cell membrane synthesis function

Most agents currently in use or under investigation, with the exception of immunotherapeutic agents and other biologic response modifiers, appear to have their primary effect on either macromolecular synthesis or function. This effect means that they interfere with either the synthesis of DNA, RNA, or proteins or the appropriate functioning of the preformed molecule. When interference in the macromolecular synthesis or function of the neoplastic cell population is sufficiently great, a proportion of the cells die. (Cell death may or may not take place at the time of exposure to the drug. Often a cell must undergo several divisions before the lethal event that took place earlier finally results in the death of the cell.) Because only a proportion of the cells die with a given treatment, repeated doses of chemotherapy

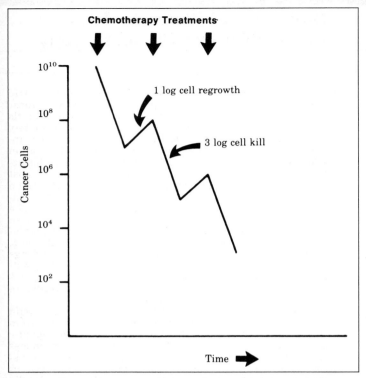

Fig. 1-1. Effect of chemotherapy on cancer cell numbers. In an ideal system, chemotherapy kills a constant proportion of the remaining cancer cells with each dose. Between doses, cell regrowth occurs. When therapy is successful, cell killing is greater than cell growth.

must be used to continue to reduce the cell number (Fig. 1-1). In an ideal system, each time the dose is repeated the same *proportion* of cells—not the same absolute number—is killed. In the example shown in Figure 1-1, 99.9% (3 logs) of the cancer cells are killed with each treatment, and there is a 10-fold (1 log) growth between treatments for a net reduction of 2 logs with each treatment. Starting at 10^{10} cells (about 10 gm or 10 cm^3 leukemia cells), it would take five treatments to reach fewer than 10^0, or one, cell. Such a model makes certain assumptions that rarely are strictly true in clinical practice.

1. All cells in a tumor population are equally sensitive to a drug.
2. Drug accessibility and cell sensitivity are independent of the location of the cells within the host and independent of local host factors, such as blood supply or surrounding fibrosis.

  3. Cell sensitivity does not change during the course of therapy.

  The lack of curability of most initially sensitive tumors is probably a reflection of the degree to which these assumptions do not hold true.

II. Tumor cell kinetics and chemotherapy. Cancer cells, unlike other body cells, are characterized by a growth process whereby their sensitivity to normal controlling factors has been partially or completely lost. As a result of this uncontrolled growth, it was once thought that cancer cells grew or multiplied faster than normal cells, and that this growth rate was responsible for their sensitivity to chemotherapy. It now is known that most cancer cells grow less rapidly than the more active, normal cells, such as bone marrow. Thus although the growth rate of many cancers is faster than that of normal surrounding tissues, growth rate alone cannot explain the greater sensitivity of cancer cells to chemotherapy.

 A. Tumor growth. The growth of a tumor depends on several interrelated factors.

  1. Cell cycle time, or the average time for a cell that has just completed mitosis to grow and again divide and pass through mitosis, determines the maximum growth rate for a tumor but probably does not determine drug sensitivity. The relative proportion of cell cycle time taken up by the DNA synthesis phase may relate to drug sensitivity of some types (S-phase specific) of chemotherapeutic agents.

  2. Growth fraction, or the fraction of cells undergoing cell division, represents the portion of cells that are sensitive to drugs whose major effect is exerted on cells that are actively dividing. If the growth fraction approaches 1 and the cell death rate is low, the *tumor doubling time* approximates the cell cycle time.

  3. Total number of cells in the population (determined at some arbitrary time at which the growth measurement is started) is clinically important because it is an index of how advanced is the cancer; it frequently correlates with normal organ dysfunction. As the total number of cells increases, so does the number of resistant cells, which in turn leads to decreased curability. Large tumors may also have greater compromise of blood supply and oxygenation, which can impair drug delivery to the tumor cells and impair drug sensitivity to both chemotherapy and radiotherapy.

  4. Intrinsic cell death rate of tumors is difficult to measure in patients but probably makes a major contribution by slowing the growth rate of many solid tumors.

 B. Cell cycle. The cell cycle of cancer cells is qualitatively the same as that of normal cells (Fig. 1-2). Each cell begins its growth during a postmitotic period, a phase called G_1, during which enzymes necessary for DNA production, other proteins, and RNA are produced. G_1 is fol-

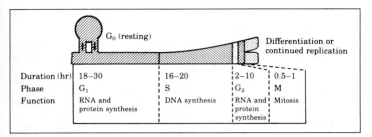

Fig. 1-2. Cell cycle time for human tissues has a wide range (16–260 hours), with marked differences among normal and tumor tissues. Normal marrow and gastrointestinal-lining cells have cell cycle times of 24–48 hours. Representative durations and the kinetic or synthetic activity are indicated for each phase.

lowed by a period of DNA *synthesis* (S) in which essentially all DNA synthesis for a given cycle takes place. When DNA synthesis is complete, the cell enters a *premitotic period* (G_2) during which further protein and RNA synthesis occur. This gap is followed immediately by *mitosis* (M), at the end of which actual physical division takes place, two daughter cells are formed, and each again enters G_1. The G_1 phase is in equilibrium with a *resting state* called G_0. Cells in G_0 are relatively inactive with respect to macromolecular synthesis and are consequently insensitive to many chemotherapeutic agents, particularly those that affect macromolecular synthesis.

C. **Phase and cell cycle specificity.** Most chemotherapeutic agents can be grouped according to whether they depend on cells being in cycle (i.e., not in G_0) and, if they depend on the cell being in cycle, whether their activity is greater when the cell is in a specific phase of the cycle. It is important to note that most agents cannot be assigned to one category exclusively. Nonetheless, these classifications can be helpful for understanding drug activity.

   1. **Phase-specific drugs.** Those agents most active against cells that are in a specific phase of the cell cycle are called *cell cycle phase-specific drugs* (Table 1-1).

      a. **Implications of phase-specific drugs.** Phase specificity has important implications for cancer chemotherapy.

         (1) **Limitation to single-exposure cell kill.** With a phase-specific agent there is a limit to the number of cells that can be killed with a single instantaneous (or very short) drug exposure because only those cells in the sensitive phase are killed. A higher dose kills no more cells.

         (2) **Increasing cell kill by prolonged exposure.** For more cells to be killed requires

Table 1-1. Cell cycle phase-specific chemotherapeutic agents

Phase of greatest activity	Class	Type	Agent
Gap 1 (G_1)	Natural product	Enzyme	Asparaginase
	Hormone	Corticosteroid	Prednisone
DNA synthesis (S)	Antimetabolite	Pyrimidine analog	Cytarabine, fluorouracil
	Antimetabolite	Folic acid analog	Methotrexate
	Antimetabolite	Purine analog	Thioguanine
	Miscellaneous	Substituted urea	Hydroxyurea
Gap 2 (G_2)	Natural product	Antibiotic	Bleomycin
	Natural product	Topoisomerase II inhibitor	Etoposide
	Natural product	Microtubule polymerization and stabilization	Taxol
Mitosis (M)	Natural product	Mitotic inhibitor	Vinblastine, vincristine, vindesine

either prolonged exposure to, or repeated doses of, the drug to allow more cells to enter the sensitive phase of the cycle. Theoretically, all cells could be killed if the blood level, or more importantly the intracellular concentration, of the drug remains sufficiently high while all cells in the target population pass through one complete cell cycle. This theory assumes that the drug does not prevent the passage of cells from one (insensitive) phase to another (sensitive) phase.

(3) **Recruitment.** A higher number of cells could be killed by a phase-specific drug if the proportion of cells in the sensitive phase could be increased (recruited).

b. **Cytarabine.** One of the best examples of a phase-specific agent is cytarabine (ara-C), which is an inhibitor of DNA synthesis and thus is active only in the S phase (at standard doses). Ara-C is rapidly deaminated in vivo to an inactive compound, ara-U; and rapid injections result in very short, effective levels of ara-C. As a result, single doses of ara-C are nontoxic to the normal hematopoietic system and are generally ineffective for treating leukemia. If the drug is given as a daily rapid injection, some patients with leukemia respond well but not nearly as well as when ara-C is given on an every 12-hour schedule. The apparent reason for the greater effectiveness of the 12-hour schedule is that the S phase (DNA synthesis) of human acute nonlymphocytic leukemia cells lasts about 18 to 20 hours. If the drug is given every 24 hours, some cells that have not entered the S phase when the drug is first administered would not be sensitive to its effect. Therefore these cells could pass all the way through the S phase before the next dose is administered and would completely escape any cytotoxic effect. However, when the drug is given every 12 hours, no cell that was "in cycle" would be able to escape exposure to ara-C, as none would be able to get through one complete S phase without the drug being present.

If all cells were in active cycle, i.e., if none were resting in a prolonged G_1 or G_0 phase, it would be theoretically possible to kill any cells in a population by a continuous or scheduled exposure equivalent to one complete cell cycle. Experiments with patients who have acute leukemia have shown that if tritiated thymidine is used to label cells as they enter DNA synthesis it may be 7 to 10 days before the maximum number of leukemia cells have passed through the S phase. This factor means that, barring permutations caused by itself or other drugs, for ara-C to have

Table 1-2. Cell cycle-specific and cell cycle-nonspecific chemotherapeutic agents

Class	Type	Agent
Cell cycle-specific		
Alkylating agent	Nitrogen mustard	Chlorambucil, cyclophosphamide, melphalan
	Alkyl sulfonate	Busulfan
	Triazine	Dacarbazine
	Metal salt	Cisplatin, carboplatin
Natural product	Antibiotic	Dactinomycin, daunorubicin, doxorubicin, idarubicin
Cell cycle-nonspecific		
Alkylating agent	Nitrogen mustard	Mechlorethamine
	Nitrosourea	Carmustine, lomustine, semustine

a maximum effect on the leukemia the repeated exposure must be continued for a 7 to 10-day period. Clinically, continuous infusion or every-12-hour dosing of ara-C for 5 days or more appears to be most effective for treating newly diagnosed patients with acute nonlymphocytic leukemia. Even with such prolonged exposure, however, a few of the cells appear not to have passed through the S phase.

2. **Cell cycle-specific drugs.** Agents that are effective while cells are actively in cycle but are not dependent on the cell being in a particular phase are called *cell cycle-specific drugs (phase-nonspecific)*. This group includes most of the alkylating agents, antitumor antibiotics, and some miscellaneous agents (Table 1-2). Some agents in this group are not totally phase-nonspecific; they may have greater activity in one phase than in another but not to the degree of the phase-specific agents. Many agents also appear to have some activity in cells that are not in cycle, although not as much as when the cells are rapidly dividing.

3. **Cell cycle-nonspecific drugs.** A third group of drugs appears to be effective whether cancer cells are in cycle or are resting. In this respect, these agents are similar to photon irradiation. Drugs in this category are called *cell cycle-nonspecific* and include mechlorethamine (nitrogen mustard) and the nitrosoureas (Table 1-2).

D. **Changes in tumor cell kinetics and therapy implications.** As cancer cells grow from a few cells to a lethal tumor burden, certain changes occur in the growth rate of the population that affect the strategies of chemotherapy. These changes have been determined by observing the characteristics of experimental tumors in animals and neoplastic cells growing in tissue culture. Such model systems readily permit accurate cell number determinations to be made and growth rates to be determined. (Because tumor cells cannot be injected or implanted into humans and permitted to grow, studies of growth rates of intact tumors in humans must largely be limited to observing the growth rate of macroscopic tumors.)

1. **Stages of tumor growth.** Immediately after inoculating a tissue culture or an experimental animal with tumor cells, there is a *lag phase* during which there is little tumor growth. Presumably, the cells in this phase are becoming accustomed to the new environment and are preparing to enter into cycle. The lag phase is followed by a period of rapid growth called *log phase,* during which there are repeated doublings of the cell number. In populations in which the growth fraction approaches 100 percent and the cell death rate is low, the population doubles within a period approximating the cell cycle time. As the cell number or tumor size becomes macroscopic, the doubling time of the tumor cell population becomes prolonged and levels off (*plateau phase*). Most clinically measurable human cancers are probably in the plateau phase; which may account, in part, for the slow doubling time observed in many human cancers (30–300 days). Because the rate of change in the slope of the growth curve during the premeasurable period is unknown for most human cancers, extrapolation from two points when the mass is measurable to estimate the onset of the growth of the malignancy is subject to considerable error. The prolongation in tumor doubling time in the plateau phase may be due to a smaller growth fraction, a change in the cell cycle time, an increased intrinsic death rate, or a combination of these factors. Factors responsible for these changes include decreased nutrients or growth promotion factors, increased inhibitory metabolites or inhibitory growth factors, and inhibition of growth by other cell–cell interactions.

2. **Growth rate and effectiveness of chemotherapy.** Chemotherapeutic agents are most effective during the period of logarithmic growth. As might be expected, this result is particularly true for the antimetabolites, which are largely S-phase-specific. As a result, when human tumors become macroscopic, the effectiveness of many chemotherapeutic agents is reduced because only part of the cell population is actively dividing. Theoretically, if the cell population could be reduced sufficiently by other means, such as surgery or radiotherapy, chemotherapy would be more effective because a higher fraction of the re-

maining cells would be in logarithmic growth. The validity of this theoretical premise is supported by the success of combined surgery plus chemotherapy or radiotherapy plus chemotherapy for breast cancer, colon cancer, Wilms' tumor, ovarian cancer, and small-cell anaplastic cell carcinoma of the lung.

III. **Combination chemotherapy.** Combinations of drugs are frequently more effective in producing responses and prolonging life than the same drugs used sequentially. There are several reasons combinations are likely to be more effective than single agents.

A. **Reasons for effectiveness of combinations**

1. **Prevention of resistant clones.** If one in 10^5 cells is resistant to drug A and one in 10^5 is resistant to drug B, it is likely that treating a macroscopic tumor (which generally would have more than 10^9 cells) with either agent alone would result in several clones of cells that are resistant to that drug. Once a resistant clone has grown to macroscopic size, and if the same mutant frequency persists for drug B, resistance to that agent would also emerge. If both drugs are used at the outset of therapy or in close sequence, however, the likelihood of a cell being resistant to both drugs (excluding for a moment the situation of pleiotropic drug resistance) is only 1 in 10^{10}. Thus the combination confers considerable advantage against the emergence of resistant clones. Compounding the problem of preexisting resistant clones is the resistance that develops through spontaneous mutation in the absence of drug exposure. The use of multiple drugs with independent mechanisms of action or alternating non-cross-resistant combinations (as well as the use of surgery or radiotherapy to eliminate macroscopic tumor) theoretically minimizes the chances for outgrowth of resistant clones and increases the likelihood of remission or cure.

2. **Cytotoxicity to resting and dividing cells.** The combination of a drug that is cell cycle-specific (phase-nonspecific) or cell cycle-nonspecific with a drug that is cell cycle phase-specific can kill cells that are slowly dividing as well as those that are actively dividing. The use of cell cycle-nonspecific drugs can also help recruit cells into a more actively dividing state, which results in their being more sensitive to the cell cycle phase-specific agents.

3. **Biochemical enhancement or effect**

a. **Combinations of individually effective drugs** that affect different biochemical pathways or steps in a single pathway can enhance each other.

b. **Combinations of an active agent with an inactive agent** potentially can result in beneficial effects by several mechanisms.

(1) **An intracellular increase** in the drug or its active metabolites, by either increasing influx or decreasing efflux (e.g., calcium channel inhibitors with multiple agents af-

fected by multidrug resistance due to P-glycoprotein over-expression).

(2) Reduced metabolic inactivation of the drug (e.g., inhibition of cytidine deaminase inactivation of ara-C with tetrahydrouridine or inhibition of 5'-nucleotidase inactivation of arabinosyl cytosine monophosphate (ara-CMP) with etidronate).

(3) Cooperative inhibition of a single enzyme or reaction (e.g., leucovorin enhancement of fluorouracil inhibition of thymidylate synthetase).

(4) Enhancement of drug action by inhibition of competing metabolites (e.g., N-phosphonacetyl-L-aspartic acid (PALA) inhibition of de novo pyrimidine synthesis with resultant increased incorporation of 5-flurouridine triphosphate (5FUTP) into RNA).

4. **Sanctuary access.** Combinations can be used to provide access to sanctuary sites for reasons such as drug solubility or affinity of specific tissues for a particular drug type.

5. **Rescue.** Combinations can be used in which one agent rescues the host from the toxic effects of another drug (e.g., leucovorin following high dose methotrexate).

B. **Principles of agent selection.** When selecting appropriate agents for use in a combination, the following principles should be observed.

1. **Choose individually active drugs.** Do not use a combination in which one agent is inactive when used alone unless there is a clear, specific biochemical or pharmacologic reason to do so, e.g., high-dose methotrexate followed by leucovorin rescue or leucovorin followed by fluorouracil. *This principle is not applicable to the combined use of biologic response modifiers (BRMs) and chemotherapeutic agents,* as cooperativity of BRMs and chemotherapy may not depend on independent cytotoxic effect of the BRMs.

2. **When possible, choose drugs in which the dose-limiting toxicities differ** qualitatively or in time of occurrence. Often, however, two or more agents that have marrow toxicity must be used, and the selection of a safe dose of each is critical. As a starting point, two drugs in combination can usually be given at two-thirds of the dose used when the drugs are given alone. Whenever a new drug combination is tried, a careful evaluation for both expected and unanticipated toxicities must be carried out.

3. **Select agents for a combination for which there is a biochemical or pharmacologic rationale.** Preferably this rationale has been tested in an animal tumor system and in the appropriate model system and has been found to be better than either agent alone.

4. **Be cautious when attempting to improve on a successful two-drug combination** by adding a third, fourth, and fifth drug simultaneously. Although this approach may be beneficial, two undesirable results may be seen:

   a. **An intolerable level of toxicity** that leads to excessive morbidity and mortality.

   b. **Unchanged or reduced antitumor effect** because of the necessity to reduce the dose of the most effective drugs to a level below which antitumor responses are not seen, despite the theoretical advantages of the combination. Therefore the addition of each new agent to a combination must be carefully considered, the principles of combination therapy closely followed, and controlled clinical trials carried out to compare the efficacy of any new regimen with a more established (standard) treatment program.

C. **Clinical effectiveness of combinations.** Combinations of drugs have been clearly demonstrated to be better than single agents for treating many, but not all, human cancers. The benefit of combinations of drugs compared with the same drugs used sequentially has been marked in diseases such as acute lymphocytic leukemia, Hodgkin's lymphoma, breast carcinoma, anaplastic small-cell carcinoma of the lung, and testicular carcinoma. The benefit is less clear in cancers such as non-small-cell carcinoma of the lung, non-Hodgkin's lymphomas with favorable prognoses, ovarian carcinoma, head and neck carcinomas, melanoma, and colorectal carcinomas, although reports exist for each of these tumors in which combinations are better in one respect or another than single agents.

IV. **Resistance to antineoplastic agents.** Resistance to antineoplastic chemotherapy is a combined characteristic of a specific drug, a specific tumor, and a specific host whereby the drug is ineffective in controlling the tumor without excessive toxicity. Resistance of a tumor to a drug is the reciprocal of selectivity of that drug for that tumor. The problem for the medical oncologist or pharmacologist is not simply to find an agent that is cytotoxic but to find one that selectively kills neoplastic cells while preserving the essential host cells and their function. Were it not for the problem of resistance of human cancer to antineoplastic agents or, conversely, the lack of selectivity of those agents, cancer chemotherapy would be similar to antibacterial chemotherapy in which complete eradication of infection is regularly observed. Such a utopian state of cancer chemotherapy has not yet been achieved for most human cancers. The problem of resistance and ways to overcome or even exploit it remains an area of major interest for the chemotherapist.

Resistance to antineoplastic chemotherapeutic agents may be either natural or acquired. *Natural resistance* refers to the initial unresponsiveness of a tumor to a given drug, and *acquired resistance* refers to the unresponsiveness that emerges after initially successful treatment. There are three basic categories of resistance to chemotherapy: kinetic, biochemical, and pharmacologic.

A. Cell kinetics and resistance. Resistance based on cell population kinetics relates to cycle and phase specificity, growth fractions and the implications of these factors for responsiveness to specific agents and schedules of drug administration. A particular problem with many human tumors is that they are in a plateau growth phase with a small growth fraction. This factor renders many of the cells insensitive to the antimetabolites and relatively unresponsive to many of the other chemotherapeutic agents. Strategies to overcome resistance due to cell kinetics include:

1. Reducing tumor bulk with surgery or radiotherapy.
2. Using combinations to include drugs that affect resting populations (with many G_0 cells).
3. Scheduling of drugs to prevent phase escape or to synchronize cell populations and increase cell kill.

B. Biochemical causes of resistance. Resistance can occur for biochemical reasons, including the inability of a tumor to convert a drug to its active form, ability of a tumor to inactivate a drug, or the location of a tumor at a site where substrates are present that bypass an otherwise lethal blockade.

Multidrug resistance (MDR), also called pleiotropic drug resistance, is a phenomenon whereby treatment with one agent confers resistance not only to that drug and others of its class but also to several other unrelated agents. MDR is commonly mediated by an enhanced energy-dependent drug efflux mechanism that results in lower intracellular drug concentrations. With this type of MDR, overexpression of a membrane transport protein called P-glycoprotein is commonly observed. Combination chemotherapy can overcome biochemical resistance by increasing the amount of active drug intracellularly as a result of biochemical interactions or effects on drug transport across the cell membrane. Calcium channel blockers, antiarrhythmics, calmodulin inhibitors, antibiotics, and lipophilic polycyclic compounds have been found to modulate the MDR effect in vitro, and some beneficial effects have been clinically observed.

The use of a second agent to rescue normal cells may also permit the use of high doses of the first agent, which can overcome the resistance caused by a low rate of conversion to the active metabolite or a high rate of inactivation. Another way to overcome resistance is to follow marrow-lethal doses of chemotherapy by autologous bone marrow transplantation. This experimental technique shows some promise for treatment of lymphomas and a few other cancers. A more widely applicable technique may be to combine high-dose chemotherapy with blood cell growth factors, e.g., granulocyte colony stimulating factor and granulocyte-macrophage colony stimulating factor. These and other marrow protective and stimulating agents are being increasingly used and may enhance the effectiveness of chemotherapy on several cancers.

C. **Pharmacologic causes of resistance.** Apparent resistance to cancer chemotherapy can result from poor or erratic absorption, increased excretion or catabolism, and drug interactions, all leading to inadequate blood levels of the drug. Strictly speaking, this result is not true resistance; but to the degree that the insufficient blood levels are not appreciated by the clinician, resistance appears to be present. The variation from patient to patient at the highest tolerated dose has led to dose-modification schemes that permit dose escalation when the toxicities of the chemotherapy regimen are minimal or nonexistent, as well as dose reduction when toxicities are great. This regulation is particularly important for some chemotherapeutic agents for which the dose-response curve is steep.

True pharmacologic resistance is caused by the poor transport of agents into certain body tissues and tumor cells. For example, the central nervous system (CNS) is a site many drugs do not reach well. Several drug characteristics favor transport into the CNS, including high lipid solubility and low molecular weight. For tumors that originate in the CNS or metastasize there, drugs of choice should be those that achieve effective antitumor concentration in brain tissue and are effective against the tumor cell type being treated.

D. **Nonselectivity and resistance.** Nonselectivity is not a mechanism for resistance but, rather, an acknowledgment that for most cancers and most drugs the reasons for resistance and selectivity are poorly understood.

Given a limited understanding of the biochemical differences between normal and malignant cells, it is gratifying that chemotherapy is successful as frequently as it is. It is to be hoped that in 20 years we will view current chemotherapy as a crude beginning, and that many more tumor target-directed agents will have been found that have a high potential for curing the human cancers that now defy treatment.

Selected Readings

Baguley, B. C., Holdaway, K. M., and Fray, L. M. Design of DNA intercolators to overcome topoisomerase II-mediated multidrug resistance. *J. Natl. Cancer Inst.* 82:398, 1990.

Baserga, R. The relationship of the cell cycle to tumor growth and control of cell division: a review. *Cancer Res.* 25:581, 1965.

Baserga, R. The cell cycle. *N. Engl. J. Med.* 304:453, 1981.

Bender, R. A., and Dedrick, R. L. Cytokinetic aspects of clinical drug resistance. *Cancer Chemother. Rep.* 59:805, 1975.

Chabner, B. (ed). *Pharmacologic Principles of Cancer Treatment*. Philadelphia: Saunders, 1982.

Clarkson, B., et al. Studies of cellular proliferation in human leukemia. *Cancer* 25:1237, 1970.

Dalton, W. S., et al. Drug resistance in multiple myeloma and non-Hodgkin's lymphoma: detection of P-glycoprotein and potential circumvention by addition of verapamil to chemotherapy. *J. Clin. Oncol.* 7:415, 1989.

DeVita, V. T., and Schein, P. S. The use of drugs in combination for the treatment of cancer: rationale and results. *N. Engl. J. Med.* 288:998, 1973.

Endicott, J. A., and Ling, U. The biochemistry of P-glycoprotein-median multidrug resistance. *Annu. Rev. Biochem.* 58:137, 1989.

Goldie, J. H., and Coldman, A. J. A mathematical model for relating drug sensitivity of tumors to their spontaneous mutation rate. *Cancer Treat. Rep.* 63:1727, 1979.

Hryniuk, W., and Bush, H. The importance of dose intensity in chemotherapy of metastatic breast cancer. *J. Clin. Oncol.* 2:1281, 1984.

Lazarus, H. M. Treatment of metastatic malignant melanoma with intensive melphalan and autologous bone marrow transplantation. *Cancer Treat. Rep.* 69:473, 1985.

Phillips, G. L., and Herzig, R. H. Treatment of resistant malignant lymphoma with cyclophosphamide, total body irradiation and transplantation of cryopreserved autologous marrow. *N. Engl. J. Med.* 310:1557, 1984.

Schabel, F. M., Jr. The use of tumor growth kinetics in planning "curative" chemotherapy of advanced solid tumors. *Cancer Res.* 29:2384, 1969.

Principles of Therapy with Biologic Response Modifiers and Their Role in Cancer Management

David R. Parkinson

I. **Definition of biologic therapy.** The term *biologic therapy* describes a variety of agents and therapeutic approaches that have evolved from advanced understanding of the biology of the immune system, the nature of tumor cells, and the relation between them. The description of cellular antitumor mechanisms, isolation and production in pharmacologic amounts of the proteins that regulate the activity of these cells, and development of monoclonal antibody technology have permitted clinical applications in humans that were derived from preclinical studies in animal tumor models.

II. **Biologic agents.** A series of proteins are responsible for the growth and development of cells of the hematopoietic and lymphoid systems. The nomenclature is confusing and misleading. A *cytokine* is a protein produced and secreted by a cell; therefore a *lymphokine* is a cytokine produced by a lymphocyte. Although many of these regulatory proteins stimulate the growth of certain cells expressing their specific cell surface receptors, they may have other widespread biologic effects as well, including antiproliferative, differentiation-inducing, or functional activation effects. These properties expand the possible applications of these proteins, but they also complicate their study and are responsible for some of the pleiotropic side effects noted when these cytokines are administered as drugs.

   A. **Cytokines.** Several of the central regulatory cytokines have been isolated, and some, e.g., interferon alpha, are now in general clinical use. Others are still under study for their possible roles in cancer medicine.

   1. **Interleukin-1 (IL-1).** The two forms of IL-1 are produced by a wide range of cells after stimulation. These cytokines, which bind to a common receptor, are among the most pleiotropic with regard to their biologic properties. IL-1 plays an important role in inflammation, inducing fever and acute-phase reactant release; and it may play a role in tissue repair following injury. Furthermore, IL-1 has immunostimulatory properties that help to activate T lymphocytes and to induce the production of other cytokines. It both induces and is a cofactor for hematopoietic growth factors such as granulocyte and monocyte colony-stimulating factors. IL-1 is both a chemoprotector and a radioprotector, protecting animals against otherwise lethal myelosuppressive doses of cytotoxic agents. For these reasons, IL-1 is under

study in wound healing, as an adjuvant in vaccine trials, and for use in association with chemotherapy and irradiation.

2. **Interleukin-2.** Originally termed T cell growth factor, IL-2 is a lymphokine product of activated T cells that binds to a specific cell surface receptor on activated T lymphocytes; the protein is central to T cell proliferation but also activates natural killer (NK) cells. Because of its powerful immunostimulatory properties, IL-2 has been widely studied for its antitumor properties. In animals IL-2 is active as a single agent in a dose- and schedule-dependent manner. For a given IL-2 treatment schedule, antitumor activity can be enhanced by the addition of other cytokines, e.g., interferon-alpha and tumor necrosis factor-alpha, or by the concomitant use of activated antitumor lymphocytes or monoclonal antibodies directed against the tumor.

IL-2 has been extensively studied in clinical trials in man. It has single agent activity against renal cell carcinoma and malignant melanoma. The greatest antitumor effects have been observed with high dose IL-2 therapy. Such intensive treatment can be administered only to patients carefully selected for cardiopulmonary status. Nevertheless, this therapy is associated with significant toxicity, as described later. IL-2 also forms the basis for adoptive cellular treatment approaches.

3. **Interleukin-4.** IL-4 is stimulatory for B cells and together with IL-2 is a growth factor for cytotoxic T cells. This wide range of immunostimulatory properties has led to its study in cancer therapy.

4. **Interleukin-6.** The IL-6 molecule possesses widespread biologic effects. In addition to playing a central role in the induction of the acute-phase response, it is important in B cell growth and differentiation and may interact with IL-2 in T cell differentiation. For these reasons and because it is active as a single agent in tumor models and may serve as an autocrine growth factor in myeloma, IL-6 and anti-IL-6 treatment strategies are being studied in patients with malignancy.

5. **Interleukin-7.** A growth factor for early lymphoid progenitors, this bone marrow stroma-derived protein may also be important in T cell activation.

6. **Interferon alpha (IFN-α).** Described initially for their antiviral properties, the alpha and beta interferons, the "type I" interferons, subserve a wide variety of biologic effects, some of which have proved useful in cancer therapy. IFN-α has been most widely studied. Its immunomodulatory effect includes activation of NK cells, modulation of antibody production by B lymphocytes, and induction on the tumor cell surface of major histocompatibility complex (MHC) antigens, making the tumor more susceptible to immune-mediated killing. However, the

principal antitumor effects of this interferon are probably related to its direct antiproliferative effects.

IFN-α is an active agent in hairy-cell leukemia and in the early phase of chronic myelogenous leukemia. It has activity as well in low grade non-Hodgkin's lymphoma, multiple myeloma, and cutaneous T cell lymphoma. Some solid tumors, principally melanoma and renal cell carcinoma, but also some squamous cell and basal cell carcinomas of the skin, have responded to interferon. Other clinical indications for the use of IFN-α include chronic infection with hepatitis C, condyloma acuminatum, and juvenile laryngeal carcinomatosis.

7. **Interferon-gamma (IFN-γ).** This interferon has weaker antiviral and a wider range of immunobiologic properties than IFN-α. It activates monocytes and macrophages, thereby upregulating FC receptors, enhancing phagocytosis, and killing intracellular organisms. It increases the surface expression of MHC and tumor-associated antigens. IFN-γ has been disappointing as an antitumor agent when used alone, and it is now being studied in combination with other biologic agents. It is effective in chronic granulomatous disease where its prophylactic use decreases the incidence and severity of infections.

8. **Tumor necrosis factor (TNF).** Originally named for their antitumor effects in animal models, TNF-α and TNF-β ("lymphotoxin") are the products of activated macrophages, share a common receptor, and subserve a wide variety of biologic effects. They serve as growth factors for fibroblasts, have some antiviral activity, activate procoagulase activity on endothelial cells, and activate osteoclasts. Immunomodulatory effects include the induction of surface MHC antigens and interaction with other cytokines such as IL-2, but TNF is directly cytotoxic to some cells, possibly through the induction of oxygen radicals. TNF may play a role in tumor cachexia. It has been shown to inhibit the enzyme lipoprotein lipase. Acute administration of TNF intravenously leads to decreased systemic vascular resistance mediated through the induction of nitric oxide in endothelial cells. The TNF generated during gram-negative shock may be responsible for the lethality of these infections, and strategies for the treatment of this condition involve blocking the effects of TNF. As a single agent, TNF has been inactive in cancer therapy in man, although toxicity, principally hypotension, has limited the doses that can be administered systemically.

B. **Hematopoietic growth factors**

1. **Erythropoietin.** Erythropoietin promotes the proliferation and differentiation of committed erythroid precursors. This factor may decrease transfusion requirements during chemotherapy and may be stud-

ied together with other factors in bone marrow failure states.

2. **Granulocyte colony stimulating factor (G-CSF)** is a growth factor with proliferative activity for bone marrow progenitors committed to the neutrophil line.

3. **Granulocyte-macrophage colony stimulating factor (GM-CSF).** Unlike G-CSF, GM-CSF exhibits its predominant proliferative effects on multipotential stem cells. However, this protein also inhibits neutrophil migration, potentiates the functions of neutrophils and macrophages, and results in production of a spectrum of cytokines from these activated cells; therefore it has been studied for its ability to reconstitute bone marrow and to activate macrophages.

4. **Interleukin-3 (IL-3).** Also known as "multi-CSF," IL-3 stimulates early multipotent marrow stem cells. The effects of both IL-3 and GM-CSF on these early stem cells can be enhanced by IL-1 and IL-6, suggesting that in the future these agents may be used in combination.

5. **Macrophage colony stimulating factor.** Also known as colony-stimulating factor 1 (CSF-1), this growth factor is relatively lineage-specific. It is responsible for proliferation and activation of monocytes.

C. **Other growth factors and regulatory proteins**

1. **Transforming growth factors (TGF).** This group of regulatory molecules have profound effects on growth and differentiation. TGF-α is related to epidermal growth factor (EGF) and binds to the EGF receptor. TGF-β, although having some growth-enhancing properties for fibroblasts, is predominantly immunosuppressive and is to be studied for its antiproliferative effects in clinical trials.

2. **Other growth and differentiation factors.** It is becoming increasingly clear that a spectrum of proteins important in the control of growth, differentiation, and function exists for all organ systems. Further understanding of these proteins and their receptors will allow greater understanding of their roles in normal and disordered biology. Some of these proteins or their receptors may ultimately find a role in therapeutics.

D. **Monoclonal antibodies (MoAb).** Antibodies binding to tumor-associated cell surface antigens can result in the destruction of tumor cells through a number of possible mechanisms, including activation of complement and antibody-dependent cell-mediated cytotoxicity (ADCC). Furthermore, these antibodies may be useful as means of targeting cytotoxic radioisotopes, toxins, or drugs to tumors, enhancing their delivery to tumors while minimizing systemic exposure. Monoclonal antibody technology has made important contributions to cancer medicine by allowing the study of differentiation-associated antigens and the phenotypic characterization of both hematopoietic and solid tumors. Antigens expressed with relative specificity on tumor cell surfaces have been defined and have served as targets for diagnostic and therapeutic applications of antibodies.

1. **Murine MoAb.** The first monoclonal antibodies used in vivo diagnostically and therapeutically were murine. Studies have pointed out the complexity of these agents. Relative distribution and densities of antigen on normal and malignant tissues, the affinity of the antibody for the antigen, and the behavior of the antigen after antibody binding are important to the success of this approach. The internal modulation of antigen from the cell surface after antibody binding is an impediment for strategies using antibody alone, a necessity for immunotoxins or chemoimmune conjugates, and irrelevant to radioisotope therapeutic strategies.

   Murine antibodies are weak activators of the human immune system; and when used alone against T or B cell lymphoid malignancies, they have generally exhibited only transient antitumor activity. The antibodies against solid tumors have been largely inactive. A problem with the repeated use of murine monoclonal antibodies has been the development of human anti-mouse antibodies (HAMA).

2. **Human MoAb.** Although human antibodies have the theoretical advantage of less immunogenicity, longer half-life, and greater immunologic activity, they have been difficult to generate in pharmacologic quantities.

3. **Chimeric MoAb.** A solution to the above problems has been the generation of genetically engineered antibodies, which combine the antigen-binding properties of the murine antibodies with the advantages of a human antibody backbone.

4. **Antibody fragments.** Small antigen-binding proteins, either antibody fragments such as F(ab')2, or single-chain antigen-binding proteins, may have shorter half-lives and greater access to tumor.

III. **Biologic strategies in cancer therapy**

A. **Single-agent therapy.** As noted above, some cytokines, principally IFN-α and IL-2, have been active as single agents in cancer therapy. In the case of IFN-α, the doses necessary for an antitumor effect range from the very low doses necessary for hairy-cell leukemia to the higher doses necessary for melanoma, which are associated with significant side effects. This problem is even more of an issue with IL-2, where the doses necessary for an antitumor effect may be associated with life-threatening toxicity. Current treatment strategies are designed to understand mechanisms of both antitumor effects and toxic effects in the expectation of developing less morbid, more effective therapy. One tenet of biologic therapy is that the optimal immunobiologic effects ("optimal biologic dose") observed with an agent may be significantly less than the maximally tolerated dose. However, the validity of this concept can be tested only through clinical trials. At least with IL-2, the maximum tolerated dose (MTD) appears to be associated with the greatest clinical activity.

B. Combination therapy. Because preclinical models suggest that combinations of biologic agents have greater therapeutic effects than single agents, clinical trials are studying the effects of immunostimulatory cytokines such as IL-2 together with monoclonal antibodies or with activated antitumor lymphocytes such as lymphokine activated killer (LAK) cells or cells generated from the tumor itself.

Preclinical studies suggest that certain combinations of biologic and cytotoxic agents may be synergistic. TNF, for example, is both a radiosensitizer and an enhancer of the antitumor effects of topoisomerase inhibitors such as etoposide. Interferon similarly enhances the antitumor activity of cisplatin and fluorouracil.

C. Adoptive cellular therapy. This treatment strategy involves the transfer of antitumor effective cells to the tumor-bearing host. To date, these cells have principally been either LAK cells generated by in vitro activation of peripheral blood lymphocytes with IL-2 or expanded populations of lymphocytes generated from the patient's own tumor. In some cases these tumor-infiltrating lymphocytes can be shown to exhibit specific cytotoxicity against the autologous tumor. This treatment approach is still experimental. An important aspect of this strategy is that it allows detailed study of the relation between tumor and host, information that may ultimately be used to activate these mechanisms in vivo.

D. Targeted therapy. As noted above, tumor-associated surface structures, either tumor-associated antigens or receptors, can be used for targeted therapy.

    1. Immunotoxins. Conjugates of plant toxins, such as ricin to monoclonal antibodies, have been used in therapeutic approaches, with responses noted in non-Hodgkin's lymphoma and chronic lymphocytic leukemia. Disadvantages of this strategy include the fact that target antigens must be internalized after antibody binding, antigen-negative cells can escape, and the plant toxin may be immunogenic.

    2. Chimeric toxins. Fusion genes composed of the cytotoxic portions of bacterial genes (e.g., diphtheria toxin or *Pseudomonas* exotoxin) and targeting ligands (e.g., the cytokines IL-2 or TGF-α) can be used to produce cytotoxic chimeric proteins that target specifically to cells expressing the respective high affinity receptor.

    3. Radioimmunotherapy. The selective targeting of radioisotopes to tumor presents many theoretical advantages over external beam radiation with regard to therapeutic index. In addition, owing to the bystander effect, even antigen-negative cells may be killed in this approach, and antibody need not be internalized for the therapy to be effective. Difficulties to date have included the necessity of developing more stable linker chemistry for the isotope attachments, the poor radiation characteristics of the iodine isotopes used in the initial studies, and the limitation of dose escalation by myelosuppression using the initial radioimmune conjugates. However, conjugates using isotopes such as yttrium 90 are under development; and together with dose fractionation and hematopoietic growth factors, they may permit delivery of therapeutic doses of radiation to solid tumors.

4. **Chemoimmunotherapy.** This potential therapeutic strategy has been hindered by a lack of good conjugation technology and appropriate chemotherapeutic agents.

E. **Reduction of chemotherapy or irradiation toxicity.** The hematopoietic growth factors show promise with regard to decreasing the length of myelosuppression, the depth of the neutrophil nadir, the number of febrile events, and the incidence of mucositis following administration of cytotoxic drugs or radiation.

F. **Increasing the effectiveness of chemotherapy or irradiation.** Less clear than the toxicity reduction issue is whether the use of myeloid growth factors allows significant increases in dose intensity for chemotherapy, through either dose escalation or a decrease in the interval between chemotherapy cycles. The agents are also being used in conjunction with bone marrow transplantation in attempts to decrease the morbidity and mortality associated with that procedure.

G. **Differentiation therapy.** Many of the myeloid growth and immune stimulating factors described above also have differentiation properties. The hematopoietic factors, including IL-3 and GM-CSF, are being studied in disorders of bone marrow differentiation, including myelodysplasia and aplastic anemia. Similarly, the interleukins may find application in certain individuals with some inherited or acquired immunodeficiency states. A group of agents active in differentiation, the retinoids, are under study for both treatment and prevention of malignancy. Tretinoin (all *trans*-retinoic acid) is active in inducing remission of acute promyelocytic leukemia. *cis*-Retinoic acid has induced remissions of advanced squamous cell carcinoma of the skin and cutaneous T cell lymphoma. β-Carotene has been shown to reduce the incidence of secondary malignancies in patients who have had squamous cell carcinoma of the head and neck. Preclinical studies suggest that these agents may be even more active when used together with some of the cytokines and growth factors discussed above.

IV. **Toxicities of biologic therapy.** In general, the predictable toxicities of biologic agents are dose- and schedule-related. Administration of the interferons on a daily basis

Table 2-1. Current status of biologic agents in cancer therapy

Agent	Status
Interferon-alpha	FDA approved for hairy-cell leukemia
	Responses also in chronic myelogenous leukemia, where 10–15% of patients with early chronic phase become Philadelphia chromosome-negative
	Responses in low grade non-Hodgkin's lymphoma, cutaneous T cell lymphomas
	Under investigation in combination with 5-fluorouracil, cisplatin, and other cytotoxic agents; also in combination with IL-2
	Activity in nonmalignant indications: condyloma acuminatum, chronic hepatitis, juvenile laryngeal papillomatosis
Interferon-beta	Still investigational: has many properties similar to IFN-α
Interferon-gamma	Investigational: active in decreasing infections in chronic granulomatous disease
	Under investigation in cancer biotherapy for macrophage-stimulating and tumor antigen-upregulating properties; little single agent activity in clinical trials to date
Interleukin-1	Investigational: under study for wound healing and chemoprotective and radioprotective properties
Interleukin-2	Investigational: single-agent activity in metastatic renal cell carcinoma and malignant melanoma
Interleukin-4	Investigational: immunostimulatory agent
Interleukin-6	Investigational: antitumor and immunostimulatory agent
Interleukin-7	Investigational: not yet in clinical trials
Transforming growth factor-beta (TGF-β)	Potential uses as an antiproliferative agent
G-CSF	Decreases length of myelosuppression following cytotoxic agents; may reduce depth of neutrophil nadir and

Table 2-1. (*continued*)

Agent	Status
	incidence of febrile episodes during neutropenia
GM-CSF	Marrow-restorative properties similar to G-CSF; also being studied for monocyte proliferation and activating characteristics
IL-3	Investigational: under study for myelorestorative properties; also being studied in aplastic anemia and myelodysplasia
M-CSF (CSF-1)	Investigational: potential uses in infections and cancer applications follow from its proliferative and activating effects on monocytes
Monoclonal antibodies	Anti-CD3 approved for treatment of allograft rejection; other antibodies remain investigational for therapeutic purposes
Immunotoxins	Investigational: demonstrate antitumor activity in refractory non-Hodgkin's lymphoma and chronic lymphocytic leukemia
Chimeric toxins	Investigational: anti-IL-2 toxin has produced antitumor activity in non-Hodgkin's lymphoma; other cytokine–toxic conjugates under development
Radioimmunoconjugates	Investigational: anti-B cell–iodine 131 conjugates have been active in refractory B cell lymphomas

is associated with systemic symptoms, e.g., fever, fatigue, and myalgia. Nonsteroidal anti-inflammatory agents and acetaminophen are useful for alleviating these symptoms, although tachyphylaxis occurs with continued therapy and these symptoms diminish over time.

The toxicities with IL-2 are dose-dependent. The importance of careful patient selection for high-dose IL-2 therapy cannot be overemphasized as the high-dose IL-2 regimens are associated with significant cardiovascular complications, including hypotension and the development of a full-blown capillary leak syndrome. Clinical manifestations include decreased serum albumin, weight gain, and development of peripheral edema in the setting of fluid support for blood pressure. This fluid overload can be associated with pulmonary compromise. Other cardiac complications of high-dose IL-2 therapy include arrhythmias, principally supraventricular and myocardial infarction. The latter complication is largely avoided by prescreening patient candidates for the presence of ischemic heart disease.

Patients on IL-2 develop a characteristic erythematous rash that may progress to desquamation. IL-2 therapy can exacerbate preexisting psoriasis and, rarely, is associated with the development of a pemphiguslike syndrome.

Patients on IL-2 characteristically have a decreased appetite, and may develop nausea and occasional diarrhea. The development of hypothyroidism has been described in association with IL-2 therapy and rarely with interferon therapy.

Development of neuropsychiatric changes, e.g., confusion, on IL-2 therapy is an indication to halt therapy. Like other IL-2 effects, these problems are reversible; but unlike the others, the neuropsychiatric changes may continue to progress for a while after discontinuation of therapy.

Although corticosteroids prevent or attenuate most IL-2-related side effects presumably by preventing the release of such IL-2-induced cytokines as TNF and IFN-γ, concern over the potential deleterious effects on the antitumor effects of IL-2 precludes their use except in life-threatening situations.

Monoclonal antibody administration has been associated with hypotension and shortness of breath. The risk of anaphylaxis, greater with repeated dosing, has led to routine administration of an intravenous test dose with anaphylactic precautions (including epinephrine, steroids, and antihistamines) on hand.

The use of ricin-conjugated immunotoxins has been associated with myalgias, elevated serum creatine phosphokinase levels, and occasional rhabdomyolysis.

V. **Current status of biologic agents in cancer therapy.** As noted in Table 2-1, biologic agents have found clinical applications in some cancer-related situations. Many more potential applications are under investigation limited only by our understanding of the biologic characteristics of these agents and their effects on normal and malignant cells.

Selected Reading

DeVita, V. T., Jr., Hellman, S., and Rosenberg, S. A. *Cancer: Principles and Practice*. Philadelphia: Lippincott, 1989.

Groopman, J. E., Molina, J-M., and Scadden, D. T. Hematopoietic growth factors: biology and clinical applications. *N. Engl. J. Med.* 321:1449, 1989.

Parkinson, D. R. Interleukin-2 in cancer therapy. *Semin. Oncol.* 15(suppl. 6):10, 1988.

Zalutsky, M. R. *Antibodies in Radiodiagnosis and Therapy*. Boca Raton: CRC Press, 1989.

Principles of Surgery in Cancer Management

Hollis W. Merrick

The traditional role of surgery in cancer management has been diagnosis and treatment of the primary disease. For many years, in fact, surgery was the only curative mode of cancer treatment. Even now more cancers are cured by surgery alone than by any other modality alone or in combination. As additional forms of treatment have become more effective, the role of surgery has evolved and is now often integrated with radiotherapy and chemotherapy. Improvement in surgical techniques and greater knowledge of the cancers often allow better surgical management of the patient with cancer. Furthermore, with longer survival there are more opportunities to perform secondary and tertiary procedures. With the increasing complexity of cancer therapy, it has become apparent that it is in the patient's best interest that the various specialties evaluate the patient and integrate the benefits of their therapy forms at an early stage. However, the involvement of the surgeon remains vital to the care of the patient through all phases of the disease.

I. **Prevention.** Because surgeons are often the primary providers of care for the patient and family with cancer, they are responsible for educating patients about cancer etiology and incidence and about prevention. For example, families of patients with polyposis coli, familial colon cancer, or ulcerative colitis require education concerning the need for frequent examination for cancer. Women with fibrocystic changes who have a history of breast cancer in a mother or sister are at high risk (12 times greater than normal risk) for cancer of the breast and must be encouraged to have regular breast examinations and mammograms when they reach the age of high risk (> 35 years). All patients should be apprised of the risks of smoking and the benefit of eating diets low in fat and high in fiber.

II. **Diagnosis.** The key to therapy of any malignant disease is accurate diagnosis. It is best gained by microscopic examination of representative tissue obtained by the surgeon by the least invasive manner possible. The diagnostic technique employed varies depending on the natural history of the tumor being investigated.

   A. **Cytology.** The use of exfoliative cytology, as with a Papanicolaou smear, has been instrumental in decreasing the morbidity due to uterine disease. Cells can also be obtained by aspiration, as from a superficial lesion, e.g., a breast tumor, or from a deep body cavity, such as a lung nodule or a pancreatic mass. Biopsies of organs or sites that are not superficial can be guided under computed tomographic (CT) or ultrasonographic control. Cytologic analysis can provide a tentative diagnosis of cancer. However, major surgical resections usually should not be undertaken on the basis of cytology alone, as the error inherent in the technique is higher than that of the standard histologic diagnosis. Techniques of making the cytologic preparation and the experience of the cytologist are critical to the reliability of this method of diagnosis.

B. Needle biopsy. The use of a cutting biopsy needle allows the surgeon to obtain a core of tissue from a suspected tumor that is sufficient for diagnosis of most tumor types. Lymphomas and sarcomas are exceptions from which a larger amount of tissue may be necessary for accurate and complete diagnosis.

C. Incisional biopsy. Incisional biopsy involves removing a wedge of tissue from a large tumor mass. It is often necessary for diagnosis of large masses before major resections and is the preferred technique for diagnosing soft tissue sarcomas. A disadvantage of this technique, however, is the opening of new tissue planes for potential contamination by tumor cells. It is important to place an incision so it is compatible with a subsequent cancer operation, such as in the extremity or with a head or neck lesion. Misplacement of an incision can often compromise subsequent surgical management.

D. Excisional biopsy. Excision of an entire tumor with little or no margin of surrounding normal tissue may be performed. This technique is acceptable when the excision can be carried out without entering new tissue planes or interfering with subsequent surgical management.

E. Comments. Although the type of diagnostic biopsy performed does not directly affect survival, it is generally advisable to avoid contaminating the adjacent normal tissue or entering new tissue planes. Attention should be paid to details of the procedure. The occurrence of a hematoma after biopsy can lead to the spread of residual tumor cells. It has been documented with breast cancer that this complication can to lead to an increased rate of local recurrence on the chest wall following primary biopsy. When multiple sites are being biopsied, it is essential to avoid contamination from one wound to another by either instruments or gloves.

   Close cooperation with the pathologist is essential to obtain the best results. The tissue must be handled appropriately if such special studies as estrogen receptor analysis, immunohistochemistry, electron microscopy, flow cytometry, or tissue culture are required from the biopsy specimen. It is important, for example, when doing a breast biopsy to prepare immediately a frozen section of a suspicious lesion. A sample from a positive lesion can be frozen for estrogen and progesterone receptor assays. Placing the specimen in formaldehyde eliminates the possibility of these assays, which may be vitally important for subsequent management of the patient.

III. Staging. The need for accurate staging prior to treatment planning has become important in a wide variety of malignancies. Detection of widespread metastatic disease in patients with breast cancer, for example, renders the standard mastectomy an inappropriate procedure. Conversely, in some patients the exact extent of the disease can be determined only through surgery. Staging laparotomy is performed for Hodgkin's disease to plan accurately for more conservative treatment modalities. The requirement for accurately staging ovarian cancer before starting therapy has been demonstrated. In addition, there is a strong case for restaging an ovarian cancer after a number of cycles of chemotherapy to determine if continued chemotherapy is required.

Staging during an operative procedure is also vitally important. For example, detection of positive parapancreatic nodal involvement secondary to cancer of the pancreas would preclude a Whipple resection with its associated high risk of mortality as being a futile procedure. Similarly, with a positive celiac axis biopsy for esophageal cancer, it is important to spare the patient the risk of the morbidity and mortality associated with a hazardous procedure. As a final step of intraoperative staging, placement of metallic clips to define the borders of a tumor (e.g., for cancer of the pancreas) or the level of dissection (e.g., the upper limits of an axillary dissection for breast cancer) facilitates future management planning by the radiotherapist.

IV. **Surgery for treatment of cancer.** Surgery is a highly effective modality for curing cancer confined to an accessible site. However, even though all visible tumor may be removed, a significant number of patients have micrometastatic disease at the time of surgery. Extension of the surgery to the regional node-bearing areas may improve survival, but positive involvement of these areas also signifies the probability of distant disease.

The development of additional forms of therapy has given hope to patients who formerly were considered incurable. Similarly, the role of surgery has expanded beyond treatment of the primary tumor to involve a wide variety of palliative, reconstructive, and rehabilitative procedures.

A. **Treatment of the primary cancer.** The use of appropriate treatment of local disease is vitally important in the management of the cancer patient in order to obtain the best possible control at the outset of the disease. The surgeon usually has the first (and thus the best) opportunity to exercise this control. Most solid tumors are best treated with en bloc resection of the primary tumor and the regional lymphatic drainage areas. It is important to take the appropriate amount of margin that is compatible with a low recurrence rate. For example, a margin of 5 cm from the tumor of colon cancer is compatible with a low recurrence rate. The surgeon must weigh the relative risks and benefits of the surgical procedure proposed with respect to adequate local control and acceptable risk of morbidity and mortality for the patient. A difficult clinical problem, for example, is management of cancer of the pancreas. A Whipple resection offers the best chance to cure the patient. However, only 4% of operated patients live 5 years, whereas the reported operative mortality in a multiple series of patients undergoing a Whipple resection is 14%.

The surgeon must be aware of the capabilities of radiotherapy, chemotherapy, or both to improve the local and systemic control of the cancer or to be the primary therapy. For example, head and neck cancers may be treated with radiotherapy in conjunction with surgery, or radiotherapy may be the preferred method for treatment of tumors in certain locations. Finally, the surgeon must be aware of improvements in other forms of treatment in the rapidly changing field of cancer therapy so the patient can be offered the optimal overall treatment.

B. Reduction of bulk residual disease. The idea of cytoreductive surgery has received much attention. Resection of bulk disease for treatment of certain cancers may well lead to increased ability to control residual disease that has not been resected. For example, removing all bulk disease to a size of 2 cm or less renders ovarian cancer tumors more responsive to chemotherapy and improves survival. Therefore there is an indication for using debulking when an additional form of effective therapy is available. However, to perform this procedure when no other effective therapy is present is of no benefit to the patient. Debulking, however, is a fertile field for investigation of new modalities. The role of intraoperative radiation therapy for control of small residual bulk tumor or microscopic disease remains to be established. If this technique proves to be effective, it may offer the benefit of significant palliation for solid tumors in conjunction with surgical debulking.

C. Resection of metastatic disease with curative intent. Patients with metastatic disease as the only site of their tumor should undergo resection if it can be accomplished with acceptable morbidity. Examples are metastases to the liver, lung, and brain, which have the potential of being cured by surgery. This method is particularly valid for slow-growing tumors not responsive to chemotherapy, e.g., adenocarcinomas and sarcomas. Pulmonary metastases from sarcoma are not infrequently the sole site of disease. Up to 30% of patients with pulmonary metastasis can be cured with resection of single or multiple lesions. Similar control rates are found with adenocarcinomas in which the lung disease is the sole site of metastasis. Similarly, hepatic metastases, particularly from colon cancer, can be resected, leading to a long-term cure rate of approximately 25%. Although this method is by far the most effective single modality, studies combining resection and infusion of chemotherapy potentially offer the prospect of improving the survival rate. Resection of solitary brain metastases should also be considered when the brain is the only site of disease. Careful consideration of the functional defect resulting from surgery should be considered in cases of solitary brain metastases.

D. Establishment of vascular access. The use of permanent right atrial catheters permits painless, reliable access for administration of chemotherapy and nutrition. These catheters have reduced the incidence of skin complications due to extravasation of drugs and have improved adherence to drug administration scheduling by providing a reliable access site. In addition, peritoneal catheters have provided ready access to the abdomen for chemotherapy of ovarian or colon cancers.

E. Treatment of oncologic emergencies. Emergency situations that call for surgical intervention may arise in cancer patients. They usually involve hemorrhage, perforation, and abscess formation. The cancer patient is often at risk because of bone marrow suppression due to chemotherapy or irradiation in addition to being at risk of hemorrhage or sepsis. Metastasis of tumor to the central nervous system, causing cord compression, may require emergency neurosurgical decompression and radiation therapy for preservation of function.

Selected Reading

Brandt, B., and Ehrenhaft, J. L. Surgical management of pulmonary metastases. *Curr. Probl. Cancer* 5:4, 1980.

Dupont, W. D., and Page, D. L. Risk factors for breast cancer in women with proliferative breast disease. *N. Engl. J. Med.* 313:146, 1985.

Griffiths, C. T., Parker, L. M., and Fuller, A. F., Jr. Role of cytoreductive surgical treatment in the management of ovarian cancer. *Cancer Treat. Rep.* 63:235, 1979.

Silberman, A. W. Surgical debulking of tumors. *Surg. Gynecol. Obstet.* 155:577, 1982.

Principles of Radiation Therapy

Ralph R. Dobelbower

I. **Irradiation as treatment for neoplastic disease.** Irradiation and surgery remain the two primary local treatment modalities for definitive management of neoplastic diseases. In contrast to systemic chemotherapy, surgery and irradiation are local modes of treatment. The choice of treatment modality is based partly on the inherent responsiveness of the neoplasm to ionizing radiation. Some neoplasms (e.g., lymphoma and seminoma) are sensitive to the effects of irradiation, whereas others (e.g., melanoma and glioblastoma multiforme) are markedly less responsive.

Irradiation is the treatment of choice for some tumors and is clearly contraindicated for others. Hodgkin's disease, regarded as nearly universally fatal just four decades ago, is highly curable in its early stages by irradiation alone. Certain cancers of the skin that tend to spread deeply along anatomic planes (inner canthus of the eye, nasolabial fold, junction of the pinna with the scalp) commonly recur after surgical treatment and are best treated primarily by irradiation. Unresectable adenocarcinoma of the pancreas is best treated with precision high-dose irradiation. The survival of patients with pancreatic cancer so treated closely parallels that of patients with resectable disease treated by total pancreatectomy or pancreaticoduodenectomy for at least the first 3 years after diagnosis.

In some clinical situations the results of surgical treatment and irradiation are comparable. For example, either modality can cure 90% of patients with stage I carcinoma of the vocal cord or the intact uterine cervix. Local control rates and survival rates of patients with early stage mammary adenocarcinoma are comparable, whether the postexcisional biopsy is followed by mastectomy or definitive irradiation. In such instances the choice of treatment modality depends on the anticipated side effects of treatment, expertise and experience of local oncologists, expense, convenience, and preference of the patient.

II. **Physical, biologic, and clinical principles of radiation treatment**
   A. **Physical principles of radiation therapy**
      1. **Types of radiation beam.** Three ionizing radiations are of importance in external beam radiation therapy: x rays, gamma rays, and electron beams.
         a. **X rays** are created through interactions of electrons with matter.
         b. **Gamma rays** are physically identical to x rays, but originate from the atomic nucleus during radioactive decay.
         c. **Electron beams** for clinical irradiation are produced by accelerators (betatrons, linear accelerators, and microtrons).
      2. **Radiation exposure.** The basic unit of radiation exposure is the Roentgen, which is defined as the

sum of all electric charges on all ions of one sign produced in air when irradiated by photons divided by
the mass of air irradiated by the photons. One Roent-
gen equals 2.58×10^{-14} coulombs/kg of air.

   3. **Radiation dose.** The unit of radiation absorbed
   dose is the rad, defined as the absorption of 100 ergs/
   gm of matter. The international unit of absorbed
   dose is the Gray (Gy), which is 1 joule/kg. One Gy is
   equivalent to 100 rad. In this handbook, the term
   centigray (cGy) centigray is used rather than rad
   (1 cGy = 1 rad).

   4. **Radiation quality.** Radiation quality defines the
   ability of radiation to penetrate matter below the
   surface. When considering radiation doses, it is important to know the depth-dose characteristics of
   the treatment beam employed. As the energy of a
   radiation beam increases, the more penetrating
   it is.

B. **Biologic principles of radiation therapy.** Factors
that affect the response of malignant (and normal) cells
to irradiation include radiation sensitivity, cellular repair capacity, multiplicity of the cell population, cellular
oxygenation, linear energy transfer, relative biologic effectiveness, and position in the cell cycle.

   1. **Radiation sensitivity** is somewhat dependent on
   histology. Some malignant cells are exquisitely
   radiosensitive (e.g., in seminoma and leukemia),
   whereas others are relatively radioresistant (e.g., in
   melanoma and glioblastoma multiforme).

   2. **Cellular repair capacity** for radiation damage is
   severely lacking in certain histologic variants (seminoma and leukemia) but seems to be enhanced in
   some neoplastic cells (melanoma).

   3. **Oxygen** is a potent radiation sensitizer, presumably
   because of its high electronegativity and its ability
   to scavenge and interact with free radicals. The *oxygen enhancement ratio,* defined as the ratio between the dose for anoxic cells and the dose for oxygenated cells to achieve isoeffect, is approximately
   2.5–3.0 for low-energy x rays. Thus the dose of radiation needed to achieve the same effect is 2.5–3.0
   times greater for anoxic cells than for oxygenated
   cells. This point is important for clinical radiotherapy, as many tumors are thought to contain central
   hypoxic cores in which cancer cells are alive but the
   oxygen supply is compromised; hence these cells are
   radioresistant.

   4. **Linear energy transfer** (LET) is defined as the
   density of ionizing events resulting from a specific
   type of radiation. Particle beams (neutrons, protons,
   stripped nuclei, and others) have higher LET than
   x rays or gamma rays. Ionizing events resulting from
   the passage of particles through tissue are closer together than for photons; and therefore more energy
   is deposited per unit length of beam path. Because of
   this increased density of energy transfer, cells are

more damaged than they would be from the passage of lower LET beams.

5. Relative biologic effectiveness (RBE) describes the observation that different radiations produce different net cellular effects. Orthovoltage (250 kV x ray) is the standard for comparison. The radiation dose for a test beam and an orthovoltage beam is determined for an isoeffect level. The ratio of the two radiation doses necessary to achieve the same effect is defined as the RBE for the test beam. For example, most neutron beams employed clinically have an RBE of approximately 3.

6. Radiosensitivity is a function of the position of a given cell in the cell cycle. Cells in mitosis are more sensitive to radiation damage than cells in interphase. Cell sensitivity in S phase is lower than in phase G_1 or G_2. If the malignant cells within a tumor could be synchronized in the cell cycle, the response of those cells to radiation could be enhanced by irradiating when most of the cells were in a radiation-sensitive phase.

C. Clinical principles of radiation therapy. Radiation treatment depends on the principle of the therapeutic ratio.

$$\text{Therapeutic ratio} = \frac{\text{normal tissue complication dose}}{\text{tumoricidal dose}}$$

If the therapeutic ratio is much greater than 1 (a large normal tissue complication dose compared to the tumoricidal dose), cure without complication can be achieved. On the other hand, if the tumoricidal dose exceeds the normal tissue complication dose in any given clinical situation, the therapeutic ratio is less than 1, and cure without complication is categorically impossible. In many clinical situations, the therapeutic ratio is empirically close to 1, and radiation oncologists use many maneuvers (fractionation of dose, protraction of dose, multiple fields, isotope implants, shaped fields, displacement of normal structures, and others) to enhance the therapeutic ratio. Most of these maneuvers either relatively increase the dose to the disease or diminish the dose to the adjacent normal tissue or transit tissues.

Complications from radiation treatment come not from irradiation of tumors but from the dose to normal tissues (Fig. 4-1). Within the treatment field of any malignant tumor, there exist malignant cells and nonmalignant cells. These cells behave differently in response to irradiation, and it is this differential response that accounts for the existence of the therapeutic ratio. Furthermore, there appear to be differences in the repair of sublethal and potentially lethal radiation injury between normal cells and malignant cells. Radiation oncologists take advantage of these inherent differences by administering repeated fractions of the radiation dose, allowing sufficient time between dose increments for re-

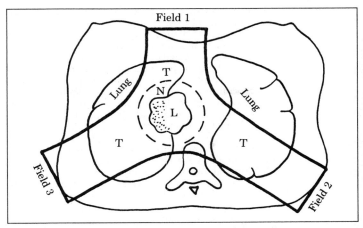

Fig. 4-1. Three-field treatment plan for a hilar lesion (*L*), illustrating the pulmonary tissue as matrix tissue (*stippled*), normal tissue (*N*) within the target volume (*broken line*), and transit tissue (*T*).

pair of radiation damage in the normal cell population. Protraction and fractionation of radiation dose are used to enhance the therapeutic ratio.

Radiation dose can be delivered by external beam therapy, intracavitary radioisotope therapy, interstitial radioisotope therapy, or systemic radioisotope administration.

1. **External beam therapy.** Radiation treatment delivered by a source external to the body is generally referred to as external beam therapy. Superficial beams (90–120 kVp) may be used to irradiate certain superficial lesions of the skin and mucous membranes. Orthovoltage beams (140–500 kVp) may be used to treat slightly deeper lesions that tend to be infiltrative (skin cancers about the inner canthus, the junction of the pinna with the scalp, and the nasolabial fold). Superficial and orthovoltage beams deliver maximum doses at the surface of irradiated tissue for these beams. The depth of the maximum dose and the penetration of the beam increase with increasing beam energy. Megavoltage beams may be generated by radioisotope decay (^{60}Co teletherapy) or electron accelerators (linear accelerators, betatrons, and microtrons). Electron beams produced by accelerators may be used in situations in which it is desirable to avoid a radiation dose to deeply situated structures while homogeneously irradiating more superficial structures. The effective depth of an electron beam is directly related to the energy of the electrons.

Linear accelerators and ^{60}Co teletherapy units are the most common radiotherapeutic devices in use in the United States today. Effective use of such equipment is enhanced by a radiation therapy simulator, an x-ray imaging device employed to help map out the radiation fields. Modern radiotherapy facilities today are equipped with a radiation therapy simulator, at least one megavoltage radiation therapy device, a source of electron beams, and a treatment planning computer.

2. **Intracavitary radioisotope therapy** is the instillation or application of radioisotope inside a body cavity. Colloidal suspensions of radioisotope (e.g., ^{32}P) may be instilled in the pleural or peritoneal cavities in situations in which pleural or peritoneal implants of disease are less than 2 mm thick (because of the limited range of penetration of the ^{32}P beta emissions) and in which there is no loculation of fluid or obliteration of the anatomic space.

   More commonly, radioisotopes are temporarily brought into immediate approximation with gynecologic malignancies with the use of specially designed applicators. Remarkably high local doses of radiation can be achieved in this manner. The isotopes commonly employed for this purpose are ^{226}Ra, ^{60}Co, and ^{137}Cs.

3. **Interstitial radioisotope therapy.** Radioactive materials may be implanted temporarily or permanently in malignant neoplasms or in tumor beds. Isotopes commonly used for this purpose include ^{192}Ir, ^{125}I, ^{226}Ra, and ^{137}Cs. Radioactive seeds are commonly employed for permanent interstitial implants, whereas seeds, wires, and needles may be used for temporary implants; the latter procedures are best accomplished using afterloading techniques to minimize radiation exposure of hospital personnel. Interstitial implantation of radioisotope may be employed as the sole treatment modality (e.g., localized prostate cancer), as a boost dose in conjunction with external beam therapy (e.g., early breast cancer, head and neck cancers), or as an adjuvant to surgery (e.g., sarcoma resection bed).

4. **Systemic radioisotope administration.** Radioisotopes may be administered systemically in certain clinical situations (e.g., disseminated thyroid cancer). This form of treatment depends on preferential concentration of radioisotope within neoplastic tissues. Improvements in the specificity of monoclonal antibodies may make this form of administration of radiotherapeutic agents more useful and more common.

III. **Definitive irradiation.** Radiation treatment is used as a single modality with curative intent in many diseases, including medulloblastoma, skin cancer, certain gynecologic cancers, many head and neck cancers, regionally localized breast cancer, nonmetastatic retinoblastoma, Hodgkin's disease, and certain non-Hodgkin's lymphomas. Depending on the clinical circumstances, definitive irradiation may be delivered with external beam therapy, interstitial therapy, intracavitary therapy, and in appropriately equipped facilities with intraoperative radiation therapy. The following are examples of diseases that may be approached with definitive radiation treatment.

A. **Hodgkin's disease.** The malignant cells of Hodgkin's disease are exquisitely radiosensitive. Patients with early-stage disease (I, II, and IIIa) are effectively treated with external beam irradiation as a single modality. Patients with more advanced disease commonly undergo irradiation to areas of bulky disease after induction chemotherapy.

Above the diaphragm, mantle fields (see Fig. 24-1) are used to treat the contiguous lymph node-bearing regions from the mediastinum to the mastoid tip. An inverted-Y field (see Fig. 24-1) is often used to irradiate the contiguous node-bearing areas from the periaortic region to the femoral triangle. Local control of Hodgkin's disease is highly dose-dependent. Doses as low as 35–40 Gy result in 95% control rates for local disease. Mantle and inverted-Y fields are not commonly treated concurrently. Usually a rest period is prescribed for marrow recovery between supradiaphragmatic and infradiaphragmatic courses of radiation therapy.

B. **Laryngeal cancer.** Laryngeal carcinoma confined to the vocal cord is highly curable with external beam irradiation. Small, coplanar opposed fields are used to deliver 60–70 Gy in 6–8 weeks. Wedges or compensators may be necessary to achieve uniform dose distribution within the treatment volume. Such treatment commonly results in preservation of voice that is of much higher quality than that resulting from voice-preserving surgical procedures for laryngeal cancer. For lesions confined to the vocal cord, the success rate is greater than 90%.

C. **Breast cancer.** Radiation therapy is effective treatment for early-stage breast cancer. It has been shown that local control of cancer in patients with primary lesions less than 4 cm in diameter is slightly superior in patients treated with tylectomy and primary radiation therapy compared to modified radical mastectomy; survival is equivalent. The breast is commonly treated with medial and lateral tangential fields to avoid irradiation of pulmonary tissue. The regional lymph nodes, if not adequately excised and if not included in the tangential portals, can be treated with anterior and posterior custom-shaped fields that mate the dose profile to the patient's cervicothoracic anatomy. A dose of 45–50 Gy is administered to the breast and often the regional lymph nodes (usually depending on the adequacy of the axillary node dissection); the tumor bed dose is boosted to 60–66 Gy using (1) reduced fields of photons or electrons or (2) interstitial implantation of radioisotope. A good cosmetic result is achieved in at least 75% of patients. Cosmetic defects are strongly related to the placement of surgical scars and the extent of surgical debulking. Surgery more extensive than complete excision of the lump generally results in a less desirable cosmetic effect and does little to decrease local recurrence.

D. Gynecologic cancer. For early cancers of the intact uterine cervix [International Federation of Gynecology and Obstetrics (FIGO) stages I and IIA], surgery and radiation therapy are equally effective. For the more advanced stages irradiation is clearly the treatment of choice. External beam radiation therapy and intracavitary therapy are integrated in the treatment of gynecologic cancer to mate the dose profile to the disease profile. Typically, the "whole pelvis" is irradiated to a dose of 40–50 Gy using external beam therapy. The anatomy of the gynecologic organs, often distorted by neoplasm, frequently returns toward normal as the tumor shrinks under the effects of fractionated ionizing external beam irradiation. This return to normal, of course, facilitates intracavitary placement of radioisotope to deliver high doses of radiation to the pelvic structures involved with tumor. Typically, the intracavitary radioisotope applications are planned with an interval of 10–14 days between 48-hour applications. Optimal interdigitation of intracavitary therapy and external beam therapy is strongly dependent on the disease stage, individual pelvic anatomy (and its distortion by tumor), tumor response to irradiation, and the experience of the radiation therapist.

E. Other tumors. Many other cancers may be successfully treated with radiation therapy as a single modality, particularly in the event that patients are medically unfit for surgery or refuse it. Generally, tumors amenable to implantation of radioisotope for interstitial therapy tend to have a better prognosis than other tumors. It remains to be seen if intraoperative radiation therapy can produce similar results in a different spectrum of tumors.

IV. Palliative irradiation. Irradiation is an effective palliative modality for symptomatic patients in many clinical situations.

A. Symptom prophylaxis. Local irradiation may be administered prophylactically in certain situations based on the known natural history of the disease and the anticipated morbidity thereof. For example, the brain is a known sanctuary site and area of frequent recurrence in patients with otherwise localized oat-cell carcinoma. Prophylactic cerebral irradiation may be administered in such instances. Patients with metastatic breast cancer found to have asymptomatic lesions in the femoral neck or shaft are at risk of sudden fracture with attendant high morbidity. This risk may be significantly reduced by local prophylactic irradiation.

B. Symptom management. Bone pain, symptoms of brain metastases, bleeding, cough, hemoptysis, visceral pain, and airway obstruction are only a few of the commonly encountered symptoms of cancer that often can be relieved or prevented by local irradiation. Treatment of patients with such problems is highly individualized. The area to be irradiated, the size of the fields, and the timing and fractionation of radiation dose are functions of the extent of disease and various other individual patient factors, including anticipated survival, performance status, and especially prior treatment with radiation and antineoplastic drugs. Palliative radiation doses generally need not be as high as those required for definitive treatment and are often administered in accelerated time-dose fractionation schemes. Radioisotope interstitial implants are generally reserved for definitive management of cancer but, in highly selected individual cases, may be indicated for palliation of symptoms. In such instances, the use of afterloading techniques, relatively low energy isotopes (e.g., ^{125}I), or both is especially important from a radiation protection point of view.

C. Radiation therapy emergencies. Certain cancer problems constitute oncologic emergencies and require the immediate attention of a radiation oncologist and other physicians.

1. Spinal cord compression
2. Severe airway compromise
3. Brain metastasis with rapid or refractory neurologic decompensation
4. Malignant cardiac tamponade
5. Superior vena cava compression (usually not a true emergency)

Radiation therapy consultation should never be delayed in such situations.

V. Combined modality therapy. Many oncologic problems are best managed by one of three treatment modalities: surgery, radiation therapy, or chemotherapy. Frequently patients with cancer present with a bulky primary lesion, macroscopically evident regional disease, and perhaps microscopic or submicroscopic systemic disease. For this reason, oncologists often adopt a multidisciplinary approach to the treatment of cancer, selecting two or perhaps three modalities of therapy for sequential or simultaneous use. This approach requires close cooperation between the surgical oncologist, radiation oncologist, and medical oncologist to provide the patient with the best treatment. Although combined-modality therapy is not effective or desirable for all kinds or stages of cancer, the regular practice of a multidisciplinary approach provides the best opportunity to exploit the advantages of each mode of treatment. Surgery and radiation therapy are local treatments. However, cancer is often not a local disease, and systemic therapy is frequently necessary to improve overall disease control.

Irradiation may be used as an adjuvant to chemotherapy or to surgery; chemotherapy may be used as an adjuvant to surgery or to irradiation; or all three modalities may be combined in a given clinical situation.

A. Irradiation as an adjuvant to surgery. When surgery and irradiation are used together simultaneously or sequentially, close cooperation between the surgical oncologist and the radiation oncologist is of key importance. If combined modality therapy is anticipated, even in the form of postoperative irradiation, it is generally in the patient's best interests to obtain a radiation oncology consultation preoperatively. In situations in which the decision to administer radiation therapy postoperatively is made at the operating table, it is best to request intraoperative consultation so that the radiation oncologist can see and palpate the extent of the tumor or tumor bed that will require irradiation postoperatively. In such situations, the appropriate placement of radiopaque localizing markers is of great importance, as is histologic confirmation of cancer, even in patients with clearly unresectable disease. A detailed operative note describing the size and extent of the neoplasm, the fixation or actual invasion of adjacent structures, and the presence of involved adjacent lymph nodes and other structures is of paramount importance.

Patients who require surgical procedures in previously irradiated fields also deserve preoperative radiation oncology consultation. Using localization films, records, previously applied fiducial marks, and the like, the radiation dose profiles can often be reestablished preoperatively. This method assists the surgical oncologist with incision placement and extent of surgery. For example, if an intestinal bypass procedure is to be performed in a previously irradiated area, it is important to know the borders of the radiation field with some precision so that nonirradiated bowel may be used for each side of the anastomosis. The skin of a previously irradiated neck tolerates J- or U-shaped incisions much better than a trifurcated incision.

Radiation therapy is an effective adjuvant to surgery for many diseases, e.g., stage II testicular seminoma, stages B2 and C rectal carcinoma, and resectable pancreatic adenocarcinoma. Radiotherapy may be delivered pre- or postoperatively, or both ("sandwich therapy"). Intraoperative irradiation is also a possibility. The advantages of preoperative, postoperative, and intraoperative irradiation are outlined in Table 4-1.

B. Chemotherapy as an adjuvant to irradiation. Chemotherapy may be employed before, during, or after a course of radiation treatment for malignant disease. Sandwich therapy may also be used with radiotherapy sandwiched between the preirradiation and postirradiation course of chemotherapy.

    1. Preirradiation chemotherapy. Chemotherapy given prior to a course of definitive irradiation (or surgery) is termed *induction chemotherapy* or *neoadjuvant chemotherapy*. The biologic advantages of such an approach are as follows.

        1. Unirradiated tumor vessels permit optimal drug delivery.

        2. Nutrition and patient condition are generally bet-

ter prior to irradiation, permitting improved tolerance to chemotherapy.

3. There is no delay in institution of systemic treatment.

The disadvantages are as follows.

1. Radiation therapy is delayed.
2. Nutrition and patient condition are generally worse after chemotherapy, often resulting in impaired tolerance of definitive radiotherapy.

2. **Concurrent chemotherapy.** Chemotherapy administered during a course of irradiation presents the following theoretic advantages.

1. Systemic chemotherapeutic agents [dactinomycin, doxorubicin (Adriamycin), bleomycin, cisplatin, fluorouracil, hydroxyurea, and methotrexate] may act as radiosensitizers.
2. There is no delay in institution of systemic therapy.

Concurrent combined modality therapy is associated with increased treatment morbidity, and doses of radiation and drug must be scaled down appropriately.

3. **Postirradiation chemotherapy.** Postirradiation chemotherapy is generally used as an adjuvant in situations in which micrometastases are suspected (e.g., breast cancer with demonstrated axillary node metastases, certain sarcomas).
4. **Sandwich chemotherapy.** Employing systemic chemotherapy before and after a course of definitive irradiation combines the advantages of items **1** and **3** above. The morbidity is combined as well. Several such regimens are being tested at present.
5. **Intraoperative radiation therapy.** The role of chemotherapy given prior to, during, or after intraoperative radiation therapy remains to be established by prospective controlled randomized study.

C. **Irradiation as an adjuvant to chemotherapy.** In some clinical oncologic situations in which chemotherapy is the primary treatment modality, radiation therapy can be used as an adjuvant for "consolidation." For example, the treatment of choice for advanced non-Hodgkin's lymphoma is multiple-agent chemotherapy. In this setting, the most common site of first recurrence is in areas of bulky disease, which are identified before systemic therapy is begun. With the patient in remission, such areas of bulky disease can be irradiated.

Local irradiation can be used as an adjuvant to chemotherapy to treat sanctuary sites of disease (e.g., the brain) for oat-cell carcinoma and acute lymphocytic leukemia.

D. **Morbidity of combined modality therapy.** Whenever therapeutic modalities are combined in antineoplastic treatment, it must be remembered that potential

Table 4-1. Advantages and disadvantages of preoperative, postoperative, and intraoperative irradiation

Preoperative irradiation		Postoperative irradiation		Intraoperative irradiation	
Advantages	Disadvantages	Advantages	Disadvantages	Advantages	Disadvantages
Undisturbed local vasculature, better tissue oxygenation before surgery; tumor more radiosensitive.	Definitive surgery is delayed. Postoperative recovery may be prolonged. Increased morbidity.	May better tailor radiation dose profile to disease profile.	Disturbed tumor bed vasculature; tumor may be less radiosensitive.	Small volume of normal tissue irradiated.	Only a single fraction may be delivered.
Less radical surgery may be required.	Surgical resection may become more difficult.	Accurate surgical and histopathologic staging of disease. Tissue repair and healing proceed normally.	Surgical complications may delay irradiation; tumor cells may repopulate.	Dose to normal structures is minimized. Very high doses may be delivered.	Surgical complications may be increased. Limited availability.

Unresectable tumor may become resectable. Tumor dissemination during surgery may be decreased. Tumor cells rendered nonviable before being surgically dislodged into circulatory system. *Apparent* reduction in histopathologic stage of disease.	*Apparent* reduction in histopathologic stage of disease.	Higher radiation doses may be delivered to small volumes.	Scarring may trap normally mobile structures (e.g., bowel) in radiation field.	No delay between surgery and irradiation. More accurate dose localization. Accurate surgical staging of diseases.

morbidity is also combined. In certain situations the effect can be synergistic rather than simply additive.

1. **Morbidity of surgery plus irradiation.** Radiation therapy, even in relatively low doses, impairs wound healing because of interference with fibroblastic proliferation. Therefore, impaired wound healing and even wound breakdown can result from combined-modality treatment. Lymph node dissections combined with local radiation therapy increase the incidence of distal lymphedema (in head, arm, and leg). Prior abdominal surgery increases the risk of intestinal radiation injury, probably by partially immobilizing small bowel with postoperative adhesive disease. Previously irradiated tissues should be handled delicately during subsequent surgical procedures. Attention must be directed to vascular supply and vascular integrity when planning surgery in irradiated fields.

2. **Morbidity of chemotherapy combined with radiation therapy.** Morbidity of radiation therapy may be immediate (during or immediately after a course of treatment) or delayed (months to years after therapy). Combining chemotherapy with radiation therapy can enhance both the immediate and the delayed morbidity of irradiation.

Exacerbation of radiation reactions in mucosal or dermal tissues can occur with concomitant use of dactinomycin, bleomycin, fluorouracil, hydroxyurea, or doxorubicin (Adriamycin). The latter drug has also been implicated in anamnestic responses to radiation therapy when given following a course of irradiation. The threshold dose for radiation pneumonitis is significantly lowered when the irradiation is administered in conjunction with doxorubicin, dactinomycin, hydroxyurea, vincristine, or procarbazine.

Leukoencephalopathy may result from combined cranial irradiation and methotrexate. Late development of leukemia and other malignant tumors can result from certain combinations of chemotherapy and irradiation. In Hodgkin's disease the risk may be as high as 10% for patients treated with extended-field irradiation and combination chemotherapy. Semustine has been implicated as an etiologic event in the late development of leukemia in patients treated with chemotherapy plus radiation therapy. Continuous monitoring of ongoing studies may elucidate additional risks of combined modality therapy.

VI. **New directions.** The field of radiation therapy is anything but static. New modalities of treatment are constantly coming to the fore. The following are but a few examples.

A. **Dynamic radiation treatment.** Most modern megavoltage radiation therapy machines have isocentric rotational capability: The gantry of the machine can rotate the treatment head around the patient on the supporting couch while aiming the radiation beam at a given point within the patient's body. With such an arrangement, one can irradiate deeply situated tumors with relatively high doses while limiting the dose to the transit tissues to tolerable levels. With the advent of computed tomography and magnetic resonance imaging, it is now relatively easy to construct three-dimensional images of tumors (and of surrounding normal tissues). With *dynamic radiation therapy,* the shape of the radiation beam is a function of gantry rotation angle, and it is then possible to conform the radiation dose profile to the three-dimensional shape of the tumor. It requires a computer-controlled multileaf radiation beam collimator for the treatment machine. This technology is not now widely available, but it is becoming more so. As its use becomes widespread, it will enhance the radiation oncologist's ability to tailor radiation dose profiles to tumor profiles and thereby improve the therapeutic ratio.

B. **Hyperthermia.** There has been a dramatic reawakening of interest in heat as a treatment for cancer. Hyperthermia has been used as a sole modality for cancer treatment, but it is much more effective when combined with radiation treatment as a biologic response modifier.

The *thermal enhancement ratio* (TER) is defined as the ratio between the x-ray dose given alone and the x-ray dose given with heat necessary to produce a certain effect. The TER appears to be greatest when heat and radiation are delivered simultaneously, but this situation is often not possible. Clinically, temperatures of 42–43°C are typically employed for 40–60 minutes. Heating may be local or systemic, and it may be delivered in a number of ways, e.g., waterbath, thermal blanket, ultrasound, and microwave. A number of hyperthermia treatment devices are now commercially available, and the use of heat as a biologic response modifier for radiation treatment is becoming widespread. Much of the work being done at present, however, must be regarded as investigational.

C. **High-dose remote afterloading.** Radiation exposure of medical personnel is a problem associated with intracavitary or interstitial brachytherapy (short-distance treatment). Historically, radioactive sources were placed in body cavities or directly into tumors by the surgeon or radiation therapist with attendant significant radiation exposure. In an attempt to reduce such exposure, afterloading techniques were developed so that hollow needles, hollow plastic tubes, or other applicators were placed at the time of surgery. At a later time, radioisotopes were inserted into the tubes, needles, or applicators, reducing the overall exposure of medical personnel.

High-dose remote afterloading systems have proliferated. These radiotherapy devices generally use relatively small sources of ^{137}Cs, ^{60}Co, or ^{192}Ir, which are housed in a radio-protective safe when not in use but which can be delivered *by remote control* into appropriate applicators in various body cavities or into tumor-bearing tissues. This system eliminates radiation exposure of medical personnel. Several such devices are now commercially available, and clinical experience with this relatively new treatment modality is fairly extensive in the treatment of tumors of the prostate, bladder, cervix, lung, esophagus, breast, and head and neck. This type of therapy is now being accomplished with high-LET sources also. It is often combined with external radiation treatment and occasionally with hyperthermia. The high doses employed with this therapeutic modality necessitate better understanding of altered fractionation schemes, and much clinical research remains to be done.

D. Radiation sensitizers. Radiation sensitizers are drugs or other agents that possess the ability to enhance the effects of ionizing radiation when administered before, during, or after radiation treatment. In this regard, they act as biologic response modifiers. Many drugs possess these properties, e.g., fluorouracil, mitomycin, cisplatin, doxorubicin, and misonidazole. The ideal radiation sensitizer is nontoxic and selectively enhances the radiosensitivity of cancer cells (but not that of normal cells). Such an ideal sensitizer, of course, has yet to be found.

With the use of radiation sensitizers, major advances have occurred in the treatment of cancers of the esophagus, anus, and bladder. As late as 1975, abdominoperineal resection was routinely used for anal cancer. Today, most such cancers can be treated effectively with radiation therapy and radiosensitizing doses of fluorouracil and mitomycin without the loss of anal function, which generally remains good to excellent.

E. Exotic radiation beams. Generating high-LET radiation beams (especially negative pi mesons and stripped nuclei) is expensive and requires elaborate high-energy equipment that is not generally available; however, a few clinical research centers are actively studying such beams in the treatment of cancer. High-LET neutron beams are available at lower cost, but such equipment is still much more expensive than conventional radiation therapy equipment.

Neutron beam therapy is at least twice as effective as conventional photon beam therapy for treating unresectable salivary gland cancers. It is clearly the treatment choice for such tumors. Neutron beam therapy also seems to be more effective than conventional x-ray treatment for locally advanced prostatic cancer. Limited availability of high-LET beams precludes widespread employment of this therapeutic modality.

Clearly, the use of exotic radiation beams and combinations thereof with conventional radiation therapy, surgery, and biologic response modifiers requires a great deal of basic and clinical investigation.

Selected Reading

Abe, M., Takahashi, M., and Sugahara, T. *Hyperthermia in Cancer Therapy*. Tokyo: Cosmos, 1985.

Anghileri, L. J., and Robert, J. *Hyperthermia in Cancer Treatment* (Vols. I, II, III). Boca Raton: CRC Press, 1986.

Brady, L. W. *Radiation Sensitizers*. New York: Masson, 1983.

Brady, L. W., and Perez, C. A. *Principles and Practice of Radiation Oncology*. Philadelphia: Lippincott, 1987.

Catterall, M., and Bewley, D. *Fast Neutrons in the Treatment of Cancer*. Orlando: Grune & Stratton, 1979.

Coia, L. R., and Moylan, D. J. *Therapeutic Radiology for the House Officer*. Baltimore: Waverly, 1984.

DeVita, V. T., Hellman, S., and Rosenberg, S. A. *Cancer Principles & Practice of Oncology*. Philadelphia: Lippincott, 1989.

Dobelbower, R. R., Jr., and Abe, M. *Intraoperative Radiation Therapy*. Boca Raton: CRC Press, 1989.

Hall, E. J. *Radiobiology for the Radiologist*. Philadelphia: Lippincott, 1988.

Halperin, E. C., et al. *Pediatric Radiation Oncology*. New York: Raven Press, 1989.

Hornback, N. B. *Hyperthermia and Cancer: Human Clinical Trial Experience* (Vols. I and II). Boca Raton: CRC Press, 1984.

Mansfield, C. M. *Therapeutic Radiology*. New York: Elsevier, 1989.

Moosa, A. R. *Comprehensive Textbook of Oncology*. Baltimore: Williams & Wilkins, 1990.

Moss, W. T., and Cox, J. D. *Radiation Oncology Rationale Technique Results*. St.Louis: Mosby, 1989.

Pierquin, B., Wison, J. F., and Chassagne, D. *Modern Brachytherapy*. New York: Masson, 1987.

Wang, C. C. *Clinical Radiation Oncology: Indications, Techniques, and Results*. Littleton, MA: PSG Pub, 1988.

Ethical Considerations in Cancer Chemotherapy

Joy D. Skeel

Consideration of ethical principles in the practice of cancer chemotherapy presupposes the need for a high degree of sensitivity by the physician for the fears and anxieties of the patient about the seriousness of the diagnosis of cancer and the need for chemotherapy. In addition to being aware of the emotional factors involved when caring for patients who require chemotherapy, physicians should also be aware of the ethical issues involved. This chapter does not deal with the emotional aspects of the disease and its treatment; discussion is restricted to ethical principles, informed consent, refusal of treatment, and decisions at the end of life.

I. **Basic concepts**
   A. **Respect for persons.** The respect for persons is an umbrella principle in medical ethics. Other principles, rules, and concepts, such as autonomy and nonmaleficence, in medical ethics are derived from this concept.
   B. **Autonomy.** Patient autonomy means that patients are self-governing, i.e., free from controlling outside influences, when making decisions regarding their own bodies. Since the early 1960s the concept of patient autonomy has become increasingly important, ethically and legally, in the practice of medicine. Needless to say, this principle plays an important role in all areas of medicine but particularly in informed consent related to research protocols and choice of other therapies.
   C. **Nonmaleficence** means not harming the patient. This principle requires that a patient not be injured or put at serious risk of harm.
   D. **Beneficence** means doing what is perceived to be good for the patient. This principle involves actively doing good, which includes preventing harm, removing harm, and providing benefits.
   E. **Paternalism.** This concept (or attitude) is the opposite of respecting another person's autonomy. It conveys the image of the strong, domineering father who assumed he knew what was best for his children. (In medicine, physicians and patients are substituted, respectively, for fathers and children.) For many years physicians made decisions they considered to be in the best interest of their patients without involving the patients substantively in the decision-making process. Paternalism is ostensibly less prevalent today than during the pre-1970s.

II. **Informed consent.** According to Jonsen, Siegler, and Winslade, informed consent is the willing and uncoerced acceptance of a medical intervention by the patient after adequate disclosure of the nature of the intervention and its risks and benefits, as well as disclosure of alternative interventions and their risks and benefits.

A. **Functions of informed consent.** The functions of informed consent are the following.

1. Promote individual autonomy and rational decision making
2. Protect patients and research subjects
3. Avoid coercive practices in medicine
4. Encourage health care professionals to examine their practice of giving information to patients
5. Help to maintain trust

B. **Five essential elements of informed consent.** Beauchamp and Childress stated that there are five elements involved in the process for a patient to give informed consent: competence (decision-making capacity), disclosure of information, comprehension of the information disclosed, voluntariness and authorization.

1. **Competence** refers to the ability to make reasonable decisions, usually within a specific sphere of a person's life. It is essential to note that persons may be capable of making reasonable decisions in some, but not all, areas of their lives. For example, although individuals may no longer be capable of running the family business, they may well be competent to say what they do (or do not) want done to their bodies (i.e., what treatments they will or will not accept).

   a. **Three general standards of competence** may be applied.

      1. Capacity to reach a decision based on rational reasons
      2. Capacity to reach a reasonable result through a decision
      3. Capacity to make a decision at all

   b. **Application to chemotherapy decisions.** In the context of making decisions regarding chemotherapy, the three standards mentioned above could be interpreted to mean that a patient would be able to:

      1. Decide whether to accept or refuse the chemotherapy and give the reasons for their choice
      2. Understand its potential risks and benefits
      3. Understand the purpose of the chemotherapy

   c. **Problems.** Occasionally attempts are made to label patients incompetent when they choose to refuse therapy a physician deems the treatment of choice. Although there are troublesome cases where competence to decide about therapy may be borderline, it is inappropriate to label a patient incompetent merely because he or she disagrees with the physician's recommendation(s). It is also necessary to acknowledge that patients sometimes make choices their physicians consider unwise.

2. **Disclosure of information** to the patient. The pa-

tient should be told what the planned method of treatment is, with its risks and benefits, along with the alternative possible treatments and their attendant risks and benefits. Some physicians also mention the possibility of unforeseen risks. The patient should be told the purpose of the treatment and be given the opportunity to ask questions. Three standards for disclosure have been developed.

  a. **Professional practice standard** relies heavily on what the physician thinks is appropriate for the patient to know. There are several problems with this standard, including the fact that it can be paternalistic and thus undermine the concept of patient autonomy.

  b. **Reasonable person standard** is based on what the hypothetical reasonable person, in contrast to the real individual person sitting in front of the physician, would want or need to know to make a reasonable, informed decision.

  c. **Subjective standard** incorporates the specific situation of the individual person and what he or she would want or need to know based on physical and emotional needs.

  d. **A compromise** between the reasonable person standard and the subjective standard probably offers the best solution. Physicians often do not have time to have a detailed psychologic history of their patients; thus a totally subjective standard would be difficult to apply. However, a physician can provide the information a reasonable person would want or need to know and then encourage the patient to ask additional questions. The questions should be answered truthfully and simply, with care being taken to avoid medical jargon.

3. **Comprehension of information disclosed.** Beauchamp and Childress noted that this element may be the most important part of the informed consent process. It is sometimes difficult to assess the degree of understanding a patient possesses, but a patient should be able, at the least, to state the risks and benefits of the treatment proposed and to acknowledge if there are alternative treatments available.

4. **Voluntariness** refers to an individual's ability to make a decision free of coercion or undue influence by others.

  a. **Voluntariness includes** having adequate information regarding the options available. For example, if a patient has information only regarding therapy A and none regarding therapy B, the decision to accept therapy A is not truly voluntary.

  b. **Voluntariness is impeded** if the patient feels coerced by the physician (whether intentionally or unintentionally) to accept one therapy over another.

      5. Authorization simply means that a person actively and autonomously authorizes a professional to perform some medical procedure or to involve the patient in a research protocol.

C. Problems with informed consent

    1. Standard of disclosure. As noted above, problems occur when trying to devise a standard of disclosure that allows a patient to make an informed decision regarding treatment options. The best alternative seems to be the compromise as discussed in **B.2.d.**

    2. Abdicating patient's rights. There are occasional (rare) circumstances when patients prefer to have the physician make the decisions for them, but it ought to be the rare exception rather than the rule, as it opens the door to potential abuse.

    3. Remote risks. Whether to disclose the possibility of remote risks seems to depend on the severity of the risk (e.g., death versus loss of hair) and how remote it is (1:100,000 versus 1:1000). If the risk is severe, e.g., death, it might be disclosed to the patient if it occurs in an approximately 1:10,000 incidence, but its remoteness ought to be emphasized.

D. Nondisclosure is occasionally built into research protocols. These protocols should be carefully reviewed by institutional review boards.

E. Practical application

    1. Competence. If a patient is known by the physician, assessment of the person's capacity to make decisions is usually straightforward. If the patient's ability to make decisions is in question, a mini mental status examination may be utilized or a psychiatry consultation requested. If it is determined that the patient's decision-making capacity is diminished and the patient is incapable of making decisions, it is necessary to identify a surrogate decision-maker, either by designating a family member or instituting guardianship proceedings.

    2. Disclosure of information. Simple, straightforward language is recommended for describing the proposed therapy. When a research protocol includes a lengthy consent form, it is wise to read through it slowly with the patient and provide opportunities for questions. It is sometimes helpful, if the patient agrees, to have a close family member or friend present for these discussions so informed discussion can continue after the physician leaves the room. A word of caution regarding the presence of other persons during disclosure of information: A physician should pay primary attention to the patient, as patients occasionally complain that their physician seems to find it easier to talk to their families than to them. Therefore, although family members may be included in these discussions, the patient should be the primary focus. A physician should disclose his or her role in research protocols to patients in a straightforward manner. Patients should also be informed that research protocols allow them to make a contribution to society if they choose to be involved (particularly in phase I or II trials) and provide them with the newest therapies available. At the same time, patients should not be made to feel that their physician will be angry or will abandon them if they choose not to participate.

Cautionary note to the physician-researcher: There is a fine line between encouraging patients to participate in research protocols and (1) subtly coercing them by displays of physician disappointment if the patients choose not to participate, or (2) excessively raising patient expectations about the potential benefit to them from the protocol. When the physician finds him- or herself in the dual roles of physician and researcher, the physician's primary obligation is to benefit the patient unless it is stated otherwise to the patient.

3. **Understanding.** The most practical way for a physician or other health professional to assess a patient's comprehension of information disclosed is to ask them questions about the risks and benefits of the proposed treatment. They should also be able to state what the alternative treatment(s) would be as well as their general awareness of the risks and benefits of the other options.

4. **Voluntariness.** Patients should not feel that excessive pressure is being put on them to accept one form of treatment over another. This statement is not meant to imply that physicians ought not make recommendations; because they should. However, a physician must be cautious when filling the dual roles of researcher and physician so as not to coerce patients to participate in a research protocol when that is not truly their choice.

5. **Authorization.** A patient authorizes a physician to proceed with a specific therapy when the individual has made an autonomous choice regarding the available treatments.

III. **Refusal of treatment** by a patient and informed consent go hand in hand. Refusal of treatment, like informed consent, ought to be informed, competent, voluntary, and authorized.

A. **Principles involved in refusal of treatment**

1. **The issue of patient autonomy** is at the center of discussions regarding refusal of treatment by the competent patient.

2. **The principle of nonmaleficence** is equally important for incompetent patients.

B. **Refusals of treatment** should be respected in cases involving competent persons unless such nontreatment would cause significant harm to other persons, particularly young children. It does not mean that there should not be serious conversations to learn why a person is refusing treatment; misperceptions regarding treatment should be clarified. It is appropriate for physicians to counsel, advise, and persuade a patient to accept treatment, particularly when the patient's disease is believed to be treatable or curable. The physician is also obligated to listen—and to hear—the patient's reasons for refusing treatment. Sometimes it is reasonable to negotiate a specific time period during which treatment will be tried and then reassessed.

C. Physician response

    1. Frustration. This response is understandable if the physician believes the patient could benefit from the treatment being refused. Nonetheless, if autonomy is a value to be preserved, competent persons should be allowed to make their own decisions.

    2. Paternalism. The physician may be tempted to override the patient's refusal of treatment, but this behavior is difficult or impossible to justify when the patient is competent.

    3. Changing physicians. If the physician is strongly opposed to the patient's decision to refuse treatment, he or she may suggest that the patient change physicians. The physician, however, must be careful not to be perceived as abandoning the patient. If the physician is gravely concerned that the patient is making a wrong decision, a consultation may be requested from an ethicist, if there is one in the institution, or from an ethics committee.

D. Incompetent patients. Treatment may be refused for incompetent patients by proxy decision makers, who are usually family members or court-appointed guardians.

    1. The principle of nonmaleficence requires that the best interests of these patients be protected.

    2. Hospital ethicists or ethics committees may be helpful in resolving disputes that arise in these circumstances, particularly when the proxy decision-maker and physician disagree as to the appropriate course of treatment.

IV. Decisions at the end of life

A. Giving information. This time is no different from any other time in the physician–patient relationship; patients deserve to know what is occurring over the course of the illness so they can get their lives in order. However, information should be given in a compassionate manner so the patient does not feel badgered or as if all hope has been destroyed.

B. Decisions regarding how aggressively to treat

    1. Options must be presented clearly and openly.

        a. Some patients may want to be **treated aggressively,** including intubation and perhaps even cardiopulmonary resuscitation, even if there is only minimal hope for a meaningful quality of life.

        b. Other patients may wish to be involved in **clinical research studies** to provide a contribution to society and medicine.

        c. Still other patients may opt for **palliative care** and no further treatment.

2. Options regarding where care will be provided should be discussed.

 a. Some patients prefer to die in the **hospital setting** or in an extended care facility.

 b. Others may choose to become part of a **hospice program** (where available), which may mean dying at home or in a hospice unit.

C. Continued caring. During this time, when aggressive treatment is usually curtailed, the patient and family need to feel cared for by the medical team. Although treatment, except for palliation, may stop, caring must not.

D. Advance directives, such as the Living Will, Durable Power of Attorney for Health Care, and other documents usually called medical directives provide varying degrees of assistance to health care professionals regarding patients' wishes if they are no longer able to communicate them to their physician. The states vary widely in how liberal or how restrictive the formal documents are. For example, Ohio's Durable Power of Attorney for Health Care is so restrictive in its prohibitions on individual freedom to choose to have nutrition and hydration or other life support withdrawn or withheld that many individuals are choosing not to sign it. Instead, they are choosing to sign other medical directives in an attempt to protect their autonomy. Advance directives are meant to provide direction to physicians and other health care professionals; and they can be best utilized if discussed in advance by patient and physician. It means that physicians should ask patients if they have signed such a document and discuss it before it becomes necessary to use it. Once again, if the physician is concerned about the document, a consultation with the ethicist or the ethics committee may be useful.

Selected Reading

Beauchamp, T., and Childress, J. *Principles of Biomedical Ethics* (3rd ed.). New York: Oxford University Press, 1983.

Cantor, N. The permanently unconscious patient. *Am. J. Law Med.* 15:381, 1989.

Emanuel, E., and Emanuel, L. Living wills: past, present, and future. *J. Clin. Ethics* 1:9, 1990; see copy of the Medical Directive, p. 17.

Graber, J., Beasley, A., and Eaddy, J. *Ethical Analysis of Clinical Medicine.* Baltimore: Urban & Schwarzenberg, 1985.

Jonsen, A., Siegler, M., and Winslade, W. *Clinical Ethics.* New York: Macmillan, 1982.

Lidz, C., et al. *Informed Consent: A Study in Decision-making in Psychiatry.* New York: Guilford Press, 1984.

Reich, W. T. (eds.). *Encyclopedia of Bioethics.* New York: Free Press, 1978.

Roth, L., Meisel, A., and Lidz, C. Tests of competency to consent to treatment. In R. B. Edwards (ed.), *Psychiatry and Ethics.* Buffalo: Prometheus Books, 1982. Pp. 201–211.

6

Systemic Assessment of the Patient with Cancer

Roland T. Skeel

I. **Establishing the diagnosis**
   A. **Pathologic diagnosis is critical.** Although it is a truism to state that the diagnosis of cancer must be firmly established before chemotherapy or any other treatment is administered, the critical nature of accurate diagnosis warrants a reminder. As a rule, there must be cytologic or histologic evidence of neoplastic cells, together with a clinical picture consistent with the diagnosis of the cancer under consideration.

   Most commonly, patients present to their physician with a complaint such as a cough or a lump; through a logical sequence of evaluation, the presence of cancer is revealed on a cytologic or histologic specimen. Less frequently, lesions are discovered fortuitously during routine examination, systematic screening for cancer, or evaluation of an unrelated disorder. With some types of cancer, pathologists can establish the diagnosis on small amounts of material obtained from needle biopsies, aspirations, or tissue scrapings. Other cancers require larger pieces of tissue for special staining, immunohistologic evaluation, flow cytometry, examination by electron microscopy, or more sophisticated studies such as evaluation for gene rearrangement.

   It is often helpful to confer with the pathologist prior to obtaining a specimen in order to determine what kind and size of specimen is adequate to establish the complete diagnosis. When a tissue diagnosis of cancer is made by the pathologist, it is incumbent on the clinician to review the material with the pathologist. This practice is not only good medicine (and good learning), it helps to be able to tell the patient you have seen the cancer with your own eyes when you give the diagnosis. It also prevents the physician from administering chemotherapy without a pathologic diagnosis. The pathologist often gives a better consultation—not just a tissue diagnosis—if the clinician shows a personal interest.

   B. **Pathologic and clinical diagnosis must be consistent.** Once the tissue diagnosis is established, the clinician must be certain that the pathologic diagnosis is consistent with the clinical findings. If the two are not consistent, a search must be made for additional information, clinical or pathologic, that allows the clinician to make a unified diagnosis. It must be remembered that a pathologic diagnosis, like a clinical diagnosis, is also an opinion with varying levels of certainty. The first part of the pathologic diagnosis—and usually the easier part—is an opinion whether the tissue examined is neoplastic. Because most pathologists rarely render a diagnosis of cancer unless the degree of certainty is high, a positive diagnosis of cancer is generally reliable. Absence of definitively diagnosed cancer in a specimen does not mean that cancer is not present, however. It only means that it could not be diagnosed on the tissue obtained, and clinical circumstances must establish if additional tissue sampling is necessary. The second part of the pathologist's diagnosis is an opinion about the type of cancer. This determination is not necessary in all circumstances but nearly always is helpful for selecting the most appropriate therapy and making a determination of prognosis.

C. **Treatment without a pathologic diagnosis.** There are rare circumstances in which treatment is undertaken before a pathologic diagnosis is established. Such circumstances are clearly exceptions, however, and involve fewer than 1% of all patients with cancer. Therapy is begun without a pathologic diagnosis only when:

1. Withholding prompt treatment or carrying out the procedures required to establish the diagnosis would greatly increase a patient's morbidity or risk of mortality
2. The likelihood of a benign diagnosis is remote

Two examples of such circumstances are (1) a patient with a primary tumor of the midbrain, and (2) a patient with superior vena cava syndrome with no accessible supraclavicular nodes and no endobronchial disease found on bronchoscopy in whom the risk of bleeding from mediastinoscopy is deemed greater than the risk from radiotherapy for a disease of uncertain nature.

II. **Staging.** Once the diagnosis of cancer is firmly established, it is important to determine the anatomic extent or stage of the disease. The steps taken for staging vary considerably among cancers because of the differing natural histories of these tumors.

A. **Staging system criteria.** For most cancers, a system of staging has been established based on the following.

1. Natural history and mode of spread of the cancer
2. Prognostic import for the staging parameters used
3. Value of the criteria used for decisions about therapy

B. **Staging and therapy decisions.** In the past, surgery and radiotherapy were used to treat patients with cancer in "early" stages, and chemotherapy was used when surgery and radiotherapy were no longer effective or when the disease was in an advanced stage at presentation. In such circumstances, chemotherapy was only palliative (except for gestational choriocarcinoma); and in the absence of exquisitely sensitive tumors or strikingly potent drugs, the likelihood of increasing the survival was low. As we have learned more about cancer growth and tumor cell kinetics, the value of early intervention with chemotherapy has been transposed from animal models to human cancers. To plan this intervention and evaluate its effectiveness, careful staging has become increasingly important. Only when the exact extent of disease has been established can the most rational plan of treatment for the individual patient be devised, whether it be surgery, radiotherapy, chemotherapy, or biologic therapy alone or in combination. No single staging system is universally used for all cancers, and none of the several systems is presented here in detail. When relevant to the specific cancers whose chemotherapy is discussed in Part III of this *Handbook,* the staging system most commonly used for that cancer is discussed.

III. **Performance status.** The performance status refers to the level of activity of which a patient is capable. It is an independent measurement (independent from the anatomic extent or histologic characteristics of the cancer) of how much the cancer has affected the patient and a prognostic indicator of how well the patient is likely to do with treatment.

A. **Types of performance status scales.** Two performance status scales are in wide use.

1. **Karnofsky Performance Status Scale** (Table 6-1) has 10 levels of activity. It has the advantage of allowing discrimination over a wide scale but the disadvantages of being difficult to remember easily and perhaps making discriminations that are not clinically useful.

2. **Eastern Cooperative Oncology Group (ECOG) Performance Status Scale** (Table 6-2) has the advantages of being easy to remember and making discriminations that are clinically useful.

3. **Using the criteria of each scale,** patients who are fully active or mildly symptomatic respond more frequently to treatment and survive longer than do patients who are less active or severely symptomatic. A clear designation of the performance status distribution of patients in therapeutic clinical trials is thus critical in determining comparability of trials and effectiveness of the treatments used.

B. **Use of performance status for choosing treatment.** In the individualization of therapy, the performance status is often a useful parameter for helping the clinician decide whether the patient will benefit from treatment or will be made worse. For example, unless there is some reason to expect a dramatic response of a cancer to chemotherapy, treatment is often withheld from patients with an ECOG performance status of 4, as responses to therapy are infrequent and toxic effects of the treatment are likely to be great.

IV. **Response to therapy.** Response to therapy may be measured by (1) survival, (2) objective change in tumor size or in tumor product (e.g., immunoglobulin in myeloma), and (3) subjective change.

A. **Survival.** One goal of cancer therapy is to allow patients to live as long and with the same quality of life as they would have if they did not have the cancer. If this goal is achieved, it can be said that the patient is cured of the cancer (though biologically the cancer may still be present). From a practical standpoint we do not wait to

Table 6-1. Karnofsky Performance Status Scale

Functional capability	Level of activity
Able to carry on normal activity; no special care needed	100%—normal; no complaints, no evidence of disease 90%—able to carry on normal activity; minor signs or symptoms of disease 80%—normal activity with effort; some signs or symptoms of disease
Unable to work; able to live at home; cares for most personal needs; varying amount of assistance needed	70%—cares for self; unable to carry on normal activity or to do active work 60%—requires occasional assistance but is able to care for most of own needs 50%—requires considerable assistance and frequent medical care
Unable to care for self; requires equivalent of institutional or hospital care	40%—disabled; requires special medical care and assistance 30%—severely disabled; hospitalization indicated, although death not imminent 20%—very sick; hospitalization necessary; active supportive treatment necessary 10%—moribund; fatal processes progressing rapidly 0%—dead

see if patients live a normal life-span before saying that a given treatment is capable of achieving a cure, but we follow a cohort of patients to see if their survival within a given time span is different from a comparable cohort without the cancer. For the evaluation of response to adjuvant therapy (additional treatment that is given to treat potential nonmeasurable, micrometastatic disease), survival analysis (rather than tumor response) must be used as the objective measure of antineoplastic effect.

It is, of course, possible that a patient may be cured of the cancer but die early owing to complications associated with the treatment. Even with complications (unless they are acute ones such as bleeding or infection) survival of patients who have been cured of the cancer is

Table 6-2. ECOG Performance Status Scale

Grade	Level of activity
0	Fully active, able to carry on all predisease performance without restriction (Karnofsky 90–100%)
1	Restricted in physically strenuous activity but ambulatory and able to carry out work of a light or sedentary nature, e.g., light house work, office work (Karnofsky 70–80%)
2	Ambulatory and capable of all self-care but unable to carry out any work activities; up and about more than 50% of waking hours (Karnofsky 50–60%)
3	Capable of only limited self-care, confined to bed or chair more than 50% of waking hours (Karnofsky 30–40%)
4	Completely disabled; cannot carry on any self-care; totally confined to bed or chair (Karnofsky 10–20%)

likely to be longer than if the treatment had not been given but shorter than if the patient never had the cancer.

If cure is not possible, the reduced goal is to allow the patient to live longer than if the therapy under consideration were not given. It is important for physicians to know if, and with what likelihood, any given treatment will result in a longer life. Such information helps the physician to choose whether to recommend treatment and the patient to decide whether to undertake the recommended treatment program.

B. Objective response. Although survival is important to the individual patient, it is not easy to predict how long a patient is going to live; thus survival does not give an early measurement of treatment effectiveness. Tumor regression, on the other hand, frequently occurs early in the course of effective treatment and is therefore a readily used measurement of treatment benefit. Tumor regression can be determined by the reduced size of a tumor or the reduction of tumor products.

    1. Tumor size. When tumor size is measured, responses are usually classified as follows.

        a. Complete response is the disappearance of all evidence of the cancer for at least two measurement periods separated by at least 4 weeks.

        b. Partial response is a decrease of 50% or more in the sum of the products of the largest diameter and the diameter perpendicular to the largest (diameter product) of all measurable lesions with no appearance of any new lesions for at least 4 weeks. When there are more than three or four measurable lesions, representative lesions are usually measured, rather than all lesions.

   c. **Stable disease** is a decrease of less than 50% to an increase of less than 25% in the diameter product of any measurable lesions.

   d. **Progression** is an increase of more than 25% in the diameter product or the appearance of any new lesions.

   If survival curves of patient populations having different categories of response are compared, those patients with a complete response frequently survive longer than those with a lesser response. If a sizable number of complete responses occur within a treatment regimen, the survival rate of patients treated with that regimen is likely to be significantly greater than that of patients who are untreated. When the number of complete responders in a population rises about 50%, the possibility of cure for a small number of patients begins to appear. With increasing percentages of complete responders, the frequency of cures is likely to increase correspondingly.

   Although patients who have partial response to a treatment usually survive longer than those who have stable disease or progression, it is often not easy to demonstrate that the overall survival of the treated population is better than a comparable untreated group. In part, this difficulty may be due to a phenomenon of small numbers. If only 15–20% of a population respond to therapy, the median survival rate may not change at all, and the numbers may not be high enough to demonstrate a significant difference in the 5 or 10% survival duration for treated and untreated populations. It is also possible that the patients who achieve a partial response to therapy are those who have less aggressive disease at the outset of treatment and thus will survive longer than the nonresponders regardless of therapy. These caveats notwithstanding, most clinicians and patients welcome a partial response and are little concerned at that point with the vagaries of survival statistics.

2. **Tumor products.** For many cancers, objective tumor size changes are difficult or impossible to document. For some of these neoplasms, tumor products (hormones, antigens, antibodies) may be measurable and may provide a good, objective way to evaluate tumor response.

   Two examples of such markers are the abnormal immunoglobulins produced in multiple myeloma and the human chorionic gonadotropin (β-hCG) produced in choriocarcinoma, both of which closely reflect tumor cell mass.

3. **Evaluable disease.** Other objective changes may occur but are not easily quantifiable. When these changes are not easily measurable, they may be

termed *evaluable*. For example, neurologic changes secondary to primary brain tumors cannot be measured with a caliper, but they can be evaluated using neurologic testing. An arbitrary system of grading the degree of severity of the neurologic deficit can be devised that permits objective evaluation of tumor response.

4. **Performance status** changes may also be used as a measure of objective change, although in many respects the performance status is more representative of the subjective than the objective status of the disease.

C. **Subjective change and quality of life (QOL) considerations.** A subjective change is one that is perceived by the patient but not necessarily by the physician or others around the patient. Subjective improvement and an acceptable QOL are often of far greater importance to the patient than objective improvement: If the cancer shrinks but the patient feels worse than before treatment, he or she is not likely to believe that the treatment was worthwhile. It is not valid to look at subjective change in isolation, however, because temporary worsening in the perceived state of well-being may be necessary to achieve subsequent long-term improvement.

This point is particularly well illustrated by the combined-modality treatment in which chemotherapy is used to treat micrometastases after surgical removal of the macroscopic tumor. In such a circumstance, the patient is likely to feel entirely well after the primary surgical procedure, but the side effects of chemotherapy increase the symptoms and make the patient feel subjectively worse for the period of treatment. The winner's stakes are valuable, however, because if the chemotherapy treatment of the micrometastases is successful the patient will be cured of the cancer and can be expected to have a normal or near-normal life expectancy rather than dying from recurrent disease. Most patients agree that the temporary subjective worsening is not only tolerable but well worth the price if cure of the cancer is a distinct possibility. This judgment depends on the severity and duration of symptoms, functional impairment, and perceptions of illness, as well as on the expected benefit (increased likelihood of survival) anticipated as a result of the treatment.

When chemotherapy is given with a palliative intent, patients (and less often physicians) may be unwilling to tolerate significant side effects or subjective worsening. Fortunately, subjective improvement often accompanies objective improvement, so that patients in whom there is measurable improvement of the cancer also feel better. The degree of subjective worsening each patient is willing to tolerate varies, and the patient and physician together must discuss and evaluate whether the chemotherapy treatment program is worth continuing. Such discussions should include a clear presentation of the scientific facts that include objective survival and

		0	1	2	3	4
Leukopenia	WBC x 10	≥4.0	3.0 - 3.9	2.0 - 2.9	1.0 - 1.9	<1.0
	Granulocytes/Bands	≥2.0	1.5 - 1.9	1.0 - 1.4	0.5 - 0.9	0.5
	Lymphocytes	≥2.0	1.5 - 1.9	1.0 - 1.4	0.5 - 0.9	0.5
Thrombocytopenia	Plt x 10	WNL	75.0 normal	50.0 - 74.9	25.0 - 49.9	<25.0
Anemia	Hgb	WNL	10.0 normal	8.0 - 10.0	6.5 - 7.9	<6.5
Hemorrhage (Clinical)	-----	none	mild, no transfusion	gross, 1-2 units transfusion/episode	gross, 3-4 units transfusion/episode	massive, >4 units transfusion/episode
*Infection	-----	none	mild, no active Rx	moderate, localized infection requires active Rx	severe, systemic infection requires active Rx, specify site	life-threatening, sepsis, specify site
Fever in absence of infection	-----	none	37.1 - 38.0c 98.7 - 100.4F	38.1 - 40.0c 100.5 - 104.0F	>40.0c >104.0F for less than 24 hours	>40.0c (104.0F) for >24 hrs or fever with hypotension

Fever felt to be caused by drug allergy should be coded as allergy.
Fever due to infection is coded under infection only.

		0	1	2	3	4
GU	Creatinine	WNL	<1.5 x N	1.5 - 3.0 x N	3.1 - 6.0 x N	>6.0 x N
	Proteinuria	No change	1 + or <0.3g% or <3g/l	2-3+ or 0.3 - 1.0g% or 3 - 10g/l	4+ or >1.0g% or >10g/l	nephrotic syndrome
	Hematuria	neg	micro only	gross, no clots	gross + clots	requires transfusion
	*BUN	<1.5 x N	1.5 - 2.5 x N	2.6 - 5 x N	5.1 - 10 x N	>10 x N

Urinary tract infection should be coded under infection, not GU.
Hematuria resulting from thrombocytopenia should be coded under hemorrhage, not GU.

GI		none	able to eat reasonable intake	intake significantly decreased but can eat	no significant intake	-----
	Nausea	none	able to eat reasonable intake	intake significantly decreased but can eat	no significant intake	-----
	Vomiting	none	1 episode in 24 hours	2 - 5 episodes in 24 hours	6 - 10 episodes in 24 hours	>10 episodes in 24 hrs or requiring parenteral support
	Diarrhea	none	increase of 2-3 stools/day over pre-Rx	increase of 4-6 stools/day, or nocturnal stools, or moderate cramping	increase of 7-9 stools/day or incontinence, or severe cramping	increase of ≥10 stools/day or grossly bloody diarrhea, or need for parenteral support
	Stomatitis	none	painless ulcers, erythema, or mild soreness	painful erythema, edema, or ulcers, but can eat	painful erythema, edema or ulcers, and cannot eat	requires parenteral or enteral support
Liver	Bilirubin	WNL	-----	$1.5 \times N$	$1.5 - 3.0 \times N$	$>3.0 \times N$
	Transaminase (SGOT, SGPT)	WNL	$\leq 2.5 \times N$	$2.6 - 5.0 \times N$	$5.1 - 20.0 \times N$	$>20.0 \times N$
	Alk Phos or 5' nucleotidase	WNL	$\leq 2.5 \times N$	$2.6 - 5.0 \times N$	$5.1 - 20.0 \times N$	$>20.0 \times N$
	Liver - clinical	no change from baseline	-----	-----	precoma	hepatic coma
Viral Hepatitis should be coded as infection rather than liver toxicity.						

Fig. 6-1. Common toxicity criteria used by many of the National Cancer Institute-sponsored clinical trials groups. They are an example of a systematic scheme for evaluating toxicity due to chemotherapy. This kind of scoring of toxicity helps when assessing the severity of adverse effects for individual patients and for groups of patients undergoing similar or diverse treatments. WNL = within normal limits.

COMMON TOXICITY CRITERIA

		0	1	2	3	4
Pulmonary	.....	none or no change	asymptomatic, with abnormality in PFTs	dyspnea on significant exertion	dyspnea at normal level of activity	dyspnea at rest
	Pneumonia is considered infection and not graded as pulmonary toxicity unless felt to be resultant from pulmonary changes directly induced by treatment.					
Cardiac	Cardiac dysrhythmias	none	asymptomatic, transient, re-quiring no therapy	recurrent or persistent, no therapy required	requires treatment	requires monitoring, or hypotension or ventricular tachycardia or fibrillation
	Cardiac function	none	asymptomatic, decline or resting ejection fraction by less than 20% of baseline value	asymptomatic, decline or resting ejection fraction by more than 20% of baseline value	mild CHF, responsive to therapy	severe or refractory CHF
	Cardiac-ischemia	none	non-specific T-wave flattening	asymptomatic, ST and T wave changes suggesting ischemia	angina without evidence for infarction	acute myocardial infarction
	Cardiac-pericardial	none	asymptomatic effusion, no intervention required	pericarditis (rub, chest pain, ECG changes)	symptomatic effusion; drainage required	tamponade; drainage urgently required

Blood Pressure	Hypertension	none or no change	asymptomatic, transient increase by >20mm Hg (D) or to >150/100 if previously WNL. No treatment required	recurrent or persistent increase by >20 mm Hg (D) or to >150/100 if previously WNL. No treatment required		hypertensive crisis
	Hypotension	none or no change	changes requiring no therapy (including transient orthostatic hypotension)	requires fluid replacement of other therapy but not hospitalization	requires therapy and hospitalization; resolves within 48 hours of stopping the agent	requires therapy and hospitalization for >48 hours after stopping the agent
Skin	----	none or no change	scattered macular or papular eruption or erythema that is asymptomatic	scattered macular or papular eruption or erythema with pruritus or other associated symptoms	generalized symptomatic macular, papular or vesicular eruption	exfoliative dermatitis or ulcerating dermatitis
Allergy	----	none	transient rash, drug fever <38c, 100.4F	urticaria, drug fever =38C, 100.4F, mild bronchospasm	serum sickness, bronchospasm, req parenteral meds	anaphylaxis
*Phlebitis Local	----	none	arm	thrombophlebitis, leg pain and swelling, with inflammation or phlebitis	hospitalization ulceration	embolus plastic surgery indicated
	----	none	pain			
Alopecia	----	no loss	mild hair loss	pronounced or total hair loss	----	----
Weight gain/loss	----	<5.0%	5.0 - 9.9%	10.0 - 19.9%	>20.0%	----

Fig. 6-1. (continued)

COMMON TOXICITY CRITERIA

		0	1	2	3	4
Sensory	neuro-sensory	none or no change	mild paresthesias loss of deep tendon reflexes	mild or moderate objective sensory loss; moderate paresthesias	severe objective sensory loss or paresthesias that interfere with function	-----
	neuro-vision	none or no change	-----	-----	symptomatic subtotal loss of vision	blindness
	neuro-hearing	none or no change	asymptomatic, hearing loss on audiometry only	tinnitus	hearing loss interfering with function but correctable with hearing aid	deafness not correctable
Motor	neuro-motor	none or no change	subjective weakness; no objective findings	mild objective weakness without significant impairment of function	objective weakness with impairment of function	paralysis
	neuro-constipation	none or no change	mild	moderate	severe	ileus >96 hours
Psych	neuro-mood	no change	mild anxiety or depression	moderate anxiety or depression	severe anxiety or depression	suicidal ideation
Clinical	neuro-cortical	none	mild somnolence or agitation	moderate somnolence or agitation	severe somnolence or agitation, confusion, disorientation or hallucinations	coma, seizures, toxic psychosis
	neuro-cerebellar	none	slight incoordination, dysdiadokinesis	intention tremor, dysmetria, slurred speech, nystagmus	locomotor ataxia	cerebellar necrosis
	neuro-headache	none	mild	moderate or severe but transient	unrelenting and severe	-----

NEUROLOGIC

Metabolic		<116	116 - 160	161 - 250	251 - 500	>500 or ketoacidosis
	Hyperglycemia	<116	116 - 160	161 - 250	251 - 500	>500 or ketoacidosis
	Hypoglycemia	>64	55 - 64	40 - 54	30 - 39	<30
	Amylase	WNL	<1.5 x N	1.5 - 2.0 x N	2.1 - 5.0 x N	>5.1 x N
	Hypercalcemia	<10.6	10.6 - 11.5	11.6 - 12.5	12.6 - 13.5	≥13.5
	Hypocalcemia	>8.4	8.4 - 7.8	7.7 - 7.0	6.9 - 6.1	≤6.0
	Hypomagnesemia	>1.4	1.4 - 1.2	1.1 - 0.9	0.8 - 0.6	≤0.5
Coagulation	Fibrinogen	WNL	0.99 - 0.75 x N	0.74 - 0.50 x N	0.49 - 0.25 X n	≤0.24 X N
	Prothrombin time	WNL	1.01 - 1.25 x N	1.26 - 1.50 x N	1.51 - 2.00 x N	>2.00 x N
	Partial thromboplastin time	WNL	1.01 - 1.66 x N	1.67 - 2.33 x N	2.34 - 3.00 x N	>3.00 x N

*Denotes ECOG specific criteria.

Fig. 6-1. (continued)

tumor response data together with whatever QOL information has been documented for the treatment proposed. Moreover the expressed desires and the social, economic, psychologic, and spiritual situation of the patient and his or her family must be sensitively considered.

V. Toxicity

A. Factors affecting toxicity.
One of the characteristics that distinguishes cancer chemotherapeutic agents from most other drugs is the frequency and severity of anticipated side effects at usual therapeutic doses. Because of the severity of the side effects, it is critical to carefully monitor the patient for adverse reactions so therapy can be modified before the toxicity becomes life-threatening. Most toxicities vary with the following.

1. Specific agent
2. Dose
3. Schedule of administration
4. Route of administration
5. Predisposing factors in the patient, which may be known and predictive for toxicity or unknown and result in unexpected toxic effects

B. Clinical testing of new drugs for toxicity.
Before the introduction of any agent into wide clinical use, the agent must undergo testing in carefully controlled clinical trials. The first set of clinical trials are called *phase I* trials. They are carried out with the express purpose of determining toxicity in humans and establishing the maximum tolerated dose, although they are done only in patients who potentially might benefit from the drug. Such trials are undertaken only after extensive tests in animals have been completed. Many human toxicities are predicted by animal studies; but because of significant species' differences, initial doses used in human studies are several times lower than doses at which toxicity is first seen in animals. Phase I trials are carried out using several schedules, and the dose is escalated in successive groups of patients once the toxicity of the prior dose has been established.

At the completion of phase I trials, there is usually a great deal of information about the spectrum and anticipated severity of acute drug effects (toxicity). However, because patients on phase I trials often do not live long enough to undergo many months of treatment, chronic or cumulative effects may not be discovered. Discovery of these toxicities may occur only after widespread use of the drug in *phase II* trials (to establish the spectrum of effectiveness of the drug) or *phase III* trials (to compare the new drug or combination with standard therapy).

C. Common toxicities.
Some toxicities are relatively common among cancer chemotherapeutic agents. Common toxicities include the following.

1. Myelosuppression with leukopenia, thrombocytopenia, and anemia
2. Nausea and vomiting
3. Mucous membrane ulceration
4. Alopecia

Aside from nausea and vomiting, these toxicities occur because of the cytotoxic effects of chemotherapy on rapidly dividing normal cells of the bone marrow and epithelium (mucous membranes, skin, hair follicles).

D. Selective toxicities. Other toxicities are less common and are specific to individual drugs or classes of drugs. Examples of these toxicities include the following.

1. Vinca alkaloids: neurotoxicity
2. Ifosfamide and cyclophosphamide: hemorrhagic cystitis
3. Anthracyclines: cardiomyopathy
4. Bleomycin: pulmonary fibrosis
5. Asparaginase: anaphylaxis (allergic reaction)
6. Cisplatin: renal toxicity, neurotoxicity

E. Recognition and evaluation of toxicity. Anyone who administers chemotherapeutic agents *must be* familiar with the expected and the unusual toxicities of the agent the patient is receiving, be prepared to avert severe toxicity when possible, and be able to manage toxic complications when they cannot be avoided.

For the purpose of reporting toxicity in a uniform manner, criteria are often established to grade the severity of the toxicity. Figure 6-1 shows the criteria used by several National Cancer Institute-supported clinical trial groups for the most common toxic manifestations. The specific toxicities of the most commonly used individual chemotherapeutic agents are detailed in Chapter 8.

Selected Reading

American Joint Committee on Cancer. *Manual for Staging Cancer* (3rd ed.). Philadelphia: Lippincott, 1988.

Bailar, J. C., III, and Smith, E. M. Progress against cancer? *N. Engl. J. Med.* 314:1226, 1986.

Bonfiglio, T. A., and Terry, R. Pathology of cancer. In P. Rubin and R. F. Bakemeier (eds.), *Clinical Oncology for Medical Students and Physicians* (6th ed.). Rochester: American Cancer Society, 1983.

Cadman, E. Toxicity of chemotherapeutic agents. In F. F. Becker (ed.), *Cancer, A Comprehensive Treatise* (Vol. 5). New York: Plenum Press, 1977.

Coates, A., et al. Improving the quality of life during chemotherapy for advanced breast cancer. *N. Engl. J. Med.* 317:1490, 1987.

Feinstein, A. R., Sosin, D. M., and Wells, C. K. The Will Rogers phenomenon: stage migration and new diagnostic techniques as a source of misleading statistics for survival in cancer. *N. Engl. J. Med.* 312:1604, 1985.

Goldhirsch, A., et al. Costs and benefits of adjuvant therapy in breast cancer: a quality adjusted survival analysis. *J. Clin. Oncol.* 7:36, 1989.

Kennealey, G. T., and Mitchell, M. S. Factors that influence the therapeutic response. In F. F. Becker (ed.), *Cancer, A Comprehensive Treatise* (Vol. 5). New York: Plenum Press, 1977.

Oken, M. M., et al. Toxicity and response criteria of the Eastern Cooperative Oncology Group. *Am. J. Clin. Oncol.* 5:649, 1982.

Rubin, P. Statement of the clinical oncologic problem. In P. Rubin and R. F. Bakemeier (eds.), *Clinical Oncology for Medical Students and Physicians* (6th ed.). Rochester: American Cancer Society, 1983.

Selection of Treatment for the Patient with Cancer

Roland T. Skeel

I. **Treatment goals.** Before deciding on a course of treatment for a patient with cancer, the goal of treatment must be clearly defined. If the goal is to cure the patient of cancer, the strategy of therapy may be different from the strategy chosen if the purpose is to prolong useful life or to relieve symptoms. To set the goal of therapy, the physician must be acquainted with the principles of therapy in each of the treatment modalities, well grounded in the ethical principles of the treatment of patients with cancer, knowledgeable about antineoplastic agents, familiar with the particular therapy for the cancer in question, and aware of the patient's individual circumstances, including stage, performance status, social situation, and concurrent illnesses.

Armed with this information the physician can plan a course of treatment and make a recommendation to the patient. Although most often it is accepted, some patients reject the recommendation as inappropriate for them for a variety of reasons. Some ask the physician for another recommendation, and others seek the opinion of a second physician. The physician must clearly present the reasons for the treatment recommendations and why they seem to be the best way to achieve the treatment objective. At the same time, it is important for the physician to allow the patient to share in setting treatment goals, as it is the patient who must undergo the treatment and be willing to abide its consequences. The physician has the obligation to make a treatment recommendation, but the patient always has the right to reject that advice without fear that the physician will be "upset," dislike the patient, or refuse to continue to give him or her care.

II. **Choice of treatment modality**
   A. **Surgery.** The oldest, most established, and still most effective way to cure most cancers is surgery. Surgery is selected as the treatment if the cancer is limited to one area and if it is anticipated that all cancer cells can be removed without unduly compromising vital structures. If it is believed that the patient can survive the operation and return to a worthwhile life, surgery is recommended. Surgery is not recommended if the risk of surgery is greater than the risk of the cancer, if metastasis always occurs despite complete removal of the primary tumor, or if the patient will be left so debilitated that although cured of cancer he or she feels life is not worthwhile.

   Most commonly, surgery is reserved for treatment of the primary neoplasm, although at times it may be used effectively to remove isolated metastases (e.g., in lung, brain, liver) with curative intent. Surgery is also used palliatively, e.g., for decompression of the brain in patients with gliomas or biliary bypass in patients with carcinoma of the pancreas. In nearly all nonhematologic cancers, a surgeon should be consulted to determine the role of surgery in the optimal treatment of the patient. Principles of surgery in cancer management are discussed in Chapter 3.

B. Radiotherapy. Radiotherapy is used for the treatment of local or regional disease when surgery cannot completely remove the cancer or it would unduly disrupt normal structures or functions. In the treatment of some cancers, radiotherapy is as effective as surgery for eradicating the tumor. In this circumstance, factors such as the anticipated side effects of the treatment, the expertise and experience of local oncologists, and the preference of the patient may influence the choice of treatment.

One determinant of the appropriateness of radiotherapy is the inherent sensitivity of the cancer to ionizing radiation. Some kinds of cancer, e.g., the lymphomas and seminomas, are sensitive to radiotherapy. Other kinds, e.g., melanomas and sarcomas, tend to be less sensitive. Such considerations do not preclude the use of radiotherapy, however, and it is helpful to obtain the evaluation of the radiotherapist prior to initiating treatment so that treatment planning can take into consideration the possible contribution of this modality.

Although radiotherapy is frequently used as the primary or curative mode of therapy, it is also well suited to palliative management of problems, e.g., bony metastases, superior vena cava syndrome, and local nodal metastases. The use of radiotherapy in the management of bony metastases and superior vena cava syndrome is discussed in Chapters 29 and 30. Principles of radiotherapy in cancer management are discussed in Chapter 4.

C. Chemotherapy. Chemotherapy has as its primary role the treatment of disease that is no longer confined to one site or region and has spread systemically. In the earliest days of chemotherapy, this interpretation directed its use to diseases that regularly presented in a disseminated form, e.g., leukemia, or after disease recurred following primary management with surgery or radiotherapy. It is now understood that widespread systemic micrometastases commonly occur early in cancer. These metastases are associated with certain predictive factors, such as the axillary node metastases of carcinoma of the breast and the large tumor size and poorly differentiated histologic features of sarcomas. Therefore chemotherapy is now applied earlier to treat systemic disease. When this treatment is used for micrometastases, the response of an individual patient cannot be measured. Rather, the effectiveness of therapy must be determined by comparing the survival of high-risk patients who receive therapy with similar (control) patients who do not receive therapy for the micrometastases.

Chemotherapy also has a role in the treatment of localized or regional disease. These specialized uses are discussed in Chapters 31 and 38.

D. Biologic response modifiers. It has long intrigued cancer biologists that cancer does not occur randomly but preferentially selects specific populations: the young, the elderly, the immunosuppressed (certain types of cancer only), and those with a strong family history of cancer. These observations have led cancer biologists to postulate that some kind of biologic control over the emergence of cancer exists, which some people have and others do not, at least at the time the cancer becomes established. One prime candidate for the mechanism of biologic control of cancer has been immunity. That immunity plays some role in controlling the development of cancer has been clearly demonstrated in animal models and a few, though not most, human neoplasms. Other biologic factors, although less well defined at the present, may be equally or more important than immunity in the development of cancer.

In an attempt to exploit and enhance the biologic control that is presumed to exist to some degree in everyone, a variety of agents called *biologic response modifiers* have been used in the treatment of cancer. Two classes of biologic response modifiers, the interferons and lymphokines (of which interleukin-2 is an example), have been intensively studied, and there is evidence of their substantial activity in some types of cancer. This area of intensive research promises to provide an important component of effective cancer therapy. Principles of biologic response modification are discussed in Chapter 2.

E. Combined modality therapy. Neither surgery, radiotherapy, biotherapy, nor chemotherapy alone is appropriate for the treatment of all cancers. Frequently patients present with cancer in which there is a bulky primary lesion, macroscopically evident regional disease, and presumed microscopic or submicroscopic systemic disease. For this reason, oncologists have turned to a multidisciplinary approach to the treatment of cancer, selecting two or more modalities of therapy for sequential or simultaneous use. This approach requires close cooperation among the surgical oncologist, radiation oncologist, and medical oncologist to provide the patient with the best overall treatment plan. Although combined modality therapy is not effective or desirable for all kinds or stages of cancers, the regular practice of a multidisciplinary approach provides the best opportunity to exploit the advantages of each mode of treatment.

Chemotherapeutic and Biologic Agents

8

Antineoplastic Drugs and Biologic Response Modifiers: Classification, Use, and Toxicity of Clinically Useful Agents

Roland T. Skeel

I. **Classes of drugs.** Chemotherapeutic agents are customarily divided into several classes. For two of the classes, the *alkylating agents* and the *antimetabolites,* the names indicate the mechanism of cytotoxic action of the drugs in their class. For *hormonal agents* the name designates the physiologic type of drug, and for the *natural products* the name reflects the source of the agents. The *biologic response modifiers,* agents that mimic, stimulate, enhance, inhibit, or otherwise alter the host responses to the cancer, are discussed extensively in Chapter 2. Data for individual agents are given in section **III** of this chapter.

Within each class are several types of agents (Table 8-1). As with the criteria for separating into class, the types are also grouped according to the mechanism of action, biochemical structure or derivation, or physiologic action. In some instances these groupings into classes and types are arbitrary, and some drugs seem to fit into either more than one category or none. However, the classification of chemotherapeutic agents in this fashion is helpful in several respects. For example, because the antimetabolites interfere with purine and pyrimidine metabolism and the formation of DNA and RNA, they are all at least cell cycle-specific and in some instances primarily cell cycle phase-specific. The nitrosourea group of alkylating agents, on the other hand, contains drugs that are predominantly or entirely cell cycle-nonspecific. Such knowledge can be helpful in planning therapy for tumors when sufficient kinetic information permits a rational selection of agents and when drugs are selected for use in combination.

The classification scheme also may help to predict cross-resistance between drugs. Tumors that are resistant to one of the nitrogen-mustard types of alkylating agents thus would be likely to be resistant to another of that same type, but not necessarily to one of the other types of alkylating agents, such as the nitrosoureas or the metal salts (cisplatin). The classification system does not help in predicting multidrug resistance, which may have several phenotypes.

A. **Alkylating agents**

1. **General description.** The alkylating agents are a diverse group of chemical compounds capable of forming molecular bonds with nucleic acids, proteins, and many molecules of low molecular weight. The compounds either are electophiles or generate electrophiles in vivo to produce polarized molecules with positively charged regions. These polarized

Table 8-1. Useful Chemotherapeutic Agents

Class and type	Agent
Alkylating agents	
Nitrogen mustard	Chlorambucil, cyclophosphamide, ifosfamide, estramustine, mechlorethamine, melphalan
Ethylenimine derivative	Thiotepa (triethylenethiophosphoramide)
Alkyl sulfonate	Busulfan
Nitrosourea	Carmustine, lomustine, semustine,* streptozocin
Triazine	Dacarbazine
Metal salt	Cisplatin, carboplatin
Antimetabolites	
Folic acid analog	Methotrexate
Pyrimidine analog	Azacytidine,* cytarabine, floxuridine, fluorouracil
Purine analog	Mercaptopurine, thioguanine, deoxycorformycin, 2-chlorodeoxyadenosine,* fludarabine

Natural products
Mitotic inhibitor — Vinblastine, vincristine, vindesine*
Podophyllum derivative — Etoposide, teniposide
Antibiotic — Bleomycin, dactinomycin, daunorubicin, amsacrine,* doxorubicin (Adriamycin), idarubicin, mithramycin, mitomycin, mitoxantrone
Enzyme — Asparaginase

Hormones and hormone antagonists
Androgen — Halotestin and others
Corticosteroid — Prednisone, dexamethasone
Estrogen — Diethylstilbestrol
Progestin — Megestrol acetate, medroxyprogesterone acetate
Estrogen antagonist — Tamoxifen
Androgen antagonist — Flutamide
Luteinizing hormone-releasing hormone (LHRH) agonist — Leuprolide, goserelin

Miscellaneous agents
Substituted urea — Hydroxyurea
Methylhydrazine derivative — Procarbazine
Adrenocortical suppressant — Mitotane
Steroid synthesis inhibitor — Aminoglutethemide
Substituted melamine — Altretamine (Hexamethylmelamine)

*Investigational agents, not yet approved by the FDA for general use.

molecules then can interact with electron-rich regions of most cellular molecules. The cytotoxic effect of the alkylating agents appears to relate primarily to the interaction between the electrophiles and DNA. This interaction may result in substitution reactions, cross-linking reactions, or strand-breaking reactions. The net effect of the alkylating agent's interaction with DNA is to alter the information coded in the DNA molecule. This alteration results in inhibition of, or inaccurate DNA replication with, resultant mutation or cell death. One implication of the mutagenic capability of alkylating agents is the possibility that they are teratogenic and carcinogenic. Because they interact with preformed DNA, RNA, and protein, the alkylating agents are not phase-specific, and at least some are cell cycle-nonspecific.

2. **Types of alkylating agents**
   a. **Nitrogen mustards.** This group of compounds produce highly reactive carbonium ions that react with the electron-rich areas of susceptible molecules. They vary in reactivity from mechlorethamine, which is highly unstable in aqueous form, to cyclophosphamide, which must be biochemically activated in the liver.
   b. **Ethylenimine derivatives.** Triethylenethiophosphoramide (thiotepa) is the only compound in this group that has much clinical use. Ethylenimine derivatives are capable of the same kinds of reactions as the nitrogen mustards.
   c. **Alkyl sulfonates.** Busulfan is the only clinically active compound in this group. It appears to interact more with cellular thiol groups than with nucleic acids.
   d. **Triazine.** Dacarbazine, the only agent of this type, was originally thought to be an antimetabolite because of its resemblance to 5-aminoimidazole-4-carboxamide (AIC). Dacarbazine is now known to act as an alkylator after AIC is cleaved from active diazomethane.
   e. **Nitrosoureas.** The nitrosoureas undergo rapid spontaneous activation in aqueous solution to form products capable of alkylation and carbamoylation. They are unique among the alkylating agents with respect to being non-cross-resistant with other alkylating agents, highly lipid soluble, and having delayed myelosuppressive effects (6–8 weeks).
   f. **Metal salts.** Cisplatin and carboplatin inhibit DNA synthesis probably through the formation of intrastrand cross-links in DNA. They also react with DNA through chelation or through binding to the cell membrane.

B. **Antimetabolites**
   1. **General description.** The antimetabolites are a group of low-molecular-weight compounds that exert

their effect by virtue of their structural or functional similarity to naturally occurring metabolites involved in nucleic acid synthesis. Because they are mistaken by the cell for a normal metabolite, they either inhibit critical enzymes involved in nucleic acid synthesis or become incorporated into the nucleic acid and produce incorrect codes. Both mechanisms result in inhibition of DNA synthesis and ultimate cell death. Because of their primary effect on DNA synthesis, the antimetabolites are most active in cells that are actively growing and are largely cell cycle phase-specific.

2. Types of antimetabolites

a. Folic acid analogs. These drugs, of which methotrexate is the only member in wide clinical use, inhibit the enzyme dihydrofolate reductase. This inhibition blocks the production of the reduced N^5-N^{10}-methylenetetrahydrofolate, the coenzyme in the synthesis of thymidylic acid. Other metabolic processes in which there is one carbon unit transfer are also affected but are probably of less importance in the cytotoxic action of methotrexate.

b. Pyrimidine analogs. These compounds inhibit critical enzymes necessary for nucleic acid synthesis and may become incorporated into DNA and RNA.

c. Purine analogs. The specific site of action for the purine analogs is less well defined than for most pyrimidine analogs, although it is well demonstrated that they interfere with normal purine interconversions and thus with DNA and RNA synthesis. Some of the analogs also are incorporated into the nucleic acids. The adenosine deaminase inhibitors, deoxycoformycin and chlorodeoxyadenosine increase the intracellular concentration of deoxyadenosine triphosphates in lymphoid cells. Among the metabolic alterations is nicotinamide adenine dinucleotide (NAD) depletion, which may result in cell death. For deoxycorformycin there is also interference with transmethylation reactions.

C. Natural products

1. General description. The natural products are grouped together not on the basis of activity but because they are derived from natural sources. The clinically useful drugs are (1) plant products, (2) fermentation products of various species of the soil fungus *Streptomyces,* and (3) bacterial products.

2. Types of natural products

a. Mitotic inhibitors. Vincristine, vinblastine, and its semisynthetic derivative vindesine are derived from the periwinkle plant (*Catharanthus roseus*), a species of myrtle. They appear to act primarily through their effect on microtubular protein with a resultant metaphase arrest and inhibition of mitosis.

   b. ***Podophyllum*** **derivative.** Etoposide, a semi-synthetic podophyllotoxin derived from the root of the mayapple plant (*Podophyllum peltatum*), forms a complex with topoisomerase II, an enzyme that is necessary for the completion of DNA replication. This interaction results in DNA strand breakage and arrest of cells in late S and early G_2 phases of the cell cycle.

   c. **Antibiotics.** The antitumor antibiotics are a group of related antimicrobial compounds produced by *Streptomyces* species in culture. Their cytotoxicity, which limits their antimicrobial usefulness, has proved to be of great value in treating a wide range of cancers. All of the clinically useful antibiotics affect the function and synthesis of nucleic acids.

      (1) Dactinomycin, the anthracyclines, doxorubicin, daunorubicin, and the anthracenedione mitoxantrone cause topoisomerase II-dependent DNA cleavage and intercalate with the DNA double helix.

      (2) Bleomycins cause DNA-strand scission. The resulting fragmentation is believed to underlie the drug's cytotoxic activity.

      (3) Mitomycin causes cross-links between complementary strands of DNA that impair replication.

      (4) Mithramycin complexes with Mg^{2+} to DNA and blocks RNA synthesis.

   d. **Enzymes.** Asparaginase, the one example of this type of agent, catalyzes the hydrolysis of asparagine to aspartic acid and ammonia and deprives selected malignant cells of an amino acid essential to their survival.

D. Hormones and hormone antagonists

   1. General description. The hormones and hormone antagonists that are clinically active against cancer include steroidal estrogens, progestins, androgens, corticoids and their synthetic derivatives, nonsteroidal synthetic compounds with steroid or steroid-antagonist activity, hypothalamic-pituitary analogs, and thyroid hormones. Each agent has diverse effects. Some effects are mediated directly at the cellular level by the drug binding to specific cytoplasmic receptors or by inhibition or stimulation of the production or action of the hormones. These agents may also act by stimulating or inhibiting natural autocrine and paracrine growth factors, e.g., epidermal growth factor, transforming growth factor-alpha (TGF-α), and TGF-β. The relative role of the various actions of hormones and hormone antagonists is not well understood and probably varies among tumor types. Other effects are mediated through indirect effects on the hypothalamus and its anterior pituitary regulating hormones. The final common pathway in most circumstances appears to lead to the malignant cell, which has retained some sensitivity to hormonal control of its growth. An exception to this mechanism is the effect of corticosteroids on leukemias and lymphomas in which the steroids appear to have direct lytic effects on abnormal lymphoid cells that have high numbers of glucocorticoid receptors.

2. **Types of hormones and hormone antagonists**

   a. **Androgens** may exert their antineoplastic effect by altering pituitary function or directly affecting the neoplastic cell.

   b. **Corticosteroids** cause lysis of lymphoid tumors that are rich in specific cytoplasmic receptors and may have other indirect effects as well.

   c. **Estrogens** suppress testosterone production (through the hypothalamus) in males and alter breast cancer cell response to prolactin.

   d. **Progestins** appear to act directly at the level of the malignant cell receptor to promote differentiation.

   e. **Estrogen antagonists** compete with estrogen for binding on the cytosol estrogen receptor protein in cancer cells and affect the natural growth factors.

   f. **Hypothalamic hormone analogs,** such as the leutenizing hormone releasing hormone (LHRH) agonists leuprolide or goserelin can inhibit LH and follicle-stimulating hormone (FSH) (after initial stimulation) and the production of testosterone or estrogen by the gonads.

   g. **Thyroid hormones** inhibit the release of thyroid-stimulating hormone, thus inhibiting growth of well differentiated thyroid tumors.

E. **Miscellaneous agents** are listed in Table 8-1. Descriptions of specific agents are found in section **III,** below.

II. **Clinically useful chemotherapeutic and biologic agents.** Section **III** of this chapter contains an alphabetically arranged description of the chemotherapeutic and biologic agents that are recognized to be clinically useful. Each drug is listed by its generic name with other common or trade names included. A brief description is given of the probable mechanism of action, clinical uses, recommended doses and schedules, precautions, and side effects. The role of the biologic agents in the therapy of malignant disease is not as well established as it is for chemotherapy, although it is clear that their indications and use will expand greatly in the near future.

A. **Recommended doses: caution.** Although every effort has been made to ensure that the drug dosages and schedules herein are accurate and in accord with published standards, readers are advised to check the product information sheet included in the package of each Food and Drug Administration (FDA)-approved drug and to read FDA–NCI (National Cancer Institute) guidelines for drugs not yet approved for general use to verify recommended dosages, contraindications, and precautions.

B. Drug toxicity: frequency designation. The doses are listed using body surface area (square meters) as the base. Adult doses from the literature, which are expressed using a weight base, have been converted by multiplying the milligram per kilogram dose by 37 to give the milligram per square meter dose. Doses using a weight base, which have been taken from the pediatric literature, have been converted using a factor of 25. Because many of the drugs are given in combination with other agents, doses most commonly used in popular combinations may also be indicated. These data should not be used as the sole source of information for any of the drugs but, rather, used as a guide to confirm and compare dose ranges and schedules and to identify potential problems. The designation of the frequency of toxic side effects is indicated as follows (probability of occurrence equals percent of patients).

1. Universal (90–100%)
2. Common (15–90%)
3. Occasional (5–15%)
4. Uncommon (1–5%)
5. Rare (< 1%)

These designations are meant only to be guides, and the likelihood of a side effect in each patient depends on their physical and psychologic status; previous treatment; dose, schedule, and route of drug administration; and other concurrent treatment.

C. Dose modification
   1. Philosophy. The optimal dose and schedule of a drug is one that gives maximum benefit with tolerable toxicity. Most chemotherapeutic agents have a steep dose-response curve; therefore if no toxicity is seen, as a rule, a higher dose should be given to get the best possible therapeutic benefit. If toxicity is great, however, the patient's life may be threatened or the patient may decide that the treatment is worse than the disease and refuse further therapy. How much toxicity the patient and the physician are willing to tolerate depends on the likelihood that more intensive treatment will make a major therapeutic difference (e.g., cure versus no cure) and on the patient's physical and psychologic tolerance for adverse effects.
   2. Guidelines
      a. Nonhematologic toxicity
         (1) Acute effects. Acute drug toxicity that is limited to 1–2 days and is not cumulative is not usually a cause for dose modification unless it is of grade 3–4 (see Fig. 6-1). Occasionally, repeating a dose that caused intractable nausea and vomiting or a temperature

higher than 40°C (104°F) is warranted, but for any other grade 3–4 toxicity, the subsequent doses should be reduced by 25–50%. If the acute drug effects (e.g., severe paresthesias or abnormalities of renal or liver function) last longer than 48 hours, the subsequent doses should be reduced by 35–50%.

A recurrence of the grade 3–4 side effects at the reduced doses would be an indication to either reduce by another 25–50% or discontinue the drug altogether. Non-dose-related toxicity, e.g., anaphylaxis, is an indication to discontinue the offending drug.

(2) **Chronic effects.** Chronic or cumulative toxicity, e.g., pulmonary function changes with bleomycin or decreased cardiac function with doxorubicin, is nearly always an indication to discontinue the responsible agent. Chronic or cumulative neurotoxicity due to vincristine may require no dose change, reduction, or discontinuation dependent on the severity of the resultant neurologic dysfunction.

b. **Hematologic toxicity.** The degree of myelosuppression and attendant risk of infection and bleeding that are acceptable depend on the cancer, the duration of the myelosuppression, and the general health of the patient. In addition, one must consider the relative benefit of less aggressive and more aggressive therapy. For example, with acute nonlymphocytic leukemia, remission is unlikely unless sufficient therapy is given to cause profound pancytopenia for at least 1 week. Because there is little benefit with lesser treatment, grade 4 leukopenia and thrombocytopenia are acceptable toxicities in this circumstance. Grade 4 myelosuppression is also acceptable when the goal is cure of a cancer that does not involve the marrow, such as testicular carcinoma. With breast cancer, on the other hand, responses are seen with less aggressive treatment, and prolonged pancytopenia may not be acceptable, particularly if chemotherapy is being used palliatively or in an adjuvant setting in which the proportion of patients expected to benefit from chemotherapy is relatively small and excessive toxicity would pose an unacceptable risk. (Whether higher doses might increase cure is currently under investigation.)

With these caveats in mind, the dose modification schemes shown in Tables 8-2 and 8-3 can serve as a guide to reasonable dose changes for drugs whose major toxicity is myelosuppression. Separate schemes are given for the nitrosoureas and for drugs that have less prolonged myelosup-

Table 8-2. Dose Modification for Myelosuppressive Drugs With the Nadir* at Less Than 3 Weeks

WBC/μl		Platelets/μl	Dose (%)
Blood count on day of scheduled treatment			
≥4000	and	≥125,000	100
3500–4000	or	100,000–125,000	75
2500–3500	or	75,000–100,000	50
<2500	or	< 75,000	0‡

*If the nadir WBC count is less than 1500/μl or platelets are less than 40,000/μl, decrease the dose by 25% in subsequent cycles.
‡If the WBC count is less than 2500/μl or platelets are less than 75,000/μl, perform the blood count weekly and resume treatment when the counts are above this level.

Table 8-3. Dose Modification for Myelosuppressive Drugs* With the Nadir at More Than 3 Weeks

WBC/μl		Platelets/μl	Dose (%)
Blood count at nadir			
>3500	and	>100,000	125
2000–3500	and	> 75,000	100
2000–3500	and	< 75,000	50
<2000	and	> 75,000	75
<2000	and	< 75,000	50
Blood count on day of scheduled treatment			
<4000	or	<100,000	0†

*Nitrosoureas or other agents whose nadir is prolonged.
†Perform weekly blood counts and withhold treatment until counts are normal; then treat with dosage adjustment based on the data in this table.

pression. Lesser dose reductions are justifiable for drugs with which myelosuppression is not a major effect.

III. **Data for clinically useful chemotherapeutic and biologic agents**
Note: Although every effort has been made to ensure that the drug dosage and schedules herein are accurate and in accord with published standards, users are advised to check the product information sheet included in the package of each FDA-approved drug and FDA–NCI guidelines for drugs that are not yet approved for general use (Table 8-1) to verify recommended dosages, contraindications, and precautions.

Agents that have not yet been approved by the FDA are included, either because they have some demonstrated usefulness or are widely used in investigational studies. As their efficacy and toxicity are more firmly established, it is expected that some will be approved by the FDA for general use, whereas others will remain investigational or be dropped from further study.

Aminoglutethemide

Other names. Cytadren, Elipten, AG

Mechanism of action. Inhibits aromatization and cytochrome P-450 hydroxylating enzymes, thereby blocking the conversion of androgens to estrogens and the biosynthesis of all steroid hormones. This drug causes, in effect, a reversible chemical adrenalectomy.

Primary indications. Breast carcinoma (investigational), adrenocortical carcinoma, ectopic Cushing's syndrome.

Usual dosage and schedule. 1000 mg daily in 4 divided doses.

Special precautions. Hydrocortisone must be given concomitantly (particularly for breast cancer) to prevent adrenal insufficiency. Suggested dose is 100 mg daily in divided doses for 2 weeks, then 40 mg daily in divided doses.

Toxicity

1. *Myelosuppression.* Leukopenia and thrombocytopenia are rare, and if they occur they resolve rapidly when the drug is stopped.
2. *Nausea and vomiting* are occasional and usually mild.
3. *Mucocutaneous effects.* A morbilliform rash is commonly seen during the first week of treatment, but it usually disappears within 1 week.
4. *Hormonal effects*
   a. Adrenal insufficiency—common without replacement hydrocortisone in patients with normal adrenal glands.
   b. Hypothyroidism—uncommon.
5. *Neurologic effects*
   a. Lethargy is common. Although usually mild and transient, it is occasionally severe.
   b. Vertigo, nystagmus, and ataxia—uncommon.
6. *Miscellaneous effects*
   a. Facial flushing—uncommon.
   b. Periorbital edema—uncommon.
   c. Cholestatic jaundice—rare.

Amsacrine (Investigational)

Other names. m-AMSA; AMSA.

Mechanism of action. Binds to DNA through intercalation and external binding. Interaction with topoisomerase II to increase DNA strand breakage.

Primary indications. Pediatric and adult acute leukemias.

Usual dosage and schedule

1. 120 mg/m^2 IV over 1–2 hours in 500 ml 5% dextrose and water for 5 days.
2. 100 mg/m^2 IV over 1–2 hours in 500 ml 5% dextrose and water on days 7, 8, and 9 (in combination regimens).

Special precautions. Use caution if patient was given prior anthracycline, as it may have additive cardiotoxicity. Solution physically incompatible with sodium chloride solutions. Avoid direct contact with skin.

Toxicity

1. *Myelosuppression.* Universal and dose-limiting.
2. *Nausea and vomiting.* Common.
3. *Mucocutaneous effects.* Mucositis is common and dose-related; occasional skin rash.
4. *Liver.* Common transient liver function abnormalities.
5. *Renal effects.* Rare.
6. *Diarrhea.* Occasional.
7. *Cardiac effects.* Possible. May be affected by prior anthracyclines, e.g., daunorubicin or doxorubicin.
8. *Neurologic effects.* Seizures, neuropathy, headache, dizziness, central nervous system (CNS) depression—uncommon.
9. *Phlebitis and local pain.* Common.

Androgens

Other names. Fluoxymesterone (Halotestin), testolactone (Teslac), others.

Mechanism of action. Mechanism of antitumor effects is not clear.

Primary indications

1. Breast carcinoma (in combination with other agents).
2. Anemia of myelodysplastic syndromes.

Usual dosage and schedule

1. Fluoxymesterone: 20–40 mg PO daily in 4 divided doses.
2. Testolactone: 1000 mg PO daily in 4 divided doses.

Special precautions. Hypercalcemia may occur with initial therapy.

Toxicity

1. *Myelosuppression.* None. Erythropoiesis is stimulated.
2. *Nausea and vomiting.* Mild and dose-related.
3. *Mucocutaneous effects.* Acne.
4. *Miscellaneous effects*
   a. Masculinization—including an increase in facial and body hair, deepening of voice, acne, baldness, and clitoral hypertrophy—is common in females but may be minimized by dose attenuation.
   b. Intrahepatic biliary stasis with hyperbilirubinemia

is uncommon but may occur at high androgen doses
(17-methyl derivatives only).

c. Fluid retention may occur, although it is less severe
with androgens than with estrogens—occasional.

Asparaginase

Other names.   L-Asparaginase, Elspar.

Mechanism of action.   Hydrolysis of serum asparagine
occurs, which deprives leukemia cells of the required amino
acid and inhibits protein synthesis. Normal cells are spared
because they generally have the ability to synthesize their
own asparagine.

Primary indication.   Acute lymphocytic leukemia, primarily for induction therapy.

Usual dosage and schedule.   Both schedules are usually
used in combination with other drugs (see under Special
precautions, item 2, below). The schedules listed are only
two of many acceptable dosing schedules (see Chapter 21).

1. 10,000 IU/m^2 IV on days 1 and 8 *or*
2. 6000 IU/m^2 IM 3 times weekly for 9 doses beginning
   day 3.

Special precautions

1. Be prepared to treat anaphylaxis at each administration
   of the drug. Epinephrine, antihistamines, corticosteroids,
   and life-support equipment should be readily available.
2. Giving concurrently with or immediately before vincristine may increase vincristine toxicity.

Toxicity

1. *Myelosuppression.* Occasional.
2. *Nausea and vomiting.* Occasional and usually mild.
3. *Mucocutaneous effects.* No toxicity occurs except as a
   sign of hypersensitivity.
4. *Anaphylaxis.* Mild to severe hypersensitivity reactions,
   including anaphylaxis, occur in 20–30% of patients.
   Such reaction is less likely to occur during the first few
   days of treatment. It is particularly common with intermittent schedules or repeat cycles. If the patient develops hypersensitivity to the *Escherichia coli*-derived enzyme (Elspar), *Erwinia*-derived asparaginase may be
   safely substituted because the two enzyme preparations
   are not cross-reactive. Note that hypersensitivity may
   also develop to *Erwinia*-derived asparaginase, and continued preparedness to treat anaphylaxis must be maintained.
5. *Miscellaneous effects*
   a. Mild fever and malaise is common and occasionally
      progresses to severe chills and malignant hyperther-
      mia.

b. Hepatotoxicity is common and occasionally severe. Abnormalities observed include elevations of serum GOT, alkaline phosphatase, and bilirubin; depressed levels of hepatic-derived clotting factors and albumin; and hepatocellular fatty metamorphosis.

c. Renal failure is rare.

d. Pancreatic endocrine and exocrine dysfunction, often with manifestations of pancreatitis, occasionally occurs. Nonketotic hyperglycemia is uncommon.

e. CNS effects (depression, somnolence, fatigue, confusion, agitation, hallucinations, or coma) are seen occasionally. They are usually reversible following discontinuation of the drug.

Azacytidine (Investigational)

Other names.   5-Azacytidine, 5 aza-C, ladakamycin.

Mechanism of action.   A pyrimidine analog antimetabolite that causes interference with nucleic acid synthesis and is incorporated into both DNA and RNA, where it acts as a false pyrimidine.

Primary indication.   Acute nonlymphocytic leukemia.

Usual dosage and schedule

1. 100 mg/m^2 IV push q8h for 5 days *or*
2. 150–200 mg/m^2 IV daily as continuous infusion for 5 days.

Special precautions.   Because of drug instability the dose should be prepared immediately before use and discarded after 8 hours. Infusions should be freshly prepared with Ringer's lactate solution and changed every 8 hours.

Toxicity

1. *Myelosuppression.* Severe in all patients, with the leukocyte nadir occurring at 12–14 days. Occasionally, suppression is prolonged beyond several weeks.
2. *Nausea and vomiting.* Common. Continuous infusion lessens nausea and vomiting.
3. *Mucocutaneous effects.* Stomatitis and rash—occasional.
4. *Miscellaneous effects*
   a. Diarrhea—common.
   b. Neurologic problems with muscle pain, weakness, lethargy, and coma—uncommon.
   c. Hepatotoxicity—rare.
   d. Transient fever—occasional.

Bleomycin

Other name.   Blenoxane.

Mechanism of action.   Bleomycin binds to DNA, causes single- and double-strand scission, and inhibits further DNA, RNA, and protein synthesis.

Primary indications

1. Testis, head and neck, penis, cervix, vulva, anus, skin, and lung carcinomas.
2. Hodgkin's and non-Hodgkin's lymphomas.

Usual dosage and schedule

1. 10–20 units/m^2 IV or IM once or twice a week *or*
2. 30 units IV push weekly for 9–12 weeks in combination with other drugs for testis cancer.
3. 60 units in 50 ml of normal saline instilled intrapleurally.

Special precautions

1. In patients with lymphoma, a test dose of 1 or 2 units should be given IM prior to the first dose of bleomycin because of the possibility of anaphylactoid, acute pulmonary, or severe hyperpyretic responses. If no acute reaction occurs within 4 hours, regular dosing may begin.
2. Reduce dose for renal failure.

Serum creatinine	Full dose (%)
2.5–4.0	25
4.0–6.0	20
6.0–10.0	10

3. The cumulative lifetime dose should not exceed 400 units because of the dose-related incidence of severe pulmonary fibrosis. Smaller limits may be appropriate for older patients or those with preexisting pulmonary disease. Frequent evaluation of pulmonary status, including symptoms of cough or dyspnea, rales, infiltrates on chest x-ray film, and pulmonary function studies are recommended to avert serious pulmonary sequelae.
4. Glass containers are recommended for continuous infusion to minimize drug instability.

Toxicity

1. *Myelosuppression.* Significant depression of counts is uncommon. This factor permits bleomycin to be used in full doses with myelosuppressive drugs.
2. *Nausea and vomiting.* Occasional and self-limiting.
3. *Mucocutaneous effects.* Alopecia, stomatitis, erythema, edema, thickening of nail bed, and hyperpigmentation and desquamation of skin are common.
4. *Pulmonary effects*
   a. Acute anaphylactoid or pulmonary-edema-like response—occasional in patients with lymphoma (see Special precautions, above).
   b. Dose-related pneumonitis with cough, dyspnea, rales, and infiltrates, progressing to pulmonary fibrosis.
5. *Fever.* Common. Occasionally severe hyperpyrexia, diaphoresis, dehydration, and hypotension have occurred and resulted in renal failure and death. Antipyretics help control fever.
6. *Miscellaneous effects*
   a. Lethargy, headache, joint swelling—rare.
   b. IM or SQ injection may cause pain at injection site.

Busulfan

Other name. Myleran.

Mechanism of action. Bifunctional alkylating agent. Its effect may be greater on cellular thiol groups than on nucleic acids.

Primary indication. Chronic granulocytic leukemia.

Usual dosage and schedule. 3–4 mg/m² PO daily for remission induction in adults until the leukocyte count is 50% of the original level, then 1–2 mg/m² daily. Busulfan may be given continuously or intermittently.

Special precautions. Obtain complete blood count weekly while patient is on therapy. If leukocyte count falls rapidly to less than 15,000/;μl, discontinue therapy until nadir is reached and rising counts indicate a need for further treatment.

Toxicity

1. *Myelosuppression.* Dose-limiting. A fall in the leukocyte count may not begin for 2 weeks after starting therapy, and it is likely to continue for 2 weeks after therapy has been stopped. Recovery of marrow function may be delayed for 3–6 weeks after the drug has been discontinued.
2. *Nausea and vomiting.* Rare.
3. *Mucocutaneous effects.* Hyperpigmentation occurs occasionally, particularly in skin creases.
4. *Pulmonary effects.* Interstitial pulmonary fibrosis is rare and is an indication to discontinue drug. Corticosteroids may improve symptoms and minimize permanent lung damage.
5. *Metabolic effects.* Adrenal insufficiency syndrome is rare. Hyperuricemia may occur when the leukemia cell count is rapidly reduced. Ovarian suppression and amenorrhea are common.
6. *Miscellaneous effects.* Secondary neoplasia is possible.

Carboplatin

Other names. Paraplatin, CBDCA.

Mechanism of action. Covalent binding to DNA.

Primary indictions. Ovarian carcinoma, endometrial carcinoma, and other cancers in which cisplatin is active.

Usual dosage and schedule. 300–400 mg/m² IV by infusion over 15–60 minutes or longer, repeated every 4 weeks.

Special precautions. Much less renal toxicity than cisplatin, so there is no need for a vigorous hydration schedule or forced diuresis. Reduce dose to 250 mg/m² for creatinine clearance of 41–59 ml/minute, reduce to 200 mg/m² for clearance of 16–40 ml/minute.

Toxicity

1. *Myelosuppression.* Anemia, granulocytopenia, and thrombocytopenia are common and dose-limiting. Red blood cell transfusions may be required. Thrombocytopenia may be delayed (days 18–28).
2. *Nausea and vomiting.* Common; but vomiting (65%) is not as frequent or as severe as with cisplatin and can be controlled with combination antiemetic regimens.
3. *Mucocutaneous effects.* Alopecia is uncommon. Mucositis is rare.
4. *Renal tubular abnormalities.* Elevation in serum creatinine or blood urea nitrogen occurs occasionally. More common is electrolyte loss with decreases in serum sodium, potassium, calcium, and magnesium.
5. *Miscellaneous effects*
   a. Abnormal liver function tests—common.
   b. Gastrointestinal pain—occasional.
   c. Peripheral neuropathies or central neurotoxicity—uncommon.
   d. Allergic reactions—uncommonly seen with rash, urticaria, pruritus, and rarely bronchospasm and hypotension.
   e. Cardiovascular (cardiac failure, embolism, cerebrovascular accidents)—uncommon.
   f. Hemolytic uremic syndrome—rare.

Carmustine

Other names.   BCNU, BiCNU.

Mechanism of action.   Alkylation and carbamoylation by carmustine metabolites interfere with the synthesis and function of DNA, RNA, and proteins. Carmustine is lipid-soluble and easily enters the brain.

Primary indications

1. Hodgkin's and non-Hodgkin's lymphomas.
2. Brain tumors.
3. Multiple myeloma.
4. Melanoma.

Usual dosage and schedule.   200–240 mg/m^2 IV as a 30- to 45-minute infusion every 6–8 weeks. Dose often is divided and given over 2–3 days. Some recommend limiting the cumulative dose to 1000 mg/m^2 to limit pulmonary and renal toxicity.

Special precautions.   Because of delayed myelosuppression (3–6 weeks), do not administer drug more often than every 6 weeks. Await a return of normal platelet and granulocyte counts before repeating therapy.

Toxicity

1. *Myelosuppression.* Delayed and often biphasic, with the nadir at 3–6 weeks, it may be cumulative with succes-

sive doses. Recovery may be protracted for several
months.
2. *Nausea and vomiting.* They begin 2 hours after therapy
and last 4–6 hours—common.
3. *Mucocutaneous effects*
    a. Facial flushing and a burning sensation at the IV site
    may be due to alcohol used to reconstitute the drug—
    common with rapid injection.
    b. Hyperpigmentation of skin following accidental con-
    tact—common.
4. *Miscellaneous effects*
    a. Hepatotoxicity—uncommon but can be severe.
    b. Pulmonary fibrosis—uncommon at low doses, but fre-
    quency increases at doses over 1000 mg/m^2.
    c. Secondary neoplasia—possible.
    d. Renal toxicity is uncommon at doses less than 1000
    mg/m^2.

Chlorambucil

Other name.   Leukeran.

Mechanism of action.   Classic alkylating agent, with
primary effect on preformed DNA.

Primary indications
1. Chronic lymphocytic leukemia.
2. Non-Hodgkin's lymphoma of favorable histologic type.

Usual dosage and schedule

1. 3–4 mg/m^2 PO daily until a response is seen or cytopenias
occur; then, if necessary, maintain with 1–2 mg/m^2 PO
daily.
2. 30 mg/m^2 PO once every 2 weeks (usually with prednisone 80 mg/m^2 PO on days 1–5).

Special precautions.   Increased toxicity may occur with
prior barbiturate use.

Toxicity

1. *Myelosuppression.* Dose-limiting and may be prolonged.
2. *Nausea and vomiting.* May be seen with higher doses
but are uncommon.
3. *Mucocutaneous effects.* Rash—uncommon.
4. *Miscellaneous effects*
    a. Liver function abnormalities—rare.
    b. Secondary neoplasia—possible.
    c. Amenorrhea and azoospermia—common.
    d. Drug fever—uncommon.
    e. Pulmonary fibrosis—rare.

2-Chlorodeoxyadenosine (Investigational)

Other names.   None.

Mechanism of action.   Deoxyadenosine analog with high

cellular specificity for B cells. Resistant to effect of adenosine deaminase. Cell death probably caused by nicotinamide adenine dinucleotide (NAD) depletion. Effect is independent of cell division.

Primary indications. Hairy-cell leukemia, chronic lymphocytic leukemia, and possibly other B cell neoplasms.

Usual dosage and schedule. 0.05–0.2 mg/kg (2–8 mg/m^2) IV daily as a continuous 7-day infusion.

Special precautions. Give allopurinol 300 mg daily as prophylaxis against hyperuricemia.

Toxicity

1. *Myelosuppression.* Moderate granulocyte suppression is common. No other hematologic toxicity has been seen.
2. *Nausea and vomiting.* None.
3. *Mucocutaneous effects.* None.
4. *Other effects.* Fever, possibly due to release of pyrogens from tumor cells.

Cisplatin

Other names. *cis*-Diamminedichloroplatinum (II), DDP, CDDP, Platinol.

Mechanism of action. Similar to alkylating agents with respect to binding and cross-linking strands of DNA.

Primary indications. Usually used in combination with other cytotoxic drugs.

1. Testis, ovary, endometrial, cervical, bladder, head and neck, gastrointestinal, and lung carcinomas.
2. Soft-tissue sarcomas.

Usual dosage and schedule

1. 40–120 mg/m^2 IV on day 1 as infusion every 3 weeks.
2. 15–20 mg/m^2 IV on days 1–5 as infusion every 3–4 weeks.

Special precautions. Do not administer if creatinine level is more than 1.5 mg/dl. Irreversible renal tubular damage may occur if vigorous diuresis is not maintained, particularly with higher doses (>40 mg/m^2) and with additional concurrent nephrotoxic drugs, such as the aminoglycosides. At higher doses, diuresis with furosemide or mannitol (or both) plus vigorous hydration are mandatory.

1. An acceptable method for hydration in patients without cardiovascular impairment for cisplatin doses up to 80 mg/m^2 is as follows.
   a. Have the patient void and begin an infusion of 2 liters of 5% dextrose in half-normal saline with potassium chloride 10–20 mEq/liter and magnesium sulfate 0.5–1.0 gm/liter (4–8 mEq/liter); run at the rate of 1000 ml/hour.

b. As soon as the infusion is started, give furosemide 40 mg IV push.

c. After 30 minutes, if the patient has voided at least 250 ml, give mannitol 12.5 gm IV push. If the patient is unable to void at a rate of 500 ml/hour, no cisplatin should be given.

d. Following the mannitol, give the cisplatin IV as a 15- to 30-minute infusion through the sidearm of the first IV line or by a second infusion.

e. Give additional mannitol or furosemide, if necessary, to maintain a urine flow of more than 500 ml/hour for the first 2 hours or if the patient shows any evidence of congestive heart failure.

f. At the end of the 2-liter infusion, the IV line may be withdrawn if the patient is to go home, or it is kept open at a rate of 150 ml/hour until the vomiting stops if the patient is to remain hospitalized.

2. For doses of more than 80 mg/m^2, the following schedule is recommended.

a. Have the patient void and begin an infusion of 2 liters of 5% dextrose in 0.5 N saline with potassium chloride 10–20 mEq/liter and magnesium sulfate 0.5–1.0 gm (4–8 mEq/liter) to run at 1000 ml/hour.

b. As soon as the infusion is started, give furosemide 40 mg IV push.

c. At 2 hours, if the patient has voided at least 1000 ml, give mannitol 12.5 gm IV push and furosemide 40 mg IV push. If the patient has been unable to void at a rate of 500 ml/hour, no cisplatin should be given.

d. Following the mannitol and additional furosemide, give cisplatin by a 30-minute infusion.

e. At the end of the cisplatin infusion, restart an infusion of 5% dextrose in 0.5 N saline with potassium chloride 10–20mEq/liter at 500 ml/hour for another 4 hours. For the next 24 hours, give at least 4 liters of fluid PO or IV.

3. For patients with known or suspected cardiovascular impairment (ejection fraction < 45%) a less vigorous rate of hydration may be used, provided the dose of cisplatin is limited (e.g., 60 mg/m^2). For example, the 2-liter infusion of 5% dextrose with potassium chloride 10–20 mEq/liter and magnesium sulfate 0.5–1.0 gm (4–8 mEq/liter) may be given at a rate of 500 to 750 ml/hour, with the cisplatin being given after the first 750 ml has infused. An alternative is to give carboplatin.

Toxicity

1. *Myelosuppression.* Mild to moderate, depending on the dose. Relative lack of myelosuppression allows cisplatin to be used in full doses with more myelosuppressive drugs. *Anemia* is common and may have a hemolytic component.

2. *Nausea and vomiting.* Severe and often intractable vomiting regularly begins within 1 hour of starting cisplatin and lasts 8–12 hours. Prolonged nausea and vomiting occur occasionally. Higher than usual doses of antiemet-

ics may partially ameliorate these symptoms. Nausea and vomiting may be minimized by the use of a combination antiemetic regimen, e.g., dexamethasone, ondanseton or metaclopramide, and lorazepam (see Chap. 37).

3. *Mucocutaneous effects.* None.
4. *Renal tubular damage and electrolyte abnormalities.* Irreversible nephrotoxicity may occur, particularly if adequate attention is not given to achieving sufficient hydration and diuresis.
5. *Ototoxicity.* High-tone hearing loss is common, but significant hearing loss in vocal frequencies occurs only occasionally. Tinnitus is uncommon.
6. *Severe electrolyte abnormalities.* These abnormalities, e.g, marked hyponatremia, hypomagnesium, hypocalcemia, and hypokalemia, may be seen up to several days after treatment.
7. *Anaphylaxis.* May occur after several doses. Responds to epinephrine, antihistamines, and corticosteroids.
8. *Miscellaneous effects*
   a. Peripheral neuropathies—clinically significant signs and symptoms are common at cumulative doses >300 mg/m².
   b. Hyperuricemia—uncommon, parallels renal failure.
   c. Autonomic dysfunction with hypotension.

Colony Stimulating Factors

Other names. Granulocyte Colony Stimulating Factor (G-CSF, rhuG-CSF filgrastin, Neupogen), Granulocyte-macrophage Colony Stimulating Factor (GM-CSF, rGM-CSF, rhuGM-CSF Sargramostin, Leukine, Prokine).

Mechanism of action. Promotes growth and differentiation of myeloid progenitor cells. May improve survival and function of granulocytes.

Primary indications

1. Granulocytopenia secondary to intensive chemotherapy.
2. Granulocytopenia from primary marrow disorders, such as idiopathic neutropenia or aplastic anemia.
3. Granulocytopenia associated with acquired immunodeficiency syndrome and its therapy.

Usual dosage and schedule. 40–500 µg/m² SQ, IM, or IV daily. Dose and duration are dependent on the purpose of administration. As an adjunct to chemotherapy, commonly 200–400 µg/m² daily SQ for 10 to 20 days.

Special precautions. Potentially antigenic and serious hypersensitivity reactions could occur.

Toxicity

1. *Myelosuppression.* None (leukocytosis).
2. *Nausea and vomiting.* Occasional.
3. *Mucocutaneous.* Hair thinning with prolonged administration. Mucositis is uncommon.

4. *Miscellaneous effects*
   a. Usually mild and short lived.
   b. Exacerbation of pre-existing dermatologic conditions—occasional.
   c. Rash—common, but often resolves spontaneously, despite continuing the drug.
   d. Bone pain, musculoskeletal symptoms such as cramps, and back or leg pain—common.
   e. Pericarditis—dose related and uncommon.
   f. Flu like symptoms (fever, chills, aches, headache)—common.
   g. Local phlebitis—common if IV.
   h. Local erythema—common if SQ.
   i. Capillary leak syndrome—rare at usual doses.
   j. Hepatic or renal dysfunction—rare.
   k. Altered mental status or hallucinations—rare.
   l. Diarrhea—uncommon.

Corticosteroids

Other names. Prednisone, dexamethasone (Decadron), and others.

Mechanism of action. Unknown but apparently related to the presence of glucocorticoid receptors in tumor cells.

Primary indications

1. Carcinoma of the breast.
2. Acute and chronic lymphocytic leukemia.
3. Hodgkin's and non-Hodgkin's lymphomas.
4. Multiple myeloma.
5. Cerebral edema.
6. Nausea and vomiting with chemotherapy. (**Note:** There have been reports of subcapsular cataracts after high-dose Decadron for nausea and vomiting. Caution is urged, particularly when used in patients who may be cured.)

Usual dosage and schedule

1. *Prednisone*: dose varies with neoplasm and combination. Typical regimen, *except* for acute lymphocytic leukemia, is as follows.
   a. 40 mg/m^2 PO days 1–14 every 4 weeks *or*
   b. 100 mg/m^2 PO days 1–5 every 4 weeks.
2. *Prednisone*: for acute lymphocytic leukemia: 40–50 mg/m^2 PO daily for 28 days.
3. *Dexamethasone*: for cerebral edema: 16–32 mg PO daily to start, then reduce to lowest dose at which symptoms remain controlled.

Special precautions. None.

Toxicity

1. *Myelosuppression.* None.
2. *Nausea and vomiting.* None.
3. *Mucocutaneous effects.* Acne; increased risk for oral,

rectal, and vaginal thrush. Thinning of skin and striae develop with continuous use.
4. *Suppression of adrenal-pituitary axis.* May lead to adrenal insufficiency when corticosteroids are withdrawn. This problem is not common on intermittent schedules.
5. *Metabolic effects.* Potassium depletion, sodium and fluid retention, diabetes, increased appetite, loss of muscle mass, myopathy, weight gain, osteoporosis, and development of cushingoid features. Their frequency depends on dose and duration of therapy.
6. *Miscellaneous effects*
   a. Epigastric pain, extreme hunger, and occasional peptic ulceration with bleeding may occur. Antacids are recommended as prophylaxis.
   b. CNS effects, including euphoria, depression, and sleeplessness, are common and may progress to dementia or frank psychosis.
   c. Increased susceptibility to infection is common.
   d. Subcapsular cataracts in patients are uncommon but have been seen even when used for prophylaxis and treatment of drug-induced emesis.

Cyclophosphamide

Other names. CTX, Cytoxan, Neosar.

Mechanism of action. Metabolism of cyclophosphamide by hepatic microsomal enzymes produces active alkylating metabolites. Cyclophosphamide's primary effect is probably on DNA.

Primary indications

1. Breast, lung, ovary, testis, and bladder carcinomas.
2. Bone and soft tissue sarcomas.
3. Hodgkin's and non-Hodgkin's lymphomas.
4. Acute and chronic lymphocytic leukemias.
5. Neuroblastoma and Wilms' tumor of childhood.
6. Multiple myeloma.

Usual dosage and schedule

1. 1000–1500 mg/m^2 IV every 3–4 weeks *or*
2. 400 mg/m^2 PO days 1–5 every 3–4 weeks *or*
3. 60–120 mg/m^2 PO daily.

Special precautions. Give dose in the morning, maintain ample fluid intake, and have patient empty bladder several times daily to diminish the likelihood of cystitis.

Toxicity

1. *Myelosuppression.* Dose-limiting. Platelets are relatively spared. Nadir is reached about 10–14 days after IV dose with recovery by day 21.
2. *Nausea and vomiting.* Frequent with large IV doses; less common after oral doses. Symptoms begin several hours after treatment and are usually over by the next day.

3. *Mucocutaneous effects.* Reversible alopecia is common, usually starting after 2–3 weeks. Skin and nails may become darker. Mucositis is uncommon.
4. *Bladder damage.* Hemorrhagic or nonhemorrhagic cystitis may occur in 5–10% of patients treated. It is usually reversible on discontinuation of the drug, but it may persist and lead to fibrosis or death. Frequency is diminished by ample fluid intake and morning administration of the drug.
5. *Miscellaneous effects*
    a. Immunosuppression—common.
    b. Amenorrhea and azoospermia—common.
    c. Inhibition of antidiuretic hormone—only of significance with very large doses.
    d. Interstitial pulmonary fibrosis—rare.
    e. Secondary neoplasia—possible.

Cytarabine

Other names.   Cytosine arabinoside, ara-C, Cytosar-U.

Mechanism of action.   A pyrimidine analog antimetabolite that, when phosphorylated to arabinosyl-cytosinetriphosphate (ara-CTP), is a competitive inhibitor of DNA polymerase.

Primary indication.   Acute nonlymphocytic leukemia.

Usual dosage and schedule

1. *Induction*: 100–200 mg/m^2 IV daily as a continuous infusion for 5–7 days (in combination with other drugs).
2. *Maintenance*: 100 mg/m^2 SQ every 12 hours for 4 or 5 days every 3–4 weeks (with other drugs).
3. *Intrathecally*: 40–50 mg/m^2 every 4 days in preservative-free buffered isotonic diluent.
4. *High dose*: 3.0 gm/m^2 IV over 1 hour every 12 hours for 12 doses. *Not recommended outside of investigational settings.*

Special precautions.   None for standard doses. High dose, give in *1 hour infusion.* Longer infusion enhances toxicity.

Toxicity (standard dose only)

1. *Myelosuppression.* Dose-limiting leukopenia and thrombocytopenia occur, with nadir at 7–10 days after treatment has ended and with recovery during the following 2 weeks, depending on the degree of suppression. Megaloblastosis is common.
2. *Nausea and vomiting.* Common, particularly if the drug is given as a push or rapid infusion.
3. *Mucocutaneous effects.* Stomatitis is seen occasionally.
4. *Miscellaneous effects*
    a. Flulike syndrome with fever, arthralgia, and sometimes a rash—occasional.
    b. Transient mild hepatic dysfunction—occasional.

Toxicity (high dose)

1. *Myelosuppression.* Universal.
2. *Nausea and vomiting.* Common.
3. *Mucocutaneous effects.* Occasional to common mucositis.
4. *Neurotoxicity.* Cerebellar toxicity is common, particularly in the elderly, but is usually mild and reversible. However, on occasion it has been severe and permanent or fatal. It is probably not prevented or ameliorated by pyridoxine supplementation 300 mg/day PO in divided doses or 150 mg IV every 12 hours for 10 days).
5. *Conjunctivitis.* Hydrocortisone 2 drops OU qid for 10 days may ameliorate or prevent keratitis.
6. *Hepatic toxicity with cholestatic jaundice.*
7. *Diarrhea.* Common.

Dacarbazine

Other names.   Imidazole carboxamide, DIC, DTIC-Dome.

Mechanism of action.   Uncertain but probably interacts with preformed macromolecules by alkylation.

Primary indications

1. Melanoma.
2. All soft-tissue sarcomas.
3. Hodgkin's lymphoma.

Usual dosage and schedule

1. 150–250 mg/m^2 IV push or rapid infusion on days 1–5 every 3–4 weeks *or*
2. 400–500 mg/m^2 IV push or rapid infusion on days 1 and 2 every 3–4 weeks.
3. 200 mg/m^2 IV daily as a continuous 96-hour infusion.

Special precautions

1. Administer cautiously to avoid extravasation, as tissue damage may occur.
2. Venous pain along the injection site may be reduced by diluting dacarbazine in 100–200 ml of 5% dextrose in water and infusing over 30 minutes rather than injecting rapidly. Ice application may also reduce pain.

Toxicity

1. *Myelosuppression.* Mild to moderate. This factor allows dacarbazine to be used in full doses with other myelosuppressive drugs.
2. *Nausea and vomiting.* Common and severe but decrease in intensity with each subsequent daily dose. Onset is within 1–3 hours, with duration up to 12 hours.
3. *Mucocutaneous effects*
   a. Moderately severe tissue damage if extravasation occurs.
   b. Alopecia—uncommon.
   c. Erythematous or urticarial rash—uncommon.

4. *Miscellaneous effects*. Flulike syndrome with fever, myalgia, and malaise lasting several days is uncommon.

Dactinomycin

Other names.   Actinomycin D, act-D, Cosmegen.

Mechanism of action.   Binds to DNA and inhibits DNA-dependent RNA synthesis. Inhibition of topoisomerase II.

Primary indications

1. Gestational trophoblastic neoplasms.
2. Wilms' tumor, rhabdomyosarcoma, and Ewing's sarcoma of childhood.

Usual dosage and schedule

1. *Children*: 0.40–0.45 mg/m^2 (up to a maximum of 0.5 mg) IV daily for 5 days every 3–5 weeks.
2. *Adults*
   a. 0.40–0.45 mg/m^2 IV on days 1–5 every 2–3 weeks.
   b. 0.5 mg IV daily for 5 days every 3–5 weeks.

Special precautions

1. Administer by slow IV push through the sidearm of a running IV infusion, being careful to avoid extravasation, which causes severe soft-tissue damage.
2. If given at or about the time of infection with chickenpox or herpes zoster, a severe generalized disease may occur that sometimes results in death.

Toxicity

1. *Myelosuppression*. May be dose-limiting and severe. It begins within the first week of treatment, but the nadir may not be reached for 21 days.
2. *Nausea and vomiting*. Severe vomiting often occurs during the first few hours after drug administration and lasts up to 24 hours.
3. *Mucocutaneous effects*
   a. Erythema, hyperpigmentation, and desquamation of the skin potentiation by previous or concurrent radiotherapy are common.
   b. Oropharyngeal mucositis is potentiated by previous or concurrent radiotherapy.
   c. Alopecia is common.
   d. Moderately severe tissue damage occurs with extravasation.
4. *Miscellaneous effects*. Mental depression is rare.

Daunorubicin

Other names.   Daunomycin, rubidomycin, DNR, Cerubidine.

Mechanism of action.   DNA strand breakage mediated by anthracycline effects on topoisomerase II.

Primary indication. Acute nonlymphocytic leukemia, acute lymphocytic leukemia.

Usual dosage and schedule

1. 60 mg/m^2 IV push on days 1, 2, and 3 every 2 weeks as induction therapy for 1 or 2 cycles in combination with other drugs.
2. 45 mg/m^2 IV push on days 1 and 2 every 4 weeks as consolidation therapy for 1 or 2 cycles in combination with other drugs.

Special precautions

1. Administer over several minutes into the sidearm of a running IV infusion, taking precautions to avoid extravasation.
2. Do not give if patient has significantly impaired cardiac function (ejection fraction < 45%), angina pectoris, cardiac arrhythmia, or recent myocardial infarction.
3. Do not exceed cumulative dosage of 550 mg/m^2 (400 mg/m^2 if given previous radiation therapy that has encompassed the heart).
4. Reduce dose if patient has impaired liver or renal function.

Serum bilirubin (mg/dl)		Serum creatinine (mg/dl)	Full dose (%)
1.2–3.0		—	75
> 3.0	*or*	> 3.0	50

Toxicity

1. *Myelosuppression.* Dose-limiting pancytopenia with nadir at 1–2 weeks.
2. *Nausea and vomiting.* Occurs on the day of administration in one-half of patients.
3. *Mucocutaneous effects.* Alopecia is common, but stomatitis is rare. Severe local tissue damage may progress to skin ulceration, and necrosis may occur with subcutaneous extravasation.
4. *Cardiac effects.* Potentially irreversible congestive heart failure may occur owing to cardiomyopathy. The incidence is highly dependent on the lifetime cumulative dose, which should not exceed 550 mg/m^2 (400 mg/m^2 if patient was given previous radiotherapy that encompassed the heart). Congestive heart failure may be predicted by serial measurement of left ventricular function or endomyocardial biopsy. Discontinue drug if there is clinical congestive heart failure or if the ejection fraction falls on the radionuclide angiogram,
   a. To less than 45% *or*
   b. To less than 50% if the total decrease is 10% or more (e.g., falls from 59% to 49%).
   If repeat EF determination shows return of function, drug may be cautiously restarted, but EF should be

measured before each dose. Transient electrocardiographic (ECG) changes are common and are not usually serious.
5. *Miscellaneous effects*
    a. Red urine caused by the drug and its metabolites—common.
    b. Chemical phlebitis and phlebothrombosis of veins used for injection—common.

Dibromodulcitol (Investigational)

Other names. DBD, mitolactol.

Mechanism of action. A halogenated hexitol, dibromodulcitol acts, at least in part, as an alkylating agent with effects on DNA, RNA, and protein synthesis.

Primary indications

1. Breast and lung carcinomas.
2. Melanoma.
3. Hodgkin's and non-Hodgkin's lymphomas.

Usual dosage and schedule

1. *As a single agent*: 100–130 mg/m^2 PO daily until mild hematologic suppression develops.
2. *In combination with other drugs*: 130–135 mg/m^2 PO daily for 10 days every 28 days.

Special precautions. Use with caution in patients with impaired renal function, as renal excretion is the primary mode of elimination of the drug and its metabolites.

Toxicity

1. *Myelosuppression.* Usually dose-limiting with thrombocytopenia predominating.
2. *Nausea and vomiting.* Uncommon.
3. *Mucocutaneous effects.* Skin pigmentation—uncommon.
4. *Miscellaneous effects*
    a. Dyspnea—occasional.
    b. Transient liver enzyme elevation—occasional.
    c. Somnolence or other neurologic problems—uncommon.

Doxorubicin

Other names. ADR, Adriamycin.

Mechanism of action. DNA strand breakage mediated by anthracycline effects on topoisomerase II.

Primary indications

1. Breast, bladder, liver, lung, prostate, stomach, and thyroid carcinomas.
2. Bone and soft tissue sarcomas.

3. Hodgkin's and non-Hodgkin's lymphomas.
4. Acute lymphocytic and acute nonlymphocytic leukemias.
5. Wilms' tumor, neuroblastoma, and rhabdomyosarcoma of childhood.

Usual dosage and schedule

1. 60–75 mg/m^2 IV every 3 weeks.
2. 30 mg/m^2 IV on days 1 and 8 every 4 weeks (in combination with other drugs).
3. 15–20 mg/m^2 IV weekly.
4. 50–60 mg instilled into the bladder weekly for 4 weeks, then every 4 weeks for 6 cycles.

Special precautions

1. Administer over several minutes into the sidearm of a running IV infusion, taking care to avoid extravasation.
2. Do not give if patient has significantly impaired cardiac function (ejection fraction < 45%), angina pectoris, cardiac arrhythmia, or recent myocardial infarction.
3. Do not exceed a lifetime cumulative dose of 550 mg/m^2 (450 mg/m^2 if patient was given prior chest radiotherapy or concomitant cyclophosphamide).
4. Reduce or hold dose if patient has impaired liver function.
   a. For serum bilirubin of 1.2–3.0 mg/dl: give one-half the normal dose.
   b. For serum bilirubin of more than 3.0 mg/dl: give one-fourth the normal dose.

Toxicity

1. *Myelosuppression.* Dose-limiting for most patients. Nadir white blood cell (WBC) and platelet counts occur at 10–14 days; recovery by day 21.
2. *Nausea and vomiting.* Mild to moderate in about one-half of patients.
3. *Mucocutaneous effects*
   a. Stomatitis that is dose-dependent.
   b. Alopecia beginning 2–5 weeks from start of therapy with recovery following completion of therapy—common.
   c. Recall of skin reaction due to prior radiotherapy—common.
   d. Severe local tissue damage possibly progressing to skin ulceration and necrosis if subcutaneous extravasation occurs—common.
   e. Hyperpigmentation of skin overlying veins used for drug injection in which chemical phlebitis has occurred—common.
4. *Cardiac effects.* Potentially irreversible congestive heart failure may occur owing to cardiomyopathy. The incidence is highly dependent on the lifetime cumulative dose, which should not exceed 550 mg/m^2. This limit is lower (450 mg/m^2) if patient has received prior chest radiotherapy or is taking cyclophosphamide concomi-

tantly. Congestive heart failure may be predicted by serial measurement of left ventricular function or endo-myocardial biopsy. Discontinue drug if there is clinical congestive heart failure or if the ejection fraction (EF) falls on the radionuclide angiogram

a. To less than 45% *or*
b. To less than 50% if the total decrease is 10% or more (e.g., falls from 59% to 49%).

If repeat EF determination shows return of function, drug may be cautiously restarted, but EF determination should be done before each dose. Transient ECG changes are common and are not usually serious.

5. *Miscellaneous effects*
   a. Red urine caused by drug and its metabolites—common.
   b. Chemical phlebitis and phlebosclerosis of veins used for injection, particularly if a vein is used repeatedly—common.
   c. Fever, chills, and urticaria—uncommon.

Epirubicin (Investigational)

Other names.   4'Epi-doxorubicin, EPI.

Mechanism of action.   DNA strand breakage, mediated by anthracycline effects on topoisomerase II.

Primary indications.   Breast carcinoma.

Usual dosage and schedule.   70–90 mg/m^2 IV every 3 weeks administered through the sidearm of a freely flowing IV infusion.

Special precautions

1. Take care to avoid extravasation.
2. Do not exceed a lifetime cumulative dose of 1000 mg/m^2 (use a reduced dose for patients with prior chest radiotherapy or prior anthracycline or anthracene therapy).

Toxicity

1. *Myelosuppression.* Dose-limiting leukopenia with recovery by day 21.
2. *Nausea and vomiting.* Common.
3. *Mucocutaneous effects*
   a. Stomatitis that is dose-dependent.
   b. Alopecia beginning approximately 10 days after the first treatment with regrowth when cessation of drug treatment occurs—common.
   c. Severe local tissue damage possibly progressing to skin ulceration and necrosis if subcutaneous extravasation occurs—common.
4. *Cardiac effects*
   a. Potentially irreversible congestive heart failure may occur owing to cardiomyopathy. The incidence depends on the lifetime dose, which should not exceed 1000 mg/m^2. This limit is lower if patient has received

prior chest radiotherapy or prior anthracycline or anthracene therapy. Congestive heart failure may be predicted by serial measurement of left ventricular function or endomyocardial biopsy.
  b. Transient ECG changes are similar in type and frequency to those observed after doxorubicin.
5. *Miscellaneous effects*
  a. Red-orange urine for 24 hours after injection owing to drugs and its metabolites—common.
  b. Diarrhea—uncommon.

Estramustine

Other name.   Emcyt.

Mechanism of action.   A chemical combination of mechlorethamine and estradiol phosphate, estramustine is believed to selectively enter cells with estrogen receptors, where it acts as an alkylating agent.

Primary indication.   Metastatic prostate carcinoma.

Usual dosage and schedule.   600 mg/m^2 PO daily in 3 divided doses.

Special precautions.   Take with meals and antacids to lessen gastrointestinal disturbances.

Toxicity

1. *Myelosuppression.* Occurs only occasionally.
2. *Nausea and vomiting.* Commonly seen soon after starting treatment but usually lessen with continued therapy and antiemetics. If persistent and severe, it may be necessary to discontinue the drug.
3. *Mucocutaneous effects.* Rash with fever is rare.
4. *Miscellaneous effects*
  a. Congestive heart failure—must be watched for in patients with preexisting cardiac disease.
  b. Gynecomastia—occasional.

Estrogens

Other names.   Diethylstilbestrol (DES), chlorotrianisene (TACE), diethylstilbestrol diphosphate (Stilphostrol), and others.

Mechanism of action.   Suppresion of testosterone production via negative feedback on hypothalamus.

Primary indications.   Prostate carcinoma

Usual dosage and schedule

1. DES, 1–3 mg PO daily.
2. Chlorotrianisene, 12–25 mg PO daily.
3. Diethylstilbestrol diphosphate, 500–1000 mg IV daily for 5–7 days, then 250–500 mg IV 1 or 2 times weekly.

Special precautions

1. Acute fluid retention and pulmonary edema are possible, particularly with high-dose IV therapy.
2. Hypercalcemia may occur with initial therapy.

Toxicity

1. *Myelosuppression*. None.
2. *Nausea and vomiting*. Common at the beginning of therapy but diminish or stop with continued treatment. Severity may be lessened by beginning treatment with doses lower than those recommended.
3. *Mucocutaneous effects*. Darkening of nipples—common.
4. *Miscellaneous effects*
   a. Peripheral edema due to sodium retention is common, but congestive heart failure occurs in fewer than 5% of patients.
   b. Diarrhea is uncommon.
   c. Any patient on estrogens may be at higher risk than normal for thromboemboli. An increase in cardiovascular deaths has been seen in male patients given DES 5 mg daily for prostate carcinoma.
   d. Increased bone pain, tumor pain, and local disease flare are associated with both good tumor response and tumor progression.
   e. Feminization occurs in male patients.

Etoposide

Other names. Epipodophyllotoxin, VP-16, VP-16–213, VePesid.

Mechanism of action. Interaction with topoisomerase II produces single-strand breaks in DNA. Arrests cells in late S phase or G_2 phase.

Primary indications

1. Small-cell anaplastic and non-small-cell lung carcinoma.
2. Germ cell cancers.
3. Lymphomas (refractory).

Usual dosage and schedule

1. 50–100 mg/m^2 IV on days 1–5 every 2–4 weeks.
2. 125–140 mg/m^2 IV on days 1, 3, and 5 every 3–5 weeks.
3. 50 mg/m^2 PO daily for 21 days. Repeat after 1–2 weeks' rest.

Special precautions

1. Administer as a 30- to 60-minute infusion to avoid severe hypotension. Monitor blood pressure during infusion.
2. Take care to avoid extravasation.
3. Must be diluted in 20–50 volumes (100–250 ml) of isotonic saline before use.

Toxicity

1. *Myelosuppression*. Dose-limiting leukopenia and less severe thrombocytopenia have a nadir at 16 days with recovery by days 20–22.
2. *Nausea and vomiting*. Usually mild to moderate problems in about one third of patients. Anorexia is common.
3. *Mucocutaneous effects*
   a. Alopecia—common.
   b. Stomatitis—uncommon.
4. *Miscellaneous effects*
   a. Hepatotoxicity—rare.
   b. Diarrhea—uncommon.
   c. Peripheral neurotoxicity—rare.
   d. Allergic reaction—rare.

Floxuridine

Other name. FUDR.

Mechanism of action. A pyrimidine antimetabolite that, when converted to the active nucleotide, inhibits the enzyme thymidylate synthetase.

Primary indications. Hepatic metastasis of gastrointestinal carcinoma, primary hepatic carcinoma.

Usual dosage and schedule. 3.5–4.0 mg/m^2 into the hepatic artery daily for 2 weeks, then off for 2 weeks. Administered an via implanted continuous infusion pump.

Special precautions

1. Reduce dose in patients with compromised liver function.
2. Ulcerlike pain or other significant gastrointestinal symptoms are indications to discontinue intraarterial therapy, as hemorrhage or perforation may occur.

Toxicity

1. *Myelosuppression*. Uncommon.
2. *Nausea and vomiting*. Uncommon unless the hepatic artery catheter has become displaced and the stomach and duodenum are being infused.
3. *Mucocutaneous effects*
   a. Stomatitis is an early sign of severe toxicity. It progresses from soreness and erythema to frank ulceration, which may become hemorrhagic in a small number of patients. Esophagitis, proctitis, and diarrhea may also occur.
   b. Partial alopecia is uncommon.
   c. Hyperpigmentation of skin over face, hands, and the vein used for the infusion—occasional.
   d. Maculopapular rash is uncommon.
   e. Sun exposure tends to increase skin reactions.
4. *Miscellaneous effects*
   a. Neurotoxicity, including headache, minor visual disturbances, and cerebellar ataxia—rare.

     b. Increased lacrimation—uncommon.
     c. Abdominal cramps and pain are common if the catheter is displaced and the stomach and duodenum are being infused. Can progress to frank gastritis or duodenal ulcer.
     d. Liver function abnormalities and jaundice—common when given by hepatic arterial infusion. Dose should be reduced during subsequent cycle.
     e. Sclerosing cholangitis when given by hepatic artery infusion—uncommon.

Fludarabine

Other names. FAMP, Fludara.

Mechanism of action. Inhibition of DNA polymerase and ribonucleotide reductase.

Primary indications

1. Chronic lymphocytic leukemia.
2. Macroglobulinemia.
3. Indolent lymphomas.

Usual dosage and schedule. 25–30 mg/m^2 IV as a 15- to 30-minute infusion daily for 5 days. Repeat every 4 weeks.

Special precautions. If there is the potential for tumor lysis syndrome, administer allopurinol and ensure good hydration and close clinical monitoring.

Toxicity

1. *Myelosuppression.* Granulocytopenia and thrombocytopenia are common but appear to become less common in patients who are responding. Infection is common during early courses; uncommon after sixth course.
2. *Nausea and vomiting.* Uncommon at usual dosage.
3. *Mucocutaneous effects.* Occasional mucositis, no alopecia.
4. *Neurotoxicity.* Uncommon at usual dosage. Somnolence or fatigue, paresthesias, and twitching of extremities may be seen. Severe neurologic symptoms, including visual disturbances, have been common at higher doses than those recommended.

Fluorouracil

Other names. 5-FU, Fluorouracil, Adrucil, 5-fluorouracil.

Mechanism of action. A pyrimidine antimetabolite that, when converted to the active nucleotide, inhibits the enzyme thymidylate synthetase and thereby blocks DNA synthesis.

Primary indications

1. Breast, colorectal, stomach, pancreas, esophagus, liver, head and neck, and bladder carcinomas.
2. Basal and squamous cell carcinomas of skin (topically).

Usual dosage and schedule

1. *Systemic*
   a. 500 mg/m^2 IV on days 1–5 every 4 weeks *or*
   b. 450–600 mg/m^2 IV weekly.
   c. 200–400 mg/m^2 daily as a continuous intravenous infusion.
2. *Intracavitary*: 500–1000 mg for pericardial effusion; 2000–3000 mg for pleural or peritoneal effusions.
3. *Intraarterial* (liver): 800–1200 mg/m^2 as a continuous infusion on days 1–4, followed by 600 mg/m^2 as a continuous infusion on days 5–21.

Special precautions

1. Reduce dose in patients with compromised liver function.
2. For intraarterial infusion, add 5000 units of heparin to 1 liter of 5% dextrose in water together with the daily dose of fluorouracil. The catheter position should be checked with dye injection every few days to ensure that it has not moved and that the hepatic artery has not thrombosed. Ulcerlike pain or other significant gastrointestinal symptoms are indications to discontinue intraarterial therapy, as hemorrhage or perforation may occur.

Toxicity

1. *Myelosuppression.* Dose-limiting with a nadir at 10–14 days after the last dose and recovery by 21 days.
2. *Nausea and vomiting.* May occur but are not usually severe.
3. *Mucocutaneous effects*
   a. Stomatitis is an early sign of severe toxicity. It progresses from soreness and erythema to frank ulceration, which becomes hemorrhagic in a small number of patients. Esophagitis, proctitis, and diarrhea may also occur.
   b. Partial alopecia—uncommon.
   c. Hyperpigmentation of skin over face, hands, and the veins used for infusion—occasional.
   d. Maculopapular rash—uncommon.
   e. Sun exposure tends to increase skin reactions.
   f. "Hand-foot syndrome" with painful, erythematous desquamation and fissures of palms and soles—common with continuous infusion, occasional with other schedules or combinations.
4. *Miscellaneous effects*
   a. Neurotoxicity, including headache, minor visual disturbances, and cerebellar ataxia—rare.
   b. Increased lacrimation—uncommon.
   c. Cardiac arrythmias—rare.

Flutamide

Other name.   Eulexin.

Mechanism of action.   Antiandrogen that inhibits binding of dihydrotestosterone at nuclear binding sites.

Primary indication.   Carcinoma of the prostate.

Usual doage and schedule.   250 mg tid daily.

Special precautions.   None.

Toxicity

1. *Myelosuppression.* Rare, but occasional WBC fluctuation. Aplastic anemia—6%.
2. *Nausea and vomiting.* Occasional.
3. *Mucocutaneous effects.* Rash—uncommon.
4. *Miscellaneous effects*
   a. Gastrointestinal: occasional diarrhea (rarely severe), flatulence, or mild abdominal pains.
   b. Occasional mild elevation of liver enzymes.
   c. Mild breast tenderness and gynecomastia is common in patients who have not had gonadal ablation.
   d. Impotence and loss of libido—common.

Hexamethylmelamine

Other names.   Altretamine, Hexalen, HXM.

Mechanism of action.   Unknown. Although it structurally resembles the known alkylating agent triethylenemelamine, it has some antimetabolite characteristics.

Primary indications.   Carcinoma of the ovary.

Usual dosage and schedule

1. 200–320 mg/m^2 PO daily in 3 or 4 divided doses for 14 or 21 days every 4 weeks when used as a single agent.
2. 150–200 mg/m^2 PO daily in 3 or 4 divided doses for 2 out of 3 or 4 weeks when used in combination.

Special precautions.   None.

Toxicity

1. *Myelosuppression.* Dose-limiting leukopenia and thrombocytopenia are uncommon. Anemia is common.
2. *Nausea and vomiting.* Usually dose-limiting and associated with anorexia, diarrhea, and abdominal cramps. Tolerance may develop.
3. *Mucocutaneous effects.* Alopecia, skin rash, and pruritus are rare.
4. *Miscellaneous effects*
   a. Peripheral sensory neuropathies—common. May be ameliorated by pyridoxine.
   b. CNS effects, including agitation, confusion, hallucinations, depression, and Parkinsonianlike symptoms—less common with recommended intermittent schedule than with continuous treatment.
   c. Decreased renal function—occasional.

Hydroxyurea

Other name.   Hydrea.

Mechanism of action. Interferes with DNA synthesis, at least in part by inhibiting the enzymatic conversion of ribonucleotides to deoxyribonucleotides.

Primary indications

1. Head and neck carcinomas.
2. Chronic granulocytic leukemia; acute lymphocytic and acute nonlymphocytic leukemia with high blast counts.

Usual dosage and schedule

1. 800–2000 mg/m^2 PO as a single daily dose *or*
2. 3200 mg/m^2 PO as a single dose every third day (not for leukemias).

Special precautions. The daily dose must be adjusted for blood counts.

Toxicity

1. *Myelosuppression*. Occurs at doses of more than 1600 mg/m^2 daily by day 10. Recovery is usually prompt.
2. *Nausea and vomiting*. Common at high doses.
3. *Mucocutaneous effects*. Stomatitis is rare. Maculopapular rash may be seen. Inflammation of mucous membranes caused by radiation may be exaggerated.
4. *Miscellaneous effects*
   a. Temporary renal function impairment or dysuria—uncommon.
   b. CNS disturbances—rare.

Idarubicin

Other names. 4-Demethoxydaunorubicin, IDA, Idamycin.

Mechanism of action. DNA strand breakage mediated by anthracycline effects on topoisomerase II or free radicals.

Primary indications

1. Acute nonlymphocytic leukemia.
2. Blast crisis of chronic granulocytic leukemia.
3. Acute lymphocytic leukemia.

Usual dosage and schedule. 12–13 mg/m^2 IV daily for 3 days (usually in a combination with cytarabine) during induction; 10–12 mg/m^2 IV daily for 2 days during consolidation.

Special precautions. Cardiac toxicity may be less than that with daunorubicin. Maximum dose not yet established.

Toxicity

1. *Myelosuppression*. Universal and dose-limiting.
2. *Nausea and vomiting*. Common.
3. *Mucocutaneous effects*. Alopecia—common; mucositis—uncommon.

4. *Hepatic dysfunction.* Common but usually not severe and not clearly due to the idarubicin.
5. *Renal effects.* Common but usually not clinically significant.
6. *Other gastrointestinal effects.* Diarrhea—occasional to common; bleeding—common in one study.
7. *Cardiac effects.* Uncommon during induction and consolidation (1–5%).
8. *Tissue damage.* If infiltration occurs—probable.
9. *Neurologic effects.* Occasional.

Ifosfamide

Other name.   Ifex.

Mechanism of action.   Metabolic activation by microsomal liver enzymes produces biologically active intermediates that attack nucleophilic sites, particularly on DNA.

Primary indications.   Testicular and lung cancers, bony and soft-tissue sarcomas.

Special precautions.   Must be used with mesna (Mesnex) to prevent hemorrhagic cystitis. Mesna dose is at least 20% of the ifosfamide dose (on a weight basis), administered just prior to (or mixed with) the ifosfamide dose and again at 4 and 8 hours after the ifosfamide to detoxify the urinary metabolites that cause the hemorrhagic cystitis. Higher doses of ifosfamide may require higher doses and longer durations of mesna. Neither mesna nor its only metabolite, mesna disulfide, affect ifosfamide or its antineoplastic metabolites. Mesna disulfide is reduced in the kidney to a free thiol compound, which then reacts chemically with urotoxic metabolites resulting in their detoxification. Vigorous hydration is also required with a minimum of 2 liters of oral or intravenous hydration daily. Administer as a slow intravenous infusion over a period of at least 30 minutes.

Usual dosage and schedule

1. 1.2 gm/m^2 IV over 30 minutes or more daily for 5 consecutive days every 3 or 4 weeks, usually with other agents. Mesna 120 mg/m^2 is given just before ifosfamide, then mesna 1200 mg/m^2 as a daily continuous infusion is given until 16 hours after the last dose of ifosfamide.
2. 3.6 gm/m^2 IV daily as a 4-hour infusion for 2 consecutive days, usually with other agents. Mesna is given at a dose of 750 mg/m^2 IV just prior to and at 4 and 8 hours after the start of the ifosfamide.
3. Higher dosage schedules have been used experimentally with up to 14 gm/m^2 being used per course over a 6-day period, with equal or greater doses of mesna.

Toxicity

1. *Myelosuppression.* Dose-limiting. Platelets are relatively spared. Granulocyte nadirs are commonly reached at

10–14 days, and recovery is seen by day 21. Thrombocytopenia may be seen with higher doses.

2. *Nausea and vomiting.* Common without standard antiemetics.

3. *Mucocutaneous effects.* Alopecia is common. Mucositis is rarely seen at standard doses. Dermatitis is rare.

4. *Hemorrhagic cystitis.* Common and dose-limiting unless a uroprotective agent such as mesna is used. With mesna, the incidence of hemorrhagic cystitis is 5–10%, and gross hematuria is uncommon. Increasing the duration of mesna may alleviate the problem during subsequent cycles.

5. *Miscellaneous effects*
   a. CNS toxicity (somnolence, confusion, depressive psychosis, hallucinations, disorientation, and uncommonly seizures, cranial nerve dysfunction, or coma)—occasional.
   b. Infertility—common in men and women, as with other alkylating agents.
   c. Renal impairment—occasional.
   d. Liver dysfunction—uncommon.
   e. Phlebitis—uncommon.
   f. Fever—rare.

Interferon-alpha

Other names. Roferon-A (interferon alfa-2a, recombinant alpha-A interferon), Intron A (interferon alfa-2b, recombinant alpha-2 interferon).

Mechanism of action. Believed to involve direct inhibition of tumor cell growth and modulation of the immune response of the host, including activation of natural killer cells, modulation of antibody production, and induction of major histocompatibility antigens.

Primary indications
1. Hairy-cell leukemia.
2. Chronic myelogenous leukemia.
3. Non-Hodgkin's lymphoma (low grade).
4. Multiple myeloma.
5. Melanoma.
6. Renal cell carcinoma.
7. Colon carcinoma (in combination with fluorouracil).

Usual dosage and schedule
1. 3–10 million units IM or SQ in various schedules. Daily dosing is often used for several weeks or months, followed by 3 times a week dosing.
2. Investigationally, doses have been higher (up to 50 million units/m^2 per dose), usually IV at doses higher than 10 million units/m^2.

Toxicity
1. *Myelosuppression.* Common but usually mild to moderate and transient, even with continued therapy.

2. *Nausea and vomiting.* Anorexia occurs in about one-half of all patients, nausea in about one-third, and vomiting in 10%.
3. *Mucocutaneous effects.* Rash, dryness, or inflammation of the oropharynx, dry skin or pruritus, and partial alopecia—occasional to common.
4. *Flulike syndrome* with fatigue, fever, chills, myalgias, arthralgias, and headache—common to universal with greater severity at higher doses. Tends to diminish with continuing therapy and acetaminophen.
5. *Neurologic effects*
   a. Peripheral nervous system: occasional paresthesias or numbness.
   b. Central nervous system: uncommon at lower doses, but with higher doses an increased likelihood including headache, somnolence, anxiety, depression, confusion, hallucinations, cerebellar dysfunction, and emotional lability.
6. *General systemic effects.* Fatigue, anorexia, and weight loss—common with chronic administration.
7. *Cardiovascular effects.* Mild hypotension—common but rarely symptomatic.
8. *Infectious effects.* Exacerbation of herpetic eruptions and nonherpetic cold sores—uncommon.
9. *Miscellaneous effects.* Leg cramps, constipation or diarrhea, insomnia, urticaria, hot flashes, coagulation disorders—uncommon.
10. *Laboratory abnormalities*
   a. Elevated liver function tests—common.
   b. Mild proteinuria, increase in serum creatinine—occasional.
   c. Hypercalcemia—occasional.

Interferon-gamma (Investigational)

Other names.   Interferon-γ, rIFN-γ.

Mechanism of action.   Believed to involve direct antiproliferative effects, modulation of the immune response of the host to tumor (including induction of macrophage cytotoxicity and monocyte-mediated antibody-dependent cellular cytotoxicity), and induction of major histocompatibility complex (MHC) class II antigens on the surface of tumor cells.

Primary indications

1. Renal cell carcinoma.
2. Melanoma.

Usual dosage and schedule.   0.1–0.3 mg SQ weekly.

Special precautions.   When diluted to less than 20 µg/ml, adsorption to glassware or plastic can be averted by adding human serum albumin to a final concentration of 2 mg/ml to 5% dextrose in water diluent *prior* to the addition of rIFN-γ.

Toxicity

1. *Myelosuppression.* Common but usually mild to moderate and transient, even with continued therapy.
2. *Nausea and vomiting.* Anorexia occurs in about one-half of all patients, nausea in one-third, and vomiting in 10%.
3. *Mucocutaneous effects.* Mild alopecia and stomatitis—occasional. Oral herpes simplex may be reactivated and psoriasis exacerbated.
4. *Flulike syndrome.* With fever, chills, myalgias, and headache—common. Starts within 2–8 hours of administration. Tends to be self-limiting and can be controlled with acetaminophen.
5. *Neurologic effects*
   a. Peripheral nervous system: occasional mild paresthesias.
   b. Central nervous system: decreased ability to concentrate, confusion, somnolence, and dizziness—occasional with dose-dependent frequency and severity; seizures—rare.
6. *Systemic effects.* Fatigue, anorexia, and weight loss—common with chronic administration.
7. *Cardiovascular effects.* Mild hypotension—common but rarely symptomatic at usual doses.
8. *Laboratory abnormalities*
   a. Elevated liver function tests—common.
   b. Mild proteinuria—common; increase in serum creatinine—occasional.
   c. Hypercalcemia—occasional.

Interleukin-2

Other names.   IL-2, Proleukin, Aldesleukin.

Mechanism of action.   Enhances mitogenesis of T cells, natural killer (NK) cells, and lymphokine-activated killer (LAK) cells; augments cytotoxity of NK and LAK cells; induces interferon-gamma.

Primary indications

1. Renal cell carcinoma.
2. Melanoma.

Usual dosage and schedule.   Wide range of doses and schedules have been used. Examples are given of low- to moderate-intensity regimens. (1 mg = 3×10^6 CETUS units.)

1. 0.33 mg/m^2 SQ 5 days a week for 12 weeks.
2. *Induction*: 2.0 mg/m^2 IV bolus (over 3–5 minutes) three times weekly for 4 weeks. Rest 2 weeks.
   Maintenance: 1.0 mg/m^2 IV bolus three times weekly for 2 successive weeks every 4 weeks.
3. 1 mg/m^2 IV bolus daily × 5 for 2 successive weeks.
4. 3 mg/m^2 as a 24-hour continuous infusion weekly for 6 weeks.

Schedules 1, 2, and 3 do not require hospitalization; schedule 4 does. None of the schedules listed requires intensive care unit admission.

Special precautions. With higher doses, capillary leak syndrome resulting in hypotension, pulmonary edema, myocardial infarction, arrhythmias, azotemia, and alterations in mental status may occur. Intensive care, controlled volume replacement, and intubation may be required.

Toxicity. All are dose-dependent.

1. *Myelosuppression.* Uncommon, although anemia requiring transfusion is common.
2. *Nausea and vomiting.* Common.
3. *Mucocutaneous effects.* Mucositis is occasional to common. Alopecia is uncommon. Pruritic erythematous rash is common.
4. *Cardiovascular effects*
   a. Arrhythmias are common and dose-related.
   b. Hypotension is dose-related but is occasionally seen at the lower dose schedules.
   c. Myocardial injury is seen primarily at the higher dose schedules.
   d. Pulmonary edema from capillary leak syndrome is common with intensive dose regimens.
   e. Weight gain is common from edema, particularly in more intensive dose regimens.
5. *Gastrointestinal effects*
   a. Anorexia—common.
   b. Diarrhea—occasional.
   c. Transient liver function abnormalities and hypoalbuminemia—common.
   d. Colonic perforations—rare.
6. *Neuropsychiatric effects*
   a. Mental status changes—common, with dose-related severity.
   b. Dizziness or lightheadedness—common.
   c. Blurry vision and other visual disturbances—occasional.
   d. Seizures—uncommon to rare at lower-dose regimens.
7. *Renal function impairment.* Common but reversible.
8. *Fever.* With or without chills—universal and may be severe.
9. *Bacterial infection.* Occasional. Probably related to chemotactic defect induced in granulocytes.
10. *Myalgias and arthralgias.* Occasional to common.
11. *Malaise and fatigue.* Common and dose-related.

Prophylaxis of acute toxicity

1. Acetaminophen 650–1000 mg PO 1 hour prior to therapy and q3h for two doses.
2. Indomethacin 25–50 mg PO 1 hour prior to therapy.
3. Meperidine 25–50 mg IV when chills start after first dose. For subsequent doses, meperidine 150 mg PO 1.5 hours before chills are predicated to start, based on the first treatment.

4. Diphenhydramine 50 mg PO q3h for 3 doses may be sub-stituted for meperidine in patients who tolerate the latter drug poorly.

Levamisole

Other name.   Ergamisol.

Mechanism of action.   Restores immune function, but whether this action is related to the mechanism of potentiation of fluorouracil effect in adjuvant therapy of colon cancer is unknown.

Primary indications.   Dukes' C carcinoma of the colon (with fluorouracil).

Usual dosage and schedule.   50 mg PO q8h for 3 days every 2 weeks for 1 year, beginning with first dose of fluorouracil. (Fluorouracil 450 mg/m^2 IV bolus daily for 5 days, then beginning 28 days later 450 mg/m^2 IV bolus weekly.)

Special precautions.   None.

Toxicity

1. *Myelosuppression.* Uncommon.
2. *Nausea and vomiting.* Nausea—common; vomiting—occasionally.
3. *Mucocutaneous effects.* Stomatitis and alopecia are uncommon.
4. *Miscellaneous effects*
   a. Dermatitis—occasional.
   b. Fatigue—occasional.
   c. Taste perversion—occasional.
   d. CNS problems (dizziness, somnolence, headache)—uncommon.
   e. Fever and rigors—uncommon.
   f. Musculoskeletal pain—uncommon.

Lomustine

Other names.   CCNU, CeeNU.

Mechanism of action.   Alkylation and carbamoylation by lomustine metabolites interfere with the synthesis and function of DNA, RNA, and proteins. Lomustine is lipid-soluble and easily enters the brain.

Primary indications

1. Lung and kidney carcinomas.
2. Hodgkin's and non-Hodgkin's lymphomas.
3. Brain tumors.

Usual dosage and schedule.   100–130 mg/m^2 PO once every 6–8 weeks (lower dose used for patients with compromised bone marrow function). Some recommend limiting cumulative dose to 1000 mg/m^2 to limit pulmonary and renal toxicity.

Special precautions.   Because of delayed myelosuppression (3–6 weeks), do not treat more often than every 6 weeks. Await a return of normal platelet and granulocyte counts before repeating therapy.

Toxicity

1. *Myelosuppression.* Universal and dose-limiting. Leukopenia and thrombocytopenia are delayed 3–6 weeks after therapy begins and may be cumulative with successive doses.
2. *Nausea and vomiting.* Begin 3–6 hours after therapy and last up to 24 hours.
3. *Mucocutaneous effects.* Stomatitis and alopecia are rare.
4. *Miscellaneous effects*
   a. Confusion, lethargy, and ataxia—rare.
   b. Mild hepatotoxicity—infrequent.
   c. Secondary neoplasia—possible.
   d. Pulmonary fibrosis is uncommon at doses of less than 1000 mg/m^2.
   e. Renal toxicity is uncommon at doses of less than 1000 mg/m^2.

Luteinizing Hormone-Releasing Hormone

Other names.   Leuprolide (Lupron, Lupron depot), goserelin (Zoladex, depot).

Mechanism of action.   Initial release of follicle-stimulating hormone (FSH) and luteinizing hormone (LH) from the anterior pituitary followed by diminution of gonadotropin secretion owing to desensitization of the pituitary to gonadotropin-releasing hormone (GnRH), and consequent decrease in the respective gonadal hormones. May also have direct effects on cancer cells, at least in cancer of the breast in which GnRH binding sites have been demonstrated.

Primary indications

1. Prostate carcinoma.
2. Breast carcinoma (investigational).

Usual dosage and schedule

1. Leuprolide 1 mg (0.2 ml) as a single daily SQ injection.
2. Leuprolide depot 7.5 mg IM monthly.
3. Goserelin depot 3.6 mg SQ monthly.

Special precautions.   Worsening of symptoms may occur during the first few weeks.

Toxicity

1. *Myelosuppression.* Rare, if at all.
2. *Nausea and vomiting.* Occasional.
3. *Mucocutaneous effects.* Erythema and ecchymosis at the injection site, rash, hair loss, itching—uncommon.
4. *Cardiovascular effects.* Congestive heart failure and thrombotic episodes—uncommon. Peripheral edema—occasional.

5. *Miscellaneous effects*
   a. CNS: dizziness, pain, headache, and paresthesias—uncommon.
   b. Endocrine: hot flashes—common; decreased libido—common; gynecomastia with or without tenderness—uncommon; impotence—uncommon.
   c. Bone pain—uncommon.
   d. Gastrointestinal: anorexia and constipation—uncommon.

Mechlorethamine

Other names.   Nitrogen mustard, HN2, Mustargen.

Mechanism of action.   Mechlorethamine is a prototype alkylating agent. Its action involves transfer of the alkyl group to amino, carboxyl, hydroxyl, imidazole, phosphate, and sulfhydryl groups within the cell, altering structure and function of DNA (primarily), RNA, and proteins.

Primary indications

1. Hodgkin's lymphoma.
2. Malignant pleural and, less commonly, peritoneal or pericardial effusions.

Usual dosage and schedule

1. 6 mg/m^2 IV on days 1 and 8 every 4 weeks (in MOPP regimen for Hodgkin's disease).
2. 8–16 mg/m^2 by intracavitary injection.

Special precautions

1. Administer over several minutes into the sidearm of a running IV infusion, taking care to avoid extravasation.
2. Because mechlorethamine is a potent vesicant, extreme care must be exercised while preparing and administering the drug. Gloves and eye glasses are recommended to protect the preparer. If accidental eye contact should occur, institute copious irrigation with normal saline and follow by prompt ophthalmologic consultation. If accidental skin contact occurs, irrigate the affected part immediately with water for at least 15 minutes and follow by 2.6% sodium thiosulfate solution (⅙ M).
3. Mechlorethamine should be used soon after preparation (15–30 minutes) as it decomposes on standing. It *must not* be mixed in the same syringe with any other drug.

Toxicity

1. *Myelosuppression.* Dose-limiting, with the nadir at about 1 week and recovery by 3 weeks.
2. *Nausea and vomiting.* Universal. They usually begin within the first 3 hours and last 4–8 hours.
3. *Mucocutaneous effects.* Severe painful inflammation and necrosis are likely if extravasation occurs. May be ameliorated if 2.6% thiosulfate solution (⅙ M) is instilled into the area to neutralize active drug, and ice

packs are applied locally for 6–12 hours. Maculopapular rash is uncommon.
4. *Miscellaneous effects*
   a. Phlebitis, thrombosis, or both of the vein used for the injection—common.
   b. Amenorrhea and azoospermia—common.
   c. Hyperuricemia with rapid tumor destruction.
   d. Weakness, sleepiness, and headache—uncommon.
   e. Severe allergic reactions, including anaphylaxis—rare.
   f. Secondary neoplasms—possible.

Melphalan

Other names.   Phenylalanine mustard, L-sarcolysin, L-PAM, Alkeran.

Mechanism of action.   Alkylating agent with primary effect on DNA. Amino acid type structure may result in cellular transport that is different from other alkylating agents.

Primary indications

1. Multiple myeloma.
2. Breast and ovarian carcinomas.

Usual dosage and schedule

1. 8 mg/m^2 PO on days 1–4 every 4 weeks *or*
2. 10 mg/m^2 PO on days 1–4 every 6 weeks *or*
3. 3–4 mg/m^2 PO daily for 2–3 weeks, then 1–2 mg/m^2 PO daily for maintenance.

Special precaution.   Myelosuppression may be delayed and prolonged to 4–6 weeks.

Toxicity

1. *Myelosuppression.* Dose-limiting; nadir at days 14–21.
2. *Nausea and vomiting.* Uncommon.
3. *Mucocutaneous effects.* Alopecia, dermatitis, and stomatitis—uncommon.
4. *Miscellaneous effects*
   a. Acute nonlymphocytic leukemia—rare but well documented.
   b. Pulmonary fibrosis—rare.

Mercaptopurine

Other names.   6-Mercaptopurine, 6-MP, Purinethol.

Mechanism of action.   A purine antimetabolite that, when converted to the nucleotide, inhibits the formation of nucleotides necessary for DNA and RNA synthesis.

Primary indications.   Acute lymphocytic and juvenile chronic granulocytic leukemias.

Usual dosage and schedule

1. 100 mg/m^2 PO daily if used alone.
2. 50–90 mg/m^2 PO daily if used with methotrexate.

Special precautions

1. Decrease dose by 75% when used concurrently with allopurinol.
2. Increase interval between doses or reduce dose in patients with renal failure.

Toxicity

1. *Myelosuppression.* Common but mild at recommended doses.
2. *Nausea and vomiting.* Uncommon.
3. *Mucocutaneous effects.* Stomatitis may be seen with very large doses. Dry, scaling rash is uncommon.
4. *Miscellaneous effects*
   a. Intrahepatic cholestasis and mild focal centrolobular necrosis with jaundice—uncommon.
   b. Diarrhea—rare.
   c. Hyperuricemia with rapid leukemia cell lysis—common.
   d. Fever—uncommon.

Methotrexate

Other names.   Amethopterin, MTX, Mexate.

Mechanism of action.   Inhibition of dihydrofolate reductase, which results in a block of the reduction of dihydrofolate to tetrahydrofolate. This blockage in turn inhibits the formation of thymidylate and purines, and arrests DNA (predominantly), RNA, and protein synthesis.

Primary indications

1. Breast, head and neck, gastrointestinal, lung, and gestational trophoblastic carcinomas.
2. Osteosarcomas (high-dose methotrexate).
3. Acute lymphocytic leukemia.
4. Meningeal leukemia or carcinomatosis.

Usual dosage and schedule

1. *Gestational trophoblastic carcinoma.* 15–30 mg PO or IM on days 1–5 every 2 weeks.
2. *Other carcinomas.* 40–80 mg/m^2 IV or PO 2–4 times monthly with a 7- to 14-day interval between doses.
3. *Acute lymphocytic leukemia.* 15–20 mg/m^2 PO or IV weekly (together with mercaptopurine).
4. *Osteogenic sarcoma.* Up to 10 gm/m^2 with leucovorin rescue (high-dose methotrexate). This usage is investigational and should not be applied outside of a research setting.
5. *Intrathecally.* 12 mg/m^2 (not > 20 mg) twice weekly.

Special precautions

1. High-dose methotrexate (> 80 mg/m^2) is experimental and should be administered only by individuals experienced in its use and at institutions where serum methotrexate levels can be readily measured.
2. Intrathecal methotrexate must be mixed in buffered physiologic solution containing no preservative.
3. Avoid aspirin, sulfonamides, tetracycline, phenytoin, and other protein-bound drugs that may displace methotrexate and cause an increase in free drug.
4. Oral anticoagulants, e.g., warfarin, may be potentiated by methotrexate; therefore prothrombin times should be followed carefully.
5. In patients with renal insufficiency it may be necessary to markedly reduce the dose or discontinue methotrexate therapy.

Toxicity

1. *Myelosuppression*. Occurs regularly, with nadir at 6–10 days after a single IV dose. Recovery is rapid.
2. *Nausea and vomiting*. Occasional at standard doses.
3. *Mucocutaneous effects*
   a. Mild stomatitis is common and is a sign that a maximum tolerated dose has been reached. Higher doses may result in confluent or hemorrhagic stomal ulcers and bloody diarrhea.
   b. Erythematous rashes, urticaria, and skin pigment changes are uncommon.
   c. Mild alopecia is frequent.
4. *Miscellaneous effects*
   a. Acute hepatocellular injury—uncommon at standard doses.
   b. Hepatic fibrosis—uncommon but seen at low chronic doses.
   c. Pneumonitis—rare.
   d. Polyserositis—rare.
   e. Renal tubular necrosis—rare at standard doses.
   f. Convulsions and a Guillain-Barré-like syndrome following intrathecal therapy—uncommon.

Mithramycin

Other names.   Plicamycin, Mithracin.

Mechanism of action.   Binds to DNA and inhibits DNA-dependent RNA synthesis.

Primary indications

1. Severe refractory hypercalcemia.
2. Rarely used as antineoplastic agent.

Usual dosage and schedule.   0.6–1.0 mg/m^2 IV for 1–3 days, with doses repeated if necessary and tolerated.

Special precautions

1. Administer as IV infusion over 0.5–3.0 hours to reduce severity of gastrointestinal toxicity.
2. Avoid subcutaneous extravasation.
3. Monitor platelet count, prothrombin time, partial prothrombin time, lactic dehydrogenase, SGOT, and BUN. Discontinue drug if significant abnormality occurs.

Toxicity. High doses, which were used in the past for testicular carcinoma, had severe myelo- and hepatotoxicity.

1. *Myelosuppression.* Dose-related thrombocytopenia is common but usually not severe at doses used for hypercalcemia; leukopenia is not usually significant.
2. *Nausea and vomiting.* Common.
3. *Mucocutaneous effects*
   a. Blushing of the face followed by a coarsening of skin folds, hyperpigmentation, and possible desquamation—occasional with alternate-day therapy.
   b. Stomatitis—common.
   c. Papular skin rash—uncommon.
   d. Alopecia—uncommon.
4. *Hepatic effects.* Coagulopathy due to clotting factor abnormalities and thrombocytopenia occurs occasionally and may be fatal. Prothrombin time, partial thrombin time, SGOT, and lactic dehydrogenase must be monitored during therapy.
5. *Miscellaneous effects*
   a. Diarrhea—common.
   b. CNS toxicity manifested by headache, irritability, and lethargy—dose-dependent.
   c. Phlebitis—uncommon.
   d. Renal effects—more than one-half of patients have some abnormality with proteinuria and mild azotemia.
   e. Electrolyte abnormalities (depression of serum calcium, phosphorus, and potassium)—common.

Mitomycin

Other names. Mitomycin C, Mutamycin.

Mechanism of action. Alkylation and cross-linking by mitomycin metabolites interfere with structure and function of DNA.

Primary indications. Bladder (intravesical), esophagus, stomach, anal, and pancreas carcinomas.

Usual dosage and schedule

1. 20 mg/m^2 IV on day 1 every 4–6 weeks *or*
2. 2 mg/m^2 IV on days 1–5 and 8–12 every 4–6 weeks.
3. 10 mg/m^2 IV on day 1 every 8 weeks in combination with fluorouracil and doxorubicin for stomach and pancreatic carcinomas.

4. 30–40 mg instilled into the bladder weekly for 4–8 weeks, then monthly for 6 months.

Special precaution.   Administer as slow push or rapid infusion through the sidearm of a rapidly running IV infusioin, taking care to avoid extravasation.

Toxicity

1. *Myelosuppression.* Serious, cumulative, and dose-limiting. Nadir is reached usually by 4 weeks but may be delayed. Recovery is often prolonged over many weeks, and occasionally cytopenia never disappears.
2. *Nausea and vomiting.* Common at higher doses, but severity is usually mild to moderate.
3. *Mucocutaneous effects*
   a. Stomatitis and alopecia—common.
   b. Cellulitis at injection site if extravasation occurs—common.
4. *Miscellaneous effects*
   a. Renal toxicity—uncommon.
   b. Pulmonary toxicity—uncommon but may be severe.
   c. Fever—uncommon.
   d. Secondary neoplasia—possible.
   e. Hemolytic uremic syndrome.

Mitotane

Other names.   *o,p′*-DDD, Lysodren.

Mechanism of action.   Suppresses adrenal steroid production, modifies peripheral steroid metabolism, and is cytotoxic to adrenal cortical cells.

Primary indication.   Adrenocortical carcinoma.

Usual dosage and schedule.   Begin with 2–6 gm PO daily in 3 or 4 divided doses and build to a maximum tolerated daily dose that is usually 8–10 gm, although it may range from 2 to 16 gm. Glucocorticoid and mineralocorticoid replacement during mitotane therapy are necessary to prevent hypoadrenalism. Cortisone acetate (25 mg PO in the a.m. and 12.5 mg PO in the p.m.) and fludrocortisone acetate (0.1 mg PO in the a.m.) are recommended.

Special precautions.   Patients who experience severe trauma, infection, or shock should be treated with supplemental corticosteroids. Because of the effect of mitotane on peripheral steroid metabolism, larger than usual replacement doses may be necessary.

Toxicity

1. *Myelosuppression.* None.
2. *Nausea and vomiting.* Common and may be dose-limiting.
3. *Mucocutaneous effects.* Skin rash occurs occasionally.
4. *CNS effects.* Lethargy, sedation, vertigo, or dizziness in up to 40% of patients; may be dose-limiting.

5. *Miscellaneous effects.* Albuminuria, hemorrhagic cystitis, hypertension, orthostatic hypotension, and visual disturbances—uncommon.

Mitoxantrone

Other names. Novantrone, dihydroxyanthracenedione, DHAD, DHAQ.

Mechanism of action. DNA strand breakage mediated by anthracenedione effects on topoisomerase II.

Primary indications

1. Acute nonlymphocytic leukemia ANLL.
2. Carcinoma of the breast or ovary.
3. Non-Hodgkin's and Hodgkin's lymphoma.

Usual dosage and schedule.

1. 12–14 mg/m^2 IV as a 5- to 30-minute infusion once every 3 weeks for solid tumors.
2. 12 mg/m^2 IV as a 5- to 30-minute infusion daily for 3 days for ANLL.

Special precautions. Rarely causes extravasation injury if infiltrated. Cardiotoxicity probably less than with doxorubicin; but prior anthracycline, chest irradiation, or underlying cardiac disease increases the risk.

Toxicity

1. *Myelosuppression.* Universal.
2. *Nausea and vomiting.* Common but less frequent and less severe than with doxorubicin.
3. *Mucocutaneous effects.* Alopecia is common, but its frequency and severity is less than with doxorubicin. Mucositis—occasional.
4. *Cardiac toxicity.* Probably less than with doxorubicin; there is no clear maximum dose, though the risk appears to increase at 125 mg/m^2 cumulative dose.
5. *Miscellaneous effects*
   a. Local—erythema and swelling with transient blue discoloration if extravasated, but rarely leads to severe skin damage.
   b. Diarrhea—uncommon.
   c. Green or blue discoloration of urine.
   d. Phlebitis—uncommon.

Pentostatin

Other name. 2′-deoxycoformycin.

Mechanism of action. Inhibition of adenosine deaminase, increase in deoxyadenosine triphosphates, inhibition of methylation reactions.

Primary indications.   Hairy-cell leukemia, chronic lymphocytic leukemia, other B cell neoplasms.

Usual dosage and schedule.   2–4 mg/m^2 IV push over 1–2 minutes, after hydration with 1 liter of 5% dextrose with 0.5 N saline or equivalent before pentostatin administration and 500 ml after the drug is given. Repeat every 2 weeks. Higher doses with treatment for 1–3 days may be used in chronic lymphatic leukemia and other B cell neoplasms.

Special precautions.   Hydration required to ensure urine output of 2 liters daily on the day pentostatin is administered. Patients often are hospitalized for their first drug administration. Allopurinol 300 mg bid is recommended in patients with a large tumor mass. Sedative and hypnotic drugs should be used with caution or not at all because CNS toxicity may be potentiated. Dose reduction or discontinuation needed for renal impairment (creatinine clearance < 50 ml/minute).

Toxicity

1. *Myelosuppression.* Common but severity variable.
2. *Nausea and vomiting.* Common but usually not severe.
3. *Mucocutaneous effects.* Mucositis—rare; skin rashes—occasional.
4. *Miscellaneous effects*
   a. Anorexia—common.
   b. Hepatic dysfunction—uncommon.
   c. Diarrhea—uncommon.
   d. Chills and fever—occasional.
   e. Renal insufficiency—rare at usual doses.
   f. Neuropsychiatric effects. High doses may cause serious neurologic and psychiatric symptoms, including seizures, mental confusion, irritability, and coma.

Procarbazine

Other name.   Matulane.

Mechanism of action.   Uncertain but appears to affect preformed DNA, RNA, and protein.

Primary indications

1. Lung carcinoma.
2. Hodgkin's and non-Hodgkin's lymphomas.

Usual dosage and schedule.   100 mg/m^2 PO daily for 7–14 days every 4 weeks (in combination with other drugs).

Special precautions.   Many food and drug interactions are possible, although their clinical significance may be low.

Drug or food	Possible result
Ethanol	Disulfiramlike reactions: nausea, vomiting, visual disturbances, headache

Drug or food	**Possible result**
Sympathomimetics, tricyclic antidepressants, tyramine-rich foods (cheese, wine, bananas)	Hypertensive crisis, tremors, excitation, angina, cardiac palpitations
CNS depressants	Additive depression

Toxicity

1. *Myelosuppression.* Pancytopenia is dose-limiting.
2. *Nausea and vomiting.* Frequent during first few days until tolerance develops.
3. *Mucocutaneous effects*
   a. Stomatitis and diarrhea—uncommon.
   b. Alopecia, pruritus, and drug rash—uncommon.
4. *CNS effects.* Paresthesias, neuropathies, headache, dizziness, depression, apprehension, nervousness, insomnia, nightmares, hallucinations, ataxia, confusion, convulsions, and coma have been reported with varying frequency.
5. *Miscellaneous effects*
   a. Secondary neoplasia—possible.
   b. Visual disturbances—rare.
   c. Postural hypotension—rare.

Progestins

Other names. Medroxyprogesterone acetate (Provera, Depo-Provera), hydroxyprogesterone caproate (Delalutin), megestrol acetate (Megace).

Mechanism of action. Mechanism of antitumor effects is not clear.

Primary indications. Endometrial and breast carcinomas.

Usual dosage and schedule

1. Medroxyprogesterone acetate 1000–1500 mg IM weekly or 400–800 mg PO twice weekly.
2. Hydroxyprogesterone caproate 1000–1500 mg IM weekly.
3. Megestrol acetate 80–320 mg PO daily.

Special precautions

1. Acute local hypersensitivity or dyspnea due to oil in IM preparations—uncommon.
2. Hypercalcemia with initial therapy—occasional.

Toxicity

1. *Myelosuppression.* None.
2. *Nausea and vomiting.* Rare.
3. *Mucocutaneous effects.* Mild alopecia or skin rash—uncommon.

4. *Miscellaneous effects*
    a. Mild fluid retention—occasional.
    b. Mild liver function abnormalities—occasional.
    c. Menstrual irregularities—common.
    d. Improved appetite, weight gain—common.

Streptozocin

Other names. Streptozotocin, Zanosar.

Mechanism of action. Inhibition of DNA synthesis, possibly by interference with pyridine nucleotide synthesis. Streptozocin appears to have some specificity for neoplastic pancreatic endocrine cells. Glucose moiety attached to nitrosourea appears to diminish myelotoxicity.

Primary indications
1. Pancreatic islet cell and pancreatic exocrine carcinomas.
2. Carcinoid tumors.

Usual dosage and schedule

1. 1.0–1.5 gm/m^2 IV weekly for 6 weeks followed by 4 weeks of observation.
2. 500 mg/m^2 IV on days 1–5 every 6 weeks.

Special precautions

1. A 30- to 60-minute infusion is recommended to reduce local pain and burning around the vein during treatment.
2. Avoid extravasation.
3. Have 50% glucose available to treat sudden hypoglycemia.

Toxicity

1. *Myelosuppression.* Uncommon and mild.
2. *Nausea and vomiting.* Common and severe. May become progressively worse over 5-day course of therapy. Standard antiemetics have been of little value.
3. *Mucocutaneous effects.* Uncommon.
4. *Nephrotoxicity.* Renal toxicity is common. Although it is not clearly dose-related, it may limit continued drug use in individual patients. Proteinuria, glucosuria, azotemia, and hypophosphatemia, if persistent or severe, are indications to discontinue therapy. Hydration may ameliorate the problem.
5. *Miscellaneous effects*
    a. Hypoglycemia. In patients with insulinoma, hypoglycemia may be severe (although transient) owing to a burst of insulin release.
    b. Hyperglycemia is uncommon in normal or diabetic patients, as normal β cells are usually insensitive to streptozocin's effect.
    c. Transient mild hepatotoxicity—occasional.

Suramin (Investigational)

Other names. Antrypol, Bayer 205, Germanin, Moranyl, Naganol, Naphuride NA.

Mechanism of action. Glycosaminoglycan agonist-antagonist 130t blocks the binding of growth factors to their receptors. Growth factors affected include platelet-derived growth factor, transforming growth factor-beta, and heparin binding growth factor-2 (also known as basic fibroblast growth factor). Inhibition of DNA polymerases and reverse transcriptase and other proteins. Inhibition of glycosaminoglycan metabolism.

Primary indications

1. Adrenocortical carcinoma.
2. Prostate carcinoma that is hormone-refractory.
3. Lymphoma that is refractory to standard agents.

Usual dosage and schedule. 350 mg/m^2 by continuous IV infusion daily for 7 days after an initial test dose of 200 mg over 10 minutes. The plasma level is then measured, the infusion rate adjusted, and the treatment continued until the plasma level reaches 250–300 μg/ml or the prothrombin time reaches 17.5 seconds. The infusion is then stopped for 2 months and the treatment cycle repeated.

Special precautions. Measurement of plasma levels is necessary to achieve the narrow concentration that is therapeutic and not prohibitively toxic. Therapy should be stopped when a steady-state drug level of 300 μg/ml is reached. Because of adrenal suppression, patients require hydrocortisone, 25 mg in the morning and 15 mg at bedtime. All patients should also receive vitamin K to reduce the likelihood of coagulopathy. Prothrombin time must be followed closely.

Toxicity

1. *Myelosuppression.* Common but usually not severe.
2. *Nausea and vomiting.* Uncommon.
3. *Mucocutaneous effects.* Transient erythematous rash is common.
4. *Adrenocortical insufficiency.* Common.
5. *Neurotoxicity.* Paresthesias are seen commonly and severe polyradiculopathy occasionally. The degree of toxicity appears to be related to the plasma suramin level, with serious reactions uncommon at plasma levels of less than 350 μg/ml.
6. *Miscellaneous effects*
   a. Vortex keratopathy—common.
   b. Liver function test abnormalities—common but reversible.
   c. Coagulopathy—common elevations of the prothrombin time, partial thromboplastin time, and thrombin time, with increased risk of spontaneous bleeding.

d. Renal effects: proteinuria is common; decrease in creatinine clearance is seen occasionally.

Tamoxifen

Other name.   Nolvadex.

Mechanism of action.   Tamoxifen is an estrogen agonist-antagonist that binds to cytoplasmic estrogen receptors. This complex is probably transported into the nucleus where it affects nucleic acid function. Also has effects on cellular growth factors, epidermal growth factors, and transforming growth factors (TGF-α and TGF-β).

Primary indications.   Breast and endometrial carcinomas.

Usual dosage and schedule.   10 mg PO twice daily.

Special precautions.   Hypercalcemia may be seen during initial therapy.

Toxicity

1. *Myelosuppression.* Uncommon and mild.
2. *Nausea and vomiting.* Occur early in the course of therapy in up to 20% of patients, but they abate rapidly as therapy is continued.
3. *Mucocutaneous effects.* Skin rash and pruritus vulvae are uncommon. May cause marked decrease in vaginal secretions and result in difficult or painful intercourse.
4. *Miscellaneous effects*
   a. Hot flashes—common.
   b. Vaginal bleeding and menstrual irregularity—uncommon.
   c. Lassitude, headache, leg cramps, and dizziness—uncommon.
   d. Peripheral edema—occasional.
   e. Increased bone pain, tumor pain, and local disease flare (associated both with good tumor response as well as with tumor progression)—occasional.
   f. Diarrhea—occasional.
   g. Slowed progression of osteoporosis.
   h. Reduction in serum cholesterol with favorable changes in lipid profile.
   i. Cataracts and other eye toxicity—rare.
   j. Thromboemlolic phenonema—rare.

Taxol (Investigational)

Other names.   None.

Mechanism of action.   Enhanced formation and stabilization of microtubules. Antineoplastic effect may result from nonfunctional tubules or altered tubulin-microtubule equilibrium. Mitotic arrest is seen and is associated with accumulated polymerized microtubules.

Primary indications

1. Carcinoma of the ovary.
2. Melanoma.

Usual dosage and schedule.   135–200 mg/m^2 as a single 24-hour infusion every 3 weeks. It is administered as 3 freshly prepared 8-hour infusions.

Special precautions.   Anaphylactoid reactions with dyspnea, hypotension, bronchospasm, urticaria, and erythematous rashes may occur as a result of the taxol itself or the Cremophor vehicle required to make taxol water-soluble. Such reaction is minimized but not totally prevented by pretreatment with antihistamines and corticosteroids and by prolonging the infusion rate (to 24 hours). Taxol must be filtered with a 0.2 micron in-line filter.

Toxicity

1. *Myelosuppression.* Granulocytopenia is universal and dose-limiting; thrombocytopenia is common; anemia is occasional.
2. *Nausea and vomiting.* Common but usually not severe.
3. *Mucocutaneous effects.* Alopecia is universal; mucositis is occasional at recommended doses.
4. *Hypersensitivity reactions.* Dyspnea, hypotension, bronchospasm, urticaria, and erythematous rashes are occasionally seen, despite precautions above.
5. *Miscellaneous effects*
   a. Sensory neuropathy—common (30–35%).
   b. Hepatic dysfunction—uncommon.
   c. Diarrhea—occasional and mild.
   d. Myalgias and arthralgias—common (25%).
   e. Seizures—rare.

Teniposide

Other names.   VM-26, Vumon.

Mechanism of action.   Topoisomerase II-mediated double strand DNA breaks. Causes cells cycle transit delay through S phase and arrest at late S/G$_2$.

Primary indications

1. Acute lymphocytic leukemia (refractory) in combination with cytarabine.
2. Lymphomas.
3. Neuroblastoma.
4. Brain tumors.

Usual dose and schedule

1. 50 mg/m^2 in 50–100 ml normal saline as a 30-minute infusion daily for 5 days.
2. 160 mg/m^2 in 250 ml normal saline as a 1-hour infusion on days 1, 3, and 5. Repeat cycle every 3 weeks.

Special precautions. Hypersensitivity reactions usually resolve with interruption of the infusion and often can be prevented with diphenhydramine and hydrocortisone pretreatment. Hypotension is alleviated by prolonging the infusion time. It is a possible vesicant.

Toxicity

1. *Myelosuppression.* Common and dose-limiting.
2. *Nausea and vomiting.* Occasional.
3. *Mucocutaneous effects.* Alopecia is common.
4. *Miscellaneous effects*
   a. Elevated liver enzymes—occasional.
   b. Hypersensitivity reactions with urticaria and flushing—occasional. Anaphylaxis—uncommon.
   c. Hypotension is related to drug infusion rate but should be seen only occasionally at the recommended dose schedules.
   d. Secondary leukemias—uncommon.

Thioguanine

Other names. 6-Thioguanine, 6-TG, Tabloid brand thioguanine.

Mechanism of action. A purine antimetabolite that, when converted to the active nucleotide, substitutes for the normal guanine nucleotide in DNA synthesis. Thioguanine also inhibits purine synthesis and conversion reactions.

Primary indication. Acute nonlymphocytic leukemia.

Usual dosage and schedule

1. *Induction:* 100 mg/m^2 PO twice daily for 8–21 days (with other drugs).
2. *Maintenance*
   a. 40 mg/m^2 PO twice daily on days 1–4 weekly (with other drugs) *or*
   b. 100 mg/m^2 PO twice daily on days 1–4 every 3–4 weeks (with other drugs).

Special precautions. None (no dose reduction required for concurrent use of allopurinol).

Toxicity

1. *Myelosuppression.* Major dose-limiting toxicity.
2. *Nausea and vomiting.* Occasional but not severe.
3. *Mucocutaneous effects*
   a. Stomatitis and diarrhea, which may necessitate reduction of the dose—uncommon.
   b. Drug rash—rare.
4. *Miscellaneous effects.* Hepatotoxicity—rare.

Thiotepa

Other name. Triethylenethiophosphoramide.

Mechanism of action. Alkylating agent similar to mechlorethamine.

Primary indications

1. Superficial papillary carcinoma of urinary bladder.
2. Malignant peritoneal, pleural or pericardial effusions.
3. Carcinoma of breast and ovary.
4. Neoplastic meningeal infiltrates.

Usual dosage and schedule

1. 12 mg/m^2 IV bolus every 3 weeks in combination with vinblastine and doxorubicin for breast cancer.
2. 30–60 mg in 40–50 ml water instilled into the bladder and retained for 1 hour. Dose is repeated weekly for 3–6 weeks, then every 3 weeks for 5 cycles.
3. 25–30 mg/m^2 in 50–100 ml saline solution as a single intracavitary injection. Dose may be repeated as tolerated by blood counts.

Special precaution.   Dose should be reduced in patients with impaired renal function, as the drug is primarily excreted in the urine.

Toxicity

1. *Myelosuppression.* Dose-limiting. Pancytopenia and sepsis may follow intravesical or intracavitary administration. Nadir counts are reached in 1–2; weeks, recovery by 4 weeks is usual.
2. *Nausea and vomiting.* Uncommon.
3. *Mucocutaneous effects.* Uncommon. Thiotepa is *not* a vesicant.
4. *Miscellaneous effects*
   a. Local pain, dizziness, headache, fever—uncommon.
   b. Secondary neoplasms—possible.
   c. Amenorrhea and azoospermia—common.

Trimetrexate (Investigational)

Other name.   TMQ.

Mechanism of action.   Inhibition of dihydrofolate reductase.

Primary indications

1. Head and neck squamous cell cancers.
2. Lung carcinoma.

Usual dosage and schedule.   8–15 mg/m^2 IV push daily for 5 days.

Special precautions.   None.

Toxicity

1. *Myelosuppression.* Leukopenia and thrombocytopenia are common (30–45%).
2. *Nausea and vomiting.* Common.
3. *Mucocutaneous effects.* Mucositis and skin rash are common (15–25%).

4. *Miscellaneous effects*
   a. Reversible nephrotoxocity—occasional.
   b. Elevated bilirubin—occasional.
   c. Fatigue—occasional.
   d. Diarrhea—uncommon.

Vinblastine

Other names.   VLB, Velban.

Mechanism of action.   Mitotic inhibition with reversible metaphase arrest due to action on microtubular and spindle contractile proteins.

Primary indications

1. Testicular, gestational trophoblastic, kidney, and breast carcinomas.
2. Hodgkin's and non-Hodgkin's lymphomas.

Usual dosage and schedule

1. 4–18 mg/m^2 IV weekly.
2. 6 mg/m^2 IV on days 1 and 15 in combination with doxorubicin, bleomycin, and dacarbazine for lymphomas.
3. 4.5 mg/m^2 IV on day 1 every 3 weeks in combination with doxorubicin and thiotepa for breast cancer.

Special precautions.   Administer as a slow push, taking care to avoid extravasation.

Toxicity

1. *Myelosuppression.* Dose-related leukopenia occurs with a nadir at 4–10 days and recovery in 7–10 days. Severe thrombocytopenia is uncommon.
2. *Nausea and vomiting.* Common but not usually severe.
3. *Mucocutaneous effects*
   a. Extravasation may lead to severe inflammation, pain, and tissue damage. Local infiltration with 1–6 ml of hyaluronidase (150 units/ml) may help.
   b. Mild alopecia is common.
   c. Stomatitis is occasionally severe.
4. *Miscellaneous effects*
   a. Neurotoxicity manifested by (1) constipation, adynamic ileus, and abdominal pain if very high doses are used; or (2) paresthesias, peripheral neuropathy, and jaw pain with lower doses. Neurotoxicity is less frequent with vinblastine than with vincristine.
   b. Transient hepatitis is uncommon.
   c. Depression, headache, convulsions, and orthostatic hypotension are rare.

Vincristine

Other names.   VCR, Oncovin.

Mechanism of action.   Mitotic inhibition with reversible metaphase arrest due to drug action on microtubular and spindle contractile proteins.

Primary indications

1. Breast carcinoma.
2. Hodgkin's and non-Hodgkin's lymphomas.
3. Acute lymphocytic leukemia.
4. Wilms' tumor, neuroblastoma, rhabdomyosarcoma, and Ewing's sarcoma of childhood.
5. Multiple myeloma.

Usual dosage and schedule.   1–2 mg/m^2 (maximum 2.0–2.4 mg) IV weekly.

Special precautions

1. Administer as a slow IV push, taking care to avoid extravasation.
2. Because neurotoxicity is cumulative, neurologic evaluation should be done before each dose and therapy withheld if severe paresthesias, motor weakness, or other severe abnormalities occur. Underlying neurologic problems accentuate vincristine's effect.
3. Reduce dose if liver disease is significant.
4. Stool softeners or high-fiber or bulk diets may avert severe constipation.

Toxicity

1. *Myelosuppression.* Mild and rarely of clinical significance.
2. *Nausea and vomiting.* Not seen unless paralytic ileus occurs.
3. *Mucocutaneous effects.* Severe local inflammation if extravasation occurs. Alopecia is common.
4. *Neurotoxicity.* Dose-dependent and dose-limiting. Mild paresthesias and decreased deep tendon reflexes are to be expected. More extensive peripheral neuropathies, severe constipation, or ileus are indications to reduce or hold therapy.
5. *Miscellaneous effects*
   a. Uric acid nephropathy due to rapid tumor cell lysis and release of uric acid is always a potential problem when therapy is first given.
   b. Syndrome of inappropriate antidiuretic hormone is rare.
   c. Jaw pain is uncommon.

Vindesine (Investigational)

Other name.   VDS.

Mechanism of action.   Mitotic inhibition with reversible metaphase arrest due to action on microtubule and spindle contractile protein.

Primary indications

1. Colorectal, lung, breast, and esophageal carcinomas.
2. Hodgkin's and non-Hodgkin's lymphomas.
3. Acute lymphocytic leukemia and the blast crisis of chronic granulocytic leukemia.
4. Malignant glioma.
5. Melanoma.

Usual dosage and schedule. 2–3 mg/m^2 IV bolus (2–3 minutes) weekly for induction, then every 2 weeks.

Special precautions. Take care to avoid extravasation.

Toxicity

1. *Myelosuppression.* Leukopenia is common but not usually severe.
2. *Nausea and vomiting.* Occasional.
3. *Mucocutaneous effects.* Alopecia is common.
4. *Neurotoxicity.* Dose-dependent and cumulative, consisting in constipation, paralytic ileus, paresthesia, myalgias, and weakness. Severity is intermediate between vincristine and vinblastine.
5. *Miscellaneous effects*
   a. Chills and fever—occasional.
   b. Phlebitis—occasional.
   c. Confusion and lethargy—rare.

Selected Reading

Chabner, B. A., and Collins, J. M. *Cancer Chemotherapy. Principles and Practice.* Philadelphia: Lippincott, 1990.

Chemotherapy of Human Cancer

Carcinomas of the Head and Neck

Ronald C. DeConti

Achievement of a management plan resulting in long-term control or cure for many patients with carcinomas of the head and neck remains an elusive, only partially realized goal for surgeons, radiation therapists, and medical oncologists. Important gains in understanding the natural history of these neoplasms have been made, and the individual achievements of irradiation, surgical techniques, and chemotherapy have been stressed. However, only recently have these modalities been combined to form new treatment plans; and increased patient benefit that might result from this multidisciplinary effort is now being explored.

This discussion focuses on the squamous cell carcinomas of the lining of the aerodigestive tract, which extends from the lip to the esophagus. These tumors account for approximately 5 percent of the new cancer cases seen in the United States each year. Excluded from this discussion are the melanomas, lymphomas, and sarcomas (which also occur in this area), as well as carcinoma of the thyroid, esophagus, and salivary glands. A cross-sectional view of the anatomic regions with the relative frequency of cancer is shown in Figure 9-1. The large number of potential tumor sites and some difficulty in determining the exact site of origin have led to broad use of these larger subdivision terms in an attempt to avoid confusion and to group the related sites. Table 9-1 lists the major sites within each of these anatomic subdivisions.

I. **Common and divergent characteristics.** Carcinomas of the head and neck are frequently considered together by students, generalists, and medical oncologists as though they represent a single therapeutic problem. A number of factors promote this concept.

   A. **Similarities.** In the United States more than 90% of all lesions are squamous cell carcinomas, occurring predominantly in men (3:1). Most patients share common demographic and epidemiologic risk factors. The incidence of head and neck cancer increases with the use of alcohol and tobacco and with advancing age. Head and neck cancers occur in continuity, one with another, and it is occasionally difficult to determine the precise site of origin in the close confines of the complicated interrelated structures comprising the oral cavity, pharynx, larynx, and sinuses. Furthermore, patterns of spread are similar, with local failure, local recurrence, and regional node failures predominating. For most sites, spread below the clavicle is unusual, occurring in only a few cases usually as pulmonary involvement. Bone lesions, usually the result of local extension involving the mandible or floor of the skull, are not uncommon, although widespread bone metastases are unusual. A few patients de-

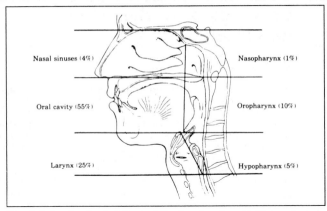

Fig. 9-1. Anatomic divisions of the head and neck. Percentages indicate the relative frequency of carcinoma in these regions.

Table 9-1. Upper aerodigestive tract sites

Region	Area	Site
Oral cavity		Lip
		Buccal mucosa
		Lower alveolar ridge
		Upper alveolar ridge
		Retromolar trigone
		Floor of mouth
		Hard palate
		Oral tongue
Pharynx	Nasopharynx	Posterior wall
		Lateral wall
	Oropharynx	Faucial arch
		Tonsillar fossa and tonsil
		Base of tongue
		Pharyngeal wall
	Hypopharynx	Piriform fossa
		Postcricoid area
		Posterior wall
Larynx	Supraglottis	Ventricular band
		Arytenoid
		Epiglottis
	Glottis	True vocal cords
	Subglottis	Subglottis
Paranasal sinuses		Antrum
		Nasal cavity
		Ethmoid
		Sphenoid
		Frontal

velop hepatic metastases. Inanition, oral ulceration, fistula formation, respiratory difficulty, and aspiration characterize the late course of the disease. Recurrence after primary treatment usually occurs within 18 months, and the patients who are not cured are usually dead within 3 years of diagnosis.

B. **Differences.** For the surgeon or radiation therapist, the differences among sites may be more significant than the similarities. Certainly, presenting signs and symptoms differ markedly. For example, patients with an anterior tongue lesion may describe pain, sensation of mass, and limited motion of the tongue. Hoarseness, dysphagia, or sore throat may predominate in patients with carcinoma of the larynx. More importantly, differences in location influence the frequency of nodal spread and the chances for contralateral node involvement. These factors frequently determine optimal treatment planning.

II. **Primary treatment.** A discussion of the complexity of treatment choices for the multitude of sites where lesions occur is beyond the scope of this chapter. In general, early lesions in most locations are suitable for treatment by surgery or irradiation, and the therapeutic choice is usually made by considering the complications of each treatment, i.e., the deformities of definitive surgery or the complications of irradiation. With increasing failure rates and the likelihood of pathologic, if not clinical, lymph node involvement as tumor bulk increases, clinicians have begun to investigate combined modality approaches. Radiation may be used electively before operation or postoperatively after a pathologic assessment of regional nodes provides the opportunity for postsurgical staging assessment. Many studies have now reported both improved local and regional node control after such multimodality approaches. Although substantial progress has been made in improving end results, with decreased morbidity and deformity, for early stage lesions in many sites, the outcome for tumors in advanced stages remains poor: For stage III disease, the 3- to 5-year survival rate is 20–40%. For stage IV disease, 5–20% long-term survivors are reported.

III. **Staging.** Any consideration of outcome in relation to treatment relies heavily on detailed pretreatment assessment of the extent of the tumor.

A. **TNM classification.** A complex site-specific staging system has been devised by the American Joint Committee for Cancer Staging. This system incorporates a TNM classification to identify, clinically and pathologically, the size of the primary tumor (T), the presence and extent of regional node metastases (N), and the presence of distant metastases (M). Table 9-2 outlines the TNM system for carcinoma of the oral cavity. For lesions of the nasopharynx, hypopharynx, or larynx, fixation or anatomic extensions are substituted for tumor size when determining the extent of the primary lesion.

B. **Stages.** The stage grouping for head and neck cancers is shown in Table 9-3. Stages I and II are determined by

Table 9-2. TNM staging system for carcinomas of the oral cavity

T stage	Primary tumor
T_X	No available information on primary tumor
T_0	No evidence of primary tumor
T_{1s}	Carcinoma in situ
T_1	Greatest diameter of tumor ≤ 2 cm
T_2	Greatest diameter of tumor $> 2 \leq 4$ cm
T_3	Greatest diameter of tumor > 4 cm
T_4	Invasion to adjacent structures such as antrum, pterygoid muscles, base of tongue, or skin of neck
N stage	Regional nodal status
N_X	Nodes cannot be assessed
N_0	No clinically positive node
N_1	Single clinically positive ipsilateral node ≤ 3 cm in diameter
N_2	Single clinically positive ipsilateral node > 3–6 cm; or multiple clinically positive nodes, none > 6 cm; or bilateral or contralateral nodes, none > 6 cm
N_3	Metastasis in a lymph node > 6 cm in greatest dimension
M stage	Distant metastasis
M_X	Not assessed
M_0	No (known) distant metastasis
M_1	Distant metastasis present

Table 9-3. Stage grouping for carcinoma of the oral cavity, pharynx, larynx, and paranasal sinuses

Stage	Groups
I	T_1, N_0, M_0
II	T_2, N_0, M_0
III	T_3, N_0, M_0 T_1 or T_2 or T_3, N_1, M_0
IV	T_4, N_0 or N_1, M_0 Any T, N_2 or N_3, M_0 Any T, any N, M_1

the size of the tumor in the absence of nodal involvement or distant metastases. Stage III comprises both large tumors and tumors of any size with early regional node involvement. Stage IV lesions may be huge with local extension or may be of any size with distant metastatic disease. This stage grouping has been uniformly applied to each tumor site to demonstrate gradations in prognosis.

IV. Chemotherapy

A. Prognostic factors. Whether chemotherapy is considered for the treatment of advanced recurrent head and neck cancer or for preoperative induction treatment, a number of similar, single prognostic variables have now been clearly identified (Table 9-4).

1. **Stage of carcinoma.** Small lesions with minimal regional node involvement respond better than the massive tumors of stage IV. Patients with stage IV, bulky nodal lesions are benefited with difficulty, and response rates are lowest for stage IV disease with pulmonary or visceral metastases. Because patients with head and neck cancers have an increased risk of developing second primary neoplasms, the finding of distant metastases in the absence of primary or regional node recurrence suggests this possibility.

2. **State of health.** Both poor ECOG performance status (see Table 6-2) and weight loss of more than 5% have been found to adversely affect prognosis. It is still unclear if aggressive attempts to improve nutrition or restore cellular immunity with hyperalimentation result in gains in the response rate.

3. **Prior treatment.** Many studies have reported the adverse effect of prior x-ray therapy on drug response. This effect has usually been attributed to an impaired tumor blood supply, a large tumor burden, and poor patient performance status. The failure to respond to irradiation or rapid relapse after radiation therapy has also been shown to adversely affect response rates.

B. **Single-agent responses.** Only methotrexate, bleomycin, fluorouracil, and cisplatin have been studied extensively as individual agents for head and neck carcinomas, and it is largely from this group that most of the combinations are derived.

1. **Methotrexate.** In efforts to improve its therapeutic index, methotrexate has been investigated in no other solid tumor as extensively as it has been investigated for the management of head and neck cancer.

a. **IV methotrexate** in doses of 40–60 mg/m^2 weekly achieves objective partial response in 25–50%

Table 9-4. Factors prognostic for response to chemotherapy

Favorable	Unfavorable
Stage III	Stage IV
No metastasis	Pulmonary metastasis
ECOG performance status 0–1*	ECOG performance status 2–3
No weight loss	Weight loss
Normal immune mechanism	Impaired delayed hypersensitivity
Prior surgery	Prior irradiation
Long disease-free interval	Short disease-free interval
No prior chemotherapy	Prior chemotherapy

*See Table 6-2.

of patients studied and is probably the most widely accepted conventional single-agent treatment for this group of tumors. Responses may occur after 1–2 weeks but usually require 4–6 weeks to become evident. Complete responses occur in approximately 7–10% of patients studied. Median response durations range from 2 to 6 months. Responders survive significantly longer than nonresponders. Treatment is usually given on an outpatient basis, and drug-related mortality is less than 4%.

  b. **Intraarterial infusions of methotrexate** have been attempted in an effort to improve drug concentrations in tumor tissue and to improve the therapeutic index of treatment, either alone or with the use of systemic leucovorin. Although these techniques have resulted in marginally superior response rates, the lack of a single predominant blood supply, the technical difficulties of the procedure, and the morbidity of problems with clot, embolus, and infection appear to have precluded widespread adoption of this approach, and it is not recommended for general use.

  c. **Leucovorin rescue** has made possible the use of moderate (240–500 mg/m^2) to high (1–3 gm/m^2) doses of methotrexate in attempts to improve response rates. Individual investigators have reported favorable rates with decreased morbidity. The duration of response is not increased, and two comparative trials have demonstrated no advantage to these treatment approaches compared to weekly IV methotrexate. The need for hydration, urinary alkalinization, careful monitoring of renal clearance, and the high cost of treatment have been important factors in limiting general use of this approach, and it is not recommended outside a research setting.

2. **Bleomycin** has attracted continued interest for treatment of head and neck cancers because of its generally mild myelosuppressant effects and the potential for its application in combination with myelosuppressive chemotherapy. Bleomycin 10–30 mg/m^2 is usually given weekly, biweekly, or on a 5-day-per-month schedule by IM and IV injections. These approaches have the advantage of being convenient for outpatient use. Tumor response rarely occurs at cumulative doses of less than 200 mg/m^2, and response most often requires a total dose of 300 mg/m^2—doses that usually produce significant mucosal toxicity. Response rates range between 15% and 25% and are generally inferior in duration to those achieved with methotrexate. In general, the mucosal toxicity that accompanies the use of bleomycin is more frequent and severe than that produced with the use of a weekly methotrexate schedule.

3. Cisplatin. Cisplatin 40–60 mg/m^2 IV is given on an every-3-week schedule. Higher doses result in an increased risk of renal toxicity unless special precautions are taken. Doses of 80–120 mg/m^2 may be tolerated if preceded by hydration and accompanied by furosemide and mannitol for diuresis to protect renal function (see Chapter 8). Cisplatin produces objective antitumor responses in approximately 25% of patients, many of whom have previously been treated with other antineoplastic drugs. Occasionally, dramatic tumor responses occur, although the frequency of complete remission is still low. Its major side effects are severe nausea, vomiting, tinnitus, occasional high-tone deafness, peripheral neuropathy, and, most significantly, renal toxicity (with progressive loss in creatinine clearance in some cases).

4. Other drugs. Of the remaining agents for which some information is available, fluorouracil may be of somewhat greater value for oral cavity lesions than other agents. Attempts have been made to demonstrate improved responses utilizing leucovorin in conjunction with fluorouracil. Its long-term value remains to be demonstrated. The 23% response rate of doxorubicin (Adriamycin) alone, although based on a small number of patients, has prompted the trial of this drug in several combinations without convincing results.

Carboplatin, a new analog of cisplatin, appears promising. To date, this drug appears as active as cisplatin with fewer side effects. Minimal nausea and vomiting allow administration without use of sedation-producing antiemetics, and the absence of nephrotoxicity allows outpatient use without intravenous hydration. It is highly likely that this drug will be increasingly substituted for cisplatin as evidence of comparable activity in combination therapies develops. Numerous biologic modifiers have been studied, but to date they have not demonstrated any value in routine clinical practice.

C. Combination chemotherapy responses. Multiple attempts have been made to improve single-agent response rates with combination chemotherapy. A number of studies using methotrexate, bleomycin, fluorouracil, and cisplatin in a variety of schedules have been reported.

The Eastern Cooperative Oncology Group, in a comparison of methotrexate, bleomycin, and cisplatin with weekly methotrexate, demonstrated a clear-cut advantage for combination chemotherapy. Forty-eight percent of patients with advanced disease responded to an outpatient program using methotrexate, bleomycin, and cisplatin compared to 35% using methotrexate alone. Complete remissions were achieved in 16% on combination chemotherapy and for 8% on methotrexate alone. The median duration of response was the same in both treatment groups, and no survival advantage was demonstrated for the combination treatment. Although neither response rate is exceptional, the careful randomization and stratification procedures used lend weight to the result. This program stands as the most controlled prospective trial to show an advantage to combination chemotherapy in the treatment of recurrent disease. Combinations of cisplatin and fluorouracil or methotrexate demonstrate similar outcomes: improved response rates but no overall gain in survival.

D. Combined-modality treatment. Attempts to increase tumor destruction with drugs prior to definitive therapy or together with radiation therapy are not new, although developments in chemotherapy have reawakened enthusiasm for this approach.

   1. Drugs before irradiation or surgery

   a. Methotrexate. In several small, single-institution studies, moderate- and high-dose methotrexate with leucovorin rescue were given for several doses or cycles in advance of irradiation or surgery. These schedules have produced response rates of approximately 75% and have avoided the problems of oral mucositis and ulceration reported by the older studies of concomitant chemotherapy. No data are available to allow comparisons of these rescue programs with weekly methotrexate schedules.

   b. Combination chemotherapy. A number of combination-drug therapy programs have been developed as initial treatment for advanced local-regional disease. These programs were intended either to reduce tumor bulk and allow more effective radiotherapy or to improve resectability of advanced lesions. In general, the programs use high-dose cisplatin in conjunction with hydration and diuretics (see Chapter 8) combined with 3–5 days of either bleomycin or fluorouracil by IV infusion. Vincristine is frequently included, and methotrexate is usually omitted. These programs produce high response rates (67–94%). In six studies composed of 215 patients, complete clinical disappearance of tumor was achieved in 19–28% of patients, and partial response was achieved in 48–74%. After 1 to 3 cycles of drug treatment, surgery, irradiation, or both followed. The number of patients with advanced local-regional disease who were made disease-free was greater than expected based on pretreatment staging expectations. Improvement in survival appeared limited to those patients who achieved complete response.

   2. Concurrent chemotherapy and radiotherapy. Bleomycin, fluorouracil, methotrexate, and cisplatin have been administered synchronously with radiation therapy in an attempt to demonstrate a synergistic effect. Most uncontrolled studies suggest improved tumor responses and some gain in survival for patients with unresectable disease. Although randomized trials have found improvement in the initial response or disease-free survival, overall survival gains have been difficult to document. As a single agent, bleomycin has been perhaps the best studied, and only one study supports an improved survival difference. Enhanced mucositis with combined treatment has been a common limitation of treatment, and split-course fractionation has frequently been used to alleviate this complication. As combination chemotherapy has shown itself to be more effective than single-agent therapy, studies are now focusing on combination chemotherapy together with radiation therapy. Once more preliminary results suggest improved short-term tumor control, though survival comparisons are difficult to quantitate. This subject continues to be an active area of clinical investigation.

    3. Drugs as posttreatment adjuvant. Whereas the most recent emphasis in head and neck cancer has been on achieving gains in early tumor control, little attention has been paid to the potential of postoperative or postirradiation therapy adjuvant drug studies. The available clinical evidence now demonstrates efficacy for two types of induction chemotherapy: (1) programs using cisplatin with 5-fluorouracil or bleomycin; and (2) drug treatment programs with methotrexate. If the lessons of tumor biology and experience in human acute leukemia and breast carcinoma apply, pursuit of a comprehensive treatment program using these agents to best kinetic and clinical advantage will offer increased opportunity to benefit larger numbers of patients with head and neck cancer than are generally benefited today, even without gains in theoretic knowledge or development of more potent drugs.

E. Pretreatment patient assessment. The extent of evaluation required to determine the suitability of a patient for chemotherapy depends, to a considerable degree, on the intent and type of program to be employed. The major organ systems affected by the antineoplastic drugs under consideration are bone marrow, lungs, and kidneys. Any pretreatment assessment should consider not only careful evaluation of the size and extent of tumor but also the presence of comorbid disease processes involving these organ systems. A careful history, review of systems, physical assessment, and routine laboratory data may provide clues in these areas.

    1. Bone marrow function. Chronic alcoholism and malnutrition or the effect of the tumor on diet may contribute to the high incidence of folate deficiency seen in this population. Because of the additive effect of this deficiency and the inhibition of folate metabolism by methotrexate, there is often increased sensitivity to even small doses of methotrexate with marked clinical toxicity.

2. **Pulmonary function.** Chronic obstructive pulmonary disease is common in this group of patients. Moderate to severe pretreatment reductions in timed forced expiratory volumes may be reduced further with treatment with bleomycin. It is recommended that if clinical assessment suggests impaired pulmonary reserve and bleomycin is to be part of the treatment program, pretreatment pulmonary function studies should be performed.

3. **Renal function.** Both cisplatin and methotrexate affect renal function. The major cumulative toxicity of cisplatin is renal. Unfortunately, there may be considerable impairment of renal function before the serum creatinine concentration rises; cisplatin doses of 80–120 mg/m^2 require serial determination of creatinine clearance to assess the cumulative effects of the drug on renal function.

Limited excretion of methotrexate prolongs the duration of high serum concentration of drugs and extends the duration of impaired DNA synthesis for normal as well as neoplastic tissues. Weekly IV methotrexate is usually given to the patients with advanced disease after it is established that the serum creatinine level is normal. A careful clinical assessment at the time of each dose is probably more reliable than serial determinations in this situation. Most episodes of serious methotrexate toxicity relate to failure to appreciate intercurrent events that limit excretion of these relatively low doses of the drug. The most common of these toxicities is probably dehydration, which is related to progressive disease, increasingly poor oral intake, nausea and vomiting, or mucositis that may have been caused by prior drug treatment. The addition of any drug that further alters renal clearance of methotrexate may tip the balance. Aspirin, sulfonamides, phenytoin, cefoxitin, and gentamicin may decrease methotrexate clearance and increase toxicity. Careful interval patient assessment with these considerations in mind helps avoid these pitfalls.

F. **Selected treatment plans.** The plans of drug administration for three types of drug treatment programs are displayed in Table 9-5.

1. **Cytoreductive induction treatment**

a. **Selection of patients.** This treatment is designed to reduce tumor bulk prior to surgery or radiotherapy in patients with advanced-stage disease and no prior therapy. The induction treatment regimen is intended for hospitalized patients following assessment of the extent of their tumor and an evaluation to exclude comorbid disease processes that might unacceptably increase the risks of treatment.

b. Administration

(1) Cisplatin + vincristine + bleomycin (COB). Oral hydration is begun the evening before treatment. On the morning of treatment an IV infusion of 5% dextrose in 0.5 N saline with potassium chloride 20 mEq/liter is begun at a rate of 200 ml/hour. Furosemide 40 mg and mannitol 12.5 gm are given IV after the first liter. The patient should be voiding freely. Immediately thereafter, cisplatin 100 mg/m^2 is added to a calibrated solution set and given over a 30-minute period, and the second liter of fluid is continued. One of a number of intensive regimens to alleviate nausea and vomiting should be begun (see Chapter 37). The volume of subsequent IV fluids for the day is judged by the extent of nausea and vomiting and the urinary excretion. On day 2, vincristine 1 mg is given by IV push, and bleomycin infusion is begun. Bleomycin 15 units is added to each of 2 liters of 5% dextrose in 0.5 N saline with potassium chloride 20 mEq/liter to be administered q24h. The continuous infusion is maintained for 4 days. On day 5, vincristine 1 mg is given by IV push. If adequate oral intake has not been resumed, additional IV fluids may be given. An infusion pump may be used to help ensure an even rate of flow.

The patient may be discharged after completion of the treatment course, depending on tolerance to the drug and the ability to eat and drink. An interim clinic visit before a second induction course is recommended as a safeguard. A second course of treatment is planned on day 21 but should be administered only after hematologic values and serum creatinine are normal and no pulmonary symptoms are reported. If tumor regression is continuing on day 42 after two cycles of treatment, a third cycle may be considered, although the cumulative risks of renal and pulmonary toxicity increase with continued treatment. At this point irradiation, surgery, or both should be considered once again.

(2) Cisplatin + fluorouracil (CF). Cisplatin 100 mg/m^2 IV on day 1 is administered with diuresis and antiemetics as described for COB in **(1)**, above. Fluorouracil 1000 mg/m^2, is divided between 2 liters of 5% dextrose in 0.5 N saline with potassium chloride 20 mEq/liter to be given q24h. Continuous infusion of fluorouracil is maintained for 5 days, usually with an infusion pump. Followup is as described in **(1)**, above, although

Table 9-5. Selected drug treatment programs in head and neck cancer

Intent	Suitability	Scheme
Cytoreductive induction treatment	Advanced stage, no prior treatment	**COB** Cisplatin 100 mg/m² IV on day 1 with induced diuresis *and* Bleomycin 30 units/day as 24-hour infusion on days 2–5 *and* Vincristine 1 mg IV on days 2 and 5 Cycle repeats in 3 weeks **CF** Cisplatin 100 mg/m² IV day 1 with induced diuresis *and* 5-Fluorouracil 1000 mg/m²/day as 24-hour infusion on days 1–5 Cycle repeats in 3–4 weeks

Concurrent radiotherapy	Advanced stage, no prior treatment	Cisplatin 75 mg/m^2 IV on day 1 with induced diuresis *and* Fluorouracil 1000 mg/m^2/day as 24-hour infusion on days 1–4 Cycle repeats in 4 weeks Radiotherapy 30 Gy/15 fractions begun day 1 Evaluate at week 9: CR or unresectable—repeat cycle with 30 Gy/15 fractions as before. PR, stable, and resectable—have surgery with a third cycle of chemotherapy and radiotherapy (30 Gy/15 fractions) 2–6 weeks after operation
Palliation	Prior treatment	Methotrexate 40 mg/m^2 IM on days 1 and 15 *and* Bleomycin 10 units IM on days 1, 8, and 15 *and* Cisplatin 50 mg/m^2 IV day 4 with induced diuresis Cycle repeats in 3 weeks
Palliation	Prior treatment and contraindications to combination drugs	Methotrexate 40–60 mg/m^2 IV weekly

CR, complete response; PR, partial response.

pulmonary toxicity is not a side effect of this program.

2. **Concurrent chemotherapy and radiotherapy.** With this program the dose of cisplatin is reduced somewhat, and fluorouracil infusion duration is limited to 4 days. Treatment is administered with hydration and antiemetics as described above.

Careful attention to fluid and nutritional support during possible periods of intense mucositis are necessary. In potentially operable patients a decision for surgery is usually made after two courses of chemotherapy and a total of 60 Gy.

3. **Combination chemotherapy for advanced recurrent disease.** With advanced recurrent disease, one of two courses of induction treatment (see **IV.F.1**) may be elected followed by an intermittent program with lesser doses of drug; or treatment is initiated on an outpatient basis using a combination drug program as described in Table 9–5. Methotrexate 40 mg/m^2 and bleomycin 10 units are given IM or IV on day 1. On day 4, cisplatin is given as an IV bolus at 50 mg/m^2. Cisplatin is given approximately 30 minutes after starting a 2-hour infusion of 2 liters of 5% dextrose in 0.5 N saline with potassium chloride 20 mEq/liter. Furosemide 40 mg is given IV at the start of the infusion, and mannitol 12.5 gm is given just before the administration of cisplatin. Antiemetics are given as necessary. On day 8 bleomycin is given at a dose of 10 units, and on day 15 methotrexate and bleomycin are repeated.

Dosages of methotrexate and cisplatin are reduced 50% for mild myelosuppression. Drugs are withheld if more severe myelosuppression occurs. Treatment is resumed as soon as peripheral blood counts recover. Methotrexate and bleomycin are withheld if stomatitis is present. Complete blood counts, including platelets, should be done on a weekly basis. Serum creatinine levels are measured on day 8 of each cycle to ensure adequate renal function before the next dose of methotrexate, and creatinine clearance should be measured if creatinine levels rise 50% or more.

4. **Methotrexate alone for advanced disease**
   a. **Selection of patients.** With a number of increased response rates reported for drug combinations compared to methotrexate alone, the latter program should probably be reserved for selected patients: patients in relapse after induction treatment programs without methotrexate, those who refuse treatment with cisplatin or bleomycin, those whose pulmonary function excludes a bleomycin treatment program, and those whose reliability and follow-up opportunities are poor.
   b. **Treatment regimens.** The usual starting dose of methotrexate is 40 mg/m^2; but if advanced age, anemia, borderline renal function, or other fac-

tors suggest sensitivity to methotrexate, the initial dose may be reduced to as low as 20 mg/m^2. Blood counts are done weekly, and if there is no evidence of mucositis or myelosuppression, the dose is escalated to a maximum of 60 mg/m^2. Most patients tolerate this treatment with minimal nausea and vomiting. A few require antiemetics. Careful attention to oral hygiene may be helpful for preventing or reducing the severity of mucositis. Candidiasis should be suspected and, if present, treated with nystatin (Mycostatin) or other anti-fungal agent. If mucositis or myelosuppression occurs, treatments are delayed until they clear and blood counts are normal.

G. Problems in supportive care

1. **Support systems.** The population of patients with head and neck cancer includes many elderly men—often social reprobates, recluses, heavy smokers and drinkers, and occasionally frank derelicts. They are frequently divorced or separated from their families, and many live alone, often in reduced circumstances. Lack of family, friends, resources, and initiative are often an impediment to adequate care, especially in advanced disease situations in which close follow-up, regular clinic visits, and adherence to treatment schedules are important. They desperately need a primary caregiver in the home or to be closely allied with the home to promote their well-being and optimal utilization of medical care and to derive advantage from the health care delivery system. Social service, ministerial help, patient care, support groups, Alcoholics Anonymous, and other social care groups should be enlisted to help the patient cope with illness.

2. **Nutrition.** Gradual, progressive weight loss and inanition are common factors in the relentless illness of many patients. Their nutrition is generally inadequate, and repetitive efforts at reinforcing the need for a high-calorie diet, as free of alcohol as possible, must be given. Depending on the location of the tumor and the particular problems with swallowing, efforts need to be extended on a regular basis to ensure adequate patient nutrition. Many patients, or their families, need to be instructed in the use of blended foods, the use of high-protein supplements, or both. Some patients benefit from the use of a pediatric feeding tube when deformities in the anatomy prevent adequate swallowing. In selected patients a gastrostomy tube feeding may be appropriate, especially early in the patient's clinical course when it is hoped that it may be only a temporary expedient. Most patients benefit from any attempts at oral hyperalimentation. The role of IV hyperalimentation is not clear and needs to be considered early in the management course during the perioperative or radiation therapy period when induction treat-

ment is taking place. Its role in maintaining patients in the advanced disease state is still unclear. Efforts to maintain nutrition must be reinforced at every opportunity with the family, the care-giver, and the patient. Dietary advice or consultation with a dietetic department should be offered freely.

3. **Mouth care** may be an important problem for some patients with head and neck cancer. Many patients have difficulty with secretions. Xerostomia may be produced by radiation therapy and may require treatment with artificial saliva. At the opposite extreme, patients with posterior tongue lesions may have edema and swelling that precludes adequate swallowing, and the pooling of secretions and subsequent aspiration become a problem. These patients may benefit from the use of suction to drain their secretions. Cleansing mouthwash may be appropriate, and efforts at dental hygiene need to be maintained. Radiation-induced bone necrosis or fistulas need to be cleaned or débrided and occasionally packed with toothpaste or other material to promote comfort.

4. **Hypercalcemia** in patients with epidermoid carcinoma of the head and neck is a common situation. As many as 23% of patients with advanced recurrent head and neck cancers may experience hypercalcemia before their death. In general, this phenomenon accompanies late-stage recurrent tumor, often with little evidence of bone involvement. Dehydration, all too common in these patients, may be a precipitating factor; in many patients hypercalcemia is mild and easily controlled with hydration, saline diuresis, or both. Although hydration, saline diuresis, or reduction in tumor achieved with irradiation, drug therapy, or surgery frequently reverses this phenomenon, a few patients require mithramycin for adequate treatment (see Chapter 28).

5. **Pneumonia.** The anatomic deformities induced by operation, recurrent tumor, or both make patients with head and neck cancer highly susceptible to aspiration of pooled secretions. Fever, tachycardia, tachypnea, rales, and infiltrates in the lung are usual findings and are often confused with bacterial pneumonia. Knowledge of the aspiration or observation of the event may be the only decisive method of proving the diagnosis. Immediate recognition of aspiration suggests treatment with steroids, antibiotics, or both.

6. **Granulocytopenia.** The greatest concern is for the need to quickly identify pulmonary infection in the presence of drug-induced granulocytopenia. The mortality due to pneumonia and sepsis is high in this situation. Appropriate cultures are needed in an effort to document infection and help distinguish the problem from aspiration. Fever in a granulocytopenic patient should be promptly treated with broad-

spectrum antibiotics without awaiting results of the cultures (see Chapter 32).

Selected Reading

Al-Kourainy, K., et al. Achievement of superior survival for histologically negative versus histologically positive clinically complete responders to cisplatin combination in patients with locally advanced head and neck cancer. *Cancer* 59:233, 1987.

Al-Sarraf, M., et al. Concurrent radiotherapy and chemotherapy with cisplatin in inoperable squamous cell carcinoma of the head and neck: an RTOG study. *Cancer* 59:259, 1987.

Adelstein, D. J., et al. Simultaneous versus sequential combined technique therapy for squamous cell head and neck cancer. *Cancer* 65:1685, 1990.

American Joint Committee in Cancer. *Staging Cancer at Head and Neck Sites. Manual for Staging Cancer.* Philadelphia: Lippincott, 1988. P. 27.

Clark, J. R., and Frei, E., III. Chemotherapy for head and neck cancer: progress and controversy in the management of patients with MO disease. *Semin. Oncol.* 4(suppl 6):44, 1989.

Decker, D. A., et al. Adjuvant chemotherapy with cis-diamminedichloroplatinum II and 120-hour infusion 5-fluorouracil in stage III and IV squamous cell carcinoma of the head and neck. *Cancer* 51:1353, 1983.

Jacobs, C., and Makuch, R. Efficacy of adjuvant chemotherapy for patients with resectable head and neck cancer: a subset analysis of the Head and Neck Contracts Program. *J. Clin. Oncol.* 8:838, 1990.

Million, R .R., and Cassisi, N. J. (eds.). *Management of Head and Neck Cancer: a Multidisciplinary Approach.* Philadelphia: Lippincott, 1984.

Vogel, S. E., et al. A randomized prospective comparison of methotrexate with a combination of methotrexate, bleomycin and cisplatin in head and neck cancer. *Cancer* 56:432, 1985.

Carcinoma of the Lung

Robert B. Livingston

I. Introduction

A. Incidence. Carcinoma of the lung is the most common malignancy seen in the United States (excluding non-melanoma skin cancer) and accounts for one of eight cancers diagnosed. With more than 140,000 deaths occurring yearly in the United States from lung cancer, it takes nearly twice the toll of any other malignancy and is responsible for one of every four cancer deaths.

B. Treatment modalities. Most of the lesions are inoperable at the time of diagnosis because of either the extent of local invasion or the presence of distant metastasis. Of those that are operable and resectable, most have local or distant recurrence. Therefore fewer than 10% of all lung cancers are curable by surgery. Although radiotherapy plays an important palliative role in lung cancer, it is infrequently curative and is effective primarily for limited regional disease or isolated metastases. For these reasons, there is a great need for effective chemotherapy to help most patients who cannot be cured with other modalities.

C. Cell types and staging. The role of chemotherapy in lung cancer differs according to the cell type. The four primary types of lung cancer are squamous cell carcinoma, adenocarcinoma, large-cell carcinoma, and small-cell carcinoma (sometimes referred to as oat-cell carcinoma, which is actually a subtype of small-cell carcinoma). Because the biologic behavior and response to treatment of the small-cell carcinomas are so different from the other three types, a separation into two broad categories—small-cell carcinoma and non-small-cell carcinoma (squamous cell, adenocarcinoma, and large cell)—is necessary for any discussion of treatment.

Chemotherapy is now the main modality of treatment for small-cell (oat-cell) carcinoma of the lung. For lesions with other histologies, chemothreapy is used in clinical practice only for palliation. For purposes of selecting treatment and comparing responses, patients who have cancers in either histologic grouping (small-cell or non-small-cell) are further subgrouped on the basis of the extent of their disease into the categories of extensive disease or limited (regional) disease. The term *extensive* is used to imply clinical evidence of dissemination beyond the hemithorax and its regional node drainage (mediastinal, scalene, and supraclavicular). The term *limited,* or *regional,* is used to describe disease that is within these boundaries clinically but is inoperable.

With the advent of a TNM-based staging system for lung cancer, it has become common to utilize its terminology for patients with more advanced disease who may be candidates for chemotherapy. "Limited" disease is stage III in the new system and is divided into "IIIA" and

"IIIB." Basically, patients with IIIA disease have (with few exceptions) tumors that are considered unresectable for cure at presentation, primarily because of mediastinal nodal involvement (N_2), which is thought to be ipsilateral. Those with IIIB disease have locally more advanced (T_4) tumors that involve extrapulmonary structures by direct extension, malignant effusion, or nodes that are positive in the supraclavicular area or contralateral mediastinum (N_3), or any combination of these findings. These patients can never be managed primarily by surgery, and they have a prognosis similar to those with *extensive* disease, now called stage IV.

II. Small-cell carcinoma of the lung (SCLC)

A. General considerations and aims of therapy. SCLC accounts for about 25% of lung cancer in the United States. Most cases are related to cigarette smoking. The tumor mass is typically central in location (mediastinal or perihilar) on the chest x-ray film. Pretreatment evaluation of the patient should include a complete blood count, liver function tests, computed tomography (CT) of the brain and abdomen, and a bone scan. If none of these tests reveal spread of the disease beyond the lung and regional nodes, the disease is deemed to be clinically limited. Such patients should undergo CT of the chest and unilateral bone marrow aspiration and biopsy to complete their staging. CT of the chest seldom reclassifies the lesion as to extent but is vital for planning radiation treatment of the primary site. The bone marrow is positive in 1 in 20 patients otherwise classed as "limited." Clinically limited disease occurs in about one-third of patients with SCLC despite the fact that microscopic hematogenous spread is almost universal at the time of diagnosis. In this group, complete response (CR) with combined chemotherapy and irradiation was formerly expected in 40–60% of patients, with long-term disease-free survival rates of 10–15%. More recent data with *concurrent* chest irradiation and cisplatin + VP-16 indicate higher CR rates and long-term disease-free survival in 25–30%. For patients with extensive disease, CR is achieved in only 10–15%, although most have a partial response (PR), symptomatic improvement, and some prolongation of survival. Median survivals are in the range of 8–18 months, respectively, for extensive and limited disease using best standard treatment; with supportive care only, the respective figures are about 6–12 weeks.

B. Remission induction. A number of combination drug programs are effective and superior to treatment with the most active single agent, cyclophosphamide, used alone. The two most common induction programs are as follows.

1. VAC

a. Vincristine 2 mg IV on day 1 *and*

b. Doxorubicin (Adriamycin) 50 mg/m^2 IV or day 1 *and*

c. Cyclophosphamide 750 mg/m^2 IV on day 1.

Repeat every 3 weeks for 4–6 cycles.

2. Cisplatin + etoposide (VP-16)
   a. Cisplatin 50–80 mg/m^2 IV on day 1 *and*
   b. Etoposide (VP-16) 60 mg/m^2 IV on days 1–5 or 100 mg/m^2 IV on days 1–3.
   Repeat every 3–4 weeks for 4–6 cycles.

Based on results of a prospective, randomized study that demonstrated a modest advantage for "alternating" VAC with cisplatin + VP-16 during the induction therapy of patients with extensive SCLC, this approach has become the most commonly used in North America, typically to a total of 3 cycles with each combination (6 in all). On the other hand, for patients with limited SCLC, cisplatin + VP-16 has become the most common induction regimen, usually with *concurrent* administration of chest irradiation. "Late intensification" with cisplatin + VP-16 was demonstrated to be of value after initial induction with VAC for limited disease. Because cisplatin + VP-16 has become the usual induction program for these patients, and because of some evidence for non-cross-resistance, it is now common to give "late intensification" with VAC for two cycles at 2–4 months after other therapy is completed. This practice was not, however, proved superior in a randomized trial.

C. **Radiation therapy and central nervous system prophylaxis.** After the maximal response to induction chemotherapy has been achieved (usually 8–12 weeks from the start of treatment), responding patients often have prophylactic whole-brain irradiation (WBI) to prevent isolated relapse at that site, which otherwise occurs in 20–40% of patients, regardless of whether chemotherapy that crosses the blood-brain barrier was employed. The usual dose has been 30 Gy in 2 weeks, but lower daily doses and more protracted fractionation are now being investigated to try to prevent late neurologic damage. Some centers no longer employ prophylactic WBI and have reported a lower incidence of isolated central nervous system (CNS) relapse than that cited. This issue remains to be settled.

The role of chest irradiation, on the other hand, has become less controversial. It now appears that radiation therapy to the primary tumor improves both local control and survival for limited-stage patients over chemotherapy alone, provided the modalities are used concurrently or in rapid alternation. The former practice of sequential chemotherapy induction, followed by radiation "consolidation" to the chest, did not prove better than chemotherapy alone and has been largely abandoned. There is some evidence that radiation to the chest provides better results if it is given in a "hyperfractionated" fashion (e.g., twice daily) at low individual doses but to a somewhat greater total dose. This approach is now being investigated in randomized trials. With extensive disease, there is no evidence that chest irradiation improves overall treatment results, as most patients relapse at multiple systemic sites.

Surgical resection has been investigated as an alternative to chest irradiation for limited disease. It is feasible in a number of responders to initial chemotherapy. However, the evidence indicates no advantage for the addition of surgical resection, except perhaps for the rare small-cell tumor with a clinical "coin lesion" on the chest x-ray film and no evidence of mediastinal involvement or other dissemination.

D. Treatment during remission. Maintenance chemotherapy is probably of no value at prolonging remission duration or survival. It appears that *reinduction* at 6 and 12 months into therapy with a single cycle of the initial induction regimen at full dose produces prolongation of response and survival, especially for patients who achieve a complete response. *Late intensification* with high-dose chemotherapy is a promising experimental approach whose ultimate value remains to be determined.

E. Complications

  1. Paraneoplastic syndromes. The most common paraneoplastic syndrome is the syndrome of inappropriate antidiuretic hormone (SIADH), which can be managed supportively with demeclocycline (300 mg tid) while induction therapy is administered. Less common paraneoplastic problems associated with small-cell carcinoma include pseudomyasthenia (Eaton-Lambert syndrome), hyperadrenocorticism due to ectopic ACTH, and galactorrhea or gynecomastia.

  2. Complications of treatment

    a. Myelotoxicity. The major risks of chemotherapy are infection related to leukopenia and bleeding due to thrombocytopenia. Nadir granulocyte and platelet counts are usually seen 10–14 days after chemotherapy has been given, and both patient and physician should be alert to the significance of an elevated temperature or, less commonly, hemorrhage during this nadir period. Any patients with a temperature of 38.2°C (101°F) or higher who is more than a few days postchemotherapy should be seen immediately in the office or the emergency room for a physical examination, chest x-ray film, complete blood count (including platelets and differential), and appropriate cultures. If the granulocyte count is less than $1000/\mu l$, the patient should be hospitalized and treated empirically with broad-spectrum antibiotics, even if no clinical site of infection is identified (see Chapter 32).

    b. Other chemotherapy-related complications

      (1) Alopecia due to cyclophosphamide and doxorubicin (Adriamycin).

      (2) Stomatitis due to methotrexate and occasionally doxorubicin.

      (3) Peripheral neuropathy and constipation due to vincristine or cisplatin. The constipation may be avoided by routine administration of psyllium hydrophilic mucilloid (Metamucil) or milk of magnesia at bedtime.

(4) Necrosis of skin with underlying slough of the soft tissue secondary to inadvertent extravasation of doxorubicin or vincristine. This disastrous complication can be avoided by meticulous care to ensure an adequate IV infusion, which should include use of a fresh site, avoidance of the dorsum of the hand or wrist veins if possible, and checking for a blood return, as well as flushing the IV line immediately after drug administration.

(5) Nausea and vomiting due to cyclophosphamide, doxorubicin, or cisplatin (especially likely to be severe with the latter, for which ondansetron or metoclopramide and dexamethasone are commonly used antiemetics).

(6) Nephrotoxicity due to cisplatin may be minimized by IV hydration and furosemide diuresis.

c. **Complications of radiation therapy**

(1) Complications of WBI include alopecia, redness and itching of the scalp, and external otitis, especially at doses of more than 30 Gy. Occasionally, patients complain of weakness or somnolence after WBI, but these symptoms are usually transient and minor. Disturbing late complications have been reported after WBI, including occasional seizures, orthostatic hypotension, and even accelerated dementia. It is not clear to what extent these problems are a function of the population being treated, but subtler cognitive defects after similar programs of cranial irradiation have been documented in children with acute lymphocytic leukemia receiving elective whole-brain "prophylaxis." It is likely that neurologic complications are more severe in patients who receive chemotherapy (especially nitrosoureas and methotrexate) concurrently or after the brain irradiation. Decisions about "prophylactic" WBI must therefore be made only after careful consideration and consultation between the medical and radiation oncologists.

(2) Complications of chest irradiation include symptomatic esophagitis (most patients), clinically significant pneumonitis (about 5–10%), and transverse myelitis. The latter complication should not occur if irradiation to a total dose of more than 45 Gy is avoided. If doxorubicin is given concomitantly with chest irradiation, esophagitis may be severe, even resulting in permanent esopha-

geal strictures, unless the doses of both drug and radiation are reduced.

F. Recurrence and treatment of refractory disease. No consistently useful chemotherapy regimen is available to treat recurrences. Occasional patients, especially if they are still fully ambulatory at the time of relapse, respond to doxorubicin, vincristine, cisplatin, mitomycin, or etoposide (VP-16) if these agents were not employed in their previous regimen. Radiation therapy is useful to palliate hemoptysis, painful bony lesions, and brain metastases, but it does not prolong survival. Median survival after relapse is only 6–12 weeks. Patients who have "chest only" recurrence may live somewhat longer.

III. Non-small cell carcinoma (NSCLC)

A. General considerations and aims of therapy. At the present time, surgery, alone or combined with subsequent radiation therapy, is the treatment of choice for resectable disease. For patients with limited inoperable disease, radiation therapy alone is the treatment of choice. The addition of chemotherapy to radiation therapy is of experimental interest but not part of routine clinical practice. Chemotherapy is used for treatment of patients with extensive disease. Its goals are to palliate symptoms (improve quality of life) and prolong survival. Extended disease-free survival (more than 2 years) with chemotherapy in this setting has been reported but remains anecdotal. At the present time, only fully ambulatory patients are appropriate candidates for chemotherapy.

B. Chemotherapy programs. No regimen of unequivocal, established benefit exists for treatment of extensive NSCLC. A Canadian study has demonstrated some benefit for the administration of CAP chemotherapy (cyclophosphamide + doxorubicin + cisplatin) or vindesine + cisplatin (VP) in patients with "advanced" NSCLC when compared to a program of supportive care alone. The following regimens were employed.

1. CAP
  a. Cyclophosphamide 400 mg/m^2 IV *and*
  b. Doxorubicin (Adriamycin) 40 mg/m^2 IV *and*
  c. Cisplatin 40 mg/m^2 IV (with prehydration and diuresis).
     Repeat every 4 weeks until progression. The cumulative dose of doxorubicin should not exceed 550 mg/m^2.

2. VP
  a. Vindesine 3 mg/m^2 IV weekly $\times$ 4, then every 2 weeks *and*
  b. Cisplatin 120 mg/m^2 IV (with prehydration and diuresis) on days 1 and 29, then every 6 weeks until progression.

The VP combination produced a median survival of 8 months compared to 6 months for CAP and 4 months for supportive care; approximately 20% of patients in the chemotherapy arms and 10% in the control group were alive at 1 year. Vindesine is not commercially available in the United States, so the related drug, vinblastine, is frequently substituted at doses of 4–6 mg/m²/week × 4, then every 2 weeks. In a randomized American trial, response rates and survival durations were comparable for the two vinca-containing programs.

Another popular program for extensive NSCLC, with response rates and survival results similar to the vinca-platinum combinations, is cisplatin + etoposide (VP-16), given in the same dose and schedule as outlined for SCLC (or with minor variations).

C. **Role of radiation therapy.** As the chance of a local response to radiation therapy is higher than the chance of a local response to systemically administered drugs in patients with non-small-cell carcinoma, radiation should be locally employed as a palliative modality. It usually is beneficial in the treatment of bony lesions and hemoptysis, but it is less often helpful for treating malignant effusions, atelectasis, or lobar collapse secondary to bronchial obstruction or brain metastasis. It should be employed in preference to decompressive laminectomy for most patients with extradural cord compression. Occasionally, anterior surgical decompression is indicated, but it requires an experienced orthopedic and neurosurgical team and should be undertaken, as a rule, only when the anticipated survival is more than 3 months.

D. **Combined modalities.** There is currently much interest in the use of cisplatin-based chemotherapy, with or without chest irradiation, as "neoadjuvant" treatment to render locally advanced NSCLC (stage III) resectable. It is clear that such treatment is feasible, and that a substantial proportion (50% in several series) of these lesions in fact become "resectable" by the usual surgical criteria. The morbidity and mortality rates there may be higher than those for patients who undergo surgery per primum for resectable disease. It is too early to assess the effect of this approach on long-term survival.

Similarly, chemotherapy and radiation therapy may be combined, concurrently or sequentially, to treat stage III patients. The results of such an approach vary from no better than with radiation alone to modest, statistically significant improvement. Randomized trials with combined-modality treatment versus irradiation are appropriate and ongoing, as are exploratory "pilot" studies. There is as yet no generally accepted, defined role of chemotherapy for stage III (limited) disease.

E. **Complications**
   1. **Paraneoplastic syndromes.** The most common of the paraneoplastic syndromes is hypercalcemia (almost never seen with small-cell carcinoma), especially if the tumor has squamous histology. This occurrence may be caused by bony metastases or ectopic parathyroid hormone-related protein, in which event it responds definitively only to measures di-

rected at the tumor. Alternatively, it may be caused by excessive prostaglandin production by the tumor. In the latter case, hypercalcemia may respond to indomethacin 50 mg tid or aspirin 600 mg qid. Intravenous hydration and oral phosphates should be administered in either case. (See Chapter 28 for a more complete discussion of hypercalcemia and its management.) Other paraneoplastic syndromes include hypertrophic osteoarthropathy and a variety of neurologic syndromes (but not Eaton-Lambert syndrome), which are likely to be alleviated only if the tumor is controlled.

   2. Treatment-related complications. Leukopenia and thrombocytopenia complications may occur, as outlined under small-cell carcinoma. Hemolytic anemia may be seen with cisplatin use, occasionally requiring blood transfusion. The vinca alkaloids and cisplatin produce constipation and peripheral neuropathy in varying degrees, with vincristine and vindesine being the worst offenders.

F. Recurrence and treatment of refractory disease. Chemotherapy of established efficacy is not available in this setting. Appropriate patients, preferably those who are fully ambulatory, may be candidates for trials of new agents in phase II studies.

Selected Reading

Einhorn, L. H., et al. Cisplatin plus etoposide consolidation following cyclophosphamide, doxorubicin and vincristine in limited small-cell lung cancer. *J. Clin. Oncol.* 6:451, 1988.

Evans, W. K., et al. Superiority of alternating non-cross-resistant chemotherapy in extensive small-cell lung cancer: the results of a multicentre randomized National Cancer Institute of Canada clinical trial. *Ann. Intern. Med.* 107:451, 1987.

Feld, R., et al. Combined modality induction therapy without maintenance chemotherapy for small cell carcinoma of the lung. *J. Clin. Oncol.* 2:294, 1984.

Kies, M. S., et al. Multimodal therapy for limited small-cell lung cancer: a randomized study of induction combination chemotherapy with or without thoracic radiation in complete responders; and with wide-field versus reduced-field radiation in partial responders: a Southwest Oncology Group study. *J. Clin. Oncol.* 5:592, 1987.

Kris, M. G., et al. Randomized trial comparing vindesine plus cisplatin with vinblastine plus cisplatin in patients with non-small cell lung cancer, with an analysis of methods of response assessment. *Cancer Treat. Rep.* 69:387, 1985.

Livingston, R. B. Treatment of advanced non-small cell lung cancer: the Southwest Oncology Group experience. *Semin. Oncol.* 6(suppl. 7):37, 1988.

Livingston, R. B., McCracken, J. D., and Crowley, J. Southwest Oncology Group trial of simultaneous chemotherapy and radiation therapy in limited small cell lung cancer. In R. J. Gralla and L. H. Einhorn (eds.), *Treatment and Prevention of*

Small Cell Lung Cancer and Non-Small Cell Lung Cancer. London: Royal Society of Medicine Services, 1989. Pp. 43–49.

Livingston, R. B., et al. Long-term survival and toxicity in small cell lung cancer: Southwest Oncology Group study. *Am. J. Med.* 77:415, 1984.

Rapp, E., et al. Chemotherapy can prolong survival in patients with advanced non-small cell lung cancer: report of a Canadian multicenter randomized trial. *J. Clin. Oncol.* 6:633, 1988.

Simes, R. J. Risk-benefit relationships in cancer clinical trials: the ECOG experience in non-small-cell lung cancer. *J. Clin. Oncol.* 3:462, 1985.

Turrisi, A. T. Brain irradiation and systemic chemotherapy for small-cell lung cancer: dangerous liaisons? *J. Clin. Oncol.* 8:196, 1990.

Carcinomas of the Gastrointestinal Tract

John C. Marsh

Cancers of the gastrointestinal (GI) tract (esophagus, stomach, small and large intestines) account for nearly 18 percent of all cancer in the United States and about 17 percent of cancer deaths. Colon cancer is by far the most common of these malignancies, with cancer of the rectum, stomach, esophagus, and small intestine occurring with decreasing frequency. Surgery continues to be the principal curative modality, but irradiation and chemotherapy have increasingly important roles and, in certain adjuvant situations, may improve the cure rate produced by surgery. Chemotherapy alone is not curative. Drugs produce objective remissions in only a 15–40 percent of patients. However, there is little question that meaningful palliation and an increase in survival can be achieved in patients who respond to chemotherapy. Controlled clinical trials, often by interinstitutional cooperative groups, have been useful in defining the natural history and therapeutic benefit of various treatment modalities. Participation in such clinical trials should be encouraged.

I. **Carcinoma of the esophagus**
   A. **General considerations and aims of therapy**
      1. **Epidemiology.** Cancer of the esophagus is predominantly of the epidermoid variety and accounts for slightly more than 1% of cancers. It is three times more common in men than women (it seems to be increasingly frequent in black men) and is often associated with excessive alcohol and tobacco use. The average patients are in their sixties. In certain parts of China it occurs with extraordinary frequency and is the most common cancer. The high incidence of cancer of the esophagus is thought to be related to dietary habits of the region, perhaps to fungal contamination of pickled vegetables. In the United States the etiology is unknown, although the epidemiology resembles that of squamous cell carcinomas of the oral cavity and upper airway. Patients with lye burns of the esophagus have an increased risk of developing esophageal cancer. A significant number of adenocarcinomas of the esophagus (up to 7% of cancers of that site) have been reported. Some of them may be gastric in origin, but most have developed in a columnar epithelium-lined lower esophagus (Barrett's esophagus). Reflux esophagitis has been implicated in the epithelial metaplasia of this condition. Chemotherapy for adenocarcinoma of the esophagus is usually the same as that for adenocarcinoma of the stomach, although trials of epidermoid cancer regimens are in progress.

   2. Clinical picture and evaluation. Carcinoma of the esophagus is usually associated with progressive and persistent dysphagia. Pain, hoarseness, weight loss, and chronic cough are unfavorable manifestations that indicate spread to regional structures (e.g., mediastinal nerves), recurrent laryngeal nerve, or fistula formation between the esophagus and the airway. The most common sites of distant metastases are the lungs and liver. Diagnosis is usually made by barium swallow, endoscopy, or lavage cytology. Careful evaluation of the lungs and liver by x-ray films and scans is needed for staging following a tissue diagnosis.

   3. Treatment and prognosis. About one-half of these tumors are operable, and one-half of the operable tumors are resectable. The overall 5-year survival is in the range of 5%, which means that most patients, if they are to benefit at all, require radiation therapy of local disease. Some surgeons believe that only lesions of the lower one-third of the esophagus are amenable to surgical resection and cure. Radiotherapy, surgery, and more recently chemotherapy are often combined. The prognosis is related to the size of the lesion and the depth of penetration of the esophageal wall. Patients are more likely to die of local disease or local recurrence than of distant metastases. The carcinoembryonic antigen (CEA) level is elevated in up to 70% of patients. The overall median survival is less than 1 year.

B. Treatment of advanced disease

   1. Standard drugs. Various single agents with modest activity are available, including cisplatin, mitomycin, fluorouracil, bleomycin, doxorubicin (Adriamycin), and methotrexate. Combination chemotherapy is probably more effective than single-agent therapy, although series from any one institution tend to be small. The following regimens are among the most active reported.

   a. Cisplatin + bleomycin + methotrexate
      (1) Cisplatin 50 mg/m^2 IV on day 4 *and*
      (2) Bleomycin 10 units IM weekly *and*
      (3) Methotrexate 40 mg/m^2 IV on days 1 and 14.
   Repeat every 21 days.

   b. Cisplatin + fluorouracil + doxorubicin
      (1) Cisplatin 75 mg/m^2 IV on day 1 *and*
      (2) Fluorouracil 600 mg/m^2 IV on days 1 and 8 *and*
      (3) Doxorubicin 30 mg/m^2 IV on day 1.
   Repeat every 28 days.

   2. Investigational drugs. Mitoguazone (methyl-GAG), on a weekly schedule, and vindesine are among the more active investigational agents. The latter is a component of an active regimen used extensively at the Memorial Sloan–Kettering Cancer Center.

C. Combined modality therapy for potentially curable patients. Because of the limited success of surgery alone, attempts have been made to combine surgery, radiotherapy, and chemotherapy in various ways. Radiotherapy alone preoperatively has added little survival benefit, and postoperative radiotherapy alone is little better. Chemotherapy added to irradiation as a preoperative regimen has been widely used with some success, but controlled data are sparse. The complete disappearance of tumor due to the preoperative regimen has been noted in 20–30% of patients, but overall survival is still low, although it appears to be better than with surgery alone. A cooperative group study suggests that preoperative chemotherapy and radiotherapy are better than preoperative radiotherapy in terms of survival, and it is possible that chemoradiotherapy without surgery may be as effective as when combined with surgery. Patients should be encouraged to enter clinical trials.

Probably the most widely used regimen is the following.

1. **Radiation therapy** 200 cGy/day 5 days/week for 15 doses *and*
2. **Cisplatin** 100 mg/m^2 IV on days 1 and 29 *and*
3. **Fluorouracil** 1000 mg/m^2 as continuous infusion on days 1–4 and 29–32.

If there is no evidence of disease progression, surgery is performed 4 weeks after chemotherapy. Postoperative radiation therapy (2000 cGy over 2 weeks) is considered if residual tumor is found in the operative specimen.

II. Gastric carcinoma
A. General considerations and aims of therapy

1. **Epidemiology.** The incidence of stomach cancer is decreasing dramatically in the United States, and it now ranks sixth as a cause of cancer death. No improvement has been seen, however, in the 5-year survival rates, which range from 5% to 15%. (The only curative modality at present is surgery.) The male–female ratio is 1.5:1.0. Stomach cancer is still the leading cause of cancer death among men in Japan and is also common in China, Finland, Poland, and Chile.

2. **Clinical picture and evaluation.** The most common symptoms are weight loss, abdominal pain, nausea, vomiting, changes in bowel habits, anorexia, and dysphagia. The diagnosis is generally made by barium swallow, endoscopy, and cytology, usually in combination. Metastases are to the liver, pancreas, omentum, esophagus, and bile ducts by direct extension and to regional and distant lymph nodes, such as those in the left supraclavicular area. Pulmonary and bone metastases are a late finding. Patients with suspected gastric cancer should undergo a careful evaluation of the liver with liver function tests and computed tomography (CT) scan.

3. **Treatment and prognosis.** Most stomach cancers are adenocarcinomas. Important prognostic factors include tumor grade and gross appearance. Diffusely infiltrating lesions are less likely to be cured than sharply circumscribed, nonulcerating ones. The pres-

ence of regional lymph node involvement or involvement of contiguous organs in the surgical specimen indicate an increased likelihood of recurrence, as does the presence of dysphagia at the time of diagnosis. Patients with proximal lesions or lesions requiring total, rather than distal subtotal, gastrectomy are also at greater risk.

B. Treatment of advanced disease

  1. Single agents with activity include fluorouracil, the nitrosoureas, doxorubicin (Adriamycin), mitomycin, cisplatin, and hydroxyurea.

  2. Combinations of these agents are more active than single drugs, and the use of combinations is associated with a higher response rate and longer duration of remission. Because the effectiveness of "standard" chemotherapy of gastrointestinal cancer is modest, better treatments, including new drugs, are greatly needed. Before treating patients with standard regimens, consideration should be given to entering the patients into clinical trials. Most new drugs being evaluated for these diseases are available only for patients previously untreated with chemotherapy. One appropriate strategy would be to use an investigational agent or regimen initially, followed by more conventional agents, such as those listed below.

  a. FAM. The FAM regimen (fluorouracil + doxorubicin + mitomycin) appears to be active (25–55% response). However, it is not clearly superior to other regimens, as a controlled study of gastric cancer patients using either fluorouracil alone, FAM, or fluorouracil + doxorubicin showed no difference in overall survival between any of the three patient groups, although response rates were higher with FAM.

  (1) Fluorouracil 600 mg/m^2 IV on days 1, 8, 29, and 36 *and*

  (2) Doxorubicin 30 mg/m^2 IV on days 1 and 29 *and*

  (3) Mitomycin 10 mg/m^2 IV on day 1.

  The cycle is repeated every 56 days.

  b. Other active regimens. A regimen with significant activity is the etoposide (VP-16) + doxorubicin + cisplatin (EAP) regimen. An overall response rate of 64% has been reported, with more responsiveness in patients with local–regional disease than with metastatic disease. This regimen was also used to treat locally advanced and nonresectable tumors, some of which were rendered resectable as a result.

  (1) Doxorubicin 20 mg/m^2 IV on days 1 and 7 *and*

  (2) Cisplatin 40 mg/m^2 IV on days 2 and 8 *and*

  (3) Etoposide 120 mg/m^2 IV on days 4, 5, and 6.

  Cycle is repeated every 3–4 weeks depending on blood counts.

A modification, allowing for weekends off, has been published in abstract form.

  (1) Doxorubicin 20 mg/m^2 IV on days 1 and 8 *and*
  (2) Cisplatin 40 mg/m^2 IV on days 2 and 8 *and*
  (3) Etoposide 100 mg/m^2 IV on days 1–3.

  Cycle is repeated every 4 weeks.

C. **Adjuvant therapy.** The Gastrointestinal Tumor Study Group (GITSG) has completed a study of adjuvant chemotherapy in patients following surgical resection suggesting that a combination of fluorouracil and semustine (methyl-CCNU) is associated with longer relapse-free survival than no chemotherapy.

  1. Fluorouracil 325 mg/m^2 IV on days 1–5 *and*
  2. Semustine 150 mg/m^2 orally on day 1 *and*
  3. Fluorouracil 375 mg/m^2 IV on days 36–40.

The cycle is repeated every 10 weeks for 2 years. Semustine is stopped after a total cumulative dose of 1000 mg/m^2. Because semustine is not commercially available, lomustine (CCNU) may be substituted at a dose of 100 mg/m^2 per cycle, with cessation after a total cumulative dose of 700 mg/m^2.

  Another study, however, has not shown benefit using the same program. Other adjuvant studies are also negative or incomplete. Chemotherapy is not yet standard following surgery. Postoperative patients should be considered for investigational trials to clarify these issues.

D. **Combined modality therapy.** A large number of patients have locally unresectable or incompletely resectable disease, and it has been known for some time that fluorouracil used in conjunction with radiotherapy adds to the survival of such patients compared with radiotherapy alone, so long as they have no evidence of metastatic disease and have disease that can be encompassed by a treatment port. The Eastern Cooperative Oncology Group (ECOG) reported that fluorouracil alone at a dose of 600 mg/m^2 IV weekly is as effective as fluorouracil combined with radiotherapy (4000 cGy) in this group of patients. Another GITSG program compared combination chemotherapy (fluorouracil + semustine) in such patients with and without radiotherapy. Short-term results were better with the combined-modality treatment, and it seems reasonable to use this treatment until more data are available.

  1. **Radiotherapy.** The local gastric lesion is treated with two courses of 2500 cGy each given over a 3-week period with a 2-week rest between courses.
  2. **Fluorouracil** 500 mg/m^2 is given IV for the first 3 days of each course of radiation.
  3. Ten weeks after completion of the radiotherapy, chemotherapy with **fluorouracil** + **semustine** (or lomustine) is begun on the schedule listed previously in **II.C.** for adjuvant chemotherapy and continued until relapse.

  A reasonable alternative would be to use radiation

therapy with fluorouracil alone at a dose of 500 mg/ m^2 IV the first and last 3 days of radiotherapy, followed by FAM (see **II.B.2.a.**) when hematologic and gastrointestinal toxicity has abated.

E. Complications. Hematologic and gastrointestinal toxicities from the chemotherapy may be accentuated by concurrent radiotherapy. If sufficiently severe, chemotherapy or radiotherapy, or both, should be withheld until improvement. Consideration is given to treating at reduced doses. In addition, the potential for leukemia arising in patients treated with the nitrosoureas (particularly semustine) must be considered.

F. Treatment of refractory disease. If the patient's disease recurs on the recommended regimens, it is reasonable to use as single agents any of the drugs noted in **II.B.** that have not been used previously. Thus for FAM relapsers, lomustine can be given in full doses, e.g., 130 mg/m^2 every 6–8 weeks. For relapsed patients on fluorouracil and semustine, the combination of mitomycin + doxorubicin (FAM without fluorouracil) is a rational choice.

III. Cancer of the small intestine
A. General considerations and aims of therapy

1. Carcinoid tumors. Carcinoid tumors are the most common tumors of the appendix and ileum. They may develop in other parts of the gastrointestinal tract but much less commonly. The usual histologic criteria of malignancy is not always applicable, and invasion and evidence of distant spread are more useful prognostic features.

In one series, the 60% of patients with intestinal carcinoids that were still confined to the wall of the gut had a 5-year survival of 85%, whereas those with tumors invading the serosa or beyond had a 5% survival at 5 years. Patients in the latter group were nearly always symptomatic, whereas patients in the former group were not. (Their tumors were discovered at surgery for appendicitis or other causes.) Tumors of the appendix are usually benign by these criteria, whereas those of the ileum are more often invasive. Surgical resection is the definitive therapy.

2. Carcinoid syndrome. About 10% of patients with carcinoid tumors are afflicted with the carcinoid syndrome, which includes diarrhea, abdominal cramps, malabsorption, and flushing. With tumors of intestinal origin, liver metastases are nearly always present. Serotonin is thought to be responsible for the abdominal symptoms, and its metabolite 5-hydroxyindoleacetic acid (5-HIAA) is excreted in large quantities in the urine and is a useful marker of disease activity. The symptoms may respond to simple antidiarrheal therapy. The flushing caused by the syndrome has been attributed to bradykinin, formed by the interaction of kallikrein (produced by the tumor) with a plasma protein. If simple symptomatic measures do not suffice, the best treatment is with the synthetic, long-acting somatostatin analog SMS-201-995, or octreotide acetate (Sandostatin). This agent, injected at a dose of 50–150 µg SQ q6–12h, effectively decreases the secretion of serotonin and other gastroenteropancreatic peptides such as insulin or gastrin. It has been helpful in ameliorating the symptoms of carcinoid tumors, e.g., flushing and diarrhea. There are even modest objective antitumor effects (14% response rate in one series).

3. **Adenocarcinomas** of the small intestine are so uncommon there is no large chemotherapy experience to report. The FAM regimen in **II.B.** is effective and a reasonable first choice.

B. **Treatment of advanced carcinoid tumors**

1. **Effective agents.** Doxorubicin (Adriamycin), fluorouracil, and streptozotocin have been shown to have some activity in this disease. Responses have also been seen with melphalan, cyclophosphamide, and methotrexate. A major advantage of using streptozotocin in combination is its lack of myelotoxicity. Response rates for combinations of fluorouracil + streptozotocin or streptozotocin + cyclophosphamide in treating carcinoids of various kinds are 25–35%, with the overall response rate for patients with tumors of intestinal origin 41%. Median durations of response of 7 months may be expected, and patients with a good performance status have the greatest likelihood of response. Tumor response correlates well with 5-HIAA excretion. One report indicated a high response rate (47%) with interferon-alpha, some of which patients were previously treated with chemotherapy.

2. **Recommended regimens**

   a. Streptozotocin 500 mg/m^2 IV on days 1–5 *and* Fluorouracil 400 mg/m^2 IV on days 1–5.
   Repeat the course every 6 weeks if the disease has responded or is stable.

   b. If the patient does not respond, doxorubicin 60 mg/m^2 IV every 3 weeks can be given with appropriate monitoring of cardiac function and leukocyte count.

   c. Interferon-alpha 3 million to 6 million units/day IM.

C. **Precautions.** Treatment of carcinoid tumors may precipitate or exacerbate the carcinoid syndrome during the first days of treatment, and the serotonin antagonists cyproheptadine and methysergide should be available.

IV. **Cancer of the large intestine**

A. **General considerations and aims of therapy.** Taken together, cancers of the colon and rectum are by far the most frequent malignancies of the gastrointestinal tract, and they account for the most deaths. Fewer than one-half of patients found to have large bowel cancers are cured by surgery, although this modality is still the only curative one available. There have been some advances in early diagnosis and in techniques of surgery, but nationwide mortality figures have not really changed appreciably. In some institutions the relative incidence of colon cancer is increasing, whereas the incidence of rectal cancer is decreasing. Local recurrence is much more common for rectal cancer (40–50%). About 50% of large bowel cancer recurrences are in the liver.

  1. **Staging.** The most commonly used staging system is that of Dukes or its modifications. This system classifies the tumor in terms of the extent to which it penetrates the bowel wall and involves regional lymph nodes. Dukes A lesions are confined to the mucosa and submucosa and are associated with a 5-year survival of more than 80%. B_1 lesions penetrate the muscularis but do not reach the serosa; patient survival is 60–80%. B_2 lesions penetrate to the serosa or through it into the pericolic fat; patient survivals range from 40% to 70%. Dukes C lesions indicate nodal involvement. If the serosa has not been penetrated (in one system of classification) it is called a C_1 lesion, with an associated 35–60% 5-year survival; the C_2 lesions are through the serosa, have positive nodes, and are associated with a 15–30% survival. Dukes D lesions have distant metastases at the time of initial staging, and there are virtually no 5-year survivors. This pathologic staging method is helpful for selecting patients who are at sufficiently high risk to justify adjuvant therapy, e.g., chemotherapy or irradiation.
  2. **Serum carcinoembryonic antigen (CEA)** level may parallel disease activity, although it is not increased in all patients with colon cancer. It is worth measuring preoperatively and, if elevated, postoperatively, as failure of an elevated value to return to normal may signify incomplete removal of the tumor. Likewise, a return to elevated values after an initial fall to normal often indicates recurrence. CEA values may also be an indicator of response during chemotherapy treatment, with a fall signifying improvement and a rise heralding regrowth of tumor.
B. **Treatment of advanced disease**
  1. **Effective agents and combinations.** For more than 30 years fluorouracil has been the standard agent in the treatment of advanced colorectal disease not amenable to surgical or radiotherapeutic control. Response rates have varied widely, but a generally agreed-on figure is 20%. Several institutions have reported rates of about 40% when fluorouracil was combined with semustine (methyl-CCNU) and, in some instances, vincristine and dacarbazine. However, when these combinations were tested by large cooperative groups, the reported improved response rates did not hold up and survival was not improved. Increased toxicity, particularly myelosuppression, was often observed.

   In recent years, several combinations of other

agents with fluorouracil have been reported to have improved response rates and, in some instances, improved survival. They include leucovorin, methotrexate, interferon-alpha, and cisplatin. The methotrexate–fluorouracil and leucovorin–fluorouracil combinations have been shown to be superior to fluorouracil alone in controlled trials. Although fluorouracil with a high-dose leucovorin regimen should be superior to a low-dose regimen on the basis of in vitro data, the current clinical data suggest that the low-dose regimen is superior in efficacy, toxicity, and expense; and it is similar in terms of survival. At present, the low-dose regimen is recommended. Moderate-dose methotrexate requiring leucovorin rescue combined with fluorouracil has produced excellent survival in our experience, but only when the fluorouracil and methotrexate are separated by a 24-hour interval (compared to 1 hour). A high response rate has been reported in a small group of patients with the fluorouracil–interferon combination. All responders in that study had previously been untreated with chemotherapy. The best of these regimens remains to be determined by controlled studies.

2. **Liver metastasis.** If the patient's disease is primarily in the liver, the response rate with IV fluorouracil alone is only about 10%. Intermittent hepatic artery infusion with fluorouracil, which is associated with a response rate of about 50%, should also be considered. Continuous infusion with floxuridine, either by continuous external infusion with permanent catheters or by an implanted or portable pump, has also been used, with response rates averaging 50%. The impact on survival is controversial.

3. **Recommended regimens**

   a. **Fluorouracil + leucovorin.** Leucovorin 20 mg/m^2, IV is followed in 1 hour by fluorouracil 425 mg/m^2 IV. The combination is given daily for 5 days. Courses are repeated at 4 and 8 weeks and at every 5 weeks thereafter.

   b. **Fluorouracil + leucovorin + methotrexate.** Methotrexate 200 mg/m^2 IV is given over 30 minutes after hydration with 1500 ml 5% dextrose in 0.5 N saline. At 24 hours fluorouracil 600 mg/m^2 IV bolus is given followed by leucovorin 10 mg/m^2 to the nearest 5 mg PO q6h × 6. Repeat every 2 weeks.

   c. **Fluorouracil + interferon.** Fluorouracil 750 mg/m^2 by continuous IV infusion is given daily for 5 days followed by 1 week at rest, then weekly IV bolus of 750 mg/m^2. Interferon-alpha 9 million units SQ 3 times weekly is given beginning on day 1; it is subsequently given on the day of the fluorouracil bolus. Acetaminophen 650 mg PO is given 30 minutes before the interferon and q4h × 3.

d. Hepatic artery infusion. The catheter must be carefully positioned by an experienced angiographer through the axillary or femoral artery. A continuous IV heparin infusion of 5000 units/day is given with fluorouracil 800 mg/m^2/day for 4 days, then 600 mg/m^2 for a maximum of 17 days as tolerated. Weekly doses of 600 mg/m^2 IV can then be given to maintain whatever response has occurred, or the hepatic artery infusion can be repeated in the hospital in 4–6 months if the IV therapy does not prevent relapse. The position of the catheter must be checked twice weekly.

For the implanted pump, the dose of floxuridine is 0.1–0.15 mg/kg/day in heparinized saline given for 2 weeks, alternating with 2 weeks of heparinized saline without floxuridine. Heparin is used in a dose of 200 units/ml. Most patients can tolerate a daily floxuridine dose of 0.1 mg/kg for repeated cycles of 14 days every 4 weeks.

C. Combined modality treatment

1. Colon cancer. For many years surgical adjuvant studies with chemotherapy have shown either marginal benefit or no benefit, and such therapy could not be recommended routinely. The combination of fluorouracil and levamisole has been shown to significantly improve the disease-free as well as the overall survival of patients with node-positive (Dukes C) resectable colon cancer, but not yet those with stage B$_2$ disease. Although other chemotherapy regimens have continued to be reported and appear to be of slight benefit, this combination serves as a current standard of comparison. A current clinical trial compares fluorouracil + levamisole to fluorouracil with either high- or low-dose leucovorin (which regimens seem to be more active in advanced disease) or to a regimen with fluorouracil + levamisole + low-dose leucovorin. There are no controlled clinical trials yet available that demonstrate the efficacy of postoperative radiotherapy in colon cancer. The *recommended regimen* is as follows.

Fluorouracil 450 mg/m^2 IV bolus daily × 5. At 28 days, begin 450 mg/m^2 IV weekly × 48 weeks *and* Levamisole 50 mg PO q8h × 3 days every 2 weeks starting day 1 for 1 year.

2. Rectal cancer

a. Preoperative irradiation. Several studies have shown that preoperative irradiation benefits patients with rectal cancer, although there are disadvantages in terms of accuracy of staging, delay before surgery, incomplete knowledge of the extent of tumor for treatment planning, and inappropriate administration of radiation to patients with early (Dukes A or B$_1$) or advanced (Dukes D) lesions. Accordingly, major attention has been given to trials of postoperative irradiation with and without chemotherapy.

b. Postoperative irradiation, with and without chemotherapy. A GITSG trial of Dukes B_2 and C rectal cancer has shown that treatment with combined chemotherapy and radiotherapy is significantly better than no treatment after surgical resection in terms of recurrence or survival. Use of either modality alone was inferior to the combined-modality regimen. The chemotherapy used was a combination of semustine (methyl-CCNU) + fluorouracil for 18 months. The same group has observed similar results with a shorter fluorouracil regimen for 6 months, thereby avoiding the use of a drug that is not routinely available and that is associated with a small but significant risk of leukemia. The following regimen is therefore recommended.

  (1) Radiotherapy 4320 cGy in 5 weeks *with* fluorouracil 500 mg/m^2 IV bolus on days 1, 2, and 3 and the last 3 days of radiotherapy *and*

  (2) Fluorouracil 350 mg/m^2/day × 5 days, beginning week 11. Repeat every 4 weeks, escalating the dose by 50 mg/m^2 as tolerated to a maximum of 500 mg/m^2 for a total of 6 courses.

D. Complications of therapy or disease. The complications of chemotherapy are those attributable to the individual drugs. Myelosuppression, nausea, vomiting, and diarrhea are common and require dose modification.

E. Treatment of refractory disease. No satisfactory treatment exists for the patient who fails treatment with fluorouracil. Some patients with liver disease failing IV therapy may respond to fluorouracil or floxuridine given as a hepatic artery infusion. The combination cyclophosphamide + methotrexate + vincristine has produced some responses, but response rates are of the order of 10% and are usually brief. The regimen is as follows.

Cyclophosphamide 300 mg/m^2 IV weekly *and*
Vincristine 1.4 mg/m^2 IV weekly (maximum dose 2.0) *and*
Methotrexate 25 mg/m^2 IV weekly.

V. Cancer of the anal canal These cancers, comprising only 1–3% of large bowel cancers, were historically treated by abdominoperineal resection with an approximately 50% cure rate. They have been seen more commonly in women but, in recent years, have shown an increase in men, particularly homosexuals. The human papilloma virus has been implicated in such patients, and anal warts are sometimes seen as well. Human immunodeficiency virus (HIV)-infected patients also have an increased incidence of anal cancer. It has been found that combined-modality treatment with chemotherapy and irradiation is curative in 75–

80% of patients and thus allows avoidance of abdominoperineal resection with retention of anal function. The following regimen is recommended.

Radiotherapy 4500 cGy in 25 fractions (5 weeks) *and*
Fluorouracil 1000 mg/m² by continuous IV infusion daily ×
    4 days (days 1–4 and 28–31) *and*
Mitomycin C 10 mg/m² IV on days 1 and 28.

Biopsy again 4 weeks after radiation therapy. If negative, no further treatment is needed; if positive, consider an additional 900 cGy (5 fractions) and 4-day course of fluorouracil and cisplatin 100 mg/m² IV on day 2. If biopsy is persistently positive, perform abdominoperineal resection.

D. Metastatic disease
    1. Mitomycin 10 mg/m² IV every 4 weeks × 2, then every 10 weeks *and*
    2. Doxorubicin 30 mg/m² IV every 4 weeks × 2, then every 5 weeks *and*
    3. Cisplatin 60 mg/m² IV, every 4 weeks × 2, then every 5 weeks.

Selected Reading

Cullinan, S. A., et al. A comparison of chemotherapeutic regimens in the treatment of advanced pancreatic and gastric carcinoma. *J.A.M.A.* 253:2061, 1985.

Flam, M. S., et al. Definitive combined modality therapy of carcinoma of the anus: a report of 30 cases including results of salvage therapy in patients with residual disease. *Dis. Colon Rectum* 30:495, 1987.

Gastrointestinal Tumor Study Group: A comparison of combination chemotherapy and combined modality therapy for locally advanced gastric carcinoma. *Cancer* 49:1771, 1982.

Gastrointestinal Tumor Study Group (Holyoke, E. D., et al.). Adjuvant chemotherapy and radiotherapy following rectal surgery. *N. Engl. J. Med.* 312:1465, 1985.

Gisselbrecht, C., et al. Fluorouracil, adriamycin and cisplatin combination chemotherapy of advanced esophageal carcinoma. *Cancer* 52:974, 1983.

Klassen, D. J., et al. Treatment of locally unresectable cancer of the stomach and pancreas: a randomized comparison of 5-fluorouracil alone with radiation plus concurrent and maintenance 5-fluorouracil—an Eastern Cooperative Oncology Group study. *J. Clin. Oncol.* 3:373, 1985.

Kvols, L. K., et al. Treatment of the malignant carcinoid syndrome: evaluation of a long-acting somatostatin analogue. *N. Engl. J. Med.* 315:663, 1986.

Leichman, L. Cancer of the esophagus. *Invest. New Drugs* 7:91, 1989.

Leichman, L., et al. Cancer of the anal canal: model for preoperative adjuvant combined modality therapy. *Am. J. Med.* 78:211, 1985.

Marsh, J. C., et al. The influence of drug interval on the effect of methotrexate and fluorouracil in the treatment of metastatic colorectal cancer. *J. Clin. Oncol.* (in press).

Mayer, R. J., et al. Status of adjuvant therapy for colorectal cancer. *J. Natl. Cancer Inst.* 81:1359, 1989.

Moertel, C. G., and Hanley, J. A. Combination chemotherapy trials for metastatic carcinoid tumor and the malignant carcinoid syndrome. *Cancer Clin. Trials* 2:327, 1979.

Moertel, C. G., et al. Levamisole and fluorouracil for adjuvant therapy of resected colon carcinoma. *N. Engl. J. Med.* 322:352, 1990.

Oberg, K., et al. Treatment of malignant carcinoid tumors with human leukocyte interferon: long-term results. *Cancer Treat. Rep.* 70:1297, 1986.

O'Connell, M. J. Current status of chemotherapy for advanced pancreatic and gastric cancer. *J. Clin. Oncol.* 3:1032, 1985.

Poon, M. A., et al. Biochemical modulation of fluorouracil: evidence of significant improvement of survival and quality of life in patients with advanced colorectal carcinoma. *J. Clin. Oncol.* 7:1407, 1989.

Preusser, P., et al. Phase II study with the combination etoposide, doxorubicin, and cisplatin in advanced measurable gastric cancer. *J. Clin. Oncol.* 7:1310, 1989.

Reed, M. I., et al. The practicality of chronic hepatic artery infusion therapy of primary and metastatic hepatic malignancies: ten-year results of 124 patients in a prospective protocol. *Cancer* 47:402, 1981.

Shepard, K., et al. Therapy for metastatic colorectal cancer with hepatic artery infusion chemotherapy using a subcutaneous implanted pump. *J. Clin. Oncol.* 3:161, 1985.

Vogl, S. E., et al. Effective chemotherapy for esophageal cancer with methotrexate, bleomycin, and cis-diamminedichloroplatinum II. *Cancer* 48:2555, 1981.

Wadler, S., et al. Fluorouracil and recombinant alpha-2a-interferon: an active regimen against advanced colorectal carcinoma. *J. Clin. Oncol.* 7:1769, 1989.

Wilke, H., et al. Preoperative chemotherapy in locally advanced and nonresectable gastric cancer: a phase II study with etoposide, doxorubicin, and cisplatin. *J. Clin. Oncol.* 7:1318, 1989.

Carcinomas of the Pancreas, Liver, Gallbladder, and Bile Ducts

David J. Schifeling

Carcinomas of the pancreas, liver, and biliary passages account for approximately 4 percent of all cancers and 7 percent of all cancer-related deaths in the United States. Virtually all patients with these cancers die. However, recent advances in diagnostic techniques offer hope for early diagnosis and improved survival.

I. **Adenocarcinoma of the pancreas**

   A. **Epidemiology and etiology.** Pancreatic cancer has occurred with increasing incidence over the last several decades and currently is the fourth leading cause of cancer-related death. Risk factors for pancreatic cancer include age, male sex, race (Polynesians, Blacks), and tobacco exposure. It is rare before age 30, and the incidence rises throughout life, with peak occurrence during the seventh decade. Smokers have 1.6–3.9 times the risk of developing pancreatic cancer compared to nonsmokers. Pancreatitis is commonly associated with carcinoma of the pancreas in pathologic specimens. Whether patients with chronic pancreatitis are at greater risk for developing pancreatic cancer is uncertain. Patients with familial pancreatitis appear to have a greater risk. Diabetes mellitus is often discovered just prior to the diagnosis of pancreatic cancer, but patients with diabetes mellitus do not have a greater risk of pancreatic cancer.

   B. **Presenting signs and symptoms.** Pain is the most common presenting symptom. It occurs in three-fourths of patients with carcinoma of the head of the pancreas and virtually all patients with carcinoma of the body or tail. Usually the pain is a dull ache in the epigastrium that radiates to the right upper quadrant when the tumor is in the head of the pancreas or to the left upper quadrant when the tumor is in the body or tail. It may be an atypical sharp or intermittent epigastric pain, or it may be located in the lumbar region of the back. As many as one-fifth of patients present with nonspecific symptoms including weight loss, anorexia, nausea, vomiting, and constipation. Seventy percent of patients with carcinoma of the head of the pancreas have jaundice, whereas fewer than 15% of patients with carcinoma of the pancreatic body have jaundice. Physical findings are generally associated with advanced carcinomas and include weight loss, hepatomegaly, and abdominal mass.

   C. **Diagnostic evaluation.** Ultrasonography and computed tomography (CT) demonstrate masses in the pancreas or dilatation of the pancreatic duct or the common bile duct. Sensitivity and specificity of CT are approximately 90%. Sensitivity and specificity of ultrasonography are somewhat less. Both tests are limited to detecting relatively large mass lesions of the pancreas and usually miss 1- to 2-cm carcinomas. Endoscopic retrograde cholangiopancreatography (ERCP) demonstrates subtle ductal abnormalities; sensitivity and specificity are in excess of 90%. Endoscopy-directed biopsies of pancreatic ducts have diagnosed tumors less than 1–2 cm in diameter. Percutaneous transhepatic cholangiography may be performed if ERCP is unsuccessful and yields similar information. Percutaneous fine needle aspiration of suspicious abnormalities identified on CT scan can confirm the diagnosis of pancreatic cancer, with 80–90% sensitivity and 100% specificity. The role of magnetic resonance imaging in carcinoma of the pancreas has not been defined, although, it appears to have the same limitations as ultrasonography and CT.

D. Laboratory tests. CA 19-9 is a cell surface glycoprotein associated with pancreatic cancer. Elevated serum levels raise the index of suspicion of pancreatic cancer in patients with a suggestive history. Rising serum levels are a useful early indicator of recurrent disease.

E. Primary therapy

   1. Surgery. Three-fourths of patients with pancreatic cancer are operative candidates, but only 15–20% have resectable tumors. Of the patients whose tumors are resected for cure, 5–10% survive 5 years. Obstructive jaundice and gastric outlet obstruction may be palliated by bypass procedures.

   2. Radiation therapy. External beam radiation therapy has been used to palliate unresectable carcinomas. Newer techniques include ^{125}I implantation and intraoperative irradiation of advanced, unresectable carcinomas. Irradiation may also be used as an adjuvant to surgical resection.

   3. Combined-modality therapy

   a. Resectable carcinomas. On the basis of a randomized study by the Gastrointestinal Study Group (GITSG), postoperative combined-modality therapy is recommended for patients with resected carcinoma of the pancreas. Radiation (40 Gy) is applied to the pancreatic bed, in split courses of 20 Gy, in combination with fluorouracil 500 mg/m^2 given as an IV bolus on days 1–3, 29–31, and 71 and then weekly thereafter for 2 years. Two-year and 5-year survivals of 43% and 25%, respectively, may be anticipated with combined-modality therapy, compared with 18% and 5% with irradiation alone.

   b. Localized unresectable carcinoma. Patients with localized but unresectable pancreatic carcinoma may be treated with 40 Gy, in split courses of 20 Gy, in combination with fluorouracil 500 mg/m^2 given as an IV bolus on days 1–3 every 4 weeks during radiation therapy, then 500 mg/m^2 once weekly for 2 years. On the basis of a GITSG study, median survivals of 10 months may be anticipated for patients treated with this regimen, compared with 5 months for those who receive radiotherapy alone. Studies of chemotherapy alone versus combined-modality therapy demonstrate a survival advantage to combined-modality therapy. Quality of life studies have not been reported.

F. **Chemotherapy of advanced disease.** Patients with pancreatic cancer are often poor candidates for chemotherapy because of severe weight loss, poor performance status, severe pain, lack of measurable or evaluable disease, and the presence of jaundice or hepatic involvement, which may interfere with clearance of therapeutic agents.

   1. **Single agents.** A number of single agents have demonstrated activity (Table 12-1). Most active are fluorouracil and mitomycin, with 20–30% response rates. Many other agents have been evaluated with disappointing activity. Ifosfamide has a response rate of 10–25% in various studies.

   2. **Combination chemotherapy.** Combination chemotherapy has been intensively investigated. The most commonly used regimens have been fluorouracil + doxorubicin + mitomycin (FAM) and streptozocin + mitomycin + fluorouracil (SMF) with response rates reported between 13% and 43%. A variety of other combination regimens have been investigated, but none has shown advantage over fluorouracil alone.

   3. **Current recommendations.** Single-agent therapy with fluorouracil 500 mg/m^2 IV on days 1–5 every 4 weeks or 500–600 mg/m^2 IV weekly or mitomycin 20 mg/m^2 IV on day 1 every 4–6 weeks is recommended for patients with disseminated pancreatic cancer and a good performance status who are not eligible for clinical trials. Because of limited effectiveness of current therapy, participation in clinical trials should be encouraged, particularly with phase II trials of new agents or combinations.

II. **Malignant islet cell carcinomas**

A. **Epidemiology and natural history.** Islet cell neoplasms occur in approximately 1 in 100,000 persons per year. Eighty percent of these tumors secrete one or more hormones excessively: most commonly insulin or gastrin; less commonly glucagon, serotonin, or adrenocorticotropic hormone (ACTH); and rarely vasoactive intestinal peptides (VIP), growth hormone-releasing hormone (GHRH), and somatostatin. Twenty percent are nonfunctional. Islet cell tumors may occur with the multiple endocrine neoplasia (MEN-I) syndrome. In families with this autosomal dominant syndrome, 80% of affected members develop islet cell tumors, most commonly gastrinoma (54%), insulinoma (21%), glucagonoma (3%), or VIPoma (1%). Other endocrine manifestations of MEN-I include parathyroid hyperplasia, pituitary adenomas (often a prolactinoma), and occasionally adrenal or thyroid adenomas. Approximately one-fourth of gastrino-

Table 12-1. Single-agent chemotherapy in pancreatic cancer

Drug	No. of patients	Response rate ± 95% confidence interval (%)
Fluorouracil	251	25 ± 3
Mitomycin	53	21 ± 6
Streptozocin	27	11 ± 6
Semustine (methyl-CCNU)	91	4 ± 2
Doxorubicin	28	7 ± 5
Ifosfamide	113	22

mas are associated with MEN type I. Eighty to ninety percent of gastrinomas occur in the head of the pancreas. Insulinomas are common equally in the head, body, and tail. Gastrinomas tend to be multiple small tumors, whereas insulinomas tend to be single tumors and glucagonomas and VIPomas single large tumors. The median age of patients is in the sixth decade. There are no sex or race associations.

Islet cell tumors generally present with symptoms caused by hormone hypersecretion, most commonly fasting hypoglycemia, or the Zollinger-Ellison syndrome followed by others. VIPomas are associated with episodic severe secretory diarrhea with hypokalemia, hypochlorhydria, and metabolic acidosis. Classically, glucagonomas are associated with necrolytic migratory erythema, mild diabetes, severe muscle wasting, and marked hyperaminoaciduria.

Sixty percent of gastrinomas are malignant. Histologic appearance and tumor size do not predict malignancy; only the presence of metastatic disease confirms malignancy. Ninety percent of malignant gastrinomas have liver metastases. Other sites of spread include abdominal nodes, peritoneum, bone, and lung. Median survival from time of diagnosis of metastatic disease is approximately 2.5 years. Only 10% of insulinomas are malignant. They are usually larger than 2.5 cm, whereas benign insulinomas are generally smaller than 2.5 cm. Most glucagonomas and VIPomas are malignant (60–80%).

B. Treatment of advanced disease

    1. Endocrine syndromes. The first goal of treatment must be to control endocrine syndromes.

        a. Gastric acid suppression. H_2 receptor antagonists with or without H_1 antagonists are successful for most patients with gastrinoma. The optimal dose must be individualized and periodically reevaluated. Gastric acid secretion should be monitored during the hour preceding the doses of H_2 antagonists and should be limited to 10 mEq. The median doses of cimetidine and ranitidine that achieve suppression of acid production are 3.6 and 1.2 gm daily, respectively.

b. Insulin suppression. Diazoxide 3–8 mg/kg/day PO divided in 3 doses (e.g., 50–150 mg PO tid) is the therapy of choice for hypoglycemia associated with insulinoma when dietary measures fail. A diuretic should be given with diazoxide to prevent water retention.

c. Octreotide acetate. A somatostatin analog (SMS-201-995 Sandostatin) that inhibits gut hormone secretion has been released for use by the Food and Drug Administration. It is clearly useful for treating carcinoid and VIPoma syndromes and possibly useful for controlling symptoms in patients with glucagonomas, GHRH tumors, and gastrinomas. It may exacerbate symptoms of insulinomas. Measurable shrinkage of the tumor by octreotide has been reported in 10–15% of patients with islet cell tumor. Moreover, the median survival may be prolonged, particularly in patients with malignant carcinoid. The usual starting dose of octreotide is 50 μg SQ bid; thereafter the dose and frequency of injections can be increased to 100 μg tid.

2. Chemotherapy of advanced islet cell tumors. Streptozocin is the most active single agent with a 50% response rate. It is a nonmyelosuppressive nitrosourea with diabetogenic effects in animals.

a. Streptozocin 500 mg/m² IV on days 1–5 + fluorouracil 400 mg/m² IV on days 1–5 have produced the highest response rates.

b. Streptozocin 500 mg/m² IV on days 1–5 + doxorubicin 50 mg/m² IV on days 1 and 22, repeated every 6 weeks, is also effective.

Renal impairment occurs in approximately 30% of patients receiving a streptozocin-based regimen; approximately one-third of those with renal insufficiency have creatinine levels higher than 2 mg/dl. Nausea and vomiting occur in approximately 60% of patients. Leukopenia occurs in approximately 75%, but only 10% have a white blood cell count of less than a 1000/μl. Stomatitis is uncommon. Liver function test abnormalities may also occur. Deaths caused by treatment are rare.

c. Interferon may diminish excess hormone secretion and induce shrinkage of tumors, and some trials have reported 50% response rates.

III. Ampullary carcinomas. In up to 80% of people, the common bile duct and main pancreatic duct empty into a common channel, the ampulla of Vater. Periampullary carcinomas can be classified according to their site of origin. Type I tumors originate in the ampulla of Vater or the duodenal portion of the common bile duct. Type II carcinomas are duodenal tumors involving the ampulla of Vater. Type III are mixed ampullary-periampullary carcinomas, and type

IV are pancreatic head carcinomas involving the ampulla. Type IV tumors carry a much worse prognosis and should be distinguished from the ampullary or periampullary carcinomas. Type I–III periampullary and ampullary carcinomas generally can be extirpated surgically. Large tumors require a Whipple resection, whereas local excision may be curative of small tumors. The overall 5-year survival is 40–50% for types I–III. The roles of irradiation and chemotherapy are uncertain. Advanced disease should be treated as adenocarcinoma of the pancreas.

IV. Carcinoma of bile ducts (cholangiocarcinoma)

    A. Epidemiology and natural history. Incidence of primary biliary tree carcinoma is approximately 2 per 100,000. Men are affected more commonly than women. Tumors occur most often in late-middle-aged or elderly patients. They are associated with cholelithiasis as well as ulcerative colitis, obesity, and liver flukes. Patients present with obstructive jaundice, except for the occasional patient with a carcinoma identified at laparotomy for cholelithiasis. Approximately one-half of bile duct tumors are located proximally. Ten percent have multicentric involvement of the bile ducts. Local invasion is common. Liver involvement occurs in nearly one-half of these patients. Surgical cure is uncommon. Bypass procedures or intubation of the biliary tree may offer palliation to patients whose tumors cannot be resected. Radiation therapy may relieve proximal obstruction without intubation or a bypass procedure.

    B. Chemotherapy of advanced disease. Few reports are available for this unusual tumor, but its response rate to fluorouracil, alone or in combination with streptozocin, is about 10%. Outside the context of a clinical trial one of the following is recommended.

        1. Fluorouracil 500 mg/m^2 IV push on days 1–5 every 4 weeks *or* 500 mg/m^2 IV weekly *or*

        2. Fluorouracil 400 mg/m^2 IV on days 1–5 *and* streptozocin 500 mg/m^2 IV on days 1–5. Repeat every 6 weeks.

V. Gallbladder carcinoma

    A. Epidemiology and natural history. Carcinomas of the gallbladder are seen predominantly in late-middle-aged or elderly women, with the highest incidence in American Indians and the population of central and eastern Europe and Israel. These areas of high frequency also report a high incidence of cholelithiasis. Patients with "porcelain" or calcified gallbladders on x-ray film have a 12–62% risk of cancer. Carcinoma of the gallbladder most commonly presents with pain, nausea and vomiting, and weight loss. Jaundice occurs in only one-third of patients. Anorexia, abdominal distension, pruritus, and melena occur in some patients. One percent of patients undergoing cholecystectomy are found to have carcinoma of the gallbladder. Overall survival is poor, as fewer than 5% of patients with resections survive 5 years. However, if the tumor is histologically confined to the mucosa or submucosa, survival rates of 64% at 5 years and 44% at 10 years have been reported. These carcinomas may invade locally into the bile ducts, liver, pancreas, stomach, or duodenum, or they may spread to regional lymph nodes and distantly to liver.

B. Chemotherapy of advanced disease. Few reports are available for review. Seven of 40 patients (18%) responded to 5-fluorouracil (5-FU). Seven of 25 patients (28%) responded to mitomycin. Four of 14 patients (31%) treated with 5-FU + doxorubicin (Adriamycin) + mitomycin responded. Choices of therapy are as follows.

1. Fluorouracil, 500 mg/m^2 IV on days 1–5 every 4 weeks *or* 500–600 mg/m^2 IV weekly *or*

2. FAM, a three-drug combination of Fluorouracil 600 mg/m^2 IV on days 1, 8, 29, 36 *and* Doxorubicin 30 mg/m^2 IV on days 1 and 29 *and* Mitomycin 10 mg/m^2 IV on day 1. Repeat every 8 weeks.

Although there may be a slightly improved response rate with FAM, the toxicity is significant and no survival or quality of life benefit has been demonstrated.

VI. Primary carcinoma of the liver

A. Epidemiology. Primary carcinoma of the liver is rare in the United States with fewer than 10,000 new patients annually, accounting for fewer than 2% of all malignancies. However, it is the leading cause of cancer death in parts of Africa and Asia. Ninety percent of primary carcinomas of the liver are hepatocellular carcinomas or hepatoma; the remaining carcinomas include cholangiocarcinomas (about 7%), hepatoblastomas, angiosarcomas, and other sarcomas. Histologic subsets of hepatocellular carcinoma have been recognized. Fibrolamellar carcinomas occur in young patients and are more likely to be resectable and cured. Hepatocellular carcinomas are more common in men than women. The peak occurrence is during the sixth decade, with the highest incidence during the ninth decade.

There appear to be three major factors associated with hepatocellular carcinoma: (1) hepatitis B; (2) alcohol abuse; and (3) aflatoxin exposure. Seventy-five percent of patients with hepatocellular carcinoma have concomitant cirrhosis, and 4–20% of patients with cirrhosis have hepatocellular carcinoma at autopsy depending on the population studied. Among the patients with hepatocellular carcinoma, 15–80% have hepatitis B surface antigenemia. In China the incidence of hepatocellular carcinoma parallels the incidence of hepatitis B infection. The introduction of an effective hepatitis B vaccine may reduce the risk of hepatocellular carcinoma in these areas. In Africa the increased risk appears to be related to exposure to aflatoxin, which is produced by the fungi *Aspergillus flavus* and *Aspegillus parasiticus* during improper food storage. Anabolic steroids also have been associated with hepatocellular carcinoma. These tumors may retain hormone dependence and regress after withdrawal of the steroid.

B. **Presentation.** Patients with primary carcinoma of the liver commonly complain of right upper quadrant pain, abdominal distension, or weight loss. The pain is usually dull or aching but may be acute and radiate to the right shoulder. Fatigue, loss of appetite, and unexplained fever may occur. Patients with underlying cirrhosis may present with hepatic decompensation: new ascites, variceal bleeding, jaundice, or encephalopathy. Rarely, patients present with paraneoplastic syndromes: Erythrocytosis is most common; and hypercalcemia, hyperthyroidism, and carcinoid syndrome have been described. Physical findings include nodular hepatomegaly with an arterial bruit and hepatic rub. Extrahepatic spread occurs in approximately 50% of patients during the course of the illness. Twenty percent of patients have lung metastases.

C. **Diagnostic evaluation.** An elevated α-fetoprotein in more than 70% of patients is associated with a poor prognosis and may be used to screen high-risk patients. Carcinoembryonic antigen (CEA) is elevated in more than 70% of patients. Ultrasonography and CT have a high sensitivity when lesions are larger than 2 cm. However, small lesions are frequently missed by both procedures. The role of magnetic resonance imaging is uncertain at this time. Fine needle aspiration usually confirms the diagnosis.

D. **Primary therapy.** At presentation 25% of patients with hepatocellular carcinoma have potentially resectable lesions. At laparotomy, only 10–12% are resected. Operative mortality is 10–30%. Cirrhosis and advanced lesions are the factors limiting resection. Long-term survival is achieved in 15–30% of patients whose tumors were resected. Recurrences appear in liver, regional lymph nodes, lungs, and bone.

E. **Therapy of advanced hepatocellular carcinoma**

1. **Single agents.** Numerous single agents have been tested in primary hepatocellular carcinoma: Alkylating agents, antimetabolites, plant alkaloids, and cisplatin have been ineffective. Doxorubicin 60 mg/m^2 IV every 21 days in recommended. This regimen results in a partial response rate of about 16%.

2. **Combination chemotherapy and other modes of treatment.** Combination chemotherapy has not had better success than single agents. Hepatic artery infusion has been studied, but there is no evidence that it significantly improves response compared to systemic administration. To date, there have been no responses to α-, β-, or γ-interferon. Irradiation has had a limited role in treating liver tumors because of hepatic intolerance to radiation. One study of radiation therapy (21 Gy in 7 fractions) plus chemotherapy (fluorouracil by hepatic artery infusion + doxorubicin IV + mitomycin IV) improved response rates (8 of 22) when compared to radiotherapy alone (2 of 11), but this regimen cannot

be recommended except in an investigational setting. Radioactive polyclonal antibodies to ferritin
have received substantial attention. Antiferritin antibodies used in combination with chemotherapy and
external beam radiation therapy have permitted resection of a few previously unresectable tumors. Current clinical trials are using yttrium 90-labeled and
antiferritin antibody. It is recommended that all patients with hepatocarcinoma be offered the opportunity to participate in a clinical trial. If none is available at their own hospital, referral to a center that is
studying this refractory cancer should be considered.

Selected Reading

Andrews, W. B., and Smith, F. P. Chemotherapy for cholangiocarcinoma and gallbladder cancer. *Sci. Pract. Surg.* 8:453,
1987.

Gastrointestinal Tumor Study Group. Further evidence of effective adjuvant combined radiation and chemotherapy following curative resection of pancreatic cancer. *Cancer* 59:
2006, 1987.

Gorden, P., et al. Somastatin and somatostatin analogue (SMS
201-995) in treatment of hormone-secreting tumors of the pituitary and gastrointestinal tract and non-neoplastic diseases of the gut. *Ann. Intern. Med.* 110:35, 1989.

Kalser, M. H., and Ellenberg, S. S. Pancreatic cancer: adjuvant
combined radiation and chemotherapy following curative resection. *Arch. Surg.* 120:899, 1985.

Moertel, C. G., Hahn, R. G., and O'Connell, M. S. Therapy of
locally unresectable pancreatic carcinoma: a randomized
comparison of high dose (6000 rads) radiation alone, moderate dose radiation (4000 rads + 5-fluorouracil), and high
dose radiation + 5-fluorouracil: Gastrointestinal Tumor
Study Group. *Cancer* 48:1705, 1981.

Moertel, C. G., Hanley, J. A., and Johnson, L. A. Streptozocin
alone compared with streptozocin plus fluorouracil in the
treatment of advanced islet-cell carcinoma. *N. Engl. J. Med.*
303:1189, 1980.

Order, S. E., et al. Iodine 131 antiferritin, a new treatment modality in hepatoma: a Radiation Therapy Oncology Group
study. *J. Clin. Oncol.* 3:1573, 1985.

Pleskow, D. K., et al. Evaluation of a serologic marker, CA 19-
9, in the diagnosis of pancreatic cancer. *Ann. Intern. Med.*
110:704, 1989.

Carcinoma of the Breast

Roland T. Skeel

I. Natural history, evaluation, and modes of treatment

A. Epidemiology and etiology. Carcinoma of the breast gave way to carcinoma of the lung as the most common cause of cancer deaths among women in the United States in 1986. Nonetheless, in 1990 more than 150,000 new cases of breast cancer were diagnosed, and there were approximately 44,000 deaths. The incidence of breast cancer varies widely among different populations. Women in western Europe and the United States have a higher incidence than women in most other parts of the world, probably in part because of the high intake of animal protein and fat. Although discrete causes of breast cancer are not known, many factors increase a woman's risk for developing the disease. Among the strongest of the risk factors is family history, particularly if more than one family member has developed breast cancer at an early age. Other factors that increase the risk are early menarche, late age at first birth, and prior benign breast disease (particularly if there is a high degree of benign epithelial atypia). Lactation was once thought to protect from breast cancer, but it is now no longer believed to have that benefit. Prior or present use of birth control pills appears to play little or no role in the risk for developing breast cancer. Although breast cancer may occur among men, such cases represent fewer than 1% of all breast cancers and is uncommonly seen in most hospitals.

B. Detection, diagnosis, and pretreatment evaluation

1. Screening. Because more lives can be saved if breast cancer is diagnosed at an early stage, many programs have been designed to detect small, early cancers. Monthly breast self-examination for all women after puberty and yearly breast examinations by a physician or other trained professional after age 30 are recommended. Mammography, when done on a regular basis, can reduce mortality due to breast cancer by 30%. It is recommended once between the ages of 35 and 40 as a baseline, once every 1–2 years (depending on risk factors) between the ages of 40 and 50, and yearly after age 50. Although each method can be of some help in detecting early lesions that can be successfully removed before metastasis has occurred, mammography is capable of detecting the smallest and therefore the most curable lesions. Thus despite the high cost of screening mammography ($75–140 in many areas of the United States), it is highly recommended that the above guidelines be followed. As an incentive to patients to follow these recommendations, physicians may inform patients that lesions amenable to tumo-

Table 13-1. Abridged TNM classification of breast cancer

Stage	Description
Primary tumor (T)	
Tis	Carcinoma in situ: intraductal carcinoma, lobular carcinoma in situ, or Paget's disease of the nipple with no tumor
T_1	Tumor $\leq$ 2 cm
T_{1a}	$\leq$ 0.5 cm
T_{1b}	$>$ 0.5 to $\leq$ 1.0 cm
T_{1c}	$>$ 1.0 to $\leq$ 2.0 cm
T_2	Tumor $>$ 2.0 to $\leq$ 5 cm
T_3	Tumor $>$ 5 cm
T_4	Any size with extension to chest wall or skin. Chest wall includes ribs, intercostal muscles, and serratus anterior muscle, but not pectoral muscles
T_{4a}	Extension to chest wall
T_{4b}	Edema, skin ulceration, or satellite skin nodules confined to same breast
T_{4c}	Both (T_{4a} and T_{4b}) criteria
T_{4d}	Inflammatory carcinoma
Nodal involvement (N)—pathologic	
pN_0	No regional lymph node metastasis
pN_1	Metastasis to movable ipsilateral axillary nodes
pN_{1a}	Only micrometastasis ($\leq$ 0.2 cm) (prognosis of patients with pN_{1a} similar to that of patients with pN_0)
pN_{1b}	Macrometastasis ($>$ 0.2 cm)
i	To 1–3 nodes, any $>$ 0.2 cm, all $<$ 2.0 cm
ii	To 4 or more nodes, any $>$ 0.2 cm, all $<$ 2.0 cm
iii	Extension of tumor ($<$ 2.0 cm) beyond capsule of node
iv	Any metastatic focus $\geq$ 2.0 cm
pN_2	Fixed metastasis to ipsilateral axillary nodes
pN_3	Metastasis to ipsilateral internal mammary nodes
Distant metastasis (M)	
M_0	None known
M_1	Metastases present, including to ipsilateral supraclavicular lymph nodes

rectomy (followed by irradiation) are more likely to be found, avoiding the necessity for mastectomy.

2. **Presenting signs and symptoms.** Although increasing numbers of nonpalpable cancers are being found by mammography, breast cancer is still most often discovered by a woman herself as an isolated, painless lump in the breast. If the mass has gone unnoticed or ignored for a time, there may be fixation to the skin or underlying chest wall, ulceration, pain, or inflammation. Some early lesions present with discharge or bleeding from the nipple. At times the primary lesion is not discovered, and the woman presents with symptoms of metastatic disease, e.g., pleural effusion, nodal disease, or bony metastases. About one-half of all lesions are in the upper outer quadrant of the breast (where most of the glandular tissue of the breast is). About 20% are central masses, and 10% are in each of the other quadrants. One-half of all women with breast cancer have axillary node metastasis unless the primary tumor has been detected by screening mammography or other screening method.

3. **Staging.** Carcinoma of the breast is staged according to the size and characteristics of the primary tumor (T), the involvement of regional lymph nodes (N), and the presence of metastatic disease (M). An abridged version of the commonly used TNM classification of breast cancer is shown in Table 13-1, and the stage grouping is outlined in Table 13-2. Although preliminary staging is commonly done prior to surgery, definitive staging that can be used for prognostic and further treatment planning purposes

Table 13-2. Stage grouping of breast cancer

Stage	T	N	M
0	Tis	N_0	M_0
I	T_1	N_0	M_0
IIA	T_0, T_1	N_1	M_0
	T_2	N_0	M_0
IIB	T_2	N_1	M_0
	T_3	N_0	M_0
IIIA	T_{0-2}	N_2	M_0
	T_3	N_1, N_2	M_0
IIIB	T_4	Any N	M_0
	Any T	N_3	M_0
IV	Any T	Any N	M_1

Note: Patients are staged in the highest group possible for their composite TNM. For example, a patient with $T_{1a}N_2M_0$ would be a stage IIIA because of the N_2 status.

usually must await postsurgical pathologic evaluation when the primary tumor size and the histologic involvement of the lymph nodes are established. It is important to note that in 30% of the patients without clinical evidence of axillary lymph node involvement the histologic evaluation reveals cancer; and in a somewhat smaller number nodes that clinically appear positive contain no cancer when examined histologically.

4. **Diagnostic evaluation**
   a. **Prior to biopsy** the woman should have a careful **history,** during which attention should be paid to *risk factors,* and a **physical examination,** with a focus not only on the involved breast but also on the opposite breast, all regional lymph node areas, the lungs, bone, and liver. This examination should be followed by bilateral mammography to help assess the extent of involvement and to look for additional homolateral or contralateral disease.
   b. **Excisional biopsy** of the primary lesion is performed, and the specimen is given intact (not in formalin) to the pathologist, who can divide the specimen for histologic examination, hormone receptor assays, or other tests. The tissue for receptor studies must be rapidly frozen with either dry ice or liquid nitrogen to preserve receptor activity.
   c. **After confirmation of the histology,** the patient is evaluated for possible metastatic disease.
      (1) **Mandatory studies** include a chest x-ray film, complete blood count, blood chemistry profile, and estrogen and progesterone receptor assays on the primary breast carcinoma and grossly cancerous nodal tissues.
      (2) **Other studies,** including radionuclide scan of the bones, skeletal survey (usually obtained only if the radionuclide scan is positive), and computed tomography (CT) scan of the liver (abdomen) are optional unless the history, physical examination, or blood studies suggest a poor prognosis or point to specific organ involvement. A carcinoembryonic antigen (CEA) assay is also often performed. Additional studies that may impart clinically useful prognostic information include evaluation of the ploidy of the malignant cells, their DNA synthesis rate (percent in S phase), and the content of other markers such as cathepsin D and the *HER-2/neu* oncogene and its protein product.

5. **Histology.** About 75–80% of all breast cancers are infiltrating ductal carcinomas, and 10% are infiltrating lobular carcinomas; these two types have similar biologic behavior. The remainder of the histologic types of invasive breast carcinoma may have

a somewhat better prognosis but are usually managed more according to the stage than to the histologic type.

C. Approach to therapy

1. **Surgery** has been and remains the most frequently utilized mode of primary therapy for most women with carcinoma of the breast. The role of surgery in the primary management of carcinoma of the breast has been evolving with a trend to lesser surgery, e.g., wide local excision, together with axillary dissection. This step is then followed by radiotherapy to control the microscopic cancer remaining in the breast.

For most women this therapy yields therapeutic results just as good as mastectomy without the need for amputating the breast and its attendant physical deformity and psychological trauma. These therapeutic changes notwithstanding, the operation that is probably most commonly performed is some version of the modified radical mastectomy in which the breast, pectoralis fascia (with or without the pectoralis minor muscle), and lymph nodes are removed. For most women operations more extensive than the modified radical mastectomy are probably of no benefit, and lesser operations, unless combined with radiotherapy, are insufficient in terms of providing important prognostic information regarding the status of the axillary lymph nodes and controlling the local disease (40% of women treated with excisional biopsy alone have recurrence in the ipsilateral breast).

For patients who have had mastectomy, reconstruction is being done with increasing frequency. It may be done at the time of mastectomy or delayed for a period (usually 1–2 years). Options include insertion of a silicone implant or transposition of a rectus muscle flap. Neither procedure has resulted in worsening of the prognosis from the breast cancer or increased the difficulty in detecting local recurrences.

2. **Radiotherapy's** role in the management of carcinoma of the breast has been expanded since the early 1970s. Radiotherapy is now commonly used in conjunction with excisional biopsy of varying degree as part of the primary therapy. In this circumstance the radiotherapy is commonly delivered using external beam therapy to the entire breast and a boost of therapy to the tumor bed with either external beam therapy or implantation of radioactive substances. Radiotherapy may also be given after mastectomy in women who have a high likelihood of local recurrence, and it is highly effective in preventing the reappearance of disease in the treated fields. Local recurrences and distant metastases also are frequently treated successfully with radiotherapy. This mode of treatment is particularly critical to the management of painful bony lesions or sites of impending pathologic fracture.

3. **Chemotherapy and endocrine therapy** are used for the treatment of early disease to reduce the likelihood of recurrence as well as for the treatment of advanced disease with distant metastasis. *Endocrine therapy* may consist in surgical, chemotherapeutic, or radiotherapeutic ablation or inhibition of the ovaries, adrenal glands, or anterior pituitary gland; or it may consist in additive therapy with estrogens, progestins, androgens, antiestrogens, or luteinizing hormone-releasing hormone (LHRH) agonists. Endocrine therapy is generally ineffective (as sole therapy) for the treatment of metastatic disease in those patients with low levels of estrogen and progesterone receptors (ERs and PRs) in their cancer and increasingly effective as the level of receptors rises. The best responses can be expected in women in whom the ER is high and PRs are present. Chemotherapy is apparently equally effective regardless of the level of hormone receptors in the cancer cell.

4. **Multimodal therapy** has had more impact on carcinoma of the breast than on any other common cancer affecting adults.

   a. **Postoperative chemotherapy or hormonal therapy** for women with a high risk of recurrence owing to positive axillary nodes (i.e., nodes containing cancer) has varying effects, depending on the menopausal status of the woman and the hormone receptor status of the tumor. In a National Institutes of Health Consensus Conference held in 1985 on adjuvant chemotherapy for breast cancer, it was noted that optimal therapy has yet to be defined for any subset of patients, and all patients and their physicians were strongly urged to participate in controlled clinical trials. *Outside the context of clinical trials,* the following was concluded.

      (1) **For premenopausal women with positive nodes,** regardless of hormone receptor status, treatment with established combination chemotherapy was recommended as standard care.

      (2) **For premenopausal women with negative nodes,** adjuvant therapy was not recommended, although consideration of adjuvant chemotherapy was recommended for certain high-risk patients within this group.

      (3) **For postmenopausal women with positive nodes and positive hormone receptor levels,** tamoxifen was recommended as the treatment of choice.

      (4) **For postmenopausal women with positive nodes and negative hormone receptor levels,** chemotherapy was not recommended as standard practice, al-

though consideration of chemotherapy was an option.

(5) For postmenopausal women with negative nodes, regardless of hormone receptor levels, there was no indication for routine adjuvant therapy. However, for certain high-risk patients in this group, adjuvant therapy was again suggested as a consideration.

Studies have shown that women with negative nodes may also benefit from adjuvant chemotherapy or hormonal (tamoxifen) therapy, at least in terms of disease-free survival, although the gain in terms of improved survival is not yet established. Current clinical trials use tumor size, hormone receptor status, and DNA synthesis rate (percent of cells in S phase) to aid in determining the patients, among those with negative nodes, who are most likely to relapse and thus most likely to benefit from adjuvant therapy.

b. Radiotherapy to the breast and nodal areas following excisional biopsy or quadrantectomy of the breast cancer appeared in several series to be as effective a treatment as mastectomy in terms of local recurrence and survival. The place of this mode of combined therapy in the management of carcinoma of the breast is not yet defined, but for most patients it is not only equivalent but preferable treatment.

c. Consultation with a surgeon, radiotherapist, and medical oncologist is critical once the diagnosis of carcinoma is highly suspected or histologically confirmed. It is important to have all of these oncology specialists see the patient *before any decisions regarding therapy are made,* so the primary physician and the patient can have opinions from several perspectives about optimal management.

It is critical to have the patient (and her family if she desires) share in the therapy decisions after she has heard the options, the relative advantages and disadvantages of each option, *and the recommendations* of the consultants. The patient should be given an opportunity to hear why the recommended treatment is thought by the physicians to be best and to decide whether that is acceptable to her.

D. Prognosis. There is a broad spectrum in the biologic behavior of breast carcinoma from the aggressive, rapidly fatal, inflammatory carcinoma to the relatively indolent disease with late-appearing metastasis and survival of 10–15 years. The likelihood of relapse and survival are influenced by the state of the disease and the hormone receptor status at diagnosis, pathologic characteristics of the tumor, measures of proliferative activity of the cancer cell, and age and general health of the patient.

1. **Stage.** Axillary node involvement and the size of the primary tumor are determinants of the likelihood of survival.

   a. **Nodes.** In one large National Surgical Adjuvant Breast Project study, 65% of all patients who had a radical mastectomy survived 5 years and 45% survived 10 years. If no axillary nodes were positive, the 5-year survival was nearly 80% and the 10-year survival 65%. If any axillary nodes were positive, the 5-year survival was less than 50% and the 10-year survival 25%. If four or more nodes were positive, the 5-year survival was 30% and the 10-year survival less than 15%.

   b. **Primary tumor.** Patients with large primary tumors do not do as well as patients with small tumors, irrespective of the nodal status, although those patients with a large primary tumor are more likely to have node involvement. Tumors that are fixed to the skin or to the chest wall do worse than those that are not. Inflammatory carcinomas have a particularly poor prognosis with a median survival of less than 2 years and a 5-year survival of less than 10%.

2. **Estrogen and progesterone receptors.** Patients without estrogen or progesterone receptors (or with very low levels) are twice as likely to relapse during the first 2 years after diagnosis as those who are receptor-positive. This observation is true for both premenopausal and postmenopausal patients within each major node group (0, 1–3, ≥4).

3. **Other prognostic factors** are emerging as independent prognostic factors, include the ploidy of the breast cancer cells (diploid better than aneuploid) and the percent of cells in DNA synthesis (low percent S better than high percent). Additional tumor markers that may have predictive value include cathepsin D, *HER-2/neu* oncogene amplification, and haptoglobin-related protein epitopes. One intriguing study carried out an immunohistologic assessment of CEA and found that patients who had CEA-negative tumors had significantly higher 5- and 10-year survival rates.

II. Chemotherapy and endocrine therapy

   A. **General considerations and aims of therapy.** Carcinoma of the breast is responsive to many cytotoxic chemotherapeutic agents, hormonal agents, and other endocrine manipulations.

   1. **Endocrine therapy** is presumed to be effective because the breast cancer tissue retains some of the endocrine sensitivity of the normal breast tissue. In the premenopausal woman, if the breast cancer growth is supported by estrogen production by the ovary, antiestrogen therapy or removal of endogenous estrogen by oophorectomy logically results in regression of the cancer, at least those tumor cells that are

dependent on the estrogen. (The dependent cells seem to be those that have the estrogen receptors.) Other mechanisms of action of the antiestrogen include inhibition of the epithelial growth factor, transforming growth factor alpha (TGF-α), and stimulation of the epithelial inhibitory factor TGF-β.

2. **Chemotherapy.** As with other cancers, the basis for the effectiveness of cytotoxic drugs in the treatment of carcinoma of the breast is not well understood. It is clear, however, that combinations of drugs are considerably more effective than single agents (although how many is enough is not as clear), and nearly all treatment programs use the drugs in various combinations.

3. **Aims of therapy** differ depending on the stage of disease being treated.

   a. **For early disease** the aim is to eradicate micrometastases in order to render the patient free of disease and prevent recurrence of the disease. Coincident with this aim is the goal of avoiding unnecessarily excessive drug-induced toxicity, both short- and long-term. Of particular theoretical concern is the possibility of second cancers arising many years after the completion of chemotherapy. Thus a goal of investigational studies has been to try to determine the minimum therapy that is effective for preventing the maximum number of recurrences.

   b. **For advanced disease** the aim is usually to temporarily reduce the tumor burden and the resultant disability in order to alleviate the patient's symptoms, improve performance, and prolong meaningful survival. Whereas long-term toxicity is not usually of great import, short-term toxicity is a major area of concern for both physician and patient, as the aim of therapy is to improve how the patient feels (quality of life) as well as to prolong the time of her remaining life.

B. **Effective agents** for treating carcinoma of the breast can be found among the alkylating agents, antimetabolites, natural products (antibiotics and vinca alkaloids), hormones, and hormone antagonists.

   1. **Among the cytotoxic drugs,** the most commonly used agents include doxorubicin (Adriamycin), cyclophosphamide, methotrexate, fluorouracil, thiotepa, mitoxantrone, and vincristine. Each of these agents has response rates of 20–40% when used as a single agent. Because combinations are so much more effective (60–80% responses) than single agents, these drugs are rarely used alone.

   2. **Among the hormones and antihormones,** the most commonly used agents are tamoxifen, various progestins (e.g., megestrol acetate), aminoglutethemide, fluoxymesterone, and prednisone. The first four may be used alone, in combination with cyto-

toxic drugs or sequentially with cytotoxic drugs; prednisone is nearly always used together with cytotoxic agents.

C. Treatment of early disease. As indicated above, standard treatment of early disease depends on primary tumor size, nodal status, menopausal status of the woman, hormone receptor status of the tumor, and other tumor characteristics. Because there is not yet optimal therapy for any subset of women with breast cancer, the women and their physicians should be encouraged to participate in a clinical trial. If none is available or the woman declines, Table 13-3 can be used as a guide for assessing risk. Table 13-4 may be used as a guide to select the type of therapy, depending on menopausal state, age, and other risk factors.

   1. Cytotoxic therapy is recommended for premenopausal women with positive nodes, irrespective of hormone receptor status. It may also be considered for certain high-risk premenopausal patients with negative nodes and high-risk postmenopausal women with negative hormone receptors. We are less in-

Table 13-3. Prognostic factors for assessing risk of recurrence of breast cancer

Parameter	Value
Lymph node involvement	Risk increased with presence of metastasis and numbers of nodes involved
Tumor size	Risk increases with tumor size independent of nodal status
Estrogen and progesterone receptors	Positive receptors confer better prognosis
Age	Complex factor. Women age 45–49 have best prognosis, with increasing likelihood of deaths from their breast cancer in older and younger age groups
Morphology	Higher nuclear and histologic grade tumors have worse prognosis
DNA content and proliferative capacity	Tumors that are diploid and have low S-phase fraction do better than those that are aneuploid or have a high S-phase fraction (by flow cytometry)
Oncogene expression	*Neu* (or *erb B-2* or *HER-2*) amplification has possible association with earlier relapse and shorter survival

Table 13-4. Adjuvant therapy of breast cancer

	Premenopausal women	Postmenopausal women	
		≤ 70 years	> 70 years
Node-positive			
ER-positive	CT → ± TAM	TAM	TAM
ER-negative	CT	CT → ± TAM	TAM
Node-negative			
ER-positive			
≤ 2 cm	Low risk*	TAM	TAM
	None		
	High risk*		
	CT → ± TAM		
> 2 cm	CT → ± TAM	TAM	TAM
ER-negative	CT	CT → ± TAM	TAM

Key: CT: CAF, CMF, or CMFP for six cycles. TAM: tamoxifen for at least 5 years, alone or after completion of chemotherapy. ER, estrogen receptor.
*Based on factors such as proliferative capacity (% S phase) as in Table 13-3.

clined to use cytotoxic therapy in the adjuvant treatment of women over age 70. The *recommended regimens* are as follows.
  a. CAF
    Cyclophosphamide 100 mg/m^2 PO daily on days 1–14 (given as a single daily dose) *and*
    Doxorubicin 30 mg/m^2 IV push on days 1 and 8, through the side arm of a free-flowing IV infusion of normal saline *and*
    Fluorouracil 500 mg/m^2 IV push on days 1 and 8.
    Repeat every 28 days for 6 cycles.
  b. CMFP
    Cyclophosphamide 100 mg/m^2 PO on days 1–14 *and*
    Methotrexate 40 mg/m^2 IV on days 1 and 8 *and*
    Fluorouracil 600 mg/m^2 IV on days 1 and 8 *and*
    Prednisone 40 mg/m^2 PO on days 1–14 (as a single dose).
    Repeat cycle every 28 days for 6 cycles.
  c. Dose modifications are outlined in Table 13-5.
2. Tamoxifen 10 mg PO bid is recommended in hormone receptor-positive postmenopausal women with positive nodes. It should be continued for at least 2 years and perhaps for life, so long as the woman remains disease-free. It is probably also beneficial in hormone receptor-positive postmenopausal women with negative nodes and may be of greater benefit than chemotherapy or no therapy in all women over age 70. It may also benefit other groups of women following cytotoxic chemotherapy, though this benefit is not yet certain. It does appear to present low

Table 13-5. Dose modification for chemotherapy of breast carcinoma

Dysfunction	Percent of full dose		
Hematologic toxicity	**All myelosuppressive drugs**		
$\geq$4000 WBC/μl *and*			
$\geq$100,000 platelets/μl	100		
<4000 WBC/μl *or*			
<100,000 platelets/μl	50*		
<2500 WBC/μl *or*			
<75,000 platelets/μl	0*		
Renal dysfunction (serum creatinine, mg/dl)	**M**	**T**	**Others**
<1.5	100	100	100
1.5–2.0	50	75	100
2.0–3.5	0	50	100
>3.5	0†	0†	0†
Hepatic dysfunction (serum bilirubin, mg/dl)	**A, VLB, VCR**		**C, M, F, T**
<1.5	100		100
1.5–3.0	50		100
3.1–5.0	25		100
>5.0	0†		0†
Hemorrhagic cystitis	Discontinue cyclophosphamide and substitute melphalan 4 mg/m² PO on days 1–5 of each cycle		
Gastrointestinal toxicity	For debilitating vomiting or diarrhea, reduce doses of C, M, F, and A by 25% for one cycle. For severe mucositis (ulcerations that inhibit eating), reduce subsequent F, M, and A by 50%. Reescalate if possible		
Cardiotoxicity	Discontinue doxorubicin		
Hypercorticism	If side effects such as hypertension, severe insomnia, psychosis, or uncontrolled diabetes occur, reduce or stop prednisone		

Table 13-5. (continued)

Dysfunction	Percent of full dose
Neurotoxicity	Reduce vincristine or vinblastine dose by 50% for moderate paresthesias or severe constipation. Discontinue for severe paresthesias, decreased strength, difficulty walking, cranial-nerve palsies, etc.

Abbreviations: A = doxorubicin (Adriamycin); C = cyclophosphamide; F = fluorouracil; M = methotrexate; T = thiotepa; VCR = vincristine; VLB = vinblastine.
*If the WBC count is <4000/μl or the platelet count is 100,000/μl on day 1 of any cycle, delay therapy and repeat these tests in 1 week. After a maximum of 2 weeks' delay, give a reduced dose according to this table. If the nadir WBC count is <1600/μl or the platelet count is <50,000/μl, reduce subsequent doses by 25%. If the nadir WBC count is >3500/μl and the platelet count is >125,000/μl, increase the dose by 25%.
†Safe guidelines cannot be given, and expert evaluation is required before therapy is applied.

risk, and our current recommendations generally include tamoxifen where it is indicated as an option in Table 13-4.

3. **Response to therapy.** It is impossible to determine if individual patients have responded to treatment for micrometastatic disease unless they relapse, as there are no parameters to measure. The effectiveness of such treatment must therefore depend on population studies. Because breast cancer may have a long natural history, and the disease may recur after 5–10 years, it is critical to defer final conclusions regarding any study until at least 5 years and preferably 10 years have passed. It is possible to make some observations, however, regarding the benefits of this kind of multimodal therapy.

a. **In node-positive premenopausal women,** both disease-free survival and absolute survival are longer in women treated with various cytotoxic regimens than in those who receive no therapy after mastectomy.

b. **In node-positive postmenopausal women,** the disease-free and absolute survival benefit to tamoxifen in receptor-positive women is also clear.

It is apparent that there is a minimal effective dose and duration of drugs that are required for therapy of micrometastases to be effective. If women are arbitrarily given less therapy than they can tolerate, their likelihood of remaining disease-free seems to be less than in women who are given full doses of the drugs. This observation has led to the recommendation that if postoperative chemotherapy is to be given doses should be as high as the patient can tolerate and should be continued for the entire planned period (usually 6 months).

    c. In all node-negative women and postmenopausal node-positive women who are receptor-negative, the benefit of therapy is less certain. It does appear that the disease-free survival is improved in women who are treated, and there is reasonable expectation—by extrapolating from experience with earlier treatment groups—that this improvement translates into improved overall survival as well.

D. Treatment of advanced disease is undergoing continuing evolution with the aim of improving the quality and duration of remissions and survivals. In patients with bony metastasis or cerebral metastasis radiotherapy usually has an important role to play in their management, and a radiotherapist should participate in planning the patients' treatment. Regardless of the role of radiotherapy, however, chemotherapy or endocrine therapy is generally indicated in patients who have advanced disease.

    1. Endocrine therapy is indicated in women who have a positive test for estrogen or progesterone receptors in their tumor tissue. It is not generally recommended as the sole therapy for women who have low receptor levels or have previously been shown to be unresponsive to hormonal manipulation. It is also not appropriate therapy for women with brain metastasis, lymphangitic pulmonary metastasis, or other dire visceral disease such as extensive liver metastasis in which a slow response could jeopardize survival.

        a. Premenopausal women. Oophorectomy is the treatment of choice. If the woman is a poor surgical risk, the LHRH analogs goserelin and leuprolide are reasonable alternatives.

        b. Postmenopausal women. Tamoxifen 10 mg PO twice daily is the treatment of choice.

        c. Secondary endocrine therapy may be indicated in women who have had a good response to the primary endocrine manipulation and then relapsed. Choices for therapy in this circumstance include the following.

            (1) Tamoxifen 10 mg PO twice daily for premenopausal women who fail after responding to oophorectomy.

            (2) Megestrol acetate 40 mg PO qid.

            (3) Aminoglutethemide 250 mg PO qid + hydrocortisone 100 mg PO in divided doses daily for the first 2 weeks, then 40 mg PO in divided doses daily. Fluorohydrocortisone 0.1 mg PO may be given daily or every other drug if there is evidence of salt wasting. (Aminoglutethemide is not approved by the Food and Drug Administration for the treatment of breast cancer.)

   (4) Fluoxymesterone 10 mg PO bid.
   (5) Transsphenoidal hypophysectomy + hydrocortisone 20–30 mg PO daily in divided doses.

2. **Cytotoxic chemotherapy,** rather than endocrine therapy, is commonly used as the first treatment for advanced disease, particularly in premenopausal patients, because the responses are more rapid and the rate of response is greater when drugs are used in combination than when endocrine therapy is used alone. For patients over age 65, however, initiation of hormone therapy may be justified, with cytotoxic therapy being reserved for patients who have failed on tamoxifen.

   a. **Primary therapy** is used as the first nonendocrine therapy for patients with advanced disease. Although several regimens have been shown to be effective, two are recommended. The first is for patients in whom doxorubicin (Adriamycin) is not contraindicated, and the second is for patients with recent myocardial infarction or congestive heart failure in whom the risk of any further myocardial compromise by doxorubicin would be too great.

      (1) CAF

         Cyclophosphamide 100 mg/m^2 PO on days 1–14 *and*

         Doxorubicin 30 mg/m^2 IV on days 1 and 8 *and*

         Fluorouracil 500 mg/m^2 IV on days 1 and 8. Repeat the cycle every 4 weeks.

            When the cumulative doxorubicin dose reaches 550 mg/m^2 substitute methotrexate 40 mg/m^2.

      (2) CMFP

         Cyclophosphamide 100 mg/m^2 PO on days 1–14 *and*

         Methotrexate 40 mg/m^2 IV on days 1 and 8 *and*

         Fluorouracil 600 mg/m^2 IV on days 1 and 8 *and*

         Prednisone 40 mg/m^2 PO on days 1–14, during the first three cycles only.

         Repeat the cycle every 4 weeks.

   b. **Secondary therapy** depends on what treatment the patient has had previously. If the patient relapses while on CMF or CMFP treatment, or within 6 months after finishing CMF treatment for micrometastatic disease, it is not likely that these drugs used in combination can be helpful in achieving a second remission. Because doxorubicin is among the most effective agents against breast carcinoma, it should be used in any combination in this situation. An effective combination (VATH) is as follows.

Vinblastine 4.5 mg/m^2 IV on day 1 *and*

Doxorubicin 45 mg/m^2 IV on day 1 (maximum cumulative dose 550 mg/m^2) *and*

Thiotepa 12 mg/m^2 IV on day 1 *and*

Fluoxymesterone (Halotestin) 20 mg PO daily

Repeat cycle every 3 weeks if blood counts permit. Other agents with activity include mitomycin, mitoxantrone, and the investigational agents dibromodulcitol, epirubicin, and vindesine.

3. **Dose modifications** are outlined in Table 13-5.

4. **Response to therapy**

   a. **Endocrine therapy.** Of patients who are ER-negative, fewer than 10% have a response to either additive or ablative endocrine therapy. Among ER-positive patients, about 60% have a partial, or better, response to either additive or ablative endocrine therapy. Responses to endocrine therapy tend to last somewhat longer than responses to cytotoxic chemotherapy, frequently lasting 12–24 months.

   b. **Cytotoxic chemotherapy** produces responses in 60–80% of patients regardless of their ER status. The responses to therapy at times are durable, but the median duration in most studies is less than 1 year.

E. **Complications of therapy.** Acute toxicities are primarily hematologic and gastrointestinal. Subacute toxicities include alopecia, hemorrhagic cystitis, hypertension, edema, and psychoneurologic abnormalities. Chronic or long-term toxicities may be cardiac or neoplastic. Dose modifications for the more common problems are given in Table 13-5. These guidelines are designed to be helpful in selecting a course of therapy that will be effective with the least risk of life-threatening toxicity. Because of individual differences, toxicities that are worse than expected may occur, and the responsible physician must always be alert for special circumstances that dictate further attenuation of the drug doses. The drug data listed in Chapter 8 should be consulted for the individual precautions and toxicities of each drug.

Selected Reading

Benner, S. E., Clark, G. M., and McGuire, W. L. Review: steroid receptors, cellular kinetics, and lymph node status as prognostic factors in breast cancer. *Am. J. Med. Sci.* 296:59, 1988.

Bonanonna, G., and Valagussa, P. Adjuvant systemic therapy for resectable breast cancer. *J. Clin. Oncol.* 3:259, 1985.

Breast Cancer Trials Committee. Adjuvant tamoxifen in the management of operable breast cancer: the Scottish trial. *Lancet* 2:171, 1987.

Clark, G. M. and McGuire, W. L. Prediction of relapse or survival in patients with node-negative breast cancer by DNA flow cytometry. *N. Engl. J. Med.* 320:627, 1990.

Early Breast Cancer Trialists Collaborative Group. Effects of adjuvant tamoxifen and of cytotoxic therapy on mortality in early breast cancer. *N. Engl. J. Med.* 319:1681, 1988.

Fisher, B., et al. Ten year follow-up results of patients with carcinoma of the breast in a cooperative clinical trial evaluating surgical adjuvant chemotherapy. *Surg. Gynecol. Obstet.* 140:528, 1975.

Fisher, B., et al. Relative worth of estrogen or progesterone receptor and pathologic characteristics of differentiation as indicators of prognosis in node-negative breast cancer. *J. Clin. Oncol.* 6:1076, 1988.

Fisher, B., et al. A randomized clinical trial evaluating sequential methotrexate and fluorouracil in the treatment of node-negative breast cancer who have estrogen negative tumor. *N. Engl. J. Med.* 320:473, 1989.

Fisher, B., et al. A randomized trial evaluating tamoxifen in the treatment of patients with node-negative breast cancer who have estrogen-receptor positive tumors. *N. Engl. J. Med.* 320:479, 1989.

Fisher, B., et al. Eight-year results of a randomized clinical trial comparing total mastectomy and lumpectomy with or without irradiation in the treatment of breast cancer. *N. Engl. J. Med.* 320:822, 1989.

Harris, J. R., Hellman, S., and Kinne, D. W. Limited surgery and radiotherapy for early breast cancer. *N. Engl. J. Med.* 313:1365, 1985.

Henderson, I. C. Adjuvant chemotherapy of breast cancer: a promising experiment or standard practice? *J. Clin. Oncol.* 3:140, 1985 (editorial).

Hryniuk, W., and Bush, H. The importance of dose intensity in chemotherapy of metastatic breast cancer. *J. Clin. Oncol.* 2:1281, 1984.

Ingle, J. N., et al. Randomized trial of bilateral oophorectomy versus tamoxifen in premenopausal women with metastatic breast cancer. *J. Clin. Oncol.* 4:178, 1986.

LiVolsi, V. A., et al. Fibrocystic disease in oral contraceptive users. *N. Engl. J. Med.* 299:381, 1978.

Love, R. R. Tamoxifen therapy in breast cancer: biology, efficacy, and side effects. *J. Clin. Oncol.* 7:803, 1989.

Ludwig Breast Cancer Study Group. Prolonged disease free survival after one course of perioperative adjuvant chemotherapy for node-negative breast cancer. *N. Engl. J. Med.* 320:491, 1989.

Mansour, E. G., et al. Efficacy of adjuvant chemotherapy in high-risk node-negative breast cancer: an intergroup study. *N. Engl. J. Med.* 320:485, 1989.

Moxley, J. H., et al. Primary treatment of breast cancer: summary of the National Institutes of Health consensus development conference. *J.A.M.A.* 244:797, 1980.

Nolvadex Adjuvant Trial Organization. Controlled trial of tamoxifen as a single adjuvant agent in the management of early breast cancer. *Br. J. Cancer* 57:608, 1988.

Osborne, C. K. Heterogeneity in hormone receptor status in primary and metastatic cancer. *Semin. Oncol.* 12:317, 1985.

Osborne, C. K., et al. Review modern approaches to the treatment of breast cancer. *Blood* 56:745, 1980.

Pickle, L. W. Estimating the long-term probability of developing breast cancer. *J. Natl. Cancer Inst.* 81:1854, 1990.

Sawka, C. A., et al. Role and mechanism of action of tamoxifen in premenopausal women with metastatic breast carcinoma. *Cancer Res.* 46:3152, 1986.

Slamon, D. J., et al. Studies of HER-2/neu proto-oncogene in human breast and ovarian cancer. *Science* 244:707, 1989.

Smalley, R. V., et al. A comparison of CAF and CMFVP in patients with metastatic breast cancer. *Cancer* 40:625, 1977.

Tandon, A. K., et al. Cathepsin D and prognosis in breast cancer. *N. Engl. J. Med.* 322:297, 1990.

Taylor, S. G., et al. Combination chemotherapy compared to tamoxifen as initial therapy for stage IV breast cancer in elderly women. *Ann. Intern. Med.* 104:455, 1986.

Tormey, D. C., et al. A randomized trial of five and three drug chemotherapy and chemoimmunotherapy in women with operable node positive breast cancer. *J. Clin. Oncol.* 1:138, 1983.

Veronesi, U., et al. Comparing radical mastectomy with quadrantectomy, axillary dissection, and radiotherapy in patients with small cancers of the breast. *N. Engl. J. Med.* 305:6, 1981.

Weiss, R. B., Henney, J. E., and DeVita, V. T. Multimodal treatment of primary breast carcinoma. *Am. J. Med.* 70:844, 1981.

Gynecologic Cancer

Robert F. Ozols

Chemotherapy is playing an increasingly important role in the treatment of patients with gynecologic cancers. For epithelial tumors of the ovary, advances in chemotherapy have led to a higher response rate, longer duration of remission, and improvement in overall survival. For germ cell tumors of the ovary, chemotherapy has transformed what was once a uniformly fatal tumor into an almost completely curable disease. For cervical cancer and cancer of the endometrium, chemotherapy currently plays primarily a palliative role. Although chemotherapy results in a substantial objective response rate in these tumors, it has usually been administered only at a time when patients have failed primary therapy with surgery or irradiation, or both. In contrast, for gestational trophoblastic neoplasms, chemotherapy is used prior to other treatment modalities and has been responsible for the high cure rate.

The same chemotherapeutic approaches are not used for all gynecologic neoplasms. Consequently, specific therapy is discussed for each gynecologic cancer.

I. Epithelial ovarian cancer

A. General considerations and aims of therapy. In the United States approximately 20,000 women per year are diagnosed as having epithelial ovarian cancer. There are no well defined high-risk patients, nor are there any specific signs or symptoms. Most patients with widespread disease present with abdominal distension and discomfort. Approximately two-thirds of women with ovarian cancer have peritoneal metastases at the time of diagnosis. Thus far, screening with ultrasonographic examinations, pelvic examinations, and serum CA-125 levels have not been established to be useful in detecting women with early stage ovarian cancer. Patients with ovarian cancer can be placed in two major prognostic groups: limited stage cancer [Federation Internationale de Gynecologie et d'Obstetrique (FIGO) stages I and II], and advanced stage cancer (FIGO stages III and IV). In both groups the primary goal of therapy is curative. Indeed, most patients with limited stage disease ovarian cancer can be cured with surgery and chemotherapy. Even in patients with advanced stage disease, there is an increasing cure rate using similar treatment modalities.

B. Limited stage disease: prognostic groups and treatment. Limited stage ovarian cancer can be subdivided into two distinct prognostic categories.

1. **Low risk patients** (favorable prognosis) with limited disease have the following clinical and pathologic characteristics: disease confined to the ovaries, well differentiated or moderately well differentiated tumor, intact capsule, no extracystic disease, no

dense adhesions, no ascites, and negative peritoneal cytology.

2. **High risk patients** (unfavorable prognosis) with limited stage ovarian cancer have the following characteristics: poorly differentiated tumor, ruptured capsule, dense adhesions, extracystic tumor, ascites, malignant peritoneal cytology, or disease spread outside the ovaries to other pelvic structures (stage II). This stage is relatively rare, as it has become appreciated that the tumor spreads insidiously throughout the peritoneal cavity and that the presence of peritoneal implants within the pelvis are almost invariably associated with peritoneal metastases throughout the abdominal cavity. Careful exploration of the entire abdominal cavity often up-stages patients who are thought clinically to have disease confined to the pelvis.

3. **Treatment.** It has been demonstrated in prospective randomized trials that there is a marked difference in survival for patients with low-risk limited disease compared to patients at high risk, and that these patients should be approached with different therapeutic modalities.

    a. In patients with **low-risk limited disease,** adjuvant therapy with single-agent melphalan has not been shown to improve survival over that which can be achieved by surgery alone. Consequently, patients who have a careful staging laparotomy and have no clinical-pathologic characteristics that place them in the high-risk category require no further therapy; they have a 5-year survival of almost 90%.

    b. In contrast, patients with **high-risk limited disease** have an 80% 5-year survival. The optimum adjuvant therapy for this group of patients remains to be established. In a prospective randomized trial, intraperitoneal ^{32}P and intermittent oral melphalan produced identical survivals, although there was substantially less toxicity due to the radioisotope. A follow-up prospective randomized trial is evaluating three cycles of cisplatin plus cyclophosphamide versus intraperitoneal ^{32}P in patients with limited stage high-risk ovarian cancer. Outside a clinical trial setting, it seems prudent that these patients should be treated with the same chemotherapeutic regimens that are used for patients with advanced ovarian cancer.

C. Advanced stage disease

  1. Stage definitions

    a. **With stage III ovarian cancer** there are peritoneal implants outside the pelvis or positive retroperitoneal or inguinal nodes (or both). Stage III has further been subclassified into A, B, and C disease on the basis of volume of *residual disease* after the initial surgery.

(1) **IIIA disease:** Gross tumor is limited to the true pelvis with negative nodes but with the presence of microscopic seeding of abdominoperitoneal surfaces.

(2) **IIIB disease:** None of the residual tumor nodules on the peritoneal surfaces exceeds 2 cm in diameter, and the lymph nodes are negative.

(3) **IIIC disease:** Residual abdominal implants are more than 2 cm in diameter or there is involvement of retroperitoneal or inguinal lymph nodes (or both).

Survival of patients for stage III disease is correlated with the volume of disease after initial surgery. Patients with abdominal implants larger than 2 cm in diameter have less than a 10% chance of achieving complete remission with standard chemotherapy, whereas patients with small volume disease have an approximately 40% chance of achieving complete remission with cisplatin-based chemotherapy.

b. **With stage IV ovarian cancer,** there are distant metastases. The most common sites of involvement are pleural effusions that must be cytologically positive or parenchymal liver metastases.

2. **Chemotherapy for patients with advanced disease**

a. **Choice of agents.** Standard treatment for advanced ovarian cancer consists in a combination chemotherapy regimen combining cyclophosphamide with either cisplatin or carboplatin. There is little room for single-agent alkylating drugs, and patients should be offered aggressive combination chemotherapy regimens. It has been demonstrated in prospective randomized trials that cisplatin-containing regimens are superior to regimens without cisplatin. It has also been demonstrated that the dose of platinum drugs is an important factor in achieving optimum results. High-dose cisplatin, however, is associated with significant toxicity, including nausea and vomiting, nephrotoxicity, and dose-limiting peripheral neuropathy. However, it has been demonstrated that carboplatin, a cisplatin analog whose dose-limiting toxicity is myelosuppression, produces results equivalent to those that can be achieved with cisplatin. Furthermore, carboplatin is not associated with significant nephrotoxicity or neurotoxicity, and it produces less nausea and vomiting.

b. **Recommended regimens**

(1) Cisplatin 75–100 mg/m^2 IV + cyclophosphamide 600 mg/m^2 IV *or*

(2) Carboplatin 300–350 mg/m^2 IV + cyclophosphamide 600 mg/m^2 IV.

Cycles of chemotherapy are administered every 4 weeks. Cisplatin must be given with vigorous saline diuresis (see Chapter 8).

3. **Results of chemotherapy.** Approximately 40% of women achieve a clinical complete remission with cisplatin-based chemotherapy. Response rates are higher in stage III patients who have less than 2 cm of disease. Median survival is also correlated with the stage and volume of the disease. Stage III patients overall have a median survival of approximately 24 months. Five-year survival is 20–25%.

4. **Treatment of previously treated patients with ovarian cancer.** Approximately 30–40% of patients who achieve a surgically confirmed complete remission after cisplatin-based chemotherapy relapse. Patients who have had a prior response to cisplatin-based chemotherapy have a high likelihood of responding to carboplatin as a single agent. In contrast, patients who have disease progression while on treatment with cisplatin-based regimens or who have a short disease-free interval are unlikely to respond to retreatment with platinum-based therapy. It has been demonstrated that hexamethylmelamine, ifosfamide, and taxol have activity in previously treated patients with ovarian cancer.

5. **Intraperitoneal chemotherapy.** Ovarian cancer remains confined to the peritoneal cavity, virtually throughout its entire clinical course. During the 1980s there were numerous clinical trials evaluating the efficacy and toxicity of intraperitoneal chemotherapy. Most drugs useful in the treatment of ovarian cancer have a pharmacologic advantage when administered via the intraperitoneal route, but it remains to be determined what the impact of intraperitoneal therapy is on overall survival. It has been demonstrated, however, that intraperitoneal administration of cisplatin 100–200 mg/m^2 IP or the combination of cisplatin 100 mg/m^2 IP plus etoposide 200 mg/m^2 IP on day 1 monthly for 6 months can produce objective response in previously treated patients and can be associated with long-term survival. For doses of cisplatin larger than 100 mg/m^2, special attention must be paid to minimizing renal toxicity, such as the simultaneous intravenous administration of sodium thiosulfate 4 gm/m^2 IV over 30 minutes, then 2 gm/m^2/hour IV for a total of 6 hours.

6. **Standard approach to patients with advanced ovarian cancer.** It has been demonstrated in prospective randomized trials that more than six cycles of chemotherapy with a cisplatin-based induction regimen is not beneficial. Consequently, induction chemotherapy with carboplatin (or cisplatin) plus cyclophosphamide should be administered for 6

courses. If patients have small-volume intraperitoneal residual disease, the intraperitoneal administration of cisplatin or the combination of cisplatin plus etoposide may lead to prolonged survival. However, it has not been unequivocally demonstrated that intraperitoneal chemotherapy administered in this setting is beneficial, and this form of therapy should still be considered experimental. There is no evidence that using whole-abdomen irradiation after induction chemotherapy is beneficial. Patients who have bulky residual disease left after induction chemotherapy have a poor prognosis, and there is no evidence that secondary cytoreduction prolongs survival. These patients should be offered treatment with phase II agents, e.g., hexamethylmelamine, ifosfamide, and taxol. These patients are also candidates for investigational phase I–II trials.

7. **Experimental approaches.** Clinical trials are in progress evaluating the importance of high-dose cisplatin or high-dose carboplatin. Because the dose limiting toxicity of carboplatin is myelosuppression, it is an ideal drug with which to evaluate the role of autologous bone marrow transplantation and the impact of colony-stimulating factors upon myelotoxicity. New combinations such as carboplatin + cyclophosphamide + hexamethylmelamine and combinations of carboplatin + cisplatin are also undergoing evaluation.

8. **Biologic therapy.** Biologic response modifiers such as interferon, interleukin II, and lymphokine-activated killer cells have been administered intraperitoneally in phase I–II trials in patients with advanced disease. Additional studies are evaluating the role of intraperitoneal immunotoxins and monoclonal antibody radioisotope conjugates. Although objective responses to biologic therapies have been observed, they remain investigational and are sometimes associated with significant toxicity.

9. **Dose modifications and guidelines for administration of chemotherapy**
   a. **Carboplatin.** Carboplatin is primarily excreted in the urine. Consequently, even though the drug is nonnephrotoxic and does not require aggressive hydration for administration, it has increased myelotoxicity in patients who have decreased renal function. Doses should be modified either empirically or with the use of a formula.

   In general, full doses of carboplatin can be given if the creatinine clearance (C_{cr}) is more than 60 ml/minute. If the C_{cr} is 40–60 ml/minute, give 60% of the carboplatin. If the C_{cr} is less than 20–40 ml/minute, give 40% of the carboplatin. If the C_{cr} is less than 20 ml/minute, do not give any.

   b. **Protection from nephrotoxicity.** Cisplatin, but not carboplatin, should be administered with a program of hydration and diuresis. Combinations of hypertonic saline, vigorous saline chloruresis, and mannitol have been used to ensure a brisk diuresis (see Chapter 8).

    c. Nausea and vomiting. The nausea and vomiting associated with platinum-based therapy can be managed with metoclopramide or ondansetron and dexamethasone (see Chapter 37).

II. Endometrial cancer

    A. Approach to therapy. Endometrial cancer is the result of the action of unopposed estrogens. Ninety percent of patients with endometrial cancer present with abnormal vaginal bleeding. Most patients (75–80%) are diagnosed when their disease is still confined to the uterine cavity without cervical involvement. The primary modality of treatment for endometrial cancer is total abdominal hysterectomy with bilateral salpingo-oophorectomy. Radiation therapy is frequently administered to help prevent vaginal vault recurrences and in an attempt to sterilize involved lymph nodes. Patients who present with stage II disease, where the tumor involves the corpus and the cervix but does not extend outside the uterus, have a survival rate of approximately 60%. Patients in whom the disease has extended outside the uterus but has not metastasized outside the true pelvis (stage III disease) have a 5-year survival of approximately 10%. A series of important prognostic factors, other than stage, have also been identified: age, uterine size, histologic grade, depth of myometrial invasion, hormone receptor status, and peritoneal cytology.

    It has been demonstrated that increasing tumor grade and depth of myometrial involvement are associated with increasing risk for lymph node involvement in the pelvis and the paraaortic region. Furthermore, grade and depth of myometrial penetration are also correlated with the presence of adnexal metastases, positive peritoneal cytology, local vault recurrence, and hematogenous spread. Although adjuvant irradiation has not been shown to improve survival, it has been shown to significantly decrease the incidence of vault recurrences. Patients with grade I lesions confined to the inner one third of the myometrium have such an excellent survival, however, that no adjuvant therapy is necessary. Patients with grade III tumors, more than one-third myometrial invasion, cervical extension, positive pelvic nodes, or pelvic disease outside the uterus are treated with external pelvic irradiation. Patients with grade II histology and less than one-third myometrial invasion can be treated with vault radium alone. Patients who have positive paraaortic lymph nodes are often treated with external pelvic irradiation plus extended field radiation. Whole-abdomen irradiation has been used for patients who have upper abdominal metastases that are completely resected at initial surgery.

    B. Role of systemic therapy in recurrent and metastatic disease. Hormonal therapy and cytotoxic chemotherapy have been used for palliative management of patients with recurrent disease or distant metastases.

   1. **Hormonal therapy.** Progestins are the initial treatment of choice for patients with recurrent endometrial cancer, particularly those who have positive hormone receptors. Common regimens are the following.

      a. Megestrol acetate 40–80 mg PO 4 times daily *or*

      b. Medroxyprogesterone 400–800 mg IM weekly.

      It has also been demonstrated that the antiestrogen tamoxifen 20 mg bid can produce responses in patients with endometrial cancer. Hormonal therapy appears to produce a response rate of approximately 30% in patients with metastatic endometrial cancer.

   2. **Cytotoxic chemotherapy.** Doxorubicin (Adriamycin) 60–75 mg/m^2 IV every 3 weeks has been reported to be the most active agent in patients with metastatic recurrent endometrial cancer. The overall response rate is approximately 38%, with 26% of the patients achieving a complete clinical remission. Whereas other single agents also have been shown to have activity against endometrial cancer, combination chemotherapy has not been established to be superior to single-agent treatment. Cisplatin and carboplatin have efficacy in patients with recurrent endometrial cancer.

III. **Cancer of the uterine cervix**

   A. **General considerations.** It is estimated there are approximately 13,000 new cases of invasive cervical cancer with approximately 7000 deaths annually. The primary modalities of treatment for cervical cancer have been surgery and radiotherapy. Irradiation has been used at all stages of the disease, whereas surgery is used only for patients with stage I and IIA disease. With stage I disease the carcinoma is confined to the cervix but has not extended onto the pelvic wall. With stage II disease the carcinoma can involve the vagina but not the lower third. Stage II disease is divided into stage IIA (without obvious parametrial involvement) and stage IIB (with obvious parametrial involvement). Cure rates are approximately 80% for stage I disease; 60% for stage II; 30% for stage III (the carcinoma has extended to the pelvic wall, or on rectal examination there is no cancer-free space between the tumor and the pelvic wall or the tumor involves the lower third of the vagina); and 10% for stage IV disease where the disease has spread to adjacent organs or to distant organs.

   B. **Treatment approaches.** Treatment usually consists of combination of external beam radiation to treat the regional nodes and intracavitary brachytherapy for treatment of the central tumor. Intracavitary treatment alone is used only in those patients with early stage disease who have a low incidence of lymph node metastases. Chemotherapy has been routinely used in patients who have failed primary treatment with surgery and radiation therapy. Chemotherapy responses have been difficult to evaluate in this group of patients primarily because of the decreased vascular supply to the tumor following radiation and surgery and to the frequent development of obstructive uropathy at the time of recurrence. Objective responses have also been difficult to quantitate owing to the extent of prior treatment. It has been established, however, that cisplatin 50–75 mg/m^2 IV over 30 minutes (with appropriate hydration) is an active agent in patients with recurrent cervical cancer, producing responses in approximately 20–30% of patients. It has also been demonstrated that carboplatin has activity in this disease, although compared to historical controls it does not appear to be as active as cisplatin, which remains the chemotherapeutic agent of choice in patients with advanced disease. It has been demonstrated that as the dose of cisplatin is increased beyond 50 mg/m^2 there is a concomitant increase in response rate. However, this increase is associated with increased toxicity and is not associated with prolongation of survival. Clinical trials evaluating the use of neoadjuvant cisplatin-based chemotherapy are in progress, although there is no evidence yet to suggest that such an approach prolongs survival. It has also been demonstrated that hydroxyurea is an effective radiation-sensitizing agent in this disease.

IV. **Gestational trophoblastic neoplasms (GTN).** The term GTN refers to a spectrum of diseases, including hydatidiform mole, invasive mole, and choriocarcinoma. GTNs can be cured with chemotherapy, even in the presence of widespread metastases.

   A. **Follow-up of patients with evacuation of a hydatidiform mole.** Complete moles have a potential for local invasion and distant spread. Distant metastases occurs in about 4% of patients after a molar evacuation, and local uterine invasion develops in approximately 15% of patients. The use of prophylactic chemotherapy at the time of molar evacuation is controversial. After molar evacuation, patients should be closely monitored with serum levels of the β-subunit of human chorionic gonadotropin (β-hCG) which is a sensitive and specific marker for this disease. Chemotherapy is administered when titers cease to fall or begin to rise. It is recommended that hCG levels be monitored on a weekly basis until they are normal for 3 consecutive weeks and then monthly until they are normal for 6 consecutive months.

   B. **Metastatic GTN.** Choriocarcinoma has a tendency for early vascular invasion with widespread distant metastases primarily to the lungs, vagina, and pelvis with brain and liver involvement less frequent. Patients with GTNs are staged depending on the spread and distant metastases; they are assigned to high- or low-risk groups based on other prognostic factors, such as age, antecedent pregnancy, interval between antecedent pregnancy and start of chemotherapy, hCG titer, size of tumor, number of metastases, and prior chemotherapy. Low-risk patients are those less than 39 years of age whose antecedent pregnancy was a hydatidiform mole, who had an interval of 4 months or less between the end of the antecedent pregnancy and the start of chemotherapy, and whose hCG level was less than 10^3 IU/liter.

Risk increases when the antecedent pregnancy was an abortion and, further, if the GTN follows a term birth. A longer interval between the end of pregnancy and start of chemotherapy worsens the prognosis, as does increasing tumor size and number of metastases. The site of metastasis is also important, with a progression from lung < spleen or kidney < gastrointestinal tract or liver < brain. Previous chemotherapy increases risk.

C. **Management approaches**
   1. **Stage I disease.** In patients with stage I disease there is a persistently elevated hCG level, and the tumor is confined to the uterine corpus. The management for these patients depends on whether the patient wishes to retain fertility. If fertility is not an issue, hysterectomy with adjuvant single-agent chemotherapy is administered. Single-agent chemotherapy is the preferred treatment in patients with stage I disease who desire to retain fertility.
   2. **Stage II and III disease.** Stage II disease consists in metastases to the vagina or pelvis (or both), whereas stage III disease includes patients with pulmonary metastases with or without uterine, vaginal, or pelvic involvement. Patients with low-risk disease, using the criteria described above, are treated with primary single-agent chemotherapy, and high-risk patients are managed with primary intensive combination chemotherapy.
   3. **Stage IV disease.** Stage IV disease consists in metastasis to any other site. All patients with stage IV disease should be treated with primary intensive combination chemotherapy plus selective application of radiation therapy and surgery. Radiation therapy should be administered to patients with brain metastases to decrease the risk of intracranial hemorrhage. Cures have been reported in excess of 75% in high-risk patients, and even patients with brain metastases can be cured.
   4. **Chemotherapy**
      a. **Single-agent chemotherapy** with either dactinomycin or methotrexate is adequate for low-risk patients. The dactinomycin can be administered in a dose of 0.40–0.45 mg/m² IV on days 1–5 every 2–3 weeks. Methotrexate, when used as a single agent, can be administered in doses of 11–19 mg/m² IV or IM on days 1–5 every 2–3 weeks. Chemotherapy should be continued for 1–2 cycles beyond undetectable titers of β-hCG in the blood.

Excellent results with minimal toxicity in non-metastatic and low-risk metastatic GTNs may be achieved with the combination

Methotrexate 40 mg/m^2 IM on days 1, 3, 5, 7 *and Leucovorin* 4 mg/m^2 IM on days 2, 4, 6, 8.

A second course is given if the β-HCG plateaus for 3 consecutive weeks, becomes reelevated, or does not fall by 1 log within 18 days of the first treatment. When the level is normal for 3 consecutive weeks, the patient may be considered to be in a remission. β-hCG levels should be followed monthly for 6 months and every 2 months through 1 year from the end of therapy. If the β-HCG remains normal at this time, the likelihood for a recurrence is low. Many recommend obtaining β-HCG titers every 3 months during the second year and at 6-month intervals indefinitely thereafter. Patients must be advised not to become pregnant for at least 1 year after remission begins.

b. Combination chemotherapy regimens for medium- or high-risk patients are as follows.

(1) MAC III (for medium-risk patients)

Days	Drug
1,3,5,7	Methotrexate 40 mg/m^2 IV
1,3,5	Dactinomycin 0.45 mg/m^2 IV (not to exceed 1.0 mg)
1,3,5	Cyclophosphamide 110 mg/m^2 IV
2,4,6,8	Leucovorin 4 mg/m^2 IM (24 hours after the methotrexate)

Repeat course in 14–17 days. Continue treatment for 10–14 weeks after β-HCG value is normal.

(2) EMA CO (for high risk patients)

Course 1: EMA

Day 1:   Etoposide 100 mg/m^2 IV infusion in 200 ml of saline over 30 minutes
Dactinomycin 0.5 mg IV push
Methotrexate 100 mg/m^2 IV push followed by 200 mg/m^2 IV infusion over 12 hours

Day 2:   Etoposide 100 mg/m^2 IV infusion in 200 ml of saline over 30 minutes
Dactinomycin 0.5 mg IV push
Leucovorin 15 mg IM, IV, or PO every 12 hours for 4 doses beginning 24 hours after the start of the methotrexate

Course 2: CO

Day 8:   Vincristine 1.0 mg/m^2 IV push

Cyclophosphamide 600 mg/m^2
IV rapid infusion in saline
Methotrexate 15 mg intra-
thecally

Repeat with course 1 starting again on day 15 unless the white blood cell (WBC) count is less than 2000/µl, platelets are less than 100,000/µl, or there is severe mucositis. The fall in serum β-hCG should be 1 log or more with each course of treatment. Course 1 requires overnight hospitalization. Therapy is continued for at least 10 weeks after β-hCG is undetectable or the projected level of β-hCG is less than 10^{-4} IU/liter.

V. Vulvar cancer. This tumor represents about 4% of cancers of the female genital tract. The primary treatment modality is surgery, with the extent of the dissection based on individual characteristics. Radiation therapy is being applied more frequently in patients with vulvar cancer. Responses to chemotherapy have been reported. Among the active agents are doxorubicin (Adriamycin), bleomycin, and cisplatin.

VI. Germ cell and gonadal stromal tumors of the ovary

    A. Germ cell tumors. Germ cell malignancies account for fewer than 5% of ovarian cancers in the United States. Dysgerminoma is the most common malignant germ cell tumor. Most patients with dysgerminomas have stage I disease. Although most germ cell tumors are rarely bilateral, dysgerminoma has a 10–15% incidence of bilaterality. Treatment consists in resecting the primary lesion. When fertility is an issue, a unilateral salpingo-oophorectomy can be performed. This tumor is sensitive to radiation therapy, although it has been demonstrated that metastatic dysgerminomas can be successfully treated with systemic chemotherapy. The treatment regimen of choice is the BEP regimen.

Bleomycin 30 units IV push on days 2, 9, 16
Etoposide 100 mg/m^2 IV over 30 minutes on days 1–5
Cisplatin (Platinol) 20 mg/m^2 IV over 15–30 minutes on days 1-5

Repeat cycle every 3 weeks for four cycles, regardless of the granulocyte count. If the patient has fever associated with granulocytopenia (ANC < 1000/µl), or significant bleeding with a platelet count of less than 50,000/µl, reduce the next dose by 25%.

Patients who present with immature teratomas can be treated with unilateral salpingo-oophorectomy, as contralateral involvement is rare. In patients with a stage IA grade I lesion, there is no evidence that chemotherapy is beneficial. However, patients with stage IA and grade II and III tumors should receive chemotherapy with the BEP regimen.

Similarly, patients who have endodermal sinus tumors should be treated with unilateral salpingo-oophorectomy and removal of gross disease. All patients

with endodermal sinus tumors should receive adjuvant chemotherapy with the BEP regimen. Most patients with disseminated germ cell tumors can now be cured with this effective combination chemotherapy regimen.
B. Sex cord stromal tumors. This group of tumors includes granulosa cell tumors, thecomas, and fibromas. Granulosa cell tumors are frequently estrogen-secreting and associated with endometrial cancer and endometrial hyperplasia. Most patients are treated with surgery alone, and there is no evidence that adjuvant chemotherapy prevents recurrence of disease. Metastatic lesions and recurrences have been treated with a variety of combinations, such as the PAC regimen.

Cisplatin 50 mg/m^2 IV over 30–60 minutes or 20 mg/m^2 IV daily × 5) *and*

Doxorubicin 50 mg/m^2 IV side arm through rapidly running IV infusion *and*

Cyclophosphamide 750 mg/m^2 IV push or over 15 minutes.

Cycles are repeated every 3–4 weeks.
Other active agents are vincristine and dactinomycin.

Selected Reading

Bagshawe, K. D. Treatment of high-risk choriocarcinoma. *J. Reproduct. Med.* 29:813, 1984.

Berkowitz, R. S. Gestational trophoblastic tumors and malignant ovarian germ cell tumors. *Curr. Opin. Oncol.* 1:119, 1983.

Hainsworth, J. D., et al. Advanced ovarian cancer: long-term results of treatment with intensive cisplatin-based chemotherapy of brief duration. *Ann. Intern. Med.* 108:165, 1988.

Hamilton, T. C., Ozols, R. F., and Longo, D. L. Biologic therapy for the treatment of malignant common epithelial tumors of the ovary. *Cancer* 60:2054, 1987.

Howell, S. B., et al. Long-term survival of advanced refractory ovarian carcinoma patients with small-volume disease treated with intraperitoneal chemotherapy. *J. Clin. Oncol.* 5:1607, 1987.

Levin, L., and Hryniuk, W. M. Dose intensity analysis of chemotherapy regimens in ovarian carcinoma. *J. Clin. Oncol.* 5:756, 1987.

Neijt, J. P., et al. Randomized trial comparing two combination chemotherapy regimens (CHAP-5 v CP) in advanced ovarian carcinoma. *J. Clin. Oncol.* 5:1157, 1987.

Omura, G. A., et al. Randomized trial of cyclophosphamide plus cisplatin with or without doxorubicin in ovarian carcinoma: a Gynecologic Oncology Group study. *J. Clin. Oncol.* 7:457, 1989.

Ozols, R. F., and Young, R. C. Ovarian cancer. In C. M. Haskell (ed.), *Current Problems in Cancer.* Chicago: Year Book Medical Publishers, 1987. Pp. 59–112.

Reichman, B., et al. Intraperitoneal cisplatin and etoposide in the treatment of refractory/recurrent ovarian carcinoma. *J. Clin. Oncol.* 7:1327, 1989.

Rozencweig, M., et al. Randomized trials of carboplatin versus cisplatin in advanced ovarian cancer. In P. A. Bunn Jr. et al. (eds.), *Carboplatin: Current Perspectives and Future Directions.* Philadelphia: Saunders, 1990. Pp. 175–186.

Williams, S. D., et al. Cisplatin, vinblastine, and bleomycin in advanced and recurrent ovarian germ-cell tumors. *Ann. Intern. Med.* 111:22, 1989.

Young, R. C., et al. Adjuvant therapy in stage I and stage II epithelial ovarian cancer. *N. Engl. J. Med.* 322:1021, 1990.

Young, R. C., et al. Staging laparotomy in early ovarian cancer. *J.A.M.A.* 250:3072, 1983.

Urologic and Male Genital Malignancies

William D. DeWys

Cancers arising in the urinary and male genital systems represent a broad spectrum of biologic behavior and responsiveness to therapy. With cancer of the bladder a major objective is management of local recurrence and local invasion. With testicular or prostatic cancer a major challenge is treatment of disease metastatic to the lymph nodes and distant sites.

The spectrum of response to medical therapy ranges from a low rate of partial response of cancer of the kidney to a high rate of complete remission and cure of testicular cancer. With kidney cancer medical therapy has no impact on average survival, although it may provide symptomatic benefit for the limited number of patients who respond to therapy. With testicular cancer, treatment provides a cure in most patients.

I. Carcinoma of the kidney

A. General considerations and aims of therapy. Cancer may arise from the parenchyma of the kidney or from the transitional cell lining of the collecting system. [The behavior and response to therapy of the latter are similar to those seen with carcinoma of the bladder (see **II,** below).] Carcinomas arising from the parenchyma of the kidney include adenocarcinomas or undifferentiated carcinomas. The term hypernephroma is sometimes used because the histologic structure resembles the cortical tissue of the adrenal gland, but this term is a misnomer.

Localized cancers are best treated by radical nephrectomy (includes removal of perinephric fat). In patients with bilateral cancer localized to the kidney, partial nephrectomy may be considered instead of bilateral radical nephrectomy and dialysis or kidney transplant. Metastatic disease, e.g., a limited number of lung nodules, if localized, may also be surgically resected. Kidney cell cancers are relatively radioresistant. Postoperative irradiation does not improve the results of surgery, but palliative irradiation of a bleeding or painful kidney or painful metastases is sometimes worthwhile. Patients with inoperable metastatic disease should be considered candidates for therapy with biologic agents, chemotherapy, or hormonal therapy.

B. Treatment regimens

1. Biologic response modifiers

a. Interleukin 2 (IL-2) alone or with lymphokine activated killer (LAK) cells, although available in only a limited number of centers, has resulted in tumor regressions in 15–30% of patients treated. Some of these responses have been complete and long-lasting. Responses correlate with IL-2 dose, performance status, prior nephrectomy, and small tumor burden.

    b. Interferon (recombinant leukocyte or human lymphoblastoid interferon) has produced regressions in 15–20% of treated patients. Doses of more than 10×10^6 units daily are required for maximum response. Average response duration is 8–10 months. Response does not seem to vary with interferon type but does correlate with prior nephrectomy, good performance status, long disease-free interval, and lung-dominant disease.

  2. Cytotoxic chemotherapy. The choices include the following.

    a. Vinblastine 5–6 mg/m² IV weekly *or*

    b. Lomustine 130 mg/m² PO every 6 weeks.

Either produces responses in 10–20% of patients. The major dose-limiting toxicity of either of these drugs is hematologic, and if the white blood cell (WBC) count is less than 3000/µl or the platelet count is less than 100,000/µl, treatment should be delayed until recovery to these values.

  3. Hormonal therapy. Progesterone was initially reported to give partial remissions in 15% of patients, but subsequent studies suggest that the response rate may be lower. Tamoxifen, an antiestrogen, produces partial remission in about 5% of patients, and an additional 20% have temporary stabilization of disease. Therapy choices include the following.

    a. Medroxyprogesterone acetate (Depo-Provera) 800 mg IM weekly *or*

    b. Megestrol acetate (Megace) 160 mg PO daily *or*

    c. Tamoxifen 10 mg PO bid.

C. Complications of therapy. Complications of IL-2 and LAK include fever and a capillary leak syndrome that results in increased interstitial water in the lungs and respiratory distress. This situation usually requires management in an intensive care unit. Interferon may cause nausea, anorexia, fatigue, myalgia, headache, and fever.

    Complications of cytotoxic therapy include nausea, which can usually be controlled with antiemetics. Vinblastine may cause mucosal toxicity or myalgias, such as jaw pain, both of which can be managed with dose adjustments. Lomustine may cause pulmonary fibrosis related to cumulative doses in the range of 1 gm/m². If this cumulative dose is reached, periodic monitoring of the pulmonary diffusing capacity is suggested.

    Hormonal therapy is usually free from side effects other than the occasional fluid retention that occurs with progestins. With tumors of other sites, tamoxifen has precipitated endocrine manifestations of malignancy, and these manifestations may possibly occur with renal cell carcinoma. If an endocrine manifestation develops, e.g., hypercalcemia, hormonal therapy should be temporarily discontinued and the endocrine manifestation managed symptomatically followed by cautious reimplementation of the hormonal therapy.

II. Bladder cancer

A. General considerations and aims of therapy.
Cancer of the bladder is usually transitional cell carcinoma. Infrequently, squamous cell carcinoma or adenocarcinoma develops, but these rare cell types are outside the scope of this text. Planning treatment for bladder cancer must take into account the anatomic stage (0, A–D), the histologic grade (I–IV), and the tumor location within the bladder (related to selection of partial or total cystectomy).

1. **Superficial stage, low-grade tumors.** At one end of the spectrum of bladder cancer is carcinoma above the lamina propria (stage 0), through the lamina propria but still confined to the mucosa (stage A), or invading the superficial muscle layer (stage B_1), which can usually be treated with transurethral resection and fulguration. However, these patients are at risk of local recurrence of their cancers and of developing additional primary tumors in the bladder. This risk may be reduced by administration of intravesical chemotherapy. Diffuse carcinoma in situ may also be treated with intravesical chemotherapy.

2. **Deep stage, high-grade tumors.** Patients with tumors that inhibit deeper invasion (more than one half of the muscle layer = stage B_2; into perivesical fat = stage C) or high grade (III and IV), or both, are usually best managed with a combination of chemotherapy, radiation therapy, and surgery. Chemotherapy or radiation therapy may be given before or after surgery.

3. **Advanced and metastatic tumors.** Patients with local recurrence beyond the scope of surgery or radiation therapy and patients with metastases are candidates for systemic chemotherapy. This therapy may achieve complete remission and prolongation of survival, or partial remission with less effect on the duration of survival.

B. Treatment regimens and evaluation of response

1. **Intravesical chemotherapy**

   a. **Method of administration and follow-up.** Intravesical therapy is administered in a volume of 40–50 ml through a Foley catheter. The catheter is clamped for 1 hour and then emptied. This procedure delivers a high local concentration to the tumor area. Patients with superficial bladder cancers require lifelong surveillance with periodic cystoscopy (initially every 3 months, then every 6 months, then annually) because even with intravesical chemotherapy an increased risk of developing new primary tumors persists. Patients being treated for diffuse in situ carcinoma should have biopsy confirmation of a return of normal mucosa after a course of instillation ther-

apy. They also require lifelong cystoscopic surveillance.

**b. Selection of patients for intravesical ther-
apy.** Because only superficial tumor cells are
being treated, stage B_2 and C disease should
undergo more aggressive therapy, e.g., surgery or
irradiation. Also, grades III and IV indicate
more aggressive disease and should usually undergo more aggressive treatment than intravesical
therapy. Three possible objectives for intravesical
therapy are as follows.

  (1) Prevention of relapse in stages 0, A, and
  B_1 and grades I and II treated with transurethral resection (TUR). Tumor cells remaining in situ after TUR can grow to produce a relapse.

  **(2) Prevention of occurrence of new blad-
  der tumors.** Patients with two or more previously resected bladder tumors should be
  treated in an effort to prevent further development of new tumors.

  (3) Carcinoma in situ. Tumors in this category may involve the bladder diffusely and
  thus be beyond the scope of TUR, but they may
  be eradicated by intravesical therapy. Doxorubicin or bacillus Calmette-Guérin (BCG)
  results in complete clearance in 60–70% of
  cases.

c. Specific intravesical therapeutic regimens
include the following.

  (1) Thiotepa 30–60 mg weekly for 3–6 weeks,
  then every 3 weeks for 5 cycles *or*

  (2) Mitomycin 30–40 mg weekly for 4–8 weeks,
  then monthly for 6 months *or*

  (3) Doxorubicin (Adriamycin) 50–60 mg weekly
  for 4 weeks, then every 3–4 weeks for 6
  cycles, with dose escalation to 90 mg if there
  is no response and no toxicity *or*

  (4) Bacillus Calmette-Guérin 120 mg of lyophi-
  lized BCG weekly for 6 weeks. (Concomitant
  percutaneous BCG given in the initial studies may not be necessary.)

d. Selection of therapy. Selection between the
listed options must be based on reported response
rates for the individual agents, costs (Table 15-1),
toxicity, and the results of comparative trials.
Systemic absorption and systemic toxicity may be
seen with thiotepa and BCG administration. One
comparative trial has shown BCG (0% recurrence) to be more effective than thiotepa (46% recurrence), and another study has shown no difference between thiotepa and mitomycin C.

e. Response to therapy. Intravesical therapy causes
complete regression of small residual bladder tumors in about 40% of patients. When superficial

Table 15-1. Response to and costs of intravesical chemotherapy

Drug	Complete response	Partial response	Drug costs/treatment
Thiotepa	29	26	Low
Doxorubicin (Adriamycin)	38	35	Medium
Mitomycin	48	26	High
BCG	56	18	Low

Source: Lamm, D. L. Intravesical therapy of superficial cancer. In *AUA Update Series* (Vol. 2). Lesson 20, 1983.

bladder tumors have been completely resected, a postoperative course of intravesical chemotherapy can be expected to decrease the risk of subsequent relapse of bladder tumors by more than 50%, compared to a group not receiving intravesical therapy. In patients who have had two or more bladder tumors, intravesical therapy can be expected to decrease the risk of subsequent tumors.

   2. Adjuvant chemotherapy. Chemotherapy has been given pre- or postoperatively to patients with deeply invasive tumors or positive lymph nodes. Patients so treated may have delays in time to relapse and an improvement in overall survival, but the optimal timing and specifics of adjuvant chemotherapy are still under study.

   3. Systemic chemotherapy for advanced disease
      a. Active drugs. Drugs that have definite activity against bladder cancer include fluorouracil, cyclophosphamide, doxorubicin (Adriamycin), cisplatin, vinblastine, and methotrexate. Of them, cisplatin is probably the most active single agent, and together cisplatin, doxorubicin, vinblastine, and methotrexate (M-VAC) may be the most effective combination.

      b. Specific regimens to consider are the following.
         (1) Vinblastine 3–4 mg/m^2 + methotrexate 30–40 mg/m^2 IV weekly.
         (2) Cisplatin 60–100 mg/m^2 IV + doxorubicin 40–60 mg/m^2 IV + cyclophosphamide 400–600 mg/m^2 IV. Repeat every 3–4 weeks.
         (3) Cisplatin 40–60 mg/m^2 IV every 3 weeks (see diuresis regimen in Chapter 8).
         (4) Doxorubicin 60 mg/m^2 IV every 3 weeks.
         (5) Cyclophosphamide 1 gm/m^2 IV every 3 weeks.
         (6) Fluorouracil 500 mg/m^2 IV weekly.
         (7) M-VAC combination. This combination has been shown to be superior to cisplatin alone in a comparative trial.

Methotrexate 30 mg/m² on day 1 *and*
Vinblastine 3 mg/m² on day 2 *and*
Doxorubicin 30 mg/m² on day 2 *and*
Cisplatin 70 mg/m² on day 2 (+ 12.5 gm mannitol).

Repeat methotrexate and vinblastine on days 15 and 22 if blood counts permit.
Repeat cycle every 28 days.

c. **Response to therapy.** The M-VAC combination may be expected to produce responses (complete plus partial) in 60–70% of patients treated. The expected toxicity may be severe and must be weighed against the expected benefits when selecting of therapy. Response is more likely in previously untreated patients, but patients who respond to single-agent therapy have a good chance of responding to subsequent combination therapy. In an adjuvant setting, preoperative chemotherapy seems to improve recurrence-free survival and overall survival when compared to historical controls undergoing surgery or surgery plus radiation therapy. A randomized study of postoperative chemotherapy (cisplatin + doxorubicin + and cyclophosphamide) has shown an improvement in time to progression and in survival (4.2 years versus 2.4 years).

Response to any of the regimens is monitored by periodic measurement of tumor masses with the expectation that most patients who respond will show improvement by 6 weeks of therapy. If a patient fails to respond to one therapeutic trial, a second trial using one of the other regimens listed should be considered. However, if a patient has two successive failures, a response to any subsequent therapy is unlikely.

C. **Complications of therapy**
   1. **Intravesical therapy.** Some patients experience local discomfort, but it does not usually limit therapy. Local fibrosis may develop after repeated instillations of thiotepa, but fibrosis is infrequent if therapy is limited to the eight instillations recommended above. Some of the administered thiotepa may be absorbed systemically and may cause bone marrow toxicity. Blood counts should be monitored before each instillation and treatment delayed if the counts have decreased significantly. Because mitomycin and doxorubicin are large molecules, systemic absorption has not been a problem. Alkylating agents, e.g., thiotepa, are known to increase the risk of second malignancies. This risk is another reason for limiting the number of instillations, as outlined above.
   2. **Systemic therapy.** The major dose-limiting toxic manifestation of cisplatin is renal damage. This damage usually can be prevented by vigorous hydra-

tion and chloride diuresis, but serum creatinine should be checked before each dose. The other drugs listed cause marrow toxicity requiring periodic blood counts and dose adjustments. Doxorubicin may cause cardiac damage, but the incidence of a clinically important degree of cardiac damage is less than 10% if the total cumulative dose is less than 550 mg/m².

III. Prostatic cancer

A. General considerations and aims of therapy.
Selection of therapy for prostatic cancer is based on the extent of disease and the patient's general medical condition and age. In some patients cancer is an incidental histologic finding in a specimen removed by TUR for what was clinically thought to be benign hypertrophy (stage A). If only a few chips are involved and the tumor is well differentiated (stage A_1), no further therapy is needed. If multiple chips are involved or if the tumor is poorly differentiated (stage A_2), or both, there is a significant likelihood of residual or recurrent cancer, and additional therapy such as radical prostatectomy or high-dose radiation therapy should be considered.

For patients with a palpable nodule but no extension outside the prostate (stage B), radical prostatectomy or high-dose radiation therapy are treatment options with equal effectiveness. The choice between the two treatments can be based on patient age, general medical condition, patient preference, and a comparison of side effects, such as the trauma of surgery versus diarrhea secondary to radiation therapy. Patients with local extension beyond the prostate (stage C) are usually best treated with high-dose (70 Gy) radiation therapy.

Patients with metastases may be treated with palliative radiation therapy, hormonal therapy, or chemotherapy. The aim is maximum relief of symptoms with the least toxicity. Asymptomatic patients with metastases can have treatment delayed until symptoms develop with no decrease in likelihood of benefit from therapy.

B. Treatment of symptomatic metastatic disease

1. Hormonal therapy is usually the first therapy for symptomatic metastatic prostatic cancer, and 75% of patients treated with hormonal therapy experience subjective response lasting an average of more than 2 years. Most of these responders also have objective evidence of response. The choice among hormonal options can be based on desired rapidity of response, patient preference, existing medical conditions, and expected duration of response. Concentrations of androgen receptors in the cytoplasm of prostatic cancer cells do not correlate with the response to endocrine therapy, but nuclear androgen receptors may have some predictive value.

a. Orchiectomy. When rapid response is required, such as with spinal cord compression, orchiectomy is often the treatment of choice. It is also preferred by some patients because it avoids the nuisance of daily medication and may require less frequent follow-up visits.

b. Estrogen. This therapy is of great historical significance but is used infrequently today. Patients who have had previous thromboembolic disease or congestive heart failure probably should not receive estrogens, which may exacerbate these conditions. If the patient is to receive estrogens, 5 Gy to the breast area is recommended prior to estrogen therapy to prevent the development of painful gynecomastia. The usual agent for estrogen administration is diethylstilbestrol (DES). The dose used must strike a balance between that adequate to suppress testosterone levels (about 3 mg daily) and the concern about an increased risk of cardiovascular problems that have been observed at DES doses of 5 mg daily. Studies in an animal model suggest that castrate levels of testosterone are not required for response. A 1 mg/day dose of DES probably is adequate for most older patients, but for young patients with higher baseline testosterone levels and less risk of cardiovascular effects, a dose of 3–5 mg/day may be considered.

c. Luteinizing hormone-releasing hormone (LHRH) analogs. After an initial brief increase in serum testosterone, these agents suppress testosterone to castrate levels. Agents initially available required daily subcutaneous injection, but depot forms requiring monthly injections are now available. Treatment regimens are as follows.

(1) Leuprolide (Leupron) 1.0 mg SQ daily.

(2) Leuprolide (Lupron) depot 7.5 mg IM monthly.

(3) Goserelin (Zoladex) depot 3.6 mg SQ monthly.

In controlled trials these agents have produced responses and survival equal to those seen with DES 3 mg/day but with less risk of nausea, edema, and thromboembolism. Disadvantages of this approach include "hot flashes," which occur in more than half of patients so treated, and temporary increases in bone pain and obstructive symptoms at the start of therapy, both of which presumably are due to the initial rise in testosterone and cost.

d. LHRH analogs plus antiandrogen. A trial comparing the LHRH analog leuprolide 1.0 mg/day SQ to the analog plus the antiandrogen flutamide 250 mg tid has shown a 2.4 month longer progression-free survival and a 7 month longer survival for the combination. Combinations of this type are now thought by many oncologists to be the initial treatment of choice for most patients with symptomatic metastatic prostatic cancer.

      e. Numerous second-line hormonal therapies have been tried, including adrenalectomy, hypophysectomy, antiandrogens, progestins, and adrenal suppressants. There are generally fewer than 20% objective regressions, and most of these responses have been of short duration. Some have suggested addition of the adrenal suppressant aminoglutethemide to the LHRH + antiandrogen combination at the time of relapse, but this suggestion requires further study.

   2. Cytotoxic chemotherapy. If patients relapse or fail to respond to hormonal therapy, they should be considered for cytotoxic chemotherapy.

      a. The drug of choice is doxorubicin (Adriamycin) 60 mg/m^2 IV every 3 weeks. Patients who have received extensive radiation therapy should initially receive 40–50 mg/m^2 with subsequent escalation to 60 mg/m^2 if the initial dose is well tolerated. This drug has resulted in objective remissions in 25% of patients and in increased survival compared to fluorouracil. However, in previously treated patients given reduced doses, doxorubicin has been relatively less effective.

      b. Evaluation of response is often difficult because easily measured disease is frequently not present. However, a marker is usually present (prostate-specific antigen, prostatic acid phosphatase, alkaline phosphatase, lactic dehydrogenase, or carcinoembryonic antigen) that may provide an indicator of response. Later, reduction in the extent of disease may be seen on bone scan or x-ray film. The alkaline phosphatase level must be interpreted with care, realizing that an increasing level may reflect either increasing disease or healing of bone in response to tumor regression.

      c. Alternate regimens. If the patient fails on doxorubicin or there is a contraindication to its use, alternate regimens include the following.

         (1) Cyclophosphamide 1 gm/m^2 IV every 3 weeks *or*

         (2) Fluorouracil 500 mg/m^2 IV weekly *or*

         (3) Methotrexate 40 mg/m^2 IV weekly *or*

         (4) Cisplatin 40 mg/m^2 every 3 weeks.

      Combinations of drugs have been studied, but none is clearly better than doxorubicin as a single drug.

C. Complications of therapy. All hormonal therapies cause decreased libido and decreased potency. Orchiectomy may cause local surgical complications such as hematoma. Estrogen therapy may cause fluid retention and an increased risk of thromboembolic events. LHRH analogs may cause an initial flare of disease and frequently produce "hot flashes." The side effects of doxorubicin include mucositis, marrow suppression, and cardiotoxicity ($< 10\%$ at a cumulative dose of < 550 mg/m^2).

IV. Testicular cancer

A. General considerations and aims of therapy.
Because testicular cancer occurs most frequently during the third and fourth decades of life, its impact in terms of potential years of life lost is greater than that of other, more common cancers that occur primarily in older people. Fortunately, curative therapy is possible even for advanced disease. The strategy for cure must take into account the histology and stage of the disease. It is useful for this discussion to divide staging into clinical and surgical stages (Table 15-2). This distinction between clinical and surgical staging is necessary because the sensitivity and specificity of the noninvasive staging procedures are only 80–85%. For example, a patient may be judged clinically to have stage I disease but on surgical staging be found to have histologic involvement of retroperitoneal lymph nodes.

B. Treatment strategies.
Selection of therapy for testicular cancer after radical inguinal orchiectomy and appropriate staging is based on histologic type and stage.

1. **Seminoma** is usually not staged surgically, and stage I and non-bulky stage II (nodes < 5 cm) are treated with radiation therapy. For clinical stage I, radiation therapy is directed to a retroperitoneal field because the risk of involvement of retroperitoneal nodes is about 20%, even when the lymphangiogram is negative. For clinical stage II, nonbulky disease (nodal mass width < 5 cm), radiation is given to encompass the involved nodes. Radiation to the mediastinum and supraclavicular nodes is now of historical interest only, as it does not significantly enhance the cure rate and compromises chemotherapy in patients who relapse after radiation therapy. Bulky stage II and all stage III seminomas are usually best treated with combination chemotherapy (see **IV.C**, below).

2. **Nonseminoma** (embryonal cell carcinoma, teratocarcinoma, and mixed types). For these cell types with clinical stage I or nonbulky stage II (nodes < 5 cm), the therapeutic plan may include surgical staging of the retroperitoneal lymph nodes, or a nonsurgical strategy may be chosen. For all patients after initial treatment, frequent monitoring (every month for 1 year, then every 2 months for 1 year) is recommended including physical examination, chest x-ray film, and serum markers: (β-subunit of human chorionic gonadotropin (β-hCG), α-fetoprotein (AFP), and lactic dehydrogenase (LDH)). If any of these markers becomes abnormal, the patient should be fully evaluated and treated.

   a. **With surgical staging.** If patients undergo retroperitoneal node dissection (a nerve-sparing approach is preferred if feasible to preserve ejaculation) for staging, subsequent treatment may be based on the results of this staging. If the retroperitoneal nodes are negative, the risk of re-

Table 15-2. Clinical and surgical staging of testicular cancer

Stage	Definition	Clinical findings	Surgical findings
I	Limited to testis	Lymphangiogram and CT scan negative	Retroperitoneal nodes histologically negative
II	Spread to nodes below diaphragm	Lymphangiogram or CT scan positive	Nodes histologically positive
III	Spread beyond retroperitoneal nodes	Positive chest radiograph, liver CT scan	Same as clinical findings or serum markers positive after testis and retroperitoneal nodes removed

current disease is about 10%; the patient may be followed with frequent monitoring (see above), with the expectation that promptly detected relapse may be cured with subsequent chemotherapy. If the nodes are positive and all nodes have been removed, the risk of recurrence is about 50%; most oncologists advise two cycles of chemotherapy (see **IV.C,** below) with an expected nearly 100% cure rate. Other oncologists recommend frequent monitoring, with chemotherapy given at the time of relapse; this regimen is associated with a cure rate that is not significantly lower than that seen with immediate chemotherapy, and 50% of patients are spared chemotherapy. Alternatively, one may divide these patients into a low-risk group (histology predominantly teratoma, < 5 nodes involved, and all nodes < 2 cm in diameter) for frequent monitoring and a high-risk group (histology predominantly embryonal, > 5 nodes involved, any node > 2 cm in diameter) to be managed with adjuvant chemotherapy.

b. Without surgical staging

(1) A subgroup of stage I patients can be identified whose risk of recurrence after orchiectomy and without node dissection is about 15%. These patients may be managed with frequent monitoring and be spared node dissection and chemotherapy. Patients must meet all of these criteria—no vascular invasion in the testicular tumor, no extension along the spermatic cord, CT scan *and* lymphangiogram negative, and all markers return to normal after orchiectomy—and must be reliable in adhering to the monitoring schedule.

(2) A subgroup of patients who would be treated with chemotherapy after lymphadenectomy may be spared lymphadenectomy and begin chemotherapy immediately after orchiectomy. Patients should meet one or more of the following criteria: vascular invasion in the testicular tumor, tumor extension along the spermatic cord, or CT scan or lymphangiogram clearly showing abnormal retroperitoneal lymph nodes. The number of cycles of chemotherapy (three or four) is based on the bulk of the disease (see **IV.C,** below). These patients are reassessed after chemotherapy, including repeat CT scans and x-ray films of the abdomen to visualize retained lymphangiogram contrast material in the lymph nodes. They are considered candidates for surgical removal of any residual tumor.

c. Bulky stage II and all stage III disease. Mangement includes a choice among various chemotherapy combinations and durations based on the bulk of disease. Disease that persists after four cycles of chemotherapy should be completely excised, if possible. Salvage chemotherapy should be used if there is residual viable tumor in the resected tissue or if relapse occurs after the initial chemotherapy.

C. **Combination chemotherapy.** The number of cycles of chemotherapy is based on tumor bulk and includes 2 cycles for adjuvant (postoperative) chemotherapy, 3 cycles for minimal disease stage II and III disease (tumor masses < 2 cm), and 4 cycles for moderate bulk stage II (retroperitoneal nodes 2–10 cm transversely) and moderate bulk stage III patients (lung nodules 2–5 cm and no liver, bone, or brain metastases). Massive stage II and III (including retroperitoneal nodes > 10 cm transversely; lung nodules > 5 cm or respiratory insufficiency; or liver, bone, or brain metastases) may also require more aggressive combination chemotherapy than is used for less bulky disease (see **C.2,** below).

1. **Standard treatment regimens.** Although several drug combinations have been developed that have equal efficacy, one combination seems preferable to the others based on ease of outpatient administration and less toxicity.

Cisplatin 20 mg/m^2 IV over 30 minutes daily on days 1–5 *and*

Etoposide 100 mg/m^2 IV over 45 minutes on days 1–5 *and*

Bleomycin 30 units IV push weekly on days 2, 9, 16.

Repeat every 3 weeks.

Therapy is not delayed and doses are not reduced because of leukopenia. If the patient has fever associated with granulocytopenia (absolute neutrophil count < 1000/μl) or significant bleeding with a platelet count of less than 50,000/μl, reduce the next dose by 25%. (Consider omitting bleomycin during the fourth cycle because of the risk of pulmonary toxicity.)

2. **Aggressive combination chemotherapy.** Patients with bulky stage II and III disease (including retroperitoneal nodes > 10 cm transversely; lung nodules > 5 cm or respiratory insufficiency; or liver, bone, or brain metastases) do poorly on standard chemotherapy and should be considered for more aggressive therapy such as the following regimen.

Cisplatin 20 mg/m^2 IV over 30 minutes on days 1–5 *and*

Etoposide 75 mg/m^2 IV over 45 minutes on days 1–5 *and*

Ifosfamide 1200 mg/m^2 IV over 30 minutes on days 1–5, with bladder protection using mesna 120 mg/m^2 just before ifosfamide and 1200 mg/m^2 continuous infusion each day until 16 hours after last dose of ifosfamide.

Repeat every 3 weeks.

3. **Surgery for residual disease.** Patients who have not achieved complete remission after 4 cycles of chemotherapy should undergo complete surgical resection of residual disease. If this surgery reveals fibrous tissue or mature teratoma, no further chemotherapy is given, and follow-up is as in **IV.C.4,** below. Patients who undergo resection of viable tumor, those who have unresectable residual tumor (even if histology shows benign teratoma, fibrosis, or necrosis), and those who fail to respond to initial therapy should receive salvage chemotherapy (see **IV.C.5,** below). Patients who had incomplete resection of benign teratoma, fibrosis, or necrosis may later have tumor progression.

4. **Follow-up.** Patients who are in complete remission at the conclusion of 4 cycles receive no further chemotherapy and are followed at monthly intervals for 1 year, then every 2 months for 2 years with physical examination, serum markers, chest x-ray film, and other tests based on the initial extent of disease. The opposite testis should be examined closely because of a 1% risk of contralateral cancer.

5. **Second-line or salvage chemotherapy.** Second line chemotherapy involves use of a combination of drugs, including cisplatin and ifosfamide, and either etoposide or vinblastine, based on the patient's prior treatment. If a patient had received the standard treatment shown above and then relapsed, he could be treated with the following regimen.

Vinblastine 0.2 mg/kg IVP on day 1 *and*
Ifosfamide 1200 mg/m^2 IV over 30 minutes on days 1–5, with mesna as shown above *and*
Cisplatin 20 mg/m^2 IV over 30 minutes on days 1–5, with hydration.

Repeat every three weeks.

D. **Prognosis.** With the strategy given, we can summarize progress in the therapy of nonseminomatous testicular cancer as follows.

	Cure rate (%)	
Stage	**1970s**	**1990s**
I	90	> 98
II	50	> 95
III	10	> 80

E. **Complications.** The toxicity from the combinations listed in **IV.C.1, IV.C.2,** and **IV.C.5,** is formidable but generally acceptable because of the young age of the patients (mean age 25 years) and the clear-cut benefits. Toxicities include nausea and vomiting, mucositis, granulocytopenic fevers, kidney damage, and pulmonary fibrosis.

V. **Nontesticular germ cell tumors.** The management of nontesticular germ cell tumors (NTGCTs) in general parallels that described above for testicular cancer. The prognosis for NTGCTs is generally less favorable than that for testicular cancer, but this difference can be explained on the basis of the bulkier disease of the NTGCTs at the time of diagnosis.

Selected Reading

Kidney

Fisher, R. I., et al. Metastatic renal cancer treated with interleukin-2 and lymphokine-activated killer cells: a phase II clinical trial. *Ann. Intern. Med.* 108:518, 1988.

Foon, K., et al. A prospective randomized trial of alpha-2b-interferon/gamma-interferon or the combination in advanced metastatic renal cell carcinoma. *J. Biol. Respir. Mod.* 7:540, 1988.

Marumo, K., et al. Human lymphoblastoid interferon therapy for advanced renal cell carcinoma. *Urology* 24:567, 1984.

Rosenberg, S. A., et al. Experience with the use of high-dose interleukin-2 in the treatment of 652 cancer patients. *Ann. Surg.* 210:474, 1989.

Swanson, D. A., Quesada, J. R. Interferon therapy for metastatic renal cell carcinoma. *Semin. Surg. Oncol.* 4:174, 1988.

Bladder

Daniels, J. R., et al. The role of adjuvant chemotherapy following cystectomy for invasive bladder cancer: a prospective comparative trial. *Proc. Am. Soc. Clin. Oncol.* 9:131, 1990.

Herr, H. W., et al. Bacillus Calmette-Guérin therapy alters the progression of superficial bladder cancer. *J. Clin. Oncol.* 6:1450, 1988.

Huland, H., et al. Long-term mitomycin C instillation after transurethral resection of superficial bladder carcinoma: influence on recurrence, progression and survival. *J. Urol.* 132:27, 1984.

Khandekar, J. D., et al. Comparative activity and toxicity of cis-diamminedichloroplatinum (DDP) and a combination of adriamycin, cyclophosphamide, and DDP in disseminated transitional cell carcinomas of the urinary tract. *J. Clin. Oncol.* 3:539, 1985.

Lamm, D. L. Intravesical therapy of superficial bladder cancer. In *AUA Update Series* (Vol. 2). Lesson 20, 1983.

Loehrer, P. J., et al. Advanced bladder cancer: a prospective intergroup trial comparing single agent cisplatin versus M-VAC combination therapy. *Proc. Am. Soc. Clin. Oncol.* 9:132, 1990.

Sarosdy, M. F., and Lamm, D. L. Long-term results of intravesical bacillus Calmette-Guérin therapy for superficial bladder cancer. *J. Urol.* 142:719, 1989.

Scher, H., et al. Neo-adjuvant chemotherapy for invasive bladder cancer: experience with the M-VAC regimen. *Br. J. Urol.* 64:250, 1989.

Sternberg, C. N., et al. Methotrexate, vinblastine, doxorubicin, and cisplatin for advanced transitional cell carcinoma of the urthelium. *Cancer* 64:2448, 1989.

Zincke, H., Sen, S. E., and Benson, R. Intravesical thiotepa and mitomycin C treatment as prophylaxis: long-term follow-up to recurrence, progression, and survival. In D. E. Johnson, C. J. Logothetis, and A. C. von Eschenback (eds.), *Systemic Therapy for Genitourinary Cancers.* Chicago: Year Book Medical Publishers, 1989. Pp. 32–42.

Prostate

Citrin, D. L., Elson, P., and DeWys, W. D. Treatment of metastatic prostate cancer: an analysis of response criteria in patients with measurable soft tissue disease. *Cancer* 54:13, 1984.

Crawford, E. D., et al. A controlled trial of leuprolide with and without flutamide in prostatic carcinoma. *N. Engl. J. Med.* 321:419, 1989.

DeWys, W. D., et al. A comparative clinical trial of adriamycin and 5-fluorouracil in advanced prostatic cancer-prognostic factors and response. *Prostate* 4:1, 1983.

Leuprolide Study Group. Leuprolide versus diethylstilbestrol for metastatic prostate cancer. *N. Engl. J. Med.* 311:1281, 1984.

Peeling, W. B. Phase III studies to compare goserelin (Zoladex) with orchiectomy and with diethylstilbestrol in treatment of prostatic carcinoma. *Urology* 33(suppl. 5):45, 1989.

Testes

DeWys, W. D. Management of testicular cancer. *Curr. Concepts Oncol.* 2:10, 1980.

DeWys, W. D., for the Testicular Cancer Intergroup Study. Adjuvant chemotherapy after retroperitoneal lymphadenectomy (pathologic stage II) nonseminomatous testicular cancer. In D. E. Johnson, C. J. Logothetis, and A. C. von Eschenbach (eds.), *Systemic Therapy for Genitourinary Cancers.* Chicago: Year Book Medical Publisher, 1989. Pp. 319–325.

DeWys, W. D., et al. Adjuvant chemotherapy of testicular cancer. In S. E. Jones and S. E. Salmon (eds.), *Adjuvant Therapy of Cancer IV.* Orlando: Grune & Stratton, 1984. Pp. 529–537.

Einhorn, L. H., et al. Evaluation of optimal duration of chemotherapy in favorable-prognosis disseminated germ cell tumors: a Southeastern Cancer Study Group protocol. *J. Clin. Oncol.* 7:387, 1989.

Loehrer, P. J., et al. Salvage therapy in recurrent germ cell cancer: ifosfamide and cisplatin plus either vinblastine or etoposide. *Ann. Intern. Med.* 109:540, 1988.

Mason, B. R., and Kearsley, J. H. Radiotherapy for stage 2 testicular seminoma: the prognostic significant of tumor bulk. *J. Clin. Oncol.* 6:1856, 1988.

Medical Research Council Working Party on Testicular Tumors. Prognostic factors in advanced non-seminomatous germ-cell testicular tumours: results of a multicentre study. *Lancet* 1:8, 1985.

Ozols, R. F., et al. A randomized trial of standard chemotherapy vs. a high-dose chemotherapy in the treatment of poor prognosis nonseminomatous germ cell tumors. *J. Clin. Oncol.* 6:1031, 1988.

Williams, S. D. et al. Immediate adjuvant chemotherapy versus observation with treatment at relapse in pathological stage II testicular cancer. *N. Engl. J. Med.* 317:1433, 1987.

Williams, S. D., et al. Treatment of disseminated germ-cell tumors with cisplatin, bleomycin, and either vinblastine or etoposide. *N. Engl. J. Med.* 316:1435, 1987.

Thyroid and Adrenal Carcinomas

Samir N. Khleif and Roland T. Skeel

Endocrine cancers account for 1.5 percent of all cancers diagnosed and 0.4 percent of cancer deaths. Thyroid cancer is the most common endocrine malignancy, accounting for 90 percent of endocrine cancers and 60–70 percent of the deaths from this group of diseases. Although the role of cytotoxic chemotherapy is limited in endocrine cancers, it is beneficial in selected cases of carcinoma of the pancreatic islet cells, thyroid, and adrenal gland. The treatment of pancreatic islet cell carcinomas and other pancreatic malignancies is discussed in Chapter 12. Here we discuss the thyroid and adrenal carcinomas. The pathology, presentation, and biologic behavior of thyroid and adrenal carcinomas are important determinants of therapy, and they are briefly considered.

I. Thyroid carcinoma
A. Background
1. **Incidence.** About 12,000 new cases of thyroid carcinoma were diagnosed in 1990, and according to the American Cancer Society there were 1200 deaths due to this cancer. The incidence of thyroid carcinoma is 5.9/100,000 women and 2.2/100,000 men. The prevalence in autopsies is 5–10%. Thyroid carcinoma usually affects persons between the ages of 25 and 65 years.

2. **Etiology and prevention.** The cause of most instances of thyroid carcinoma is unknown, although experimentally prolonged stimulation by thyroid stimulating hormone (TSH) may lead to the development of thyroid carcinoma. Some cases appear to be related to a dose-dependent phenomenon involving radiation to the neck during childhood. Thyroid malignancy has been observed 20–25 years after the radiation exposure in atomic bomb survivors and in children treated with radiation therapy for benign conditions of the head and neck. The frequency increases with doses up to 12 Gy and then decreases, so that with doses over 20 Gy the risk of developing malignancy becomes relatively low. Some cases of thyroid carcinoma (usually medullary carcinoma) are familial, as seen in the multiple endocrine neoplasia (MEN) syndromes, particularly MEN-IIa or MEN-IIb. Although ionizing radiation for benign conditions of the head and neck is no longer being used, cases related to this usage are still being seen. In cases of accidental nuclear exposure, it is thought that the use of potassium iodide to block the thyroid uptake of radioactive iodine in children would be of help in reducing the incidence of subsequent thyroid cancer. This modality was used in eastern Europe following the Chernobyl accident.

3. **Histologic types.** The most common histologic types of thyroid carcinoma are as follows.
   a. **Well differentiated adenocarcinoma,** which includes papillary carcinoma (40–50%), follicular carcinoma (25%), and mixed papillary–follicular adenocarcinoma (20%).
   b. **Anaplastic or undifferentiated carcinoma** (15–20%).
   c. **Medullary carcinoma** (1–5%).
   d. **Thyroid lymphoma** (5%).
4. **Prognosis**
   a. **Cell types.** Patients with papillary or mixed papillary–follicular histology (which have a similar biologic and prognostic behavior) have an excellent prognosis, with less than 15% mortality at 20 years. Patients with pure follicular carcinoma do not do as well as those with papillary elements, at least in part because there is a tendency for the follicular carcinoma to spread via the bloodstream, whereas the papillary carcinoma spreads more by lymphatics. Medullary carcinoma arises from the parafollicular (C) cells, which normally secrete the hormone calcitonin. About 50% of the cases of medullary carcinoma are familial, as part of three clinical syndromes (MEN-IIa, MEN-IIb, and familial non-MEN medullary thyroid carcinoma). Regional lymph node and distant metastases are common in patients with medullary carcinomas and occur in early stages of the disease. The 10-year survival rate following surgical resection is 40–60%. Patients with anaplastic thyroid carcinoma have an abysmal prognosis, with a median survival of 4 months.
   b. **Other factors.** In addition to the cell type, the prognosis of thyroid carcinoma is shown to be unfavorably related to:
      (1) **Increased size** of the tumor, especially more than 4 cm.
      (2) **Patient age** more than 40 years.
      (3) **Presence of distant metastases.** (Well differentiated carcinoma tends to metastasize to the lung or bone. Patients with lung or bone metastases have survival rates at 5, 10, and 15 years of 53%, 38%, and 30%, respectively.)
      (4) **Abnormal DNA content** in tumor cells (the more pronounced the aneuploidy, the more aggressively the cancer behaves).
      (5) **Male sex.** This difference may be related to the fact that men tend to be older at the time of diagnosis and are more likely to have a worse histologic type. In contrast to most other cancers, limited regional lymph node metastasis of well differentiated thyroid carcinomas does not influence survival substantially, and radiation-induced thyroid

carcinoma is not associated with a worse prognosis.

B. **Diagnosis and staging.** Any solitary nonfunctioning thyroid nodule (cold nodule) should be considered a possible malignant tumor until proved otherwise. The overall incidence of cancer in a cold nodule is 25%. Although toxic goiters are less likely to contain carcinoma, a hyperfunctioning thyroid nodule does not automatically confer benignity. As most thyroid tumors spread primarily by local extension and regional nodal metastasis, assessment of the extent of disease is concentrated on the neck. Presurgical studies include inspection and palpation, indirect laryngoscopy, radionuclide scanning, esophagogram, computed tomography (CT) scan of the neck, and needle aspiration cytology. The accuracy of needle aspiration biopsy ranges between 50% and 97%, depending on the pathologist and the institution. Whereas the best method for the diagnosis of well differentiated thyroid and medullary carcinoma is surgical resection, large needle biopsy is the method of choice for diagnosing thyroid lymphoma and anaplastic carcinoma. Chest radiography should be performed before surgery to rule out pulmonary metastasis. If there is any clinical or laboratory suggestion of bone metastases, a radionuclide bone scan should be performed.

C. **Treatment.** The therapeutic approach to patients with thyroid carcinoma depends considerably on the histologic type.

1. **Well differentiated thyroid carcinoma.** The management approach to the patient with well differentiated thyroid carcinoma is illustrated in Table 16-1.

   a. **Surgery.** Surgery is the only definitive therapy. Although the surgical approach may differ among surgeons and institutions, many surgeons prefer a bilateral near total thyroidectomy, taking into consideration that with well differentiated thyroid carcinoma the incidence of the disease in the contralateral lobe is 20–87%. Limited lymph node involvement does not substantially influ-

Table 16-1. Guidelines for the treatment of well differentiated thyroid carcinoma

Patient age	Extent of the disease (cm)	Treatment*
< 45 years	< 2	Lobectomy or NTT + HS
	> 2	NTT + HS
	Metastasis	NTT + HS + RAI
> 45 years	< 2	NTT + HS
	> 2	NTT + HS + RAI
	Metastasis	NTT + HS + RAI

*NTT = near-total thyroidectomy; HS = TSH suppression; RAI = radioactive iodine.

ence the survival rate, but it is associated with an increase in the local recurrence. Total thyroid-ectomy with modified neck dissection is often preferred for those who have cervical lymph node involvement. Mortality after thyroidectomy in well differentiated thyroid carcinoma approaches 0%. Complications include permanent recurrent laryngeal nerve damage in 2% of patients and permanent hypoparathyroidism in 1–2% of cases.

b. **Suppressive therapy.** Because there is good evidence that well differentiated thyroid cancer cells are usually responsive to TSH, TSH suppression is an essential component in the treatment of all of these tumors (Table 16-1). Because suppression of TSH suppresses the growth of malignant as well as normal thyroid tissue, the recurrence rate is reduced; and in a few cases metastatic lesions have diminished markedly. This hormonal suppression can be achieved by the administration of exogenous thyroid hormone. Usually, 200–250 µg of thyroxine (levothy-roxine or T_4) daily is necessary to obliterate the pituitary response to thyrotropin-releasing hormone (TRH), although the dose should be individualized to a maximum tolerable level. Side effects and dose-limiting factors include symptoms of thyrotoxicosis, angina, or cardiac arrhythmias. Other alternatives include liothyronine (T_3) and desiccated thyroid preparations.

c. **Radiation therapy.** Radiotherapy depends to a large degree on the clinical practice of the institution. Treatment with radioactive iodine (RAI) (^{131}I) is usually recommended for patients with well differentiated thyroid carcinoma and known postoperative residual disease, distant metastases, or locally invasive lesions; large lesions in patients older than 45 years of age also call for RAI therapy (Table 16-1). Although the effect of RAI on survival is not well determined, it is clear that the use of RAI and T_4 markedly decreases the recurrence rate. Effective use of RAI treatment requires the following: (1) tumor cells that are capable of receiving and concentrating iodide (i.e., well differentiated papillary or follicular carcinoma); and (2) appropriate patient preparation by withholding thyroid hormone administration for 2–4 weeks to provide the iodine-concentrating cells with the highest endogenous TSH stimulation. Effective doses usually are 50–150 mCi depending on the size and extent of the disease. Isolation of the patients is required by federal regulations until the total body radiation activity decreases below 30 mCi. Potential side effects expected after therapy include temporary bone marrow depression, nausea, sialoadenitis with possible permanent cessation of salivary flow (radiation mumps), skin reaction over the tissue concentrating the radioiodine, pulmonary fibrosis, and a small risk of later development of acute leukemia (2%). Once ablation is successful, patients are placed on suppressive therapy. Patients with lung metastases treated with RAI have a 20-year survival rate of 54%. In contrast, patients with bony involvement have a 10-year survival rate of 0%. Scintigraphy should be performed 4–6 weeks after therapy to detect any residual carcinoma. Most well differentiated thyroid carcinomas grow very slowly. The rate of recurrence is 0.5–1.6% per year. Therefore lifelong annual serum thyroglobulin assays are recommended. Scintigraphy is suggested if the thyroglobulin is found to be elevated.

The role of external radiation therapy in well differentiated thyroid carcinoma is limited. It is considered for tumors that concentrate little or no iodine.

2. **Medullary thyroid carcinoma.** With familial medullary carcinoma, the disease is almost always bilateral. Regional lymph node involvement is common in early stages. Therefore total thyroidectomy and central lymph node dissection are required. The overall 10-year survival rate following surgical resection is 40–60%. Postoperative annual evaluation is recommended by measuring calcitonin and carcinoembryonic antigen (CEA) levels, both of which substances are secreted by the medullary thyroid carcinoma cells, as a follow-up for residual disease or recurrence. Suppressive therapy is of no benefit because medullary cells do not have TSH receptors. RAI and cytotoxic chemotherapy are of little utility. Cisplatin, streptozotocin, carmustine, methotrexate, and fluorouracil have shown little if any benefit. However, some studies have shown chemotherapy to produce occasional responses of metastatic disease (see below). Local radiation therapy is useful in some cases as palliative therapy.

3. **Anaplastic thyroid carcinoma.** Most anaplastic tumors are unresectable at the time of presentation. Combination chemotherapy or chemotherapy plus irradiation have shown encouraging results for local control, and some partial and complete remissions have been seen.

4. **Chemotherapy**
   a. **Single agent chemotherapy.** The most widely applied cytotoxic agents are doxorubicin (Adriamycin), bleomycin, cisplatin, and etoposide. Each of these medications has demonstrated some activity against anaplastic and medullary thyroid carcinomas. Improved survival may be achieved in those patients responding to sequential exposure to these agents.

   Doxorubicin has proved to be the best single

chemotherapeutic agent with the highest response rate. Used as 60–75 mg/m^2 IV every 3 weeks has resulted in objective responses in 20–45% (median 34%) of patients with advanced refractory metastatic thyroid carcinoma. The response rate is probably highest for the medullary type and lowest for undifferentiated thyroid carcinoma. A high single dose of doxorubicin, which should be increased in case of no response, appears to be essential for a therapeutic effect. Because of its lower cardiotoxicity 4'-epidoxorubicin (epirubicin—still investigational), although almost as effective as doxorubicin, may be given at higher doses and over longer periods and is therefore preferred by some investigators.

   b. Combination chemotherapy. This therapy is usually used in association with doxorubicin. Cisplatin 40 mg/m^2 + doxorubicin 60 mg/m^2 given every 3 weeks yielded a higher rate and quality response than doxorubicin alone. These results included complete remission in 12% of patients, several of whom survived more than 2 years. Toxicity was no worse in the combination therapy. Other combination chemotherapy used includes doxorubicin + bleomycin + vincristine + melphalan with a response rate of 36%. Doxorubicin + bleomycin + and vincristine is another combination with a 64% response rate. Doxorubicin 10 mg/m^2 IV has been used in combination with external radiotherapy 90 minutes prior to the first radiation treatment and weekly thereafter. In this combination, the radiotherapy was given at a dose of 1.6 Gy per treatment twice a day for 3 consecutive days weekly for 6 weeks. Patients with undifferentiated thyroid carcinoma who are treated in this fashion showed an improvement in the median survival compared to historical controls.

   In general, the highest response is observed in patients with pulmonary metastasis. If thyroid carcinoma responds to chemotherapy, a prolongation of the median survival from 3–5 months to 15–20 months can be achieved.

5. **Lymphoma.** Lymphoma is more thoroughly addressed in Chapter 24. The discussion here briefly highlights its significance concerning thyroid malignancies. By definition, lymphoma of the thyroid is the one that at the time of diagnosis is confined to the gland or to the gland and regional lymph nodes. The major histologic type is non-Hodgkin's lymphoma. Autoimmune thyroiditis is a predisposing factor. Lymphoma of the thyroid usually presents with rapid enlargement of the gland within a few weeks and is bilateral in 25% of the cases. If the tumor is confined to the thyroid, surgical excision alone yields a 5-year survival rate of 70–90%. However, once the lymphoma extends beyond the thyroid

gland, surgical therapy does not improve survival, and irradiation and chemotherapy are indicated.

II. Adrenal carcinoma

A. Adrenocortical carcinoma

1. **Incidence and etiology.** Adrenocortical carcinoma is a rare tumor with fewer than 200 new cases occurring yearly in the United States. It accounts for 0.05–0.20% of all cancers and 0.2% of cancer deaths. It has a prevalence of 2/1,000,000 worldwide. The peak age of adrenocortical carcinoma occurs during the fourth and fifth decades of life. The incidence in women in most reports is about 2.5 times higher than in men, who tend to be older at diagnosis. Women have a tendency to develop a functional carcinoma, whereas males usually develop a nonfunctional malignancy. There is no family predilection, and no etiologic factors have been established.

2. **Clinical picture.** Adrenal carcinoma may present with one of the following clinical pictures.

   a. A palpable abdominal mass or an abdominal mass detected incidentally by abdominal imaging for some other purpose. Approximately 50% of patients have a palpable abdominal mass at the time of diagnosis.

   b. A functioning tumor with or without endocrine signs and symptoms of Cushing's syndrome, virilization, or feminization, depending on the age and the sex of the patient. Such manifestations are due to an increase in the production of a wide variety of steroid hormones. Ten percent of adrenocortical carcinoma is associated with virilization and 12% with feminization. Adrenal carcinoma is the cause for 10% of all cases of Cushing's syndrome.

   c. Other frequent presenting symptoms include upper abdominal pain, weight loss, anorexia, and malaise. Usually these symptoms are associated with advanced disease.

3. **Pathology and diagnosis.** Most malignant adrenal masses represent carcinomatous metastatic lesions, primarily from the lung and breast. Accordingly, the coincidental finding of an adrenal mass requires complete screening of the patient for a hidden primary carcinoma. With a primary adrenal tumor there may be some difficulty distinguishing adenoma from carcinoma. Criteria for differentiating benign from malignant tumors (Table 16-2) were suggested by Page, DeLellis, and Hough of the Armed Force Institute of Pathology.

   Adrenocortical carcinoma can be distinguished according to the pathologic pattern, depending on the cellular arrangement and the pleomorphism, into: (1) well differentiated adrenocortical carcinoma, which occurs more commonly in women and usually presents with a functioning tumor; and (2) anaplastic carcinoma, which is more common in men

Table 16-2. Diagnosis of malignancy in adrenocortical neoplasms

Reliability	Clinical criteria	Pathologic criteria
Diagnostic of malignancy	Weight loss, feminization, nodal or distant metastases	Tumor weight > 100 gm tumor necrosis, fibrous bands, vascular invasion, mitoses
Consistent with malignancy	Virilism, Cushing/virilism, no hormone production	Nuclear pleomorphism
Suggestive of malignancy	Elevated urinary 17-ketosteroids	Capsular invasion
Unreliable	Hypercortisolism, hyperaldosteronism	Tumor giant cells, cytoplasmic size variation, ratio between compact and clear cells

Source: Adapted from Page, D. L., DeLellis, R. A., and Hough, A. J. Tumors of the adrenal. In *Atlas of Tumor Pathology.* Washington, DC: AFIP, 1986.

and is often associated with lack of hormone production.

4. Staging and prognosis. Most patients (70%) present with stage III or IV disease. Adrenocortical carcinoma is a highly malignant cancer with an overall 5-year mortality of 75–90%, depending on the stage and morphology of the disease. The most commonly used staging system (derived from the TNM classification system) for adrenocortical carcinoma is as follows.

Stage	Size (cm)	Node or local invasion	Metastasis
I	< 5	−	−
II	> 5	−	−
III	Any	+	−
IV	Any	+/−	+
		Both	−

Metastases of adrenocortical carcinoma most commonly occur to the lung (71%), lymph nodes (68%), liver (42%), and bone (26%). The median survival time of patients with well differentiated carcinoma is 40 months, whereas patients with anaplastic carcinoma have a more dismal median survival time of 5 months. The mean survival time of patients with stages I, II, and III disease is 24–28 months, and for stage IV disease, 12 months.

5. Treatment

    a. Surgery. Up to one-half of adrenocortical carcinomas can be resected, although incompletely in some patients; however, the remainder have either too extensive local invasion or metastases to other sites in the abdomen, liver, lung, or other locations. Of those patients whose tumors were resected for cure, 40% remain disease-free. The remainder die, usually with extensive metastatic disease, within an average of less than 1 year. Patients who undergo complete resection should be followed on a monthly basis with steroid levels to detect recurrence. Serial magnetic resonance imaging (MRI) may also be used for the same purpose.

    b. Radiation therapy. Radiotherapy provides symptomatic relief from pain due to local or metastatic disease, especially bony metastases. It has also been used to prevent local recurrence following surgical resection (40–55 Gy over 4 weeks), but the benefit is uncertain and there is no proof that it improves survival.

    c. Chemotherapy. Indications include recurrent, metastatic, and nonresectable adrenocortical carcinoma. Agents used are the following.

        (1) Adrenocortical suppressants

            (a) Mitotane (*o,p*-DDD, Lysodren). An unconventional chemotherapy and a close chemical relative of the insecticide DDT, it has been used to treat adrenocortical carcinoma since 1960.

(i) **Mechanism of action and pharmacokinetics.** Mitotane inhibits corticosteroid biosynthesis and destroys adrenocortical cells secreting cortisol. The cytotoxic effect of mitotane has been considered transient and inconsistent. The exact biochemical mechanism of mitotane's effect is not fully known. Mitotane modifies the metabolism of steroids, apparently by blocking 11β-hydroxylation within the adrenal cortex, leading to a decrease in the 17-hydroxycorticosteroid levels. Under the effect of the mitochondrial enzyme P-450 monooxygenase, mitotane probably changes to the acyl chloride, which binds to the macromolecules of the mitochondria, leading to their destruction and consequently to the destruction of the adrenocortical cells. The part that is most affected by this action is the zona reticularis and the least is the zona glomerulosa. Forty percent of the medication is absorbed from the gastrointestinal tract. The drug is highly lipid-soluble and subsequently is concentrated in both normal and malignant adrenocortical cells. Reports of its plasma half-life range from 18 to 159 days.

(ii) **Dosage and administration.** Treatment with mitotane is started at 2–6 gm/day PO in three divided doses, then gradually increased in monthly one-dose increments until 9–10 gm/day is reached or until the maximum tolerated dose is achieved with no side effects. Blood levels of o,p-DDD should be maintained at more than 14 μg/ml to demonstrate a therapeutic response. Levels more than 20 μg/ml have a higher incidence of toxicity.

(iii) **Response and follow-up.** Objective tumor regression usually occurs within 6 weeks after the initiation of therapy and is seen in 70% of patients as a decrease in excessive hormone production. However, the reduction in hor-

mone production is not regularly
accompanied by an objective tumor
response. In about 30–40% of patients, the tumor size is reduced
significantly. The median duration of response is 10.5 months,
and complete remission has not
yet been achieved. If no clinical
benefit is demonstrated at the maximum tolerated dose after 3 months,
the case may be considered a clinical failure. Postoperative adjuvant therapy with mitotane has
resulted in no improvement in
survival. The combination of mitotane and radiation therapy has
not conferred any additional benefit over mitotane alone.

(iv) **Side effects.** Nausea and vomiting occur in 80% of patients.
Severe neurotoxicity, which may
occur during long-term treatment,
presents as somnolence, depression,
ataxia, and weakness in 60% of
patients. Reversible diffuse electro-
encepholographic (EEG) changes
may also occur. Adrenal insufficiency occurs in 50% of patients
(without replacement), and 20% of
patients develop dermatitis. As
the maximal dosage is often limited by the severity of, and the patient's tolerance to, the side effects, the total dose may range
widely from patient to patient.

(v) **Glucocorticoid   replacement**
during mitotane is necessary to
prevent hypoadrenalism. Replacement can be achieved by administering cortisone acetate 25 mg
PO in the morning and 12.5 mg
PO in the evening plus fludrocortisone acetate 0.1 mg PO in the morning. Plasma cortisol rather than
17-hydroxycorticosterol should be
used to monitor adrenal function
during mitotane use. In cases of
severe trauma or shock, mitotane
should be discontinued immediately.

(vi) **Nonresponders** to mitotane can
be treated with other adrenocortical suppressants, including metyrapone (75 mg PO q4h) or aminoglutethimide (250 mg PO q6h
initially, with stepwise increase in

dosage to a total of 2 gm/day or until limiting side effects appear that resemble those of mitotane). The latter drug inhibits conversion of cholesterol to pregnenolone. Metyrapone can induce hypertension and hypokalemic alkalosis. Neither of these medications have antitumor effect, but they are effective in relieving the signs and symptoms of excessive hormonal secretion.

Another medication that can be used is ketoconazole 200–600 mg/day. It is a potent adrenal inhibitor that produces clinical alleviation of the signs and symptoms within 4–6 weeks. In addition, it may cause regression of pulmonary and hepatic metastases, though the mechanism is not clear. Other drugs that might be of benefit in controlling symptoms include those that block the action of steroids in their target tissues, e.g., anti-mineralocorticoid and antiandrogenic agents, and more recently antiglucocorticoid agents, e.g., mifepristone (RU-486). None of these medications has an effect on tumor regression.

(2) **Cytotoxic chemotherapy.** This therapy form is usually used in patients who show no response to mitotane. Because of the small number of patients who require such therapy, the experience with this treatment modality is limited despite many clinical trials. No cytotoxic drug has shown definite effectiveness in the treatment of adrenocortical carcinoma, although doxorubicin, cisplatin, and suramin have been reported to produce partial responses in patients with metastatic disease. Few combination chemotherapy regimens have been effective. Cyclophosphamide 600 mg/m^2 IV + doxorubicin 40 mg/m^2 IV + cisplatin 50 mg/m^2 IV given in cycles every 3 weeks led to partial remission in 2 of 11 patients with adrenocortical carcinoma. The only combination that induced complete remission is cisplatin 40 mg/m^2 IV + etoposide 100 mg/m^2 IV + bleomycin 30 units IV given every 4 weeks. Three of four patients responded with one complete remission. Severe side effects occurred in both of these studies.

   d. Arterial embolization is another modality used
      for palliation of adrenocortical carcinoma. It is
      used to decrease the bulk of the tumor, suppress
      tumor function, and relieve pain. Embolic agents
      used include polyvinyl alcohol foam and surgical
      gelatin.
B. Pheochromocytoma
   1. Description and diagnosis. Pheochromocytoma is
      a tumor that arises from chromaffin cells mainly in
      the adrenal medulla (90% of cases), as well as other
      places (e.g., the urinary bladder, heart, and most
      commonly the organ of Zuckerkandl). It is an uncom-
      mon tumor with an incidence of 1–2/100,000/year. It
      is found in 0.005–0.300% of autopsies and is respon-
      sible for fewer than 0.1–0.5% of all cases of hyper-
      tension. Pheochromocytoma can be hereditary, as
      part of the MEN syndrome (MEN-IIa, MEN-IIb), or
      familial, with no other manifestation of the MEN
      syndrome. Hereditary pheochromocytoma is usually
      bilateral and never malignant. The incidence of ma-
      lignant pheochromocytoma ranges between 5% and
      45%. Although it may be difficult to differentiate be-
      tween benign and malignant pheochromocytoma on
      the basis of pathologic criteria, malignant pheochro-
      mocytomas are usually larger and have more mitoses
      with greater polyploidy than benign pheochromocy-
      toma. The only definite proof of malignancy is the
      presence of tumor in secondary sites where chromaf-
      fin tissue is not normally present. The diagnosis of
      pheochromocytoma depends on a thorough history
      and physical examination, increased catecholamine
      levels in the plasma and the urine (including epi-
      nephrine, norepinephrine, dopamine, total meta-
      nephrines, and vanillylmandelic acid), an abnormal
      clonidine suppression test, cross-sectional imaging
      such as with a CT scan or MRI scan, and ^{131}I-metaio-
      dobenzylguanidine (MIBG) scintigraphy. The overall
      5-year survival with malignant pheochromocytoma
      is 36–44%. Although pheochromocytoma is a rare tu-
      mor, early detection and treatment are crucial owing
      to its high morbidity and potential mortality.
   2. Treatment
      a. Surgery is the only definitive therapy for pheo-
         chromocytoma. It requires careful preoperative
         preparation to achieve control of the blood pres-
         sure, blood volume, and heart rate. Phenoxyben-
         zamine, an α-adrenergic blocker, is started 1–2
         weeks prior to surgery in a dose of 10–20 mg PO
         3–4 times a day. Some patients require the addi-
         tion of β-blockers, e.g., propranolol 80–120 mg/
         day, which are indicated for persistent supraven-
         tricular tachycardia or the presence of angina. To
         prevent hypertensive crisis secondary to unop-
         posed vasoconstriction, the β-blocker should
         never be given prior to the α-antagonist. Other α-

adrenergic blockers are used for the same purpose, including prazosin, which is a selective α_1-antagonist. Labetalol, which is both an α- and a β-antagonist, has also been used successfully for preoperative preparation of pheochromocytoma. Because of the possibility of postoperative residual tumor, because pheochromocytoma has a 10% incidence of metastasis, and because 10% of the patients have multiple primaries, close postoperative follow-up is mandatory. It includes a history and physical examination every 3 months and catecholamine measurements for 1 year; these same studies should then be done every 6 months for 1 year, followed by a similar evaluation yearly for life. Redevelopment of signs and symptoms suggesting pheochromocytoma or a rising trend of catecholamine levels requires imaging including ^{131}I MIBG scintigraphy. Some groups recommend that ^{131}I MIBG scintigraphy be done yearly regardless of the catecholamine levels or the clinical picture. The recurrence rate of pheochromocytoma postoperatively is 5% per year.

Chemotherapy and radiation therapy are reserved for locally invasive, metastatic, and inoperable lesions. Response to both of these treatments is evaluated by regression of tumor size and a decrease in the catecholamine levels.

b. **Chemotherapy.** Owing to the small number of patients with pheochromocytoma, limited data are available regarding the effect of chemotherapy. Because streptozocin has yielded favorable results in the treatment of neuroendocrine tumors in the gastrointestinal tract, it was used as a single agent in a patient with malignant pheochromocytoma. Streptozocin has shown promising results with a 73% reduction in urinary vanillylmandelic acid level and significant tumor size regression. Because of the functional and biologic similarities between pheochromocytoma and neuroblastoma, the combination of cyclophosphamide + vincristine + dacarbazine, which induces an 80% response in neuroblastoma, was used in two series to treat pheochromocytoma. The chemotherapy regimen consisted of cyclophosphamide 750 mg/m^2 IV on day 1 + vincristine 1.4 mg/m^2 IV on day 1 + and dacarbazine 600 mg/m^2 IV on days 1 and 2; it was repeated in 21- to 28-day cycles. Tumor size regressed in 53% of patients, and the urinary catecholamine levels decreased in 79% of patients. The median response averaged 18 months. Improvement of blood pressure control and performance status occurred with minimal toxicity.

c. **Radiation therapy.** MIBG is actively taken up and concentrated by pheochromocytoma cells with high sensitivity and specificity. Consequently, a high dose of ^{131}I MIBG is to treat pheochromocytoma. This treatment has shown some evidence of response in terms of tumor size regression and decreased catecholamine levels. The uptake of MIBG by pheochromocytoma requires the presence of an active neuronal pump mechanism, which limits the use of this agent to patients with pheochromocytoma who have the ability to concentrate ^{131}I MIBG in the cells. Therefore initial screening of the ability of the pheochromocytoma to concentrate small doses of ^{131}I MIBG is necessary to determine the probable efficacy of the treatment.

d. Supportive pharmacologic therapy. α-Blockers should be used to prevent severe hypertension morbidity and mortality, especially in untreated patients or those receiving chemotherapy. Another pharmacologic agent that can be used is α-methylparathyrosine (Metyrosine), which inhibits tyrosine hydroxylase, a rate limiting step in catecholamine biosynthesis. Metyrosine allows the use of lower doses of α-blockers. Other medications include β-blockers, which are used to control arrhythmias, angiotensin converting enzyme (ACE) inhibitors, and calcium channel blockers, which are also used for hypertension control.

Selected Reading

Thyroid Carcinoma

Ahuja, S., and Ernst, H. Chemotherapy of thyroid carcinoma. *J. Endocrinol. Invest.* 10:303, 1987.

Bierwaltes, W. H., et al. An analysis of "ablation of thyroid remnants" with I-131 in 511 patients from 1947–1984 experience at University of Michigan. *J. Nucl. Med.* 25:1287, 1984.

Brown, A. P., et al. Radioiodine treatment of metastatic thyroid carcinoma: the Royal Marsden experience. *Br. J. Radiol.* 57:323, 1984.

Cady, B., and Rossi, R. An expanded view of risk group definition in differentiated thyroid carcinoma. *Surgery* 104:947, 1988.

Gottlieb, J. A., and Hill, C. S. Chemotherapy of thyroid cancer with Adriamycin. *N. Engl. J. Med.* 290:193, 1974.

Grant, C. S., et al. Local recurrence in papillary thyroid carcinoma: is extent of surgical resection important? *Surgery* 104:954, 1988.

Hay, I. D., et al. Ipsilateral lobectomy versus bilateral lobar resection in papillary thyroid carcinoma: a retrospective analysis of surgical outcome using a novel prognostic scoring system. *Surgery* 102:1088, 1987.

Hoskin, P. J., and Harmer, C. Chemotherapy for thyroid cancer. *Radiother. Oncol.* 10:187, 1987.

Leedman, P. J., et al. Combination chemotherapy as single modality therapy for stage IE and IIE thyroid lymphoma. *Med. J. Aust.* 152:40, 1990.

Schlumberger, M., et al. Long-term results of treatment of 283 patients with lung and bone metastases from differentiated thyroid carcinoma. *J. Clin. Endocrinol. Metab.* 63:960, 1986.

Shiamoka, K., et al. A randomized trial of doxorubicin versus doxorubicin plus cisplatin with advanced thyroid carcinoma. *Cancer* 56:2155, 1985.

Sizemore, G. W. Medullary carcinoma of the thyroid gland. *Semin. Oncol.* 14:306, 1987.

Adrenocortical Carcinoma

Bodie, B., et al. The Cleveland Clinic experience with adrenal cortical carcinoma. *J. Urol.* 141:257, 1989.

Haq, M. M., et al. Cytotoxic chemotherapy in adrenal cortical carcinoma. *Cancer Treat. Rep.* 64:909, 1980.

Hogan, T. F., et al. A clinical and pathological study of adreno-cortical carcinoma. *Cancer* 45:2880, 1980.

Lubitz, J. A., Freeman, L., and Okun, R. Mitotone use in inoperable adrenal cortical carcinoma. *J.A.M.A.* 223:1109, 1973.

Luton, J. P., et al. Clinical features of adrenocortical carcinoma, prognostic factors, and the effect of mitotane therapy. *N. Engl. J. Med.* 322:1195, 1990.

May, C. A., and Garnett, W. R. Treatment of adrenocortical carcinoma: a case report and review of the literature. *Drug Intell. Clin. Pharm.* 20:24, 1980.

Page, D. L., Dellelis, R. A., and Hough, A. J. Tumors of the adrenal. In *Atlas of Tumor Pathology.* Washington, DC: AFIP, 1986.

Samaan, N. A., and Hickey, R. C. Adrenal cortical carcinoma. *Semin. Oncol.* 14:292, 1987.

Venkatesh, S., et al. Adrenal cortical carcinoma. *Cancer* 64:765, 1989.

Pheochromocytoma

Auerbuch, S., et al. Malignant pheochromocytoma: effective treatment with a combination of cyclophosphamide, vincristine, and dacarbazine. *Ann. Intern. Med.* 109:267, 1988.

Bierwaltes, W. H., et al. Malignant potential of pheochromocytoma. *Proc. AACR* 27:617, 1986.

Bravo, E. L., and Gifford, R. W. Pheochromocytoma: diagnosis, localization and management. *N. Engl. J. Med.* 311:1298, 1984.

Feldman, J. M. Treatment of metastatic pheochromocytoma with streptozotocin. *Arch. Intern. Med.* 143:1799, 1983.

Keiser, H. R., et al. Treatment of malignant pheochromocytoma with combination chemotherapy. *Hypertension* 7:1, 1985.

Shapiro, B., and Sisson, J. C. *Atlas of Nuclear Medicine,* Philadelphia: Lippincott, 1988. P. 72.

Sheps, S. G., et al. Recent development in the diagnosis and treatment of pheochromocytoma. *Mayo. Clin. Proc.* 65:88, 1990.

Melanomas and Other Skin Malignancies

Larry Nathanson

I. Melanoma
A. Introduction
1. Natural history

a. Origin and occurrence. Melanoma is a malignancy originating in the melanocytes of the skin. During embryologic development these cells differentiate in the neural crest and migrate to the skin and eye. In adults they are responsible for the formation of skin pigment. About 10% of melanomas occur in some extradermal site, primarily in the eye, mucous membrane, anus, or external genitalia. The incidence of the disease has doubled since the early 1970s with a current lifetime risk in the general population of about 0.7%. This striking increase in incidence, the largest of any cancer in the United States, is presumably due to increased exposure to actinic radiation, particularly in the ultraviolet-B spectrum. Melanoma is equally prevalent in men and women, and its peak age of incidence is during the sixth decade. Early recognition and early diagnosis of this disease result in prompt and curative surgical management.

b. Precursor lesions and familial melanoma. Congenital and dysplastic nevi may be precursor lesions for melanoma. Although the dysplastic nevi may be sporadic or familial, they constitute markers of increased risk for melanoma. Attention should be paid to careful follow-up of patients and families with dysplastic nevi with or without melanoma, as early excision of either lesion may result in prevention of the disease, which may otherwise be tragically fatal.

c. Types of primary lesions. There are four major types of cutaneous lesion. In order of increasing aggressiveness, they are *lentigo maligna melanoma, superficial spreading melanoma, nodular melanoma,* and *palmar–plantar–mucosal melanoma.* These lesions vary in size from the lentigos (5 cm or more) to the smaller, palpable, nodular melanoma. Symptomatically, they share a characteristic history of growth and one or more of the following symptoms: change in pigmentation, ulceration, itching, or bleeding when the lesions become actively malignant. On examination, they share a tendency to have absent hair follicles, irregular margins, and variegated coloring of hues of blue, red, or white; these signs help distinguish them from benign nevi.

     d. Metastasis. At initial presentation, up to 30% of patients have disease spread beyond the local lesion. In about one-half of these patients, disease has spread no further than regional nodes. In the other half, there is evidence of distant metastasis. Of those patients with only primary melanoma initially, about one-sixth subsequently develop metastasis. Of these patients, one-fifth experience metastases in soft tissues alone (lymph nodes, skin, or subcutaneous tissue). In the other four-fifths, metastases appear in other tissues and organs (particularly liver, lung, brain, or bone) alone or together with soft tissue disease. Forty-five percent of patients with melanoma that is not cured develop central nervous system (CNS) metastases during the course of the disease.

     e. Ocular melanoma is the most common malignancy of the eye. Although enucleation was the standard therapy for primary ocular melanoma, studies are now under way to evaluate use of local radiotherapy with or without sight-preserving surgery. When metastatic (usually to the liver), the same therapy is employed as is described for cutaneous melanoma.

  2. Staging of melanomas is often difficult because of the poor resolution of diagnostic radiologic studies. However, in patients at high risk for advanced disease, in addition to the usual conventional roentgenograms, radionuclide scans, and sonograms, computed tomography (CT) or magnetic resonance imaging (MRI) scanning of the head and body may be helpful in staging procedures. MRI, utilizing optimal technology has been demonstrated to be a more specific and sensitive test for metastasis than is CT scanning. Gallium scanning and lymphangiography are occasionally useful.

  3. Surgical treatment and prognosis. Standard treatment for melanoma is wide excision (1–3 cm tumor-free margin) of the primary lesion. Routine prophylactic regional lymph node dissection has not proved to increase survival. Retrospective data, however, strongly suggest benefit following lymph node dissection in the patient with a primary lesion depth of 1.51–3.99 mm. The prognosis of an excised primary lesion varies inversely according to the thickness of the lesion and is better in women and for cutaneous primary lesions of the extremities (compared with trunk, head, or neck). Survival decreases sharply as the extent of disease increases (Table 17-1). Surgery is occasionally indicated in the patient with metastatic disease, especially with a symptomatic solitary lesion of the brain or elsewhere.

B. Chemotherapeutic interventions

  1. Systemic therapy

     a. Patient selection. When selecting patients with

Table 17-1. Staging and prognosis in malignant melanoma

Stage	Site	5-Year Survival (%)
I	Primary tumor only, by depth (mm)	85
	0.75	99
	0.76–1.50	92
	1.51–3.99	78
	4.0	40
II	Local metastases (< 5 cm from primary melanoma)	50
III	Regional metastases to lymph nodes or soft tissue	25
IV	Distant metastases	
	Soft tissue	10
	Visceral	5

metastatic melanomas as candidates for chemotherapy, favorable clinical factors predicting the likelihood of chemotherapeutic response must be kept in mind. These factors include the following.

1. Good performance status (initially ambulatory)
2. Soft tissue disease or a relatively small number of visceral sites (pulmonary metastases are most sensitive)
3. Youth (< 65 years of age)
4. No prior chemotherapy
5. Normal hemogram and normal hepatic and renal function
6. Absence of CNS metastases

   b. Single-agent chemotherapy. A number of single agents have been found to have antitumor activity against melanoma. The response rates to these agents vary widely as reported by various authors. It must be emphasized that, despite these reports, metastatic melanoma remains one of the neoplasms most refractory to chemotherapy, and patients lacking symptoms to palliate achieve a few months gain in survival at best.

   (1) Dacarbazine (DTIC), the standard single agent for treatment of this disease, is usually given at a dose of 200 mg/m^2 IV on days 1–5 every 3 weeks or 750 mg/m^2 IV on day 1 every 6 weeks. Response rate is 20–25%.

   (2) Nitrosoureas have each been used for melanoma and probably have similar efficacy.

   (a) Carmustine (BCNU) 150 mg/m^2 IV every 6 weeks *or*

   (b) Semustine (MeCCNU) 100–130 mg/m^2 PO every 6 weeks *or*

   (c) Lomustine (CCNU) 100–130 mg/m^2 PO every 3–6 weeks.

These regimens are the most commonly used, and each has a response rate of 15–20%.

(3) **Platinum-containing drugs**—cisplatin 100 mg/m^2 IV every 3 weeks or carboplatin 400 mg/m^2 every 3 weeks appear to have similar efficacy. Dose may be cautiously escalated for optimal response.

(4) **Dactinomycin, ifosfamide (+ mesna) alkylating agents, vinca alkaloids, and procarbazine** have response rates of 10–15%.

(5) **Very high-dose chemotherapy** with either carmustine or melphalan with or without autologous bone marrow transplantation is now being evaluated.

c. **Multiple agent chemotherapy.** A number of chemotherapeutic combinations have been used for melanoma, and some of the regimens with data on significant numbers of patients are listed in Table 17-2. The first combination listed employs cisplatin, dacarbazine, carmustine, and tamoxifen. This drug combination is associated with a 55% objective response rate and a median survival of 14 months or more in responding patients. Another combination includes the use of dactinomycin and dacarbazine together in large single-pulse doses given approximately once every 3–4 weeks. This combination has been reported by the Southwest Oncology Group to have a response rate of approximately 30–40%, but the median survival time is only 8–10 months.

A cisplatin-containing combination that has been reported to have a significant objective re-

Table 17-2. Combination chemotherapy of malignant melanoma

Regimen	Dosage
PBT-T	Cisplatin (Platinol) 25 mg/m^2 IV on days 1–3 every 3 weeks
	Dacarbazine (DTIC) 220 mg/m^2 IV on days 1–3 every 3 weeks
	Carmustine (BCNU) 150 mg/m^2 IV once every 6 weeks
	Tamoxifen 10 mg bid PO continuously
VDP	Vinblastine 5 mg/m^2 IV on days 1 and 2
	Dacarbazine 150 mg/m^2 IV on days 1–5
	Cisplatin 75 mg/m^2 IV on day 5
DTIC-ACT-D	Dacarbazine (DTIC) 750 mg/m^2 IV on day 1
	Dactinomycin (actinomycin D) 1 mg/m^2 IV on day 1
	Repeat cycle every 4 weeks

sponse rate in advanced disease employs vinblastine, dacarbazine, and cisplatin. It has achieved a 35–45% objective response rate in patients with advanced disease. Median survival is similar to those regimens previously mentioned.

Although definitive studies have not been completed, the substitution of carboplatin for cisplatin in the above combinations may give just as good results while avoiding the nephrotoxicity and neurotoxicity associated with that drug.

One of the major problems with these programs has been the high incidence of relapse in the CNS, a metastatic site that tends to respond poorly to chemotherapy. Any of the regimens in Table 17-2 should be considered if the patient has a good performance status and can be expected to tolerate an intensive chemotherapy regimen.

d. Adjuvant chemotherapy. A variety of chemotherapy programs have been used in patients with high-risk primary melanoma (lesion thickness > 1.5 mm) or patients with node metastasis. The efficacy of adjuvant chemotherapy in this setting is controversial. Although several studies have suggested that either chemotherapy or a combination of chemotherapy plus immunotherapy may be beneficial to these patients, no study has unequivocally proved the usefulness of adjuvant therapy. A prospective randomized adjuvant study of 107 hyperthermic perfusions found a statistically significant superior survival in patients with extremity primary melanoma, stages I, II, and III. If confirmed, perfusion in patients with extremity melanoma will constitute a new example of the efficacy of adjuvant chemotherapy.

2. Regional chemotherapy

a. Infusion and perfusion. Arteriovenous isolation with perfusion chemotherapy has long been used in patients with regional melanoma, particularly that confined to the lower extremities. A variety of drugs has been employed including the alkylating agents (especially nitrogen mustard and melphalan) and more recently dacarbazine and carmustine. The perfusate is heated (usually to 40°C) in most studies (see **I.B.1.d**).

Intraarterial infusion has been carried out with the previously mentioned drugs, as well as with doxorubicin or cisplatin. This treatment is technically much easier than perfusion. It may represent optimal treatment of patients with regional recurrent disease, especially when used with external tourniquet control.

b. Intracavitary chemotherapy. The use of intracavitary thiotepa, dacarbazine, or bleomycin may be of benefit in reducing the rate of development of pleural or peritoneal effusions. Colloidal gold (^{198}Au) or chromic phosphate (^{32}P) is occasionally helpful for this complication, as is tetracycline, a sclerotogenic agent. Each of these drugs should be administered through an indwelling chest tube as described in Chapter 31.

c. **Brain metastases.** Melanoma of the CNS has been a particularly difficult problem and is a relatively common occurrence. The standard approach is radiotherapy to the whole brain in one of several dosage schedules accompanied initially by corticosteroids. The use of high-dose fractions (400–800 cGy) may be somewhat superior to conventional radiotherapy but does not increase survival. No chemotherapeutic regimen, including nitrosoureas, which are known to cross the blood-brain barrier, has been effective in the control of CNS metastases. However, some patients may respond for long periods to CNS radiotherapy, particularly if no other visceral site is involved.

d. **Intralesional immunotherapy.** Intralesional immunotherapy, particularly with bacillus Calmette-Guérin (BCG), lymphokines, or interferon, has been shown in a number of reports to control both injected and uninjected regional intradermal metastases (satellitosis). Although this treatment is not applicable to patients who have distant disease or bulky regional disease, in patients with early recurrence it may produce long disease-free survivals. Occasional cases of systemic BCG infection occurring with this treatment are usually easy to control with antituberculous chemotherapy.

e. **Radiotherapy** may be helpful in controlling circumscribed and symptomatic extra-CNS lesions such as painful bony metastases. Hyperthermia simultaneous with irradiation may potentiate its efficacy in the treatment of soft tissue metastases.

3. **New treatment approaches including biologic response modifiers (BRMs).** Studies with interferons, especially recombinant interferon-alpha ($r\alpha IFN$) have yielded 5–15% objective responses, and currently the interferons have been employed alone and in combination with chemotherapy. Doses of $r\alpha IFN$ range from 3×10^6 to 10×10^6 units SQ 3 times weekly to daily. There are conflicting data on the question of additive or synergistic effects of $r\alpha IFN$ and chemotherapy.

Interleukin-2 (IL-2), a potent lymphokine, has been used with or without lymphokine activated killer (LAK) cells for melanoma. This treatment is toxic and requires special facilities for its use. The development of continuous infusion schedules for IL-2 use may diminish toxicity. Substitution of tumor-infiltrating lymphocytes for LAK cells may have more potent tumor lytic activity. Response rates in these treatments vary from 20% to 50%. The use of IL-2 plus rαIFN may be more effective, and less toxic, than use of either agent alone.

Specific immunotherapy utilizing monoclonal antibodies to melanoma-associated antigens is being actively studied in this disease.

The use of hormones for treating melanoma has been suggested by the discovery that some melanoma tumor cells contain cortisol-binding protein receptors. Although there are reported antitumor effects of tamoxifen, the use of tamoxifen with chemotherapy is the only well documented example of synergy, and may represent the ability of this drug to abrogate the multidrug resistance phenotype. The retinoids have been used as anticarcinogens in a variety of experimental melanomas, and they appear to have an effect on inhibition of pigment formation, as well as on slowing tumor growth. This technique is as yet an experimental one.

Radiopotentiating agents may have a place in the treatment of melanoma. For example, the use of cisplatin may potentiate the antitumor effects of radiation. Hyperthermia either alone or as a radiopotentiator has been shown to have antitumor effects on superficial lesions of metastatic melanomas.

Other drugs that may have promise following early testing include ifosfamide, a newly available phosphoramide mustard, and taxol, a derivative of the bark of the yew tree.

Antipigmentary chemotherapy, particularly with drugs that are tyrosinase inhibitors or that may inhibit cysteine incorporation into nucleic acid polymerases, has antitumor effects on experimental melanomas. These drugs include α-methylparatyrosine (Demser), 6-hydroxydopa, pimozide, and 4-hydroxyanisole. Their efficacy has not yet been demonstrated in any clinical study.

II. Nonmelanoma skin cancer

A. Etiology and epidemiology.
Nonmelanoma skin cancer is the most common type of malignancy in the United States, and it was estimated that there would be in excess of 450,000 new cases in the United States in 1991.

The most common types of skin cancer are basal cell carcinoma (BCC) (or epithelioma) and squamous cell carcinoma (SCC). This summary excludes other types of skin tumor such as mycosis fungoides, tumors of the skin appendages, and Kaposi sarcoma (see Chapter 27). BCC and SCC are more common in men than in women. Like melanoma, squamous carcinoma is increasing in incidence in the United States. The most frequent etiologic factor is exposure to actinic radiation. Accordingly, individuals with fair skin and light hair and eyes tend to have a high incidence of the diseases. In addition, it is more common on the lower extremities in the female than in the male subject. Individuals with chronic sun exposure are at a particular risk for this disease. Whites have a greater incidence than Orientals, who in turn have a greater incidence than Blacks. BCC is more common than SCC in Whites, and SCC is more common than BCC in Blacks. Multiple primary skin cancers can be seen in affected individuals. Other etiologic factors include exposure to x rays, chronic scarring (especially that occurring with burns), chronic inflammatory states, and exposure to arsenic.

B. Actinic keratosis

    1. Natural history. Actinic keratoses (e.g., solar keratosis) are lesions found in the exposed areas of the skin and are assumed to be precancerous, as SCC may arise from them. In the patient predisposed to the development of such lesions, use of sun protective creams (e.g., p-aminobenzoic acid) may be an important preventive medical practice.

    2. Topical chemotherapy. Fluorouracil is used as a 1% solution or cream on the face and up to a 5% concentration on the arms, applied twice daily for 2–4 weeks by the patient rubbing it in with fingertips. Care must be taken around the eyes, but individuals may be treated on the periorbital skin. Fluorouracil must be applied smoothly with avoidance of accumulated ointment in the nasolabial folds. After application, the hands must be washed. Erythema begins 3–7 days after treatment and progresses to scaling, erosion, and tenderness, at which time the application should be stopped. The reaction subsides rapidly, and lesions on the face heal within 2–6 weeks (somewhat longer on the arms). Repeated courses of fluorouracil may be used, and an overly brisk reaction may be treated locally with topical steroids. Because topical steroids protect against the inflammatory effect of fluorouracil but do not diminish its antitumor effect, it seems likely that fluorouracil exerts its effects by a cytotoxic mechanism rather than by a nonspecific inflammatory sloughing of superficial skin layers. This sloughing may be in part from a local delayed hypersensitivity reaction.

C. Basal cell carcinoma

    1. Natural history. The most common type of BCC is the noduloulcerative or "rodent ulcer" form. It presents as a well defined nodule that has rolled pearly or translucent borders traversed by telangiectases and a central concave area that is often ulcerated. A variety of histologic subtypes of this tumor exist, including solid, keratotic, cystic, and adenoid varieties. Pigmented types, which may resemble malignant melanoma (pigmented basal cell epithelioma), are important because of this differential diagnosis. These lesions have a low metastatic potential, and 85% of them are present on the skin of the head and neck. In neglected cases (0.1–0.2% of total patients) metastases may occur. When seen, such metastases occur an average of 11 years after the primary lesion was first noted. Lymph nodes, lung, and bone may be involved in decreasing order of likelihood.

2. Topical treatment. Superficial surgery, electrodesiccation, chemosurgery, or radiation therapy (especially with electron beam) may be used on these lesions. The cure rate should be above 95% regardless of the technique employed. Chemosurgery usually employs the use of zinc chloride fixative paste (Mohs' technique).

The use of fluorouracil in a topical solution or ointment, as described under the treatment of actinic keratosis (see **II.B.2**) is usually reserved for patients with multiple or widespread lesions because of the efficacy of the nonchemotherapeutic techniques. Deeply invasive tumors are not appropriately treated with fluorouracil because the drug penetrates only a few millimeters into the skin.

D. Squamous cell carcinoma

1. Natural history. Squamous cell carcinoma may occur at any site on the skin, as well as on mucous membranes, particularly on the lips, vulva, penis, and anus. The area from which it arises rarely appears normal but usually has the changes associated with actinic keratosis. The latter process may be considered an in situ state of SCC. A rough, scaly surface with thickening of the skin and often well circumscribed macular changes are frequently present. A reddish, brownish, or grayish cast to the skin may also be present. Crusting, thickening, or ulceration strongly suggests malignant change. An indurated border also is suggestive of malignancy.

The primary lesion histopathologically is in the epidermis, with cells penetrating the dermis often with keratinization and epidermal pearl formation. The degree of cellular differentiation, atypicality of cells, and depth of penetration of the tumor are prognostic factors.

About 0.2% of patients develop metastatic tumors, and 90% of these metastases are to the lymph nodes only. Only one-half of patients with lymph node metastases and 60% of patients with distant metastases die within 5 years.

The exceptional lesions that arise in normal-appearing skin or in other preexisting lesions (scars of thermal, chemical, or radiation injury) tend to be more aggressive than those that arise in actinically damaged skin. Surgery by a variety of means is the conventional treatment of SCC, as it is of BCC. The choices include curettage and desiccation. Radiation therapy, cryotherapy, and chemosurgery have also been used, and all produce cure rates in excess of 94%. Treatment of locally recurrent tumors is less satisfactory, and the importance of patients receiving prompt and adequate treatment early in the disease must be emphasized. As for BCC, the use of Mohs' chemotherapy with zinc chloride fixative paste may be highly effective in SCC.

2. **Topical chemotherapy.** Superficial SCCs may be effectively treated with 5% topical fluorouracil with relatively little toxicity and an essentially 100% cure rate. However, it is important with more invasive lesions to avoid the possibility that fluorouracil may fail to control microscopic islands of invasive SCC and therefore may delay appropriate therapy. When treatment of more invasive or noduloulcerative SCC is contemplated, 20% fluorouracil under occlusive dressings may be employed if standard therapy is refused or contraindicated. As a rule, at least 3 weeks of treatment are required, although at times it is necessary to treat for up to 12 weeks.

E. **Multifocal tumors.** In patients who have widespread multifocal superficial tumors developing, as with xeroderma pigmentosum, chronic arsenic exposure, Bowen's disease (multiple intraepidermal squamous carcinomas), extensive radiation dermatitis, or long-term extensive actinic changes, the use of surgical techniques may be impossible. In these patients, applications of dinitrochlorobenzene, purified protein derivative of tuberculin, streptokinase-streptodornase, or other agents may be clinically useful. These medications are applied in topical fashion to a large area of the skin in increasing concentrations and can produce selective lytic effects on malignant epidermal cells even when the cells are present in microscopic foci that otherwise would not be readily detectable. The allergic contact dermatitis that results from the application of these immunoadjuvants appears to destroy most microscopic BCCs. Whether these allergic reactions are directly responsible for tumor lysis or they simply result from an attraction of sensitized "killer" lymphocytes to the areas where microscopic deposits of epidermoid neoplastic epidermal cells are present is not yet known. The fact that neoplastic epidermal cells are selectively killed has an important clinical implication. Scarring rarely develops from this type of treatment because normal epidermal cells remain viable and are not replaced by proliferating fibroblasts.

Selected Reading

Ahmann, D. L., et al. Complete responses and long-term survivals after systemic chemotherapy for patients with advanced malignant melanoma. *Cancer* 63:224, 1989.

Carey, R. W., et al. Treatment of metastatic malignant melanoma with vinblastine, dacarbazine, and cisplatin: a report from the Cancer and Leukemia Group B. *Cancer Treat. Rep.* 70:329, 1986.

Clark, W. H., et al. Model predicting survival in stage I melanoma based on tumor progression. *J. Natl. Cancer Inst.* 81:1893, 1989.

Dutcher, J. P., et al. A phase II study of interleukin-2 and lymphokine-activated killer cells in patients with metastatic malignant melanoma. *J. Clin. Oncol.* 7:477, 1989.

Ghussen, F., et al. The role of regional hyperthermic cytostatic perfusion in the treatment of extremity melanoma. *Cancer* 61:654, 1988.

McClay, E. F., and Mastrangelo, M. J. Systemic chemotherapy for metastatic melanoma. *Semin. Oncol.* 15:569, 1988.

Nathanson, L. (ed.). *Medical Management of Advanced Melanoma.* New York: Churchill Livingstone, 1986. Pp. 1–268.

Patterson, J. A. K., and Geronemus, R. G. Cancers of the skin. In V. T. DeVita, S. Hellman, and S. A. Rosenberg (eds.), *Cancer: Principles and Practice of Oncology* (3rd ed.). Philadelphia: Lippincott, 1989. Pp. 1469–1498.

Pezzuto, J. M., et al. Approaches for drug development in treatment of advanced melanoma. *Semin. Oncol.* 15:578, 1988.

Von Wussow, P., et al. Intralesional interferon-alpha therapy in advanced malignant melanoma. *Cancer* 61:1071, 1988.

Wolff, S. N., et al. High-dose thiotepa with autologous bone marrow transplantation for metastatic malignant melanoma: results of phase I and II studies of the North American bone marrow transplantation group. *J. Clin. Oncol.* 7:245, 1989.

Primary and Metastatic Brain Tumors

Jane B. Alavi

I. Occurrence and tumor characteristics

A. Primary brain tumors

1. **Incidence.** Primary tumors of the brain result in 2–3% of all deaths caused by cancer. The overall incidence in the United States is about 5/100,000, but in children under age 14 the incidence is 6.5/100,000. These tumors account for about 20% of all cancers in children.

2. **Histology.** Most intracranial neoplasms arise from meningeal or neuroectodermal tissue. Meningiomas (which arise from the meninges) are generally benign and encapsulated and can be removed surgically. They are rarely malignant (sarcomatous), and chemotherapy has no role in their treatment. Gliomas account for two-thirds of primary brain tumors. They arise from astrocytes (astrocytoma and glioblastoma), oligodendroglia (oligodendroglioma), and the ependymal cells that line the ventricles (ependymoma). Medulloblastomas and primitive neuroectodermal tumors (pineoblastoma and cerebral neuroblastoma) arise from unknown precursor cells, are highly malignant, and have a propensity to spread via the cerebrospinal fluid (CSF) to the spinal cord.

   The astrocytomas occur with a broad range of histologic differentiation. The well differentiated tumors, grades I and II, can often be cured by surgery. The more highly malignant types—anaplastic astrocytoma (grade III) and glioblastoma (grade IV)—are not curable. During childhood, two-thirds of the neoplasms are found in the cerebellum or brainstem, and the common histologic types are medulloblastoma, ependymoma, and low-grade astrocytoma. Fewer than 20% are glioblastoma. In contrast, primary tumors in adults are nearly always supratentorial, more than 50% are glioblastomas, and about 18% are meningiomas.

B. Metastatic (secondary) brain tumors.

The overall incidence of metastatic tumors to the brain is higher than the incidence of primary brain tumors in adults. Approximately 20% of patients with cancer are found to have brain metastases at autopsy. The most common primary sites are the lung (all cell types) and breast. Melanoma, colorectal carcinoma, unknown primaries, and renal carcinoma primaries occur less frequently. Some rare tumors, such as choriocarcinomas, give rise to brain metastases with unusual frequency. Most brain metastases are found in the cerebral hemispheres, few are found in the cerebellum or midbrain, and most are multiple at the time of diagnosis. Meningeal metastases are seen less frequently, and the primary tumors are usually breast or lung cancers, lymphoma, or melanoma.

II. Approach to therapy: primary and metastatic brain tumors

A. Surgery. Surgical removal depends on the location of the lesion, its size, and its propensity to infiltrate surrounding areas of the brain. Because gliomas tend to infiltrate normal brain tissue surrounding the obvious tumor mass, it is unusual to cure patients with surgery alone without resultant unacceptable neurologic deficits. Metastatic cancers, on the other hand, often do not infiltrate extensively and can sometimes be resected easily. However, this measure should be attempted only when the metastasis is solitary as revealed by computed tomography (CT) or MRI scan and when the patient's cancer is under good control systemically. In these circumstances, surgery followed by radiotherapy results in a longer survival than is produced by radiotherapy alone (40 weeks versus 15 weeks).

B. Radiation therapy has a major role in the treatment of gliomas. The tumor dose must exceed 5000 cGy to achieve control. Partial brain irradiation is usually adequate. In the case of medulloblastomas, radiotherapy is applied to the entire neuraxis after surgical extirpation of the primary lesion because these tumors tend to metastasize by shedding cells into the CSF. Whole-brain irradiation is employed for metastatic cancers.

C. Chemotherapy is used to treat patients with the more malignant gliomas, including the anaplastic astrocytomas, oligodendrogliomas, and glioblastoma multiforme. Because of the highly malignant features of medulloblastoma, chemotherapy is also used to treat this tumor. Chemotherapy probably has little role in the treatment of cerebral metastases. Malignant meningeal infiltrates, also called "carcinomatous meningitis" may respond to a combination of radiation therapy and intrathecal chemotherapy.

D. Supportive care. Because of their location in the central nervous system (CNS), intracranial tumors may cause serious neurologic symptoms, including seizures, headaches, and impairment of mental, motor, and sensory function. This dysfunction is the result of the combined effects of the tumor and a variable degree of surrounding cerebral edema. Therapy is therefore directed toward reducing the edema as well as reducing the size of the malignant tumor mass.

III. Chemotherapy

A. General considerations

1. **Special characteristics of primary brain tumors.** The blood supply to brain tumors is not homogeneous owing to poorly vascularized areas of central necrosis. The tumor vessels lack the normal blood-brain barrier; but at the more rapidly growing outer edge of the tumor the blood-brain barrier is mostly intact. Therefore it has usually been assumed that the most effective chemotherapeutic agents are

those that are lipid-soluble or with a relatively low molecular weight, such that they are able to cross the normal blood-brain barrier and achieve adequate intracerebral concentration. Another requirement for the use of brain tumor chemotherapy is that it be able to achieve cell kill in a heterogeneous population of tumor cells. A large percentage of the cells in gliomas appears to be in a resting state (G_0) and thus relatively insensitive to cell cycle-active agents.

2. **Aims of treatment.** The two major aims of therapy for glioma are to reduce the neurologic deficit and to prolong a useful and comfortable life by reducing the tumor mass and associated edema. Surgical decompression, when possible, and radiation therapy are standard treatments. There is some controversy over the role of adjuvant chemotherapy. The major use of chemotherapy is to treat patients who relapse after radiation therapy.

There is little evidence that chemotherapy improves the survival for glioblastoma (median < 1 year). Survival has been shown to depend more on certain prognostic factors such as patient age, performance status at diagnosis, and extent of surgical resection.

3. **Quality of life.** Quality of life is a complex issue with neurologic tumors because it depends largely on the type of deficit induced by the tumor (e.g., hemiparesis, aphasia, inability to read or write). Treatment has been shown to improve quality of life somewhat.

4. **Response evaluation.** Responses are sometimes difficult to analyze because of symptoms due to edema, seizures, steroid therapy, and a fixed neurologic deficit from surgery. Nonetheless, regular neurologic examinations with scoring of the neurologic deficit and repeated CT or MRI scans of the brain usually enable the physician to make an objective determination of response.

B. **Specific chemotherapy agents**

1. **Nitrosoureas** have been the most effective drugs against malignant gliomas and medulloblastomas. The responses vary from 30% to 50%, with a median duration of about 6 months. When administered to glioma patients as an adjuvant to radiation therapy, carmustine or lomustine appear to prolong survival minimally, compared with radiation therapy alone. The major benefit may be to young and middle-aged adults or to those with anaplastic astrocytoma rather than glioblastoma.

   a. **Carmustine (BCNU)** is given usually at a dose of 80 mg/m^2 IV daily for 3 days every 6–8 weeks.

   b. **Lomustine (CCNU)** may be given at 130 mg/m^2 PO once every 6–8 weeks.

   c. **Duration.** Two cycles are usually administered; and if a response is observed clinically or by CT scan, the drug is continued until progression or a total dose of 1200 mg/m^2 (of either drug) has been reached.

d. **Precautions.** These drugs may produce severe and delayed myelotoxicity. Patients over age 60 should be treated with lower doses. All patients should have frequent blood counts during treatment, and subsequent doses should be lowered if there is a significant nadir: white blood cell (WBC) count < 2000/μl or platelet count < 75,000/μl). Treatment to cumulative doses in excess of 1200 mg/m^2 may be associated with pulmonary fibrosis that is usually irreversible and sometimes fatal. Less common toxicities are hepatotoxicity and phlebitis, or pain in the arm used for treatment.

2. **Combinations.** Vincristine 1–2 mg/m^2 (maximum 2 mg) IV weekly up to 4 weeks and procarbazine 100 mg/m^2/day PO for about 4 weeks are sometimes given together or with a nitrosourea. Good responses can be achieved, but combinations have not been proved to be superior to single agents.

3. **Other agents and approaches to drugs**

   a. **Advanced glioma:** Hydroxyurea, dacarbazine, methotrexate, cisplatin, and etoposide have activity. Aziridinylbenzoquinone (AZQ) and some other investigational agents are also active.

   b. **Medulloblastoma:** Cisplatin with either etoposide or CCNU has been used, but controlled trials have not yet proven benefit in the adjuvant setting. Patients with medulloblastoma should be entered in a clinical trial whenever it is possible and the patient is agreeable.

   c. **Newer approaches** to therapy of brain tumors include administration of drugs into the internal carotid artery in order to achieve higher local doses. Intracarotid BCNU has been associated with severe ophthalmic and cerebral toxicity and cannot be recommended. Cisplatin by the intraarterial route does produce a large number of responses. Very high dose systemic chemotherapy with autologous bone marrow rescue is another investigational approach. Interferons do not appear to be effective. Interleukins and LAK cells are being evaluated, but thus far there is little to suggest that biologic treatments are useful.

4. **Meningeal carcinomatosis** is treated with radiation therapy to the symptomatic areas of the CNS (e.g., to the brain for cranial nerve dysfunction) as well as intrathecal chemotherapy.

   a. The most commonly used agent is **methotrexate** 12 mg/m^2 (maximum 15 mg) per dose once or twice a week until the cytologic examination shows clearing of the CSF, then once a month as maintenance.

   b. **Alternate agents** are thiotepa 2–10 mg/m^2, and cytosine arabinoside 30 mg/m^2.

    c. Administration. Each of these chemotherapy agents should be freshly prepared in preservative-free diluent. Because drugs administered into the lumbar intrathecal space do not always reach the upper spinal cord, it is preferable to give the agents into an Ommaya reservoir, which may be implanted under the scalp and connected by a catheter, through a burr hole, to the frontal horn of the lateral ventricle. This method permits easy access to the CSF, and achieves good drug levels throughout the CSF pathways. If the lumbar intrathecal route is used, it is recommended that the volume injected be larger than the volume withdrawn (e.g., withdraw 5 ml for analysis and inject 10 ml).

    d. Complications of intrathecal chemotherapy include painful arachnoiditis or leukoencephalopathy. The latter is more likely to occur if the Ommaya catheter tip becomes lodged in the brain tissue rather than the CSF. Bone marrow suppression is not usually severe unless the patient undergoes spinal irradiation or systemic chemotherapy as well. Oral leucovorin can be given after the intrathecal methotrexate (10 mg leucovorin PO q6h × 6–8 doses, starting 24 hours after the methotrexate) to prevent marrow toxicity.

C. Treatment of cerebral edema

  1. Corticosteroids are usually started soon after the diagnosis of brain tumor is established. Dexamethasone 4–10 mg q6h PO or IV reduces or eliminates the lethargy, headache, visual blurring, and nausea caused by cerebral edema and also often reduces some of the focal neurologic signs and symptoms, e.g., hemiparesis or dysphagia.

    The corticosteroid dose may be tapered and stopped after radiation therapy is complete—and resumed if symptoms recur. The dose should be held at a level that maximizes therapeutic benefit and minimizes unwanted side effects, e.g., gastric irritation, sleeplessness, mood swings, cushingoid body features, increased appetite, and proximal myopathy. It is also advisable to suggest that patients take an antacid with the steroid and that they watch for the occurrence of oral and vaginal thrush, which can be effectively treated with nystatin (suspension or suppositories) or clotrimazole (lozenges or suppositories).

  2. Treatment of refractory cerebral edema

    a. When moderate doses of dexamethasone do not effectively control cerebral edema, the dose may be increased transiently to 40 mg IV 4–6 h. This dose should usually not be maintained longer than 48–72 hours.

    b. Mannitol diuresis. In an urgent situation, an osmotic diuretic acts more rapidly than a corticosteroid.

(1) **Mannitol** 75–100 gm (as a 15–25% solution) is given by rapid infusion over 20–30 minutes and repeated at 6- to 8-hour intervals as needed.

(2) **Cautions and duration.** Careful monitoring of electrolytes, fluid intake and output, and body weight is essential to avoid dehydration. The osmotic diuresis may be discontinued when there is an improvement in the signs and symptoms of the cerebral edema and when the corticosteroids or other measures to reduce cerebral edema have taken effect.

D. Seizure control. As the occurrence of seizures is common in patients with cerebral neoplasms, many physicians recommend starting all such patients on anticonvulsant therapy with phenytoin 300 mg/day, regardless of whether the patient has already experienced a seizure. Other oncologists treat only if the patient has had seizures or has undergone craniotomy. Anticonvulsants are used for every patient who has had a craniotomy, regardless of the seizure history. For those on long-term anticonvulsant therapy, it is important to check drug levels at intervals, especially after dosages of other medications are changed or new medications are added, because interactions between drugs occur.

Seizures are a particular problem after cisplatin therapy. They result from falling phenytoin levels and hypomagnesemia.

Selected Reading

Burger, P. C., and Vollmer, R. T. Histologic factors of prognostic significance in the glioblastoma multiforme. *Cancer* 46:1179, 1980.

Duffner, P. K., et al. Primitive neuroectodermal tumors of childhood. *J. Neurosurg.* 55:376, 1981.

Grossman, S. A., et al. Decreased phenytoin levels in patients receiving chemotherapy. *Am. J. Med.* 87:505, 1989.

Hubbard, J. L., et al. Adult cerebellar medulloblastomas: the pathological, radiographic, and clinical disease spectrum. *J. Neurosurg.* 70:536, 1989.

Kornblith, P. L., and Walker, M. Chemotherapy for malignant gliomas. *J. Neurosurg.* 68:1, 1988.

Kovnar, E. H., et al. Preirradiation cisplatin and etoposide in the treatment of high-risk medulloblastoma and other malignant embryonal tumors of the central nervous system: a phase II study. *J. Clin. Oncol.* 8:330, 1990.

Levin, V. A., et al. Modified procarbazine, CCNU, and vincristine (PCV 3) combination chemotherapy in the treatment of malignant brain tumors. *Cancer Treat. Rep.* 64:237, 1980.

Mellet, L. B. Physicochemical considerations and pharmacokinetic behavior in delivery of drugs to the central nervous system. *Cancer Treat. Rep.* 61:527, 1977.

Patchell, R. A., et al. A randomized trial of surgery in the treatment of single metastases to the brain. *N. Engl. J. Med.* 322:494, 1990.

Shapiro, W. R., et al. Randomized trial of three chemotherapy regimens and two radiotherapy regimens in postoperative treatment of malignant glioma. *J. Neurosurg.* 71:1, 1989.

Shapiro, W. R., and Shapiro, J. R. Principles of brain tumor chemotherapy. *Semin. Oncol.* 13:56, 1986.

Sposto, R., et al. The effectiveness of chemotherapy for treatment of high grade astrocytoma in children: results of a randomized trial. *J. Neurooncol.* 7:165, 1989.

Tirelli, U., et al. Etoposide (VP-16-213) in malignant brain tumors: a phase II study. *J. Clin. Oncol.* 2:432, 1984.

Trojanowski, T., et al. Quality of survival of patients with brain gliomas treated with postoperative CCNU and radiation therapy. *J. Neurosurg.* 70:18, 1989.

Walker, M. D., et al. Randomized comparison of radiotherapy and nitrosoureas for malignant glioma after surgery. *N. Engl. J. Med.* 303:1323, 1980.

Wasserstrom, W. R., Glass, J. P., and Posner, J. B. Diagnosis and treatment of leptomeningeal metastasis from solid tumors: experience with 90 patients. *Cancer* 49:759, 1982.

Weiss, R. M., Poster, D. S., and Penta, J. S. The nitrosoureas and pulmonary toxicity. *Cancer Treat. Rev.* 8:111, 1981.

Zimm, S., et al. Intracerebral metastasis in solid-tumor patients: natural history and results of treatment. *Cancer* 48:384, 1981.

Soft Tissue Sarcomas

Robert S. Benjamin

I. Classification and approach to treatment

A. Types of soft tissue sarcomas. The soft tissue sarcomas are a group of diseases characterized by neoplastic proliferation of tissue of mesenchymal origin. They differ from the more common carcinomas, which arise from epithelial tissue. Sarcomas can arise in any area of the body and from any origin; however, they most commonly arise in the soft tissue of the extremities, trunk, retroperitoneum, and head and neck area. There are at least 21 types of sarcoma, classified according to lines of differentiation toward normal tissue. For example, rhabdomyosarcoma shows evidence of skeletal muscle fibers with cross-striations; liposarcoma shows fat production; and angiosarcoma shows vessel formation. Precise characterization of the types of sarcoma is often impossible, and these tumors are called *unclassified sarcomas*. All of the primary bony sarcomas may arise from soft tissue, leading to such diagnoses as extraskeletal osteosarcomas, extraskeletal Ewing's sarcoma, and extraskeletal chondrosarcoma. An increasingly common diagnosis at present is malignant fibrous histiocytoma. This tumor is characterized by a mixture of spindle (fibrous) cells and round (histiocytic) cells arranged in a storiform pattern with frequent areas of pleomorphic appearance and frequent giant cells.

B. Metastatic spread of all sarcomas tends to be through the blood rather than through the lymphatic system. The lungs are by far the most frequent site of metastatic disease, and local metastases by direct invasion are the second most common area on involvement, followed by bone and liver. (Liver metastases are common with leiomyosarcomas of gastrointestinal origin, however.) Central nervous system (CNS) metastases are extraordinarily rare.

C. Staging of sarcomas is complex and demands an expert sarcoma pathologist.

1. The primary determinant of stage is **tumor grade.** Grade 1 tumors are stage I, grade 2 tumors are stage II, and grade 3 tumors are stage III. Any tumor with lymph node metastases is automatically stage III, and any tumor with gross invasion of bone, major vessel, or major nerve is stage IV.

2. Further division of stages I–III into A and B is based on **tumor size.** A = tumor size less than 5 cm; and B = tumor size 5 cm or more. For stage III, lymph node metastases are classified as III_C; for stage IV, local invasion is called IV_A; and IV_B represents distant metastases.

D. Primary treatment

1. **Surgery and radiotherapy.** Treatment of the primary tumor involves surgery with or without radia-

tion therapy. If radiation therapy is not used, surgery must be radical. Although it often involves amputation, more and more frequently complete excision of the involved muscle group from origin to insertion is being performed.

2. **Adjuvant chemotherapy.** The role of adjuvant chemotherapy is unclear, with both positive and negative studies reported. Other studies are currently under way in an attempt to clarify the role of adjuvant chemotherapy. Some investigators believe that adjuvant therapy is clearly indicated for patients whose histologic type, grade, or location is known to convey a poor prognosis.

E. **Prognosis** is related to stage, with a 5-year survival rate of 75% for stage I, 55% for stage II, and 29% for stage III. The survival rate for stage IV disease is less than 10%; however, a definite fraction of patients in this category can be cured. Most patients with stage IV disease, if left untreated, die within 6–12 months; however, there is great variation in actual survival, and patients may go on with slowly progressive disease for many years.

F. **Response to treatment** is measured in the standard fashion for solid tumors.

1. **Complete remission** implies complete disappearance of all signs and symptoms of disease.

2. **Partial remission** is a 50% or more decrease in measurable disease, calculated by comparing the sum of the products of perpendicular diameters of all lesions before and after therapy. When disease is not measurable in two dimensions but can be followed objectively by angiogram, x-ray films, ultrasonography, or computed tomography (CT), a definite decrease in the amount of metastatic disease confirmed by two independent investigators is the equivalent of a partial response, as calculated by a 50% decrease in measurable tumor.

3. **Lesser degrees of tumor shrinkage** are categorized by some physicians as stable disease and by others as improvement or minor response. Stable disease implies a less than 25% increase in disease for at least 8 weeks. For all response categories, no new disease must appear during response.

4. **Progression.** New disease in any area or a 25% or more increase in measurable disease constitutes progressive disease.

5. **Survival.** In all cases, patients whose disease responds objectively to chemotherapy survive longer than patients with progressive disease, and the degree of prolongation of survival is directly proportional to the degree of antitumor response that can be measured.

II. **Chemotherapy**

A. **General considerations and aims of therapy.** Although there are numerous types of soft tissue sarcoma, there are few differences among them regarding responsiveness to a standard soft tissue sarcoma regimen. Chondrosarcomas and leiomyosarcomas of gastrointestinal origin respond less frequently than the other soft tissue sarcomas. In contrast, two tumors, Ewing's sarcoma and rhabdomyosarcoma, particularly in the pediatric age group, are responsive in a fraction of cases to dactinomycin or vincristine, or both. The other tumors are not.

The goal of therapy for patients with advanced disease is primarily palliative, although a small fraction, about 20%, of patients who achieve complete remission are in fact cured. The first aim therefore is to achieve complete remission, and we have demonstrated that the prognoses are the same whether complete remission is obtained by chemotherapy alone or by chemotherapy plus adjuvant surgery, i.e., surgical removal of all residual disease. Short of complete remission, partial remission causes some palliation with relief of symptoms and prolongation of survival by approximately 1 year. Any degree of improvement or stabilization of previously advancing disease likewise increases survival.

B. **Effective drugs.** The most important chemotherapeutic agent is doxorubicin (Adriamycin), which forms the backbone of all combination chemotherapy regimens. Dacarbazine (DTIC), a marginal agent by itself, adds significantly to doxorubicin in prolonging remission duration and survival as well as increasing the response rate. Cyclophosphamide adds marginally, if at all, but is included in some effective regimens. Ifosfamide, a newly released analog of cyclophosphamide, has documented activity in patients who are refractory to combinations containing cyclophosphamide. It is usually given together with the uroprotective agent mesna to prevent hemorrhagic cystitis.

The key to effective sarcoma chemotherapy is the steep dose-response curve for doxorubicin. At a dose of 45 mg/m^2 the response rate is less than 20% compared with a 37% response rate at a dose of 75 mg/m^2. A similar dose-response relation exists with combination chemotherapy, and the regimens with the best reported results are those utilizing the highest doses.

C. **Primary chemotherapy regimen.** The most effective primary chemotherapy regimens include doxorubicin plus dacarbazine (ADIC), with or without the addition of cyclophosphamide (CyADIC) or ifosfamide and Mesna (MAID). The CyADIC regimen is a modification of the standard CyVADIC regimen, which includes vincristine. Because analysis has shown that vincristine makes no significant contribution and produces neurotoxicity, its addition at a dose of 2 mg maximum or 1.4 mg/m^2 weekly for 6 weeks and then once every 3–4 weeks is recommended only for rhabdomyosarcoma and Ewing's sarcoma. By giving doxorubicin and dacarbazine by continuous 72- or 96-hour infusion with the two drugs mixed in the same infusion pump, nausea and vomiting are markedly reduced, and the chemotherapy can be continued until a cumulative doxorubicin dose of 800 mg/m^2 is reached with less cardiac toxicity than with standard doxorubicin administration and a cumulative dose of 450 mg/m^2.

1. **Continuous-infusion CyADIC regimen** is as follows.
   a. Cyclophosphamide 600 mg/m^2 IV day 1 *and*
   b. Doxorubicin by continuous 96-hour infusion, 60 mg/m^2 IV (15 mg/m^2/24 hours for 4 days) *and*
   c. Dacarbazine, by continuous 96-hour infusion, 1000 mg/m^2 IV (250 mg/m^2/24 hours for 4 days) mixed in the same bag or pump as the doxorubicin. Doses are divided into 4 consecutive 24-hour infusions.
   d. Repeat cycle every 3–4 weeks.
2. **Continuous-infusion ADIC regimen** is as follows.
   a. Doxorubicin, by continuous 96-hour infusion, 90 mg/m^2 IV (22.5 mg/m^2/24 hours for 4 days) *and*
   b. Dacarbazine, by continuous 96-hour infusion, 900 mg/m^2 IV (225 mg/m^2/24 hours for 4 days) mixed in the same bag or pump as the doxorubicin. Doses are divided into 4 consecutive 24-hour infusions.
   c. Repeat cycle every 3–4 weeks.
3. **MAID regimen** is as follows.
   a. Mesna, by continuous 96-hour infusion, 10,000 mg/m^2 IV (2500 mg/m^2/24 hours for 4 days) *and*
   b. Doxorubicin, by continuous 72-hour infusion, 60 mg/m^2 IV (20 mg/m^2/24 hours for 3 days) *and*
   c. Ifosfamide, by continuous 72-hour infusion, 7500 mg/m^2 IV (2500 mg/m^2/24 hours for 3 days); doses divided into 3 consecutive 24-hour infusions *and*
   d. Dacarbazine, by continuous 96-hour infusion, 1000 mg/m^2 IV (250 mg/m^2/24 hours for 4 days) mixed in the same bag or pump as the doxorubicin. Doses are divided into 4 consecutive 24-hour infusions.
   e. Repeat cycle every 3–4 weeks.
4. **Dose modification.** Doses of doxorubicin, cyclophosphamide, ifosfamide, and mesna should be increased or decreased by 25% each course of therapy in order to achieve a lowest absolute granulocyte count of approximately 500/μl. Maximum doxorubicin dose is limited to 800 mg/m^2, at which point therapy should be discontinued unless cardiac biopsies indicate that it is safe to continue. For Ewing's sarcoma and rhabdomyosarcoma the therapy is continued, and dactinomycin (2 mg/m^2 single dose or 0.5 mg/m^2 daily for 5 days) may be substituted for the doxorubicin with continuation of the regimen for a total of 18 months.
5. **Alternative regimen for children with rhabdomyosarcoma** is the so-called pulse VAC regimen. Dactinomycin is given at a total dose of 2.0–2.5 mg/m^2 by divided daily injection over 5–7 days (e.g.,

0.5 mg/m^2 daily for 5 days) repeated every 3 months for a total of 5 courses. Cyclophosphamide pulses of 275–330 mg/m^2 daily for 7 days are begun at the same time but are given every 6 weeks with vincristine 2 mg/m^2 on days 1 and 8 of each cyclophosphamide cycle. Cyclophosphamide cycles are terminated prematurely if the white blood cell counts fall below 1500/µl. Chemotherapy continues for 2 years.

D. Secondary chemotherapy. Secondary chemotherapy for patients with sarcoma is relatively unrewarding, with response rates of less than 10% for almost all conventional drugs or regimens tested. The best commercially available drug is ifosfamide, which if not used for primary treatment produces a response in about 20% of patients. Methotrexate, with a response rate of about 15% regardless of schedule, is the only other active agent. When patients fail primary chemotherapy and ifosfamide, therefore, they should be entered in a phase II study of a new agent to see if some activity can be established, as other reasonably good alternatives do not exist.

E. Complications of chemotherapy. Side effects of sarcoma chemotherapy can be classified into three categories: life-threatening, potentially dangerous, and unpleasant.

  1. Life-threatening complications of chemotherapy are infection or bleeding. Because thrombocytopenia of less than 20,000/µl rarely occurs with this type of chemotherapy, bleeding is rare. Approximately 20% of patients have documented or suspected infection related to drug-induced neutropenia at some time during their treatment courses. These infections are rarely fatal if treated promptly at the onset of the febrile neutropenia episode with broad-spectrum, bactericidal antibiotics.

  2. Potentially dangerous side effects of chemotherapy include the following.

   a. Mucositis in fewer than 25% of patients, which may interfere with oral intake or may act as a source of infection.

   b. Granulocytopenia, which predisposes the patient to infection but because of its brevity rarely causes infection.

   c. Thrombocytopenia, which is usually insignificant.

   d. Cardiac damage due to doxorubicin rarely causes clinical problems at the doses recommended, with usually reversible congestive heart failure occurring in fewer than 5% of patients.

   e. Hemorrhagic cystitis, a rare complication of cyclophosphamide therapy, is the dose-limiting toxicity of ifosfamide. It can be prevented in most cases by administration of another agent, mesna, before and after each ifosfamide dose, allowing higher doses of ifosfamide to be used.

3. Unpleasant but rarely serious problems include nausea and vomiting (primarily due to dacarbazine) and alopecia (due to doxorubicin, cyclophosphamide, and ifosfamide).

Selected Reading

Antman, K. H., et al. Phase II trial of ifosfamide with mesna in previously treated metastatic sarcoma. *Cancer Treat. Rep.* 69:499, 1985.

Benjamin, R. S., et al. The chemotherapy of soft tissue sarcomas in adults. In *Management of Primary Bone and Soft Tissue Tumors.* Chicago: Year Book Medical Publishers, 1977. Pp. 309–316.

Elias, A. Response to mesna, doxorubicin, ifosfamide, and dacarbazine in 108 patients with metastatic or unresectable sarcoma and no prior chemotherapy. *J. Clin. Oncol.* 7:1208, 1989.

Lindberg, R. D., et al. Conservative surgery and radiation therapy for soft tissue sarcomas. In *Management of Primary Bone and Soft Tissue Tumors.* Chicago: Year Book Medical Publishers, 1977. Pp. 289–298.

Russell, W. O., et al. A clinical and pathological staging system for soft tissue sarcomas. *Cancer* 40:1562, 1977.

Bony Sarcomas

Robert S. Benjamin

There are four major sarcomas of bone, each differing somewhat in clinical behavior, chemotherapy responsiveness, and prognosis. All present as painful bony lesions, and all metastasize preferentially to lung and then to other bones Untreated prognosis is inversely proportional to chemotherapy responsiveness. The sarcomas are considered in order of chemotherapeutic responsiveness, which is as follows: (1) Ewing's sarcoma; (2) osteosarcoma; (3) malignant fibrous histiocytoma of bone; and (4) chondrosarcoma.

Response to treatment is evaluated according to the usual criteria used for solid tumors, identical to those reported in Chapter 19 for soft tissue sarcomas. Angiography is particularly helpful for defining response of primary bone tumors to chemotherapy, and angiographic response correlates well with pathologic tumor destruction. Often complete resection and examination of the total specimen are required to follow response to therapy of a primary lesion and to confirm complete remission.

I. Ewing's sarcoma
A. General considerations and aims of therapy
1. **Tumor characteristics.** Ewing's sarcoma is a highly malignant, small, round cell tumor of bone. It occurs most commonly during the second decade, with 90% of patients under age 30. There is a slight predominance in males. The most common locations are the pelvis or the diaphysis of long tubular bones of the extremities. Often systemic symptoms of fever and leukocytosis suggest infection. Radiographically, the predominant feature is osteolysis, although sclerosis does occur. Frequently, the periosteal reaction has the so-called onion skin pattern with layering of subperiosteal new bone, frequently with spicules radiating out from the cortex. Prognosis, until recently, was poor with a less than 10% five-year survival and almost one-half of the patients dead within 1 year of diagnosis.
2. **Primary treatment.** For this reason and because of the mutilative surgery involved in resecting the primary lesion, radiotherapy has been the primary modality for local tumor control. As techniques for limb salvage surgery have become more widely practiced, attempts to utilize surgery rather than radiation therapy are increasing.
B. Chemotherapy. The timing of chemotherapy in relation to treatment of the primary lesion varies among investigators. Commonly, chemotherapy is given initially for 3–4 months followed by treatment of the primary lesion with surgery or radiotherapy, followed by additional chemotherapy for a total of 17–18 months.
1. **CyVADIC regimen.** Perhaps the best chemotherapeutic regimen for Ewing's sarcoma is the continu-

ous-infusion CyVADIC regimen, which is mentioned elsewhere (see Chap. 19, **II.C**).

   a. Cyclophosphamide 600 mg/m^2 IV on day 1 *and*
   b. Vincristine 1.4 mg/m^2 (2 mg maximum) IV weekly for 6 weeks, then on day 1 of each cycle *and*
   c. Doxorubicin (Adriamycin) 60 mg/m^2 IV by 96-hour continuous infusion through a central venous catheter (15 mg/m^2/24 hours for 4 days) *and*
   d. Dacarbazine (DTIC) 1000 mg/m^2 IV by 96-hour continuous infusion (250 mg/m^2/24 hours for 4 days) mixed in the same bag or pump as the doxorubicin. Doses are divided into 4 consecutive 24-hour infusions.
   e. Repeat cycle every 3–4 weeks.

2. **Dose modifications.** Courses are repeated with a 25% increase or decrease in the doses of cyclophosphamide and doxorubicin depending on morbidity. Most patients can tolerate a nadir granulocyte count of 500/μl; and unless this point is reached, maximum dose and benefit may not be achieved. Courses are repeated in 3–4 weeks as soon as granulocyte recovery to 1500/μl platelet recovery to 100,000/μl occur. Complications are as described for soft tissue sarcomas (see Chap. 19, **II.C.2**), with the addition of peripheral neuropathy from vincristine. When the cumulative dose of doxorubicin has reached 800 mg/m^2, dactinomycin is substituted at a dose of 2 mg/m^2 on day 1 or 0.5 mg/m^2 daily for 5 days for a total of 18 months of chemotherapy.

3. **Alternative regimens omitting dacarbazine.** The doses of cyclophosphamide may be varied up to 1500 mg/m^2; dactinomycin is given with, or in place of, doxorubicin; and in some cases high-dose methotrexate is added. Direct comparison of the various approaches has not shown marked superiority of one regimen over another.

4. **Responses.** Most patients with metastatic disease obtain complete remission; however, almost all patients relapse and ultimately die of the disease. When chemotherapy is used to treat the primary disease along with surgery or irradiation, the prognosis depends on the size and location of the primary tumor. Patients with large flat-bone lesions have a less than 30% cure rate compared with a 60–70% cure rate for those patients with long-bone lesions, which are generally smaller. An alarming complication of the chemotherapy–irradiation combination is a high frequency of second malignancies in cured patients, with 4 of 10 patients in one series developing secondary sarcomas within their radiated fields. This complication is another reason for considering surgical intervention rather than irradiation, as chemotherapy is required for cure regardless of whether the primary lesion can be controlled with radiation.

5. **Secondary chemotherapy.** Occasional responses have been seen with etoposide (VP-16), other alkyl-

ating agents (especially ifosfamide), the nitrosoureas, and cisplatin. A combination of etoposide and ifosfamide is now frequently used. Nonetheless, secondary responses are poor, and the survival of a relapsed patient with Ewing's sarcoma is measured in weeks.

II. Osteosarcoma

A. General considerations. Osteosarcoma is a tumor with a poor prognosis in the absence of effective chemotherapy. It is the most common primary bone sarcoma. It frequently affects patients 10–25 years old and tends to be located around the knee in about two-thirds of patients, with two-thirds of those tumors involving the distal femur. As with other sarcomas of bone, pulmonary metastases are most common, followed by bony metastases.

B. Role of chemotherapy. Chemotherapy is usually employed in the adjuvant situation both pre- and postoperatively, and its value in this regard has been conclusively demonstrated by the use of preoperative chemotherapy. Patients who obtain complete response to preoperative chemotherapy with tumor destruction of 90% or more have significantly improved survival. Response rates of evaluable tumors range from 30% to 80%. Cure of primary disease with adjuvant chemotherapy is 50–80%. Preoperative chemotherapy is given for up to 4 months prior to surgery. The primary tumor is then removed, either with a limb-sparing procedure or amputation, together with all known metastatic disease. It is then followed by additional postoperative chemotherapy.

C. Effective agents. The three major standard single agents for treatment of osteosarcoma are cisplatin, doxorubicin, and high-dose methotrexate. Although there are relatively few studies of ifosfamide, impressive responses have been noted in several series, and it certainly should be considered as having the same range of activity as the other three primary drugs. In addition, the combination of bleomycin, cyclophosphamide, and dactinomycin (BCD) has been effective.

D. Recommended regimen. A variety of regimens may be recommended based on preliminary or more extensive evaluation. They are as follows.

1. Doxorubicin + cisplatin

a. Doxorubicin 75–90 mg/m^2 IV by 96-hour continuous infusion through a central venous catheter *and*

b. Cisplatin 120 mg/m^2 IA (for primary tumor) or IV on day 6.

c. Repeat the cycle every 4 weeks. Discontinue both drugs after 800 mg/m^2 cumulative doxorubicin dose. If cisplatin must be discontinued earlier, substitute dacarbazine 750 mg/m^2 IV over 96 hours.

2. Alternating cycle chemotherapy is as follows.

a. High-dose methotrexate 8–12 gm/m^2 IV weekly for 4 weeks with leucovorin rescue (see **III.E.2**).

   b. Three weeks later administer BCD for 2 consecutive days.
      (1) Bleomycin 12 units/m^2 IV daily on days 1 and 2,
      (2) Cyclophosphamide 600 mg/m^2 IV daily on days 1 and 2,
      (3) Dactinomycin 450 μg/m^2 IV daily on days 1 and 2.
   c. Three weeks later repeat high-dose methotrexate weekly for 2 weeks.
   d. One week later give doxorubicin 45 mg/m^2 IV daily for 2 consecutive days.
   e. Three weeks later repeat high-dose methotrexate weekly for 2 weeks. Repeat the cycles using the sequence of BCD, high-dose methotrexate, doxorubicin, and high-dose methotrexate for 5 courses.
   3. Following primary chemotherapy, if there is less than 90% tumor necrosis at surgery, switch to the alternative regimen.
E. Special precautions during administration
   1. Cisplatin. Prehydration is necessary, either with overnight infusion of IV fluids at 150 ml/hour or 1 liter of fluid over 2 hours (for adults), followed by at least 6 liters of fluid containing potassium chloride (at least 20 mEq/liter) and magnesium sulfate (at least 4 mEq/liter) for the first day or two following cisplatin administration. The addition of mannitol (50 ml of a 20% solution) prior to cisplatin followed by 200 ml of a 20% solution mixed with normal saline in a total volume of 1 liter to run simultaneously with the cisplatin over 2–3 hours is preferred by many investigators. Particular care about electrolyte balance, including frequent determinations of magnesium, is necessary. In the presence of severe hypomagnesemia, magnesium sulfate 10–20 mEq/m^2 may be infused over 2–4 hours.
   2. High-dose methotrexate. Pretreatment creatinine clearance should be more than 70 ml/minute.
      a. Methotrexate administration and alkalinization of urine. Before administration of high-dose methotrexate, sodium bicarbonate 0.5 mEq/kg IV is infused over 15–30 minutes in an attempt to create an alkaline urine. Allopurinol, 300 mg/day for 3 days, is given starting 1 day before the methotrexate infusion. Methotrexate is dissolved in no more than 1000 ml of 5% dextrose in water with a final concentration of approximately 1 gm/dl. The total dose ranges from 8 gm/m^2 for fully grown patients to 12 mg/m^2 for children. The dose should be increased on subsequent courses if an immediate postinfusion methotrexate level is less than 10^{-3} M. Sodium bicarbonate 50 mEq/liter is added to the methotrexate solution which is infused over 4 hours. At completion

of the infusion an IV infusion of 5% dextrose in water with bicarbonate (50 mEq/liter) is given at a dose of 10 ml/kg over 2 hours if the patient is unable to drink or if the 24-hour methotrexate levels of the previous high-dose methotrexate treatment have been more than 1.5×10^{-5}M. The IV infusion is then discontinued, and the patient is encouraged to drink sufficient fluid to produce alkaline urine: approximately 1600 ml/m^2 for the first 24 hours and 1900 ml/m^2 daily for the next 3 days. Sodium bicarbonate, 14–28 mEq PO q6 h, is administered to ensure alkaline urine. The pH of the urine is measured; and if it is less than pH7 an extra dose of bicarbonate is administered.

   b. Leucovorin rescue. Twenty-four hours after the start of the methotrexate infusion, leucovorin 15–25 mg is administered PO q6h for a least 10 doses or IM if the oral medication is not tolerated.

   c. Serum methotrexate levels should be monitored and should fall approximately 1 log/day. When methotrexate concentration falls below 5×10^{-8} M, leucovorin may be safely discontinued. Intravenous hydration is required whenever oral intake is inadequate to produce sufficient urine output as previously defined as well as for abnormal serum methotrexate concentration, persistent vomiting, or early toxicity.

F. Complications. Complications of chemotherapy depend on the drugs. For doxorubicin and cyclophosphamide, the major complication is infection due to neutropenia. Other complications include stomatitis, nausea and vomiting, and delayed cardiac toxicity, as discussed for the management of soft tissue sarcomas (see Chap. 19, **II.E**). Dactinomycin causes similar side effects except cardiac toxicity. Methotrexate predominantly causes stomatitis, but it may cause myelosuppression and renal, hepatic, and central nervous system abnormalities. Cisplatin and dacarbazine cause severe nausea and vomiting. In addition, cisplatin nephrotoxicity is primarily a tubular defect with hypomagnesemia as the most prominent manifestation, but hypocalcemia, hypokalemia, and hyponatremia also occur. Delayed cumulative nephrotoxicity can cause impaired glomerular function as well. Ototoxicity may occur but is less common. Delayed neurotoxicity also occurs. Both cisplatin and methotrexate can, by causing renal toxicity, exacerbate their other side effects.

G. Recurrence and treatment of refractory disease. Patients with osteosarcoma who are refractory to a combination of doxorubicin and cisplatin may respond to high-dose methotrexate; patients refractory to high-dose methotrexate may respond to doxorubicin + cisplatin, and patients refractory to this regimen may respond to ifosfamide or, rarely, to BCD. However, treatment of refractory disease is usually disappointing, and participation in studies of new agents are indicated for patients whose lesions cannot be resected. Surgical resection of pulmonary metastases remains the only viable secondary therapy for most patients. For this reason, careful follow-up for detection of metastases while they are still at the stage of resectability is indicated.

III. **Malignant fibrous histiocytoma of bone.** This entity, characterized by a purely lytic lesion in bone, has a exceptionally poor prognosis when treated with surgery alone, although the number of reported patients is small. It may be difficult to distinguish from fibroblastic osteosarcoma and may be best considered as a fibroblastic osteosarcoma with minimal (i.e., no detectable) osteoid production. The tumor responds well to the CyADIC regimen for soft tissue sarcomas, with more than one-half of patients obtaining at least partial remission. In addition, cisplatin at a dose of 120 mg/m^2 every 4 weeks has produced remissions, even in patients who have failed primary therapy. A particularly attractive approach for patients with large, unresectable primary tumors is the use of cisplatin given by the intraarterial route. Complete tumor destruction in one patient and a good partial remission in a second patient have been reported among three patients so treated. Systemic doxorubicin may be added as for osteosarcomas (see **III.D.1**). Alternatively, responses have been seen after high-dose methotrexate-based regimens for osteosarcomas (see **III.D.2**). After local tumor destruction, surgery may be employed to remove residual disease. Because of the primary poor prognosis, adjuvant chemotherapy with the continuous infusion CyADIC regimen is recommended until an 800 mg/m^2 cumulative doxorubicin dose has been reached.

IV. **Chondrosarcoma.** The chemotherapy for chondrosarcoma is totally inadequate, and no regimen can be recommended except for the rare patient with mesenchymal chondrosarcoma, a subtype that may respond to CyADIC chemotherapy or cisplatin. Most patients are candidates only for surgical management. Metastatic disease should be treated on phase II protocols in an attempt to determine some effective type of chemotherapy that may be recommended in the future.

Selected Reading

Benjamin, R. S., et al. Chemotherapy for metastatic osteosarcoma: studies by the M.D. Anderson Hospital and the Southwest Oncology Group. *Cancer Treat. Rep.* 62:237, 1978.

Benjamin, R. S., et al. Preoperative chemotherapy for osteosarcoma: a treatment approach facilitating limb salvage with major prognostic implications. In S. E. Jones and S. E. Salmon (eds.), *Adjuvant Therapy of Cancer IV.* Orlando: Grune & Stratton, 1984. Pp. 601–610.

Chawla, S. P., et al. Adjuvant chemotherapy of primary malignant fibrous histiocytoma of bone—prolongation of disease-free and overall survival. In S. E. Jones and S. E. Salmon (eds.), *Adjuvant Therapy of Cancer IV.* Orlando: Grune & Stratton, 1984. Pp. 621–629.

Eilber, F., et al. Adjuvant chemotherapy for osteosarcoma: a randomized prospective trial. *J. Clin. Oncol.* 5:21, 1987.

Gehan, E. A., et al. Osteosarcoma: the M. D. Anderson experience, 1950–1974. In W. D. Terry and D. Windhorst (eds.), *Immunotherapy of Cancer: Present Status of Trials in Man.* New York: Raven Press, 1978.

Hayes, F. A., et al. Metastatic Ewing's sarcoma: remission induction and survival. *J. Clin. Oncol.* 5:1199, 1987.

Miser, J. S., et al. Ifosfamide with mesna uroprotection and etoposide: an effective regimen in the treatment of recurrent sarcomas and other tumors of children and young adults. *J. Clin. Oncol.* 5:1191, 1987.

Nesbit, M. E., et al. Multimodal therapy for the management of primary, nonmetastatic Ewing's sarcoma of bone: an intergroup study. *Nat. Cancer Inst. Monogr.* 56:255, 1981.

Rosen, G. Past experiences and future considerations with T-2 chemotherapy in the treatment of Ewing's sarcoma. In *Management of Primary Bone and Soft Tissue Tumors.* Chicago: Year Book Medical Publishers, 1977. Pp. 187–240.

Rosen, G., et al. The successful management of metastatic osteogenic sarcoma: a model for the treatment of primary osteogenic sarcoma. In A. T. van Oosterom, F. M. Muggia, and F. J. Cleton (eds.), *Therapeutic Progress in Ovarian Cancer, Testicular Cancer and the Sarcomas.* Hingham: Leiden University Press, 1980. Pp. 249–365.

Rosen, G., et al. Ewing's sarcoma: ten-year experience with adjuvant chemotherapy. *Cancer* 47:2204, 1981.

Rosen, G., et al. Preoperative chemotherapy for osteogenic sarcoma: selection of postoperative adjuvant chemotherapy based on the response of the primary tumor to preoperative chemotherapy. *Cancer* 49:1221, 1982.

Acute Leukemias

Neil A. Lachant and Roland T. Skeel

The leukemias are a heterogeneous group of disorders characterized by the abnormal proliferation, accumulation, or both of hematopoietic cells and their immature precursors. Great therapeutic advances have been made since the early 1960s, so that many individuals can now be cured of these otherwise fatal illnesses. Unfortunately, however, an unacceptable high proportion of affected individuals still die from these diseases. Many questions remain unanswered as to the optimum way to treat these disorders. Therefore *all individuals with leukemia should be considered candidates for well designed experimental protocols.*

I. **Diagnosis and classification.** Acute leukemia is a clonal disorder that arises in a hematopoietic stem cell and ultimately gives rise to a state of functional bone marrow failure. The acute leukemias are divided into acute nonlymphocytic (ANLL) and acute lymphocytic (ALL) forms. Although the peripheral smear may be highly suggestive of acute leukemia, the diagnosis is made by examining the bone marrow. Classification into the ANLL and ALL categories is usually based on the morphologic, histochemical, enzymatic, and immunologic (antigenic) characteristics of the blast cells. Occasionally, electron microscopy, cytogenetics, and molecular biologic techniques aid in establishing the diagnosis. The principles used to diagnose and classify acute leukemia are presented below.

A. **Acute nonlymphocytic leukemia.** The French–American–British (FAB) system is most widely used for the diagnosis and subclassification of ANLL. Normally, myeloblasts (monoblasts cannot be distinguished morphologically from myeloblasts) and promyelocytes constitute fewer than 5% of the nucleated cells in the marrow. In general, the diagnosis of ANLL is established by demonstrating that leukemic cells (myeloblasts, promyelocytes, monoblasts, promonocytes, megakaryoblasts) constitute more than 30% of the nucleated marrow cells (or > 30% of the nonerythroid nucleated cells in the case of erythroleukemia). Classically, histochemical stains have been used to demonstrate that cells are of nonlymphoid origin. Common histochemical stains that are "positive" in nonlymphoid cells are sudan black B and peroxidase (myeloblasts, promyelocytes), "nonspecific" esterases, which are inhibited by sodium fluoride (monoblasts), and "block positive" periodic acid-Schiff (pronormoblasts in erythroleukemia). Antigens commonly demonstrated by immunologic techniques include My 7 and My 9 (myeloblasts and monoblasts) and von Willebrand factor and platelet antigen 1 (megakaryoblasts). A simplified version of the FAB classification system is as follows: M_1 = myelocytic leukemia without maturation; M_2 = myelocytic leukemia with maturation; M_3 = promyelocytic leukemia; M_4 = myelomonocytic leukemia; M_5 = monocytic leukemia; M_6 = erythroleukemia; and M_7 = megakaryoblastic leukemia.

B. Acute lymphocytic leukemia. Whereas mature lymphocytes may account for up to 25% of the nucleated cells in the adult bone marrow, recognizable lymphoblasts are not a component of normal marrow. In general, the diagnosis of ALL is established by demonstrating that leukemic lymphoblasts constitute more than 25% of the nucleated marrow cells. Because of its lack of reproducibility, the morphologic subclassification of ALL by the FAB system has been abandoned. In general, ALL is subclassified according to B cell or T cell lineage based on immunologic markers. Immunologic markers classically suggesting B cell lineage are the common ALL antigen (CALLA, CD10) ("common" or prepre-B cell ALL), intracytoplasmic μ heavy chains (pre-B cell ALL), and surface membrane immunoglobulin (B cell ALL). Ia, B4 (CD19), and B1 (CD20) are common generic B cell markers. T cell ALL arises from stage I (prothymocyte) and stage II thymocytes. Immunologic markers classically suggesting T cell lineage are T11 (CD2, sheep red blood cell receptor), T10 (panthymocyte), and T9 (transferrin receptor). The enzyme terminal deoxynucleotidal transferase (TdT) can be demonstrated in cells of early B cell (prior to pre-B cell) and T cell (through thymocyte) lineage.

C. Hybrid and stem cell acute leukemia. When nonlymphoid and lymphoid markers can be demonstrated on 10% or more of the leukemic cells, the leukemia is considered to be hybrid. With biphenotypic leukemia the individual leukemic cells express both lymphoid and nonlymphoid markers, whereas with bilineal leukemia the individual cells are heterogeneous, expressing either nonlymphoid or lymphoid markers but not both. With stem cell leukemia, the cells express only rudimentary hematopoietic markers (e.g., Ia antigen).

II. Initial support. Once the diagnosis of acute leukemia has been established, the next 24–48 hours are usually spent preparing the patient for the initiation of cytotoxic chemotherapy. The following issues need to be addressed in almost all individuals facing induction chemotherapy, as those individuals who are in the best overall shape are best able to tolerate the rigors of induction chemotherapy.

A. Hydration and correction of electrolyte imbalance. Dehydration needs to be corrected and adequate urine output maintained to prevent renal failure due to the deposition of cellular breakdown products. In the absence of cardiac disease, normal saline with or without 5% dextrose is infused to maintain the urine output at more than 100 ml/hour. The concomitant use of loop diuretics may be necessary in individuals with congestive heart failure. Although a variety of electrolyte problems may occur in individuals with acute leukemia, hypokalemia is the most troublesome, particularly in individuals with ANLL. Parenteral potassium replacement should be given even in individuals with ANLL who are normokalemic, as a normal serum potassium level does not reflect the diminished potassium stores of most of these individuals.

B. Prevention of uric acid nephropathy. Hyperuricemia is common at presentation and may also occur with the tumor lysis caused by chemotherapy. Allopurinol is the mainstay of preventing uric acid nephropathy. The usual initial adult dose is 300 mg (150 mg/m^2) bid for 2–3 days, which is then decreased to 300 mg once a day for the duration of the chemotherapy. Common side effects of allopurinol include rash and hepatic dysfunction. If chemotherapy needs to be initiated urgently, allopurinol at a dose of 600 mg bid is well tolerated for 1–2 days. With the advent of allopurinol, the role of urine alkalinization has become less clear. Although urine alkalinization increases uric acid solubility, it decreases the solubility of urinary phosphates and may promote phosphate deposition in individuals susceptible to the tumor lysis syndrome (e.g., B cell ALL and T cell lymphoblastic leukemias). A commonly employed method of urine alkalinization is to hydrate the patient with 0.5 N saline containing two syringes of sodium bicarbonate (44 mEq NaHCO$_3$/syringe) per liter.

C. Blood product support. Most individuals with acute leukemia present with bone marrow failure, so symptomatic anemia and thrombocytopenia must be corrected (see **II.H.2;** see also Chap. 33).

D. Fever or infection. Individuals frequently have a fever or an infection at initial diagnosis. The approach to fever and infection is discussed in Chapter 32. *The cardinal rule is that all individuals with acute leukemia and fever have an infection until proved otherwise.* Given the myelo- and immunosuppressive effects of chemotherapy and leukemia, severe infections should be treated aggressively prior to initiating chemotherapy but may be difficult to control.

E. Vascular access. Because of the need for several sites of venous access for at least 1 month, a multiple-lumen implantable catheter must be placed as soon as possible (see Chap. 38).

F. Suppression of menses. A serum human chorionic gonadotropin (β-hCG) assay (pregnancy test) should be done in all premenopausal women prior to initiating chemotherapy. Because menorrhagia may occur owing to the severe thrombocytopenia that is seen during induction chemotherapy, preventing menses becomes desirable. Medroxyprogesterone (Provera) may be used for hormonal support of the progestational endometrium. Medroxyprogesterone 10 mg bid PO should be started 5–7 days before the presumed starting time of the next menstrual period. It may be increased to 10 mg tid or higher if breakthrough bleeding occurs. Depo-Provera is contraindicated in the thrombocytopenic and neutropenic individual.

G. Psychosocial support. Individuals with acute leukemia are usually previously healthy individuals who have suddenly had to accept their own imminent mortality. Intensive psychologic support by the health care team, family, and religious leaders is critical for maintaining the patient's sense of well-being (see Chap. 34).

H. Optimization of comorbid disease. Individuals with good performance status are best able to tolerate chemotherapy. Comorbid disease (e.g., heart failure, diabetes, chronic lung disease) should be aggressively treated prior to initiating induction chemotherapy.

II. Therapeutic principles of and approach to therapy for acute leukemia

A. Therapeutic aim. The goals of chemotherapy are to eradicate the leukemic clone and reestablish normal hematopoiesis in the bone marrow. Two important principles need to be remembered: (1) long-term survival is seen only in individuals in whom a complete response is attained; and (2) with the exception of bone marrow transplantation as salvage therapy, the response to initial therapy predicts the fate of the individual with acute leukemia. Although leukemia therapy is toxic, and infection is the major cause of death during therapy, the median survival of untreated (or unresponsive) acute leukemia is 2–3 months, and most untreated individuals die of bone marrow failure. The doses of chemotherapy are never reduced because of cytopenias, as lowered doses still produce the unwanted side effects (further marrow suppression) without having as great a potential for eradicating the leukemic clone and ultimately improving marrow function.

B. Forms of chemotherapy

1. **Induction.** Initial intensive chemotherapy is given in an attempt to eradicate the leukemic clone and to induce a remission (complete response).

2. **Postinduction (postremission) chemotherapy.** Further chemotherapy is given after a complete response has been obtained in an attempt to further eradicate the residual, but nondetectable, leukemic cells.

   a. **Maintenance.** Low doses of drugs designed for outpatient use given for up to 3 years.

   b. **Consolidation.** Repeated courses of the same drugs at the same doses used to induce the remission, given soon after the remission has been achieved. Consolidation requires further acute hospitalization.

   c. **Intensification.** Intensive courses of putatively non-cross-resistant drugs given soon after the remission has been achieved. Early intensification requires further acute hospitalization.

C. Definition of response. The criteria are based on the peripheral blood counts and the status of the bone marrow at the time of marrow recovery, not at the time of marrow aplasia.

1. **Complete response (complete remission, CR)** is the return of the complete blood count (CBC) to "normal"—absolute neutrophil count (ANC) of more than

1500/μl, and platelet count of more than 100,000/μl in conjunction with a normal bone marrow (i.e., normal cellularity, < 5% blasts or promyelocytes/promonocytes, and an absence of obvious leukemic cells, e.g., containing Auer rods).

2. **Partial response** is the persistence of gross residual leukemia: 5–25% leukemic cells in the bone marrow.

IV. Therapy of adult ANLL

A. **General plan of therapy.** The day that induction chemotherapy is started is arbitrarily called day 1. Bone marrow aspiration and biopsy are repeated on approximately day 12–14. If the bone marrow is severely hypoplastic with fewer than 5% residual blasts or if the bone marrow is aplastic, no further chemotherapy is given and the patient is supported until bone marrow recovery occurs (usually 1–3 weeks). If there is residual leukemia at day 14 (which occurs 40% of the time), a second course of chemotherapy at attenuated doses is given. A bone marrow examination is repeated 2 weeks later (approximately day 26–28). For that 10% of patients with residual disease at day 28, a third course of chemotherapy may be given and the same evaluation process repeated. Once a complete response has been documented, the potential benefit of further postinduction therapy should be determined on an individual basis.

B. **Induction.** The same chemotherapeutic regimens are used to treat the various subtypes of ANLL (M_1–M_7). Factors that influence the choice of the chemotherapeutic program to be employed include the individual's cardiac function, age, and performance status. The initial drug doses outlined below are based on the presence of normal hepatic function but are not modified based on peripheral blood counts.

1. **De Novo ANLL.** Individuals who develop ANLL de novo have the best response to chemotherapy. Therapeutic options vary depending on the clinical situation.

a. **Normal cardiac function.** The two most commonly used programs are "7 + 3" and "DAT." Each produces a remission rate of 65–70% and they should be considered equivalent.

(1) **"7 + 3" combination**

Cytarabine 100 mg/m^2/day IV continuous infusion on days 1–7 *and*
Daunorubicin 45 mg/m^2 IV push on days 1–3.

If there is residual leukemia in the day 14 bone marrow specimen, the second course of chemotherapy is attenuated to a 5-day infusion of ara-C and 2 days of daunorubicin ("5 + 2"). There is no dose modification for the second course based on blood counts.

(2) **DAT**

Cytarabine 25 mg/m^2 IV bolus followed by 200 mg/m^2/day IV continuous infusion on days 1–5 *and*

Daunorubicin 60 mg/m^2 IV push on days 1–3 *and*

Thioguanine 100 mg/m^2 PO every 12 hours on days 1–5.

If there is residual leukemia in the day 14 bone marrow specimen, a second course of DAT is initiated at full doses. With either "7 + 3" or DAT, the dose of drugs for the second cycle is decreased to 50% of the initial dose if hepatic dysfunction (bilirubin > 2.0 mg/dl or transaminase > twice baseline) develops.

(3) **Mitoxantrone** may be substituted for daunorubicin in the "7 + 3" program at a dose of 12 mg/m^2. Mitoxantrone is cardiotoxic and should not be used in the presence of cardiac dysfunction.

(4) **Other agents.** Idarubicin, high dose ara-C, and amsacrine (m-AMSA) have been shown to be active for the induction of ANLL. None is considered to be superior to "7 + 3" or DAT. A few reports have suggested that fewer patients require a second induction course to achieve eradication of the leukemia cells when they are treated with induction regiments that substitute idarubicin, 12 mg/mg^2 daily on days 1–3, for daunorubicin. Some, therefore, use this drug as the preferred anthracycline.

b. **Impaired cardiac function.** The use of an anthracycline or an anthracenedione is contraindicated for induction therapy in individuals with severe underlying cardiac disease, particularly if the patient has had a recent myocardial infarction or has an ejection fraction of less than 50%. The choice of therapy in this situation is **high dose cytarabine** (HDAC) which consists of cytarabine 3 gm/m^2 IV infusion over 2–3 hours q12h for 12 doses. Unique complications include ulcerative keratitis and neurotoxicity. Because ara-C is secreted in tears, ulcerative keratitis can be prevented by instilling eyedrops (saline, methylcellulose, or steroid) q2h while awake and Lacri-Lube Ophthalmic Ointment (Allergan Pharmaceuticals) at bedtime starting at the time HDAC is initiated and continuing for 2–3 days after the last dose of HDAC. Neurotoxicity (e.g., cerebellar dysfunction, somnolence) occurs more frequently in older individuals and as the number of doses of HDAC increases. Some investigators add either

L-asparaginase or amsacrine (m-AMSA) to the HDAC.

2. ANLL in the elderly. Given that the median age at presentation is approximately 60 years, ANLL in the "elderly" individual is a common problem. Owing to the effects of comorbid disease and "old age" on normal physiology, elderly individuals are less able to withstand the inherent toxicity of induction chemotherapy compared to "younger adults." The decision to forgo therapy in an elderly patient with ANLL should not be made a priori based solely on age; rather, the decision to treat or not to treat should be based on more substantive factors, such as the presence of comorbid disease, performance status prior to diagnosis, quality of life prior to diagnosis, and projected long-term survival. In general, 40–50% of elderly individuals can achieve a complete response to chemotherapy. When a decision is made to treat the elderly patient with ANLL, modified doses of induction chemotherapy should be used.

a. Modified "7 + 3"

Cytarabine 100 mg/m^2/day IV continuous infusion on days 1–7 *and*
Daunorubicin 30 mg/m^2 IV push on days 1–3

b. Modified DAT

Cytarabine 100 mg/m^2/day SQ q12h on days 1–5 *and*
Daunorubicin 50 mg/m^2 IV push on day 1 *and*
Thioguanine 100 mg/m^2 PO q12h on days 1–5

c. Modified HDAC is a decrease in the cytarabine dose from 3 gm/m^2 to 2 gm/m^2 for 12 doses.

d. Low-dose cytarabine. Low-dose ara-C should not be considered as first line therapy but should be reserved for individuals who truly are not candidates for more intensive therapy. Low-dose ara-C is 10 mg/m^2 SQ bid given for 10–21 days.

3. Secondary ANLL. In general, secondary ANLL (e.g., arising after prior irradiation or alkylating chemotherapy, or evolving from a myelodysplastic syndrome or myeloproliferative disorder) does not respond as well to standard induction chemotherapy as does de novo ANLL. The advisability of chemotherapy needs to be assessed in each individual situation. Therapeutic options include supportive care, "7 + 3," and HDAC plus daunorubicin (45 mg/m^2 IV on days 1–3).

4. ANLL during pregnancy. The fortunes of both the mother and fetus must be considered when discussing the therapeutic options for a pregnant woman who develops ANLL. Therapeutic abortion must be considered if ANLL develops during the first trimester. If therapeutic abortion is not an option or if ANLL develops during the second or third trimester, induction chemotherapy should be undertaken. Except for a modest increase in fetal deaths and an increased risk of premature labor, "7 + 3" and DAT appear to be well tolerated by both the patient and the fetus. However, the long-term effects of *in utero* exposure are not yet known, as these exposed individuals are now just reaching their third decade of life.

C. **Postinduction therapy.** The fact that most patients with ANLL relapse despite attaining a complete remission suggests that further postinduction therapy is indicated to eradicate the residual but undetected leukemic clone. Although the optimum form remains controversial, almost all patients with ANLL benefit from some form of postinduction therapy. As with induction therapy, the type of postinduction therapy should be determined on an individual basis. Relative contraindications to postinduction therapy include complications during induction (e.g., posttransfusion hepatitis with persistent hepatic dysfunction, systemic fungal infection), poor tolerance of induction by the elderly, and pregnancy. Individuals with ANLL in first remission should be considered candidates for experimental protocols examining postinduction therapy.

1. **Maintenance.** Given the rigors of further intensive, cytoreductive chemotherapy, maintenance is generally the treatment of choice for elderly individuals as well as younger individuals who did not tolerate induction well. In general, remission duration is 12–15 months, and overall survival is 18–24 months with maintenance chemotherapy. Maintenance may be initiated when the peripheral blood counts have returned to normal, marrow cellularity is normal, infections have cleared, and mucositis has resolved. In general, maintenance is of no additional value after consolidation therapy. Maintenance may be alternating blocks of drugs or repetitive courses of the same drugs.

a. **Alternating courses.** A commonly used program of alternating blocks of drugs has been devised by Cancer and Acute Leukemia Group B (CALGB). Each of the four courses is given on a monthly basis during the cycle. Two cycles are given. If a bone marrow examination shows that the patient is still in a complete remission at the end of the second cycle, no further therapy is given. Minimal blood counts for initiating maintenance are an ANC of more than 2000/μl and a platelets count of more than 100,000/μl. Each cycle consists of the following four courses.

Course 1: Cytarabine 100 mg/m^2 SQ bid on days 1–5
Thioguanine 100 mg/m^2 PO bid on days 1–5

Course 2:   Cytarabine 100 mg/m² SQ bid on days 1–5
Vincristine 2 mg IV on days 1 and 8
Prednisone 40 mg/m² PO on days 1–5 (100 mg maximum)

Course 3:   Cytarabine 100 mg/m² SQ bid on days 1–5
Daunorubicin 45 mg/m² IV on days 1 and 2
This course may require support for pancytopenia.

Course 4:   Cytarabine 100 mg/m² SQ bid on days 1–5
Vincristine 2 mg IV on days 1 and 8
Prednisone 40 mg/m² PO on days 1–5 (100 mg maximum)

Once maintenance has been started, the next course may be given in 4 weeks, provided that infection, bleeding, and mucositis from the previous course have cleared, the ANC is more than 2000/μl, and the platelet count is more than 100,000/μl. If the ANC and platelet count are below the minimum, repeat them in 1 week and use the following criteria.

Dose (%)	ANC/μl	Platelets/μl
100	> 2000	> 100,000
50	1000–1999	50,000–99,999
0	< 1000	< 50,000

Dose adjustments for hematologic toxicity should also be based on nadir blood counts or the development of grade 4 bleeding or infection during the previous course.

Dose (%)	Nadir ANC/μl	Nadir platelets/μl
100	> 1000	> 50,000
50	< 1000	< 50,000

b. Repetitive courses. A program of repetitive courses of the same drugs may also be used. The course is repeated every week for 2 years. Minimal blood counts for initiating maintenance are an ANC of more than 1500/μl and a platelet count of more than 100,000/μl. The drugs used are

Thioguanine 40 mg/m² PO q12h on days 1–4
Cytarabine 60 mg/m² SQ on day 5

Once maintenance has been started, dose adjustments for hematologic toxicity may be based on blood counts obtained at the start of the course.

Dose (%)	ANC/μl	Platelets/μl
100	> 1500	> 100,000
50	1000–1499	50,000–99,999
0	< 1000	< 50,000

    c. Birth control. Given the potential teratogenic effects of cytotoxic chemotherapy, appropriate measures for preventing conception must be addressed with women who are undergoing maintenance therapy and who may still be in their reproductive years. Although there are no clear data linking maintenance chemotherapy in the male partner to teratogenic effects in the fetus, it appears prudent to suggest that appropriate birth control measures be undertaken in this situation as well.

2. Consolidation. Whether consolidation offers a survival advantage or has an improved cost/benefit ratio compared to the maintenance programs outlined above remains controversial. When taken *in toto* the current published data do not suggest that consolidation offers a distinct advantage compared to maintenance: Despite the lack of confirmatory data, some investigators recommend 1 to 3 cycles of consolidation with "7 + 3" or DAT rather than maintenance.

3. Early intensification. Although early intensification represents the best strategy devised thus far for postinduction chemotherapy, it is not without risks. Given the intensity of this further marrow ablative chemotherapy, approximately 5–10% of individuals die during intensification and another 60–70% have severe infections or extramedullary organ toxicity. Despite these risks, uncontrolled trials suggest that more than 50% of individuals are in a continuous complete remission after 24 months. Whether this finding will translate into improvement in overall survival is not yet clear. Intensification appears to be the best postinduction chemotherapeutic option currently available for individuals under the age of 30. Intensification should also be strongly considered in individuals between the ages of 30 and 50. Intensification should be initiated when the peripheral blood counts have returned to normal (ANC > 1500/μl and platelets > 100,000/μl), marrow cellularity is normal, infections have cleared, and mucositis has resolved. Most intensification programs are based on HDAC.

HDAC + daunorubicin. HDAC and HDAC plus daunorubicin are intensification programs based on commercially available drugs. A single course is given.

Cytarabine 3 gm/m^2 IV infusion over 1 hour q12h on days 1–6 (12 doses) *and*
Daunorubicin 30 mg/m^2 IV on days 7–9

D. Relapsed ANLL. Given the current state of the art, cytotoxic chemotherapy offers essentially no chance for long-term survival for the individual with relapsed ANLL. These individuals should be considered prime candidates for experimental protocols or bone marrow transplantation.

E. Role of bone marrow transplantation in ANLL

    1. Allogeneic transplantation is the use of bone marrow obtained from a sibling who is HLA-compatible with the recipient. Although bone marrow transplantation (BMT) receives much fanfare in the medical literature and the lay press, it has been estimated that at most 10% of individuals with ANLL are in reality candidates for an allogeneic BMT. Allogeneic BMT should be considered an option for individuals under the age of 40–45 years. For individuals with ANLL in second remission, allogeneic BMT is the treatment of choice, as it offers a 20–30% chance of long-term survival. BMT should probably be considered the optimal form of salvage therapy.

    2. Autologous transplantation is the use of the recipient's own bone marrow. The most obvious benefit of using the person's own bone marrow is the absence of graft-versus-host disease, and the obvious disadvantage is the potential for reinfusing leukemic cells. As methods of bone marrow purging improve and new technology (e.g., polymerase chain reaction) allows better detection of residual leukemia, autologous BMT may become the best form of early intensification.

V. Therapy of adult ALL

A. General plan of therapy for adult ALL is somewhat different from that of ANLL. The day that induction chemotherapy is started is again arbitrarily called day 1. In contrast to ANLL, the bone marrow is usually not checked at day 14 for the development of aplasia but at the end of induction for remission status. Newer, more aggressive protocols however, base therapeutic decisions on the day 14 bone marrow status. Once attainment of a complete response has been documented, the potential benefit of further postinduction therapy should be determined on an individual basis. Issues that need to be addressed in all individuals are the prophylaxis of the central nervous system (CNS) sanctuary and the role of further chemotherapy.

B. Induction therapy. By definition, all adult ALL is considered to be high risk. Therapeutic options vary depending on the clinical situation.

    1. Normal cardiac function. In the presence of normal cardiac function, adults with ALL are usually treated with an anthracycline-containing program.

        a. VPD. Vincristine, prednisone, and daunorubicin are most commonly used for induction therapy of adult ALL. The overall response rate is 75–85%. Although L-asparaginase proved to be of value during the preanthracycline era, its role in anthracycline-based programs is unclear. Given the significant toxicity of L-asparaginase, many investigators no longer recommend its use. There are a number of variations on the basic VPD program shown below. Some options are shown in parentheses.

Vincristine 2 mg IV on days 1, 8, 15, (22) *and*
Prednisone 40 or 60 mg/m^2 PO on days 1–28 or 1–35, followed by rapid taper *and*
Daunorubicin 45 mg/m^2 IV on days 1–3 (L-asparaginase 500 IU/kg IV on days 22–32)

b. DVPL. DVPL is a variation with a reported 94% response rate in young adults.

Daunorubicin 60 mg/m^2 IV on days 1–3 *and*
Vincristine 2 mg IV on days 1, 8, 15, 22 *and*
Prednisone 60 mg/m^2 PO on days 1–28 *and*
L-Asparaginase 6000 U/m^2 IM on days 17–28

If a bone marrow examination on day 14 shows residual leukemia, a single dose of daunorubicin 50 mg/m^2 in given. If a bone marrow examination on day 28 has residual leukemia, further DVPL is given.

Daunorubicin 50 mg/m^2 IV on days D29 and 30 *and*
Vincristine 2 mg IV on days 29 and 36 *and*
Prednisone 60 mg/m^2 PO on days 29–42 *and*
L-Asparaginase 6000 U/m^2 IM on days 29–35

c. "7 & 3, V & P" or DATVP. Given the unacceptably high relapse rate after VPD, which may be due in part to the underdiagnosis of hybrid leukemia, many investigators recommend the use of a hybrid program combining either "7 + 3" or DAT as used for ANLL induction with vincristine and prednisone as described above.

2. Impaired cardiac function. The use of an anthracycline is contraindicated for induction therapy in individuals with underlying cardiac disease. An active program in patients with impaired cardiac function is MOAD.

Methotrexate 100 mg/m^2 IV on day 1 *and*
Vincristine 2 mg IV on day 2 *and*
L-Asparaginase 500 IU/kg IV infusion on day 2 *and*
Dexamethasone 6 mg/m^2 PO on days 1–10

MOAD is given in sequential 10-day courses (minimum 3 courses maximum 5 courses) until a remission. Once a complete response has been attained, two additional courses of MOAD are given. *In toto,* a minimum of 5 and a maximum of 7 courses can be given.

3. ALL in the elderly. In general, full doses of induction therapy are used in elderly individuals with ALL. Some investigators decrease the dose of vincristine by 50%. Full doses of daunorubicin are usually used.

D. CNS prophylaxis. During the era prior to prophylaxis

of the CNS, more than 50% of children and adults relapsed solely in the CNS. Treatment of the CNS sanctuary after a complete remission has been attained has dramatically decreased the risk of CNS relapse. CNS prophylaxis is usually given prior to maintenance but is given as part of maintenance in some centers. If short-term consolidation is to be used, CNS prophylaxis may be delayed until after the completion of consolidation due to the marrow suppressive effects of prophylaxis. Two equivalent options exist.

1. **Cranial irradiation and intrathecal methotrexate.** Cranial irradiation (CRT) with intrathecal methotrexate (IT MTX) has been the classic method of CNS prophylaxis and is usually initiated within 2 weeks of attaining a complete remission.

   a. **CRT** (18–24 Gy in 2-Gy fractions) is usually applied to the cranial vault. The spine is not irradiated because the marrow toxicity would significantly limit the ability to give further chemotherapy. Common acute complications of irradiation include stomatitis, parotitis, alopecia, marrow suppression, and headaches. Long-term complications include dental caries. Like children, young adults may develop learning disorders, impaired growth, and leukoencephalopathy.

   b. **IT MTX** is used instead of irradiation for prophylaxis of the spinal cord. A commonly used program is a 12 mg/m^2 (maximum 15 mg) dose of *preservative-free* MTX diluted in *preservative-free* saline or Elliot's B solution given intrathecally (IT) once a week for 6 weeks. Some investigators also give 10 mg of hydrocortisone succinate IT to try to prevent lumbar arachnoiditis, which may limit the ability to give all six of the planned courses of IT MTX. After cerebrospinal fluid (CSF) is obtained for appropriate studies, 5 ml of CSF is withdrawn into a syringe containing MTX diluted in 10 ml of vehicle. This method produces a final MTX concentration of about 1 mg/ml or less (higher concentrations increase the risk of arachnoiditis). The IT MTX is then given in an "in and out" manner: 1–2 ml is injected into the spinal canal, and 0.5–1.0 ml of CSF is then withdrawn back into the syringe. This "in and out" process is repeated until all of the MTX has been given. This method is used to ensure that the MTX is actually given into the subarachnoid space. Leucovorin 5 mg may be given orally every 6 hours for 4 doses to ameliorate the mucositis, although it usually is not needed unless the patient is getting concurrent systemic methotrexate. Complications of methotrexate include chemical arachnoiditis and leukoencephalopathy.

2. **Chemoprophylaxis.** Given the toxicity of whole-brain irradiation, especially in young individuals,

other strategies of CNS prophylaxis have been developed. The combination of systemic high-dose methotrexate with IT MTX is considered to be as effective as CRT with IT MTX. The combination of a 6-day course of HDAC in combination with IT MTX is being studied as a means to accomplish both consolidation and CNS prophylaxis.

D. Postinduction therapy. Although it is generally agreed that some form of therapy is needed after remission induction for ALL, the optimum form has yet to be devised. Although maintenance, without doubt, increases both disease-free survival (approximately 12–18 months) and overall survival (approximately 18–24 months) for individuals with ALL, most patients still relapse. The results of single institution studies appear promising, but randomized prospective studies have not demonstrated that consolidation–intensification improves survival of ALL patients when compared to maintenance therapy.

Maintenance therapy for adult ALL usually consists in methotrexate and 6-mercaptopurine. Pulses of vincristine and prednisone are often given as "reinforcement" as they have relatively little toxicity. Maintenance is usually started once the marrow suppression and the oral toxicity of the CNS prophylaxis have cleared. Maintenance therapy may be given in a pulse or a continuous manner. Although allopurinol is usually not needed during maintenance, the dose of mercaptopurine should be decreased by 75% when given concomitantly with allopurinol.

   1. Pulse maintenance therapy is an 8-week cycle consisting of 3 courses of methotrexate and 6-mercaptopurine given every 2 weeks, followed by a 2-week pulse of vincristine and prednisone.

   Methotrexate 7.5 mg/m^2 PO on days 1–5, weeks 1, 3, 5 *and*

   Mercaptopurine 200 mg/m^2 PO on days 1–5, weeks 1, 3, 5 *and*

   Vincristine 2 mg IV on day 1, weeks 7 and 8 *and*

   Prednisone 40 mg/m^2, PO on days 1–7, weeks 7 and 8

   Oral methotrexate should be taken in a single daily dose, as splitting the daily dose significantly increases the mucositis. Approximately 3 doses of intrathecal methotrexate need to be given once maintenance has started. The schedule should be coordinated so that the IT MTX is given on day 1 of the 5 scheduled days of MTX. On the days when intrathecal MTX is given, the oral methotrexate is not given. Pulse maintenance is continued for 2–3 years.

   Dose adjustments for hematologic toxicity due to the methotrexate and mercaptopurine should be made based on blood counts obtained prior to the start of each course.

Dose (%)	ANC/μl	Platelets/μl
100	$\geq$ 2000	$\geq$ 100,000
75	1500–1999	75,000–99,999
50	1000–1499	50,000–74,999
0	< 1000	< 50,000

2. **Continuous maintenance therapy** consists in continuous daily mercaptopurine with weekly doses of methotrexate. Two weeks of vincristine and prednisone as described above may be added every 10–12 weeks.

   Mercaptopurine 50 mg/m^2 PO every day
   Methotrexate 20 mg/m^2 IV or PO every week

   Dose adjustments for hematologic toxicity from the methotrexate and mercaptopurine should be made based on blood counts obtained periodically during the course (WBC = white blood cells).

Dose (%)	WBC/μl	Platelets/μl
100	$\geq$ 2500	$\geq$ 100,000
66	2000–2500	75,000–99,999
33	1500–2000	50,000–74,999
0	< 1500	< 50,000

E. **Relapsed ALL.** Although a second remission can usually be achieved in adults with ALL, they tend to be short-lived. HDAC does not appear to be as effective for ALL as it is for ANLL. Commonly used programs for relapsed ALL include "7 + 3" and VM-26 (teniposide)/cytarabine (VM-26 165 mg/m^2 IV infusion over 45 minutes twice a week for 4 weeks/cytarabine 300 mg/m^2 rapid IV push twice a week for 4 weeks). Individuals with relapsed ALL should be considered prime candidates for experimental protocols or bone marrow transplantation.

F. **Role of bone marrow transplantation.** As with adult ANLL, the role of BMT in the management of adult ALL remains unclear. Allogeneic marrow transplantation during first remission has not yet been shown to offer a survival advantage. Allogeneic marrow transplantation offers the only credible hope for long-term survival for the individual in second remission. The use of autologous marrow transplantation during first remission may improve survival when compared to standard maintenance therapy. Individuals with ALL should be considered candidates for randomized, prospective studies examining the role of BMT.

VI. **Childhood ALL**

A. **Background.** The great advances made in the treatment of childhood ALL have served as a model for the approach to other malignancies. More than half of the children who develop ALL are long-term survivors after modern therapy. Although childhood ALL is now considered a "curable malignancy," the optimum management of these individuals remains to be determined. The therapeutic approach to childhood ALL is in constant evolution given our new insights into "risk factors" for long-term survival as well as the identification of iatrogenic complications in these long-term survivors. The therapeutic programs outlined below are presented as representative standard regimens that are currently in use. Given the intensity of these highly curative regimens, many dose modifications are necessary. Individuals considering the use of the following programs for childhood ALL in a setting outside of cooperative group trials should consult a reference source such as the National Cancer Institute's computerized on-line cancer reference, Physician Data Query (PDQ) for full details of dose modification. As with adult acute leukemia, all children with ALL should be considered candidates for well designed experimental protocols.

B. Definition of risk. The general plan of therapy for childhood ALL is based on "risk factors" that relate to the ability to achieve long-term survival. In general, children are grouped into perceived low-risk (standard), intermediate-risk, and high-risk categories at presentation. Many factors have been identified as putative risk factors but the most consistent are age, white blood cell (WBC) count, morphology/immunology, and cytogenetics. Given that most children attain a complete response with induction therapy, the assignment to a risk category becomes most important when planning postinduction therapy, as individuals who are perceived to be at higher risk require more intensive therapy.

C. Treatment of low risk ALL. Prognostic features associated with low risk ALL include (1) girls age 2–9 years with a WBC count of less than 10,000/µl and with any platelet count; and (2) boys age 2–9 years with a WBC count of less than 10,000/µl and with a platelet count of more than 100,000/µl. These individuals generally have prepre-B cell ("nonB/nonT,","common") ALL. Individuals with B cell (FAB L$_3$, Burkitt's) and T cell lymphoblastic leukemia/lymphoma syndromes and those with the Ph^1 chromosome are at high risk by definition and are excluded. Although vincristine and prednisone alone induce a remission in 70–80% of low-risk individuals, the addition of L-asparaginase or daunorubicin appears to improve the response rate to over 95%. In general, daunorubicin is not used in low-risk ALL patients because of its cardiac toxicity.

  1. Induction therapy. Vincristine, prednisone, and L-asparaginase are most commonly used for induction therapy of low-risk ALL. The overall response rate is better than 95%. L-Asparaginase (L-ASP) is an agent with many potential complications. Given the risk of anaphylaxis, L-ASP should be given in a setting where resuscitation can be begun immediately. If L-ASP is to be given intramuscularly, many investigators prefer to give it in an extremity rather than in the buttocks or deltoids, so a tourniquet can be applied to slow its systemic release if anaphylaxis occurs. The use of cryoprecipitate may become necessary if hypofibrinogenemia occurs. A commonly used induction program is the following.

Vincristine 1.5 mg/m² (2 mg maximum) IV on days 1, 8, 15, 22 *and*

Prednisone 40 mg/m² PO on days 1–28 *and*

L-Asparaginase 6000 IU/m² IM on days 4, 6, 8, 11, 13, 15, 18, 20, 22, *and*

Methotrexate 10 mg (age 2 years) or 12 mg (age ≥ 3 yrs) IT on days 1 and 15

A repeat bone marrow examination is often performed on day 14. Individuals who have more than 10% residual blasts are thought to have a poorer prognosis and should be switched to more intensive therapy. A bone marrow examination is again performed on day 28. If a complete remission has been attained, the individual proceeds to consolidation therapy. If the bone marrow still shows a partial response, further induction therapy is given [see below for tips on giving mercaptopurine (6-MP)].

Vincristine 1.5 mg/m² (2 mg maximum) IV on days 29 and 36 *and*

Prednisone 40 mg/m² PO on days 29–42 *and*

6-MP 75 mg/m² PO on days 29–42 *and*

Methotrexate 10 mg (age 2 years) or 12 mg (age ≥ 3 years) IT on days 29 and 36

2. Consolidation therapy is initiated when the bone marrow indicates that a complete remission has been attained. It usually occurs on the 29th day of induction for initial responders but may be on the 42nd day for those who needed additional induction therapy. Consolidation therapy is begun on the 29th day of induction. Mercaptopurine (6-MP) is begun when the ANC is more than 1000/µl and the platelet count is more than 100,000/µl. All other medications are given regardless of the ANC and platelet count. The dose of 6-MP should be decreased by 75% with the concomitant use of allopurinol. 6-MP may be more efficacious if given as a single dose in the evening.

6-MP 75 mg/m² PO on days 1–28 *and*

Vincristine 1.5 mg/m² (2 mg maximum) IV on day 1 *and*

Prednisone 20 mg/m² PO on days 1–3, 10 mg/m² PO on days 4–6, 5 mg/m² PO on days 7–10, 2.5 mg/m² PO on days 11–14 *and*

Methotrexate 10 mg (age 2 years) or 12 mg (age ≥ 3 years) IT on days 1, 8, 15, 22

3. Maintenance therapy is begun when the ANC is higher than 1000/µl and platelet count is higher than 100,000/µl. Maintenance is continued for 2 years in girls and 3 years in boys. In the schema shown below, maintenance therapy is given in 85-day cycles.

6-MP 75 mg/m^2 PO on days 1–85 *and*

Vincristine 1.5 mg/m^2 (2 mg maximum) IV on days 1, 29, 57 *and*

Prednisone 40 mg/m^2 PO on days 1–5, 29–33, 57–61 *and*

Methotrexate 20 mg/m^2 PO in the evening on days 8, 15, 22, 29, 36, 43, 50, 57, 64, 71, 78 *and*

Methotrexate 10 mg (age 2 years) or 12 mg (age $\geq$ 3 years) IT on day 1

D. Treatment of intermediate risk ALL. Prognostic features associated with intermediate risk ALL include (1) age 1–2 years with a WBC count of less than 50,000/μl, (2) age 2–10 years with a WBC count of 10,000–49,999/μl, and (3) boys age 2–10 years with a WBC count of less than 10,000/μl and platelet count of less than 100,000/μl.

1. Induction therapy. Vincristine, prednisone, and L-ASP are commonly used for the induction therapy of intermediate-risk ALL.

Vincristine 1.5 mg/m^2 (2 mg maximum) IV on days 1, 8, 15, 22 *and*

Prednisone 40 mg/m^2 PO on days 1–28 *and*

L-Asparaginase 6000 IU/m^2 IM on days 4, 6, 8, 11, 13, 15, 18, 20, 22, *and*

Methotrexate 8 mg (age 1 year), 10 mg (age 2 years) or 12 mg (age $\geq$ 3 years) IT on days 1 and 15

A bone marrow examination is performed on day 28. If a complete remission has been attained, the individual proceeds to consolidation therapy.

2. Consolidation therapy is usually initiated on the 29th day of induction therapy. If necessary, it is delayed until the ANC is more than 500/μl and the platelet count is more than 100,000/μl. The 6-MP dose should be decreased by 75% with the concomitant use of allopurinol.

6-MP 75 mg/m^2 PO on days 1–28 *and*

Vincristine 1.5 mg/m^2 (2 mg maximum) IV on day 1 *and*

Prednisone 20 mg/m^2 PO on days 1–3, 10 mg/m^2 PO on days 4–6, 5 mg/m^2 PO on days 7–10, 2.5 mg/m^2 PO on days 11–14 *and*

Methotrexate 8 mg (age 1 year), 10 mg (age 2 years) or 12 mg (age $\geq$ 3 years) IT on days 1, 8, 15, 22

3. Treatment of extramedullary disease. Irradiation of the CNS is begun as soon as possible during consolidation for individuals with documented CNS leukemia. Cranial irradiation is usually applied to a dose of 18 Gy in 1.8 Gy fractions starting during the first week of consolidation therapy. This phase is followed by spinal irradiation at a dose of 3.0 Gy/day for 3 days. Irradiation of both testes is also undertaken in the presence of testicular enlargement or for biopsy-proved testicular involvement. The dose is 24 Gy given in 8 fractions of 3 Gy.

4. **Interim maintenance therapy.** A bone marrow examination is performed on day 29 of consolidation therapy. Individuals in a complete or partial remission proceed to interim maintenance. Day 1 of interim maintenance therapy is usually the 29th day of consolidation therapy. If necessary, interim maintenance is delayed until the ANC is more than $1000/\mu l$ and the platelet count is more than $100,000/\mu l$.

6-MP 60 mg/m^2 PO on days 1–57 *and*

Methotrexate 20 mg/m^2 PO on days 8, 15, 22, 29, 36, 43, 50 *and*

Vincristine 1.5 mg/m^2 (2 mg maximum) IV on days D1 and 29 *and*

Prednisone 20 mg/m^2 PO on days 1–5, 29–33 *and*

Methotrexate 8 mg (age 1 year), 10 mg (age 2 years) or 12 mg (age $\geq$ 3 years) IT on day 1

Patients with a continuing complete or partial response proceed to delayed intensification therapy.

5. **Delayed intensification therapy** consists in two phases, reinduction and reconsolidation. Day 1 of delayed intensification therapy is usually the 57th day of interim maintenance therapy. If necessary, interim maintenance should be delayed until the ANC more than $1000/\mu l$ and the platelets count more than $100,000/\mu l$.

   a. **Reinduction therapy** is as follows.

   Vincristine 1.5 mg/m^2 (2 mg maximum) IV on days 1, 8, 15 *and*

   Dexamethasone 10 mg/m^2 PO on days 1–21, then taper on days 22–29 *and*

   L-Asparaginase 6000 IU/m^2 IM on days 4, 6, 8, 11, 13, 15 *and*

   Doxorubicin 25 mg/m^2 IV on days 1, 8, 15

   b. **Reconsolidation therapy** begins on the 29th day of reinduction.

   Dexamethasone—continue taper from reinduction *and*

   Cyclophosphamide 1 gm/m^2 IV on day D29 *and*

   Thioguanine 60 mg/m^2 PO 2 hours after the evening meal on days 29–42 *and*

   Cytarabine 75 mg/m^2 IV or SQ on days 30–33, 37–40 *and*

   Methotrexate 8 mg (age 1 year), 10 mg (age 2 years) or 12 mg (age $\geq$ 3 years) IT on days 29 and 36

6. **Maintenance therapy** is the final phase. Maintenance starts on the 50th day of delayed intensification, or when the ANC and platelet count have re-

covered. Maintenance therapy consists in 12-week cycles that are repeated so that girls receive 2 years of therapy and boys receive 3 years of therapy when measured from the beginning of interim maintenance therapy. The doses of methotrexate and 6-mercaptopurine are adjusted to maintain the ANC between 1000 and 2000/μl and the platelets at more than 100,000/μl.

Methotrexate 8 mg (age 1 year), 10 mg (age 2 years), or 12 mg (age ≥ 3 years) IT on day 1 *and*

Vincristine 1.5 mg/m² (2 mg maximum) IV on days 1, 29, 57 *and*

Prednisone 40 mg/m² PO on days 1–5, 29–33, 57–61 *and*

6-MP 75 mg/m² PO on days 1–84 *and*

Methotrexate 20 mg/m² PO on days 8, 15, 22, 29, 36, 43, 50, 57, 64, 71, 78

E. Treatment of high-risk ALL. Prognostic features associated with high-risk ALL include (1) age over 10 years, (2) age 1–9 years with a WBC of more than 50,000/μl, or (3) the presence of the Ph¹ chromosome. A number of intensive protocols have been devised for the initial treatment of high-risk ALL. The Berlin-Frankfurt-Munster (BFM) protocol shown below is representative.

  1. Induction therapy. Daunorubicin is commonly added to vincristine, prednisone, and L-asparaginase for induction therapy of high-risk ALL.

Vincristine 1.5 mg/m² (2 mg maximum) IV on days 1, 8, 15, 22 *and*

Prednisone 60 mg/m² PO on days 1–28, then taper on days 29–39 *and*

L-Asparaginase 6000 IU/m² IM on days 4, 6, 8, 11, 13, 15, 18, 20, 22 *and*

Daunorubicin 25 mg/m² IV on days 1, 8, 15, 22 *and*

Methotrexate 8 mg (age 1 year), 10 mg (age 2 years), or 12 mg (age ≥ 3 years) IT on days 15 and 29 *and*

Cytarabine 30 mg (age 1 year), 50 mg (age 2 years), or 70 mg (age ≥ 3 years) IT on day 1

A bone marrow examination is performed on day 28. If complete or partial remission has been attained, the individual proceeds to consolidation therapy.

  2. Consolidation therapy. Day 1 of consolidation therapy is usually the 35th day of induction therapy. If necessary, consolidation is delayed until the ANC is more than 500/μl and the platelet count more than 100,000/μl.

Prednisone, continue to taper from induction *and*

Cyclophosphamide 1 gm/m² IV on days 1 and 15 *and*

6-MP 60 mg/m² PO on days 1–28 *and*

Cytarabine 75 mg/m² IV or SQ on days 2–5, 9–12, 16–19, 23–26 *and*

Methotrexate 8 mg (age 1 year), 10 mg (age 2 years), or 12 mg (age $\geq$ 3 years) IT on days 2, 9, 16, 23

3. **CNS prophylaxis** consists in the intrathecal methotrexate as outlined above plus craniospinal irradiation. Cranial irradiation is usually given to a dose of 18 Gy in 1.8-Gy fractions starting during the first week of consolidation. This phase is followed by spinal irradiation at a dose of 3.0 Gy/day for 3 days. Irradiation of both testes is also undertaken in the presence of testicular enlargement or for biopsy-proved testicular involvement. The dose is 24 Gy given in 8 fractions of 3 cGy.

4. **Interim maintenance therapy.** A bone marrow examination is performed on day 34 of consolidation therapy. Individuals in a complete or partial remission proceed to interim maintenance therapy. Day 1 of interim maintenance therapy is usually the 35th day of induction therapy. If necessary, this phase is delayed until the ANC is more than 1000/μl and the platelet count more than 100,000/μl. Interim maintenance therapy consists in one course of 6-MP and methotrexate followed by a 2-week rest period.

6-MP 60 mg/m^2 PO on days 1–42 *and*
Methotrexate 15 mg/m^2 PO on days 1, 8, 15, 22, 29, 36

A bone marrow examination and lumbar puncture are performed 2 weeks after finishing the second course of 6-MP + methotrexate (day 56). Patients with a continuing complete or partial response and with a normal lumbar puncture proceed to delayed intensification therapy.

5. **Delayed intensification therapy** consists in two phases: reinduction and reconsolidation. Day 1 of delayed intensification therapy is usually the 35th day of interim maintenance therapy. If necessary, the latter is delayed until the ANC is higher than 1000/μl and platelets are more than 100,000/μl.

   a. **Reinduction therapy**

   Vincristine 1.5 mg/m^2 (2 mg maximum) IV on days 1, 8, 15 *and*
   Dexamethasone 10 mg/m^2 PO on days 1–21, then taper on days 22–30 *and*
   L-Asparaginase 6000 IU/m^2 IM on days 4, 6, 8, 11, 13, 15 *and*
   Doxorubicin 25 mg/m^2 IV on days 1, 8, 15

   b. **Reconsolidation therapy** begins on the 29th day of reinduction therapy.

   Dexamethasone, continue taper from reinduction *and*
   Cyclophosphamide 1 gm/m^2 IV on day 29 *and*
   Thioguanine 60 mg/m^2 PO on days 29–42 *and*
   Cytarabine 75 mg/m^2 IV or SQ on days 30–33, 37–40 *and*

Methotrexate 8 mg (age 1 year), 10 mg (age 2 years), or 12 mg (age $\geq$ 3 years) IT on days 30 and 37

6. Maintenance therapy is the final phase. It starts on the 50th day of delayed intensification therapy, or when the ANC and platelet count have recovered. Maintenance therapy consists in 12-week cycles that are repeated so girls receive 2 years of therapy and boys 3 years of therapy when measured from the beginning of interim maintenance therapy. The doses of methotrexate and mercaptopurine are adjusted to maintain the ANC at 1000–2000/μl and the platelets at more than 100,000/μl.

Methotrexate 8 mg (age 1 year), 10 mg (age 2 years), or 12 mg (age $\geq$ 3 years) IT on day 1 *and*

Vincristine 1.5 mg/m^2 (2 mg maximum) IV on days 1, 29, 57 *and*

Prednisone 40 mg/m^2 PO on days 1–5, 29–33, 57–61 *and*

6-MP 75 mg/m^2 PO on days 1–84 *and*

Methotrexate 20 mg/m^2 PO on days 8, 15, 22, 29, 36, 43, 50, 57, 64, 71, 78

F. Other forms of ALL. Burkitt's leukemia (FAB L$_3$, B cell) and the T cell leukemia/lymphoma syndrome are highly aggressive forms of acute leukemia. Specialized programs, which are beyond the scope of this chapter, have been designed to treat these disorders. Children less than 1 year of age also represent a high-risk population that merits a special approach.

G. Relapsed ALL. Because a second remission can usually be achieved in children with ALL, the long-term prognosis depends more on the time to relapse, the site of relapse, and prior chemotherapy exposure. For low-risk children who have a bone marrow relapse more than a year after discontinuing postinduction therapy, systemic chemotherapy may still produce long-term survival. A commonly used combination is as follows.

Vindesine (VM-26) 165 mg/m^2 as a 45-minute infusion (1 mg/ml in 5% dextrose in ⅓ N saline) twice weekly for 4 weeks *and*

Cytarabine 300 mg/m^2 IV push twice weekly for 4 weeks

Low-risk individuals who relapse within 1 year of discontinuing postinduction therapy, intermediate- or high-risk individuals who relapse at any time, or any individuals who relapse during postinduction therapy should be considered prime candidates for experimental protocols or bone marrow transplantation. Individuals who relapse in sanctuary sites (i.e., CNS or testicles) should be treated with local means followed by systemic chemotherapy.

H. Role of bone marrow transplantation. The role of BMT in childhood ALL continues to be defined. Given their excellent prognosis with chemotherapy alone, children with low-risk ALL should not be considered candidates for allogeneic BMT during their first remission. Given the unacceptably high rate of relapse of individuals with high-risk ALL, B cell ALL, and T cell lymphoblastic leukemia/lymphoma when treated with chemotherapy alone, these patients should be considered candidates for randomized, prospective protocols exploring the curative use of BMT during their first remission. BMT should also be considered a potential therapeutic option for all children in their second to fourth remission. Because chemotherapy alone is unlikely to produce long-term survival except for low-risk children who have a bone marrow relapse more than a year after discontinuing postinduction therapy, BMT should be considered potentially curative therapy, as it may produce 50% long-term survival.

VII. Hybrid and stem cell acute leukemia represent interesting management problems. Although large series of these patients are not usually reported, they are generally thought to have a poor prognosis. An intuitive approach to induction that is often used with these diseases of unclear lineage is to combine "7 + 3" as used for ANLL with vincristine and prednisone as used for adult ALL. Given the partial lymphoid nature of these cells, CNS prophylaxis should be given. The best form of postremission therapy is unclear. If chemotherapy is employed, the alternating-courses approach used for ANLL maintenance is attractive because it contains agents active against both lymphoid and nonlymphoid cells. BMT may also be an appropriate option during remission.

VIII. Management problems. Although individuals receiving therapy for acute leukemia often have a "predictable" course, certain clinical manifestations require further individualization of the therapeutic approach.

    A. CNS leukemia. Leukemic involvement of the CNS bodes poorly for the adult with acute leukemia given the morbidity of the associated neurologic dysfunction, the inability to control CNS leukemia on a long-term basis, and the common association with active marrow disease. CNS involvement occurs most frequently with hyperleukocytosis and the monoblastic, B cell, and T cell lymphoblastic leukemias.

        1. Diagnosis. Although the occurrence of CNS involvement in ALL at diagnosis is well recognized, there is a 10% risk of occult CNS involvement at the time of diagnosis in adult ANLL. Thus in all cases of acute leukemia a lumbar puncture should be performed at or shortly after the time of diagnosis. In individuals with high peripheral blast counts and no CNS symptoms, it is usually prudent to perform the lumbar puncture after chemotherapy has decreased the blast count. In this way, contamination of the CSF specimen in the event of a traumatic lumbar puncture is prevented. Common clinical features of CNS leukemia include headache, altered sensorium, and cranial nerve palsy (especially cranial nerve VI). Features suggestive of CNS involvement indicate the need for an immediate lumbar puncture because (1) neurologic dysfunction is most amenable to therapy within the first 24 hours, and (2) infectious meningitis must be excluded in the immunocompromised host. The diagnosis of CNS leukemia is made by finding 5 or more blast cells on a cytospin preparation of 1 ml of CSF. Essentially all individuals with CNS leukemia have an elevated CSF protein level as well; however, in the absence of infection, this finding by itself is suggestive but not diagnostic of CNS leukemia.

2. **Treatment.** Although the therapy of CNS leukemia is usually only palliative, it should be initiated as soon as possible. The rapid initiation of therapy may reverse or prevent cranial nerve palsies, which are a morbid complication for both patients and caretakers. The treatment for CNS leukemia is usually concomitant cranial irradiation and intrathecal chemotherapy. Cranial irradiation is usually given to a total of 30 Gy in 1.5- 2.0 Gy fractions. Intrathecal chemotherapy is given in the manner described under CNS prophylaxis. Intrathecal chemotherapy is repeated every 3–4 days with appropriate laboratory studies being done with each lumbar puncture. When blast cells are no longer seen on the cytospin preparation, two more doses of intrathecal drug are given, usually followed by a monthly "maintenance" intrathecal injection. Intrathecal methotrexate (12 mg/m^2 IT, maximum 15 mg) with oral leucovorin (5 mg PO q6h × 4 doses starting at the time of the lumbar puncture) is most commonly used for ALL. Ara-C (50 mg IT) is most commonly used for ANLL. The addition of 10 mg of intrathecal hydrocortisone succinate may ameliorate chemical arachnoiditis and have some antileukemic effect as well. Some investigators advocate instilling IT ara-C and methotrexate at the same time or alternating doses of ara-C and methotrexate. Some investigators advocate the routine use of an intraventricular reservoir for treating individuals with CNS leukemia.

C. **Hyperleukocytosis** (blast counts > 100,000/μl) predisposes to rheologic problems.

1. **Leukostasis** (vascular plugging) occurs almost exclusively with ANLL. Cerebral and cardiopulmonary dysfunction due to vascular obstruction, vessel wall necrosis with hemorrhage, or both are the most common clinical manifestations. Hyperleukocytosis is an oncologic emergency. Given the increased risk of early death with hyperleukocytosis, therapy should be rapidly initiated as soon as the diagnosis is made. If the patient is hemodynamically stable, leukapheresis is the most rapid way to lower the blast count. The goal of the leukapheretic session is to lower the blast count to less than 100,000/μl if possible. With

very high blast counts ($>200,000/\mu l$), decreasing the blast count by 50% may have to be the initial goal, as mathematic modeling suggests that prolonged leukapheresis after a "3 liter exchange" does not significantly decrease the blast count further. Leukapheresis may be repeated daily. Systemic chemotherapy should be initiated immediately after emergent leukapheresis or if leukapheresis is contraindicated. Hydroxyurea, 3–5 $gm/m^2/day$ split into 3 doses daily, is most commonly used. Hydroxyurea is stopped at the time more specific induction chemotherapy is initiated. In patients presenting with hyperleukocytosis, an allopurinol dose of 600 mg bid is well tolerated for the first 2 days followed by 300 mg bid for 2–3 days.

2. **Hyperviscosity.** Blood viscosity increases as the blast count rises. Fortunately, concomitant anemia produces a decrease in viscosity. Aggressive red blood cell (RBC) transfusion in individuals with hyperleukocytosis may precipitate symptoms of hyperviscosity. RBC transfusions should be used judiciously with a blast count of more than $200,000/\mu l$, especially in patients with ANLL. Unless the patient is symptomatic due to anemia, a packed cell volume (hematocrit) of 20–25% is a reasonable goal.

C. **Acute promyelocytic leukemia (APML).** APML is an uncommon (approximately 5%) form of ANLL that presents unique management challenges.

1. **Disseminated intravascular coagulation (DIC).** Hypergranular promyelocytic leukemia predisposes to the development of a devastating form of DIC. Under the best of circumstances, pooled data suggest that 5% of these individuals die of CNS hemorrhage within the first 24 hours of hospitalization and that another 25% die for the same reason during induction chemotherapy.

   a. **Diagnosis.** If looked for carefully, essentially all individuals with APML have clinical or laboratory features of DIC. Even with severe thrombocytopenia, bleeding stops quickly at the site of bone marrow examination in the usual patient. Prolonged oozing (1–2 hours) at the bone marrow site is a telltale sign of DIC. Subtle laboratory signs suggestive of an underlying consumptive coagulopathy in APML include prolongation of only the prothrombin time (> 1 second) or a normal fibrinogen titer (fibrinogen is an acute-phase reactant that is normally elevated in acute leukemia at presentation). The laboratory diagnosis of decompensated DIC in APML is readily apparent (prolonged prothrombin, partial thromboplastin, and thrombin times; decreased fibrinogen titer; and increased fibrin degradation products).

   b. **Treatment.** The first rule for managing DIC is to treat the underlying cause. Once the patient has been stabilized, the rapid initiation of induction chemotherapy is the cornerstone of the management of APML (ideally within 12 hours or at most within 24 hours of diagnosis). The lysis of the leukemic promyelocytes transiently exacerbates the clinical and laboratory manifestations of DIC. Intensive blood product support is usually necessary. Reasonable transfusion goals are to keep the platelet count higher than 50,000/μl (especially if heparin is used or there is a significant elevation of the fibrin degradation products) and the fibrinogen level at more than 150 mg/dl. Platelet and cryoprecipitate transfusions may be needed as often as every 2 hours to maintain hemostasis.

The most controversial aspect of the management of APML is the role of heparin in controlling the DIC. Given that APML is an uncommon form of ANLL, it is not possible to assess the efficacy of heparin in the usual randomized prospective manner. Thus all of the available data are based on retrospective analyses. The biases of retrospective studies aside, when taken in toto the published data seem to suggest that heparin indeed decreases the risk of early death due to CNS hemorrhage and increases the overall complete response rate of APML. When heparin is to be used, it should be initiated immediately if the patient has clinical or laboratory evidence of DIC. If even subtle laboratory signs of DIC are absent, heparinization probably can be delayed until the time when chemotherapy is to be initiated. The goal of heparin therapy should be to control the clinical manifestations of DIC; thus the heparin dose should be adjusted by monitoring the platelet count and the fibrinogen titer every 2–6 hours initially depending on the severity of the DIC and not by aiming for an arbitrary partial thromboplastin time as is done with thromboembolic disease. A reasonable initial heparin dose is a 500 units/hour (7 units/kg) constant infusion given without an initial heparin bolus. The duration of heparin therapy is empiric. The heparin can usually be tapered and stopped within 7–10 days as the manifestations of DIC subside. Case reports suggest that individuals with disproportionate activation of the fibrinolytic system (dramatically increased fibrin degradation products, very short euglobulin clot lysis time) may benefit from the use of ε-aminocaproic acid (EACA). Given that an underlying consumptive coagulopathy is present, EACA must be used with concomitant heparin to prevent life-threatening thrombosis.

2. **Residual disease** is not uncommonly found in the bone marrow after the second attempt at induction therapy in APML patients. Although residual disease needs further vigorous treatment in other forms

of ANLL if long-term survival is to be attained, data suggest that "promyelocytic maturation" and bone marrow recovery may occur in individuals with residual APML. Thus the benefits of further cytotoxic therapy must be addressed for each individual.

D. Extramedullary leukemia. Infiltration of organs outside the marrow may occur with acute leukemia. Diffuse organ infiltration (e.g., multiple skin nodules and gum infiltration with acute monoblastic leukemia) is best treated with systemic chemotherapy. Isolated accumulations of leukemic cells may occur with ANLL (granulocyte sarcoma, chloroma) and less often with ALL (lymphoblastoma). These foci are best treated with local irradiation at curative doses (30 Gy). Although most commonly associated with active marrow disease, chloromas and lymphoblastomas may occur as a sole site of relapse or as an initial presentation in association with a normal bone marrow. In either case, they universally herald the subsequent development of leukemic infiltration of the bone marrow. An intuitive approach is to treat these individuals with "adjuvant" induction chemotherapy.

IX. Ineffective modalities. A variety of agents and therapeutic modalities have been shown to be ineffective in the treatment of acute leukemia. They include immunotherapy [BCG, MER (methanol-extracted residue of BCG)], biologic response modifiers (interferon, IL-2), monoclonal antibodies, and maturational agents (cis-retinoic acid, low dose ara-C) Trans-retinoic acid may have benefit in acute promyelocytic leukemia.

Selected Reading

Arlin, Z., et al. Randomized multicenter trial of cytosine arabinoside with mitoxantrone or daunorubicin in previously untreated adult patients with acute nonlymphocytic leukemia (ANLL). *Leukemia* 4:177, 1990.

Benham Kahn, S., et al. Full dose versus attenuated dose daunorubicin, cytosine arabinoside, and 6-thioguanine in the treatment of acute nonlymphocytic leukemia in the elderly. *J. Clin. Oncol.* 2:865, 1984.

Bennett, J. M., et al. Proposed revised criteria for the classification of acute myeloid leukemia: a report of the French-American-British Cooperative Group. *Ann. Intern. Med.* 103:626, 1985.

Bleyer, W. A., and Poplack, D. G. Prophylaxis and treatment of leukemia in the central nervous system and other sanctuaries. *Semin. Oncol.* 12:131, 1985.

Gaynon, P. S., W.A., et al. Intensive therapy for children with acute lymphoblastic leukaemia and unfavourable presenting features early conclusions of study CCSG-106 by the Children's Cancer Study Group. *Lancet* 1:921, 1988.

Gottlieb, A. J., et al. Efficacy of daunorubicin in the therapy of adult acute lymphocytic leukemia: a prospective randomized trial by Cancer and Leukemia Group B. *Blood* 64:267, 1984.

Hoelzer, D., and Gale, R. P. Acute lymphoblastic leukemia in adults: recent progress, future directions. *Semin. Hematol.* 24:27, 1987.

Hoyle, C. F., et al. Beneficial effect of heparin in the management of patients with APL. *Br. J. Haematol.* 68:283, 1988.

Hurd, D. D. Allogeneic and autologous bone marrow transplantation for acute nonlymphocytic leukemia. *Semin. Oncol.* 14:407, 1987.

Mayer, R. J. Current chemotherapeutic treatment approaches to the management of previously untreated adults with de novo acute myelogenous leukemia. *Semin. Oncol.* 14:384, 1987.

Papalia Early, A., et al. Treatment of refractory adult acute lymphocytic leukaemic and acute undifferentiated leukaemia with an anthracycline antibiotic and cytosine arabinoside. *Br. J. Haematol.* 48:369, 1981.

Ramsay, N. K. C., and Kersey, J. H. Indications for marrow transplantation in acute lymphoblastic leukemia. *Blood* 75:815, 1990.

Steinherz, P. G. Radiotherapy vs intrathecal chemotherapy for CNS prophylaxis in childhood ALL. *Oncology* 3:47, 1989.

Wolff, S. N., et al. High-dose cytarabine and daunorubicin as consolidation therapy for acute myeloid leukemia in first remission: long-term follow-up and results. *J. Clin. Oncol.* 9:1260, 1989.

Chronic Leukemias

Neil A. Lachant and Roland T. Skeel

I. Chronic myelogenous leukemia (CML)

A. Definition and diagnosis. CML is a disorder seen in middle-age adults ($>$ 40 years). A palpable spleen (75%), anemia, and thrombocytosis (45%) are characteristic. The diagnosis of CML is established by demonstrating a persistent neutrophilic leukocytosis in which mature forms predominate over immature forms, there is low or absent leukocyte alkaline phosphatase activity, and the Ph[1] chromosome is present (90%). Of the 10% of individuals who lack the Ph[1] chromosome, one-half may be shown to have rearrangement of the *bcr-cAbl* oncogene by Western blotting. Those remaining 5% of individuals, who lack the Ph[1] chromosome and the *bcr-cAbl* rearrangement, are more likely to be classified as having a myelodysplastic syndrome rather than Ph[1]-negative CML. A bone marrow examination is done in CML patients to establish the prognosis and to obtain material for cytogenetic studies rather than for diagnosis.

B. Natural history. CML has a biphasic natural history. During the chronic phase, CML runs an indolent course with less than 10% mortality during the first 2 years. After an average 2.5–3.0 years, CML enters an aggressive phase that, if unchecked, results in the demise of the patient. CML ultimately evolves into a disease that resembles acute leukemia (blastic transformation, blast crisis).

C. Therapy. Chemotherapy remains a palliative modality for the management of CML. Although chemotherapy can improve the quality of life and to a small extent the overall survival of individuals with CML by preventing early death, chemotherapy has done little to prevent the development of the aggressive phase of CML or the development of blastic crisis. Bone marrow transplantation is the only potentially curative modality for the treatment of CML.

   1. Chronic phase. Therapy should be initiated in essentially all individuals with CML at the time of diagnosis. Select individuals with a stable, minimally elevated white blood cell (WBC) count may be initially observed only, with the institution of chemotherapy reserved for the time when disease progression occurs.

      a. Chemotherapy. The goal of initial therapy should be to lower the WBC count until it is back in the normal range ($<$10,000/µl). Once the WBC count has normalized, two approaches may be used. A common approach is to discontinue chemotherapy until the WBC count rises to 25,000–50,000/µl, at which point chemotherapy may be reinstituted. Once chemotherapy is begun for a second time, the patient is kept on a maintenance dose.

One advantage for this approach is the decreased exposure to chemotherapeutic agents. Moreover, the time to the reinstitution of therapy is a relative prognostic indicator. Another approach is to maintain the patient on small-dose chemotherapy from the start. Neither approach offers an obvious survival benefit compared to the other. Busulfan and hydroxyurea are most commonly used to treat CML. Neither has been shown to offer a survival benefit compared to the other.

(1) **Busulfan.** Because busulfan inhibits stem cell proliferation, it usually takes 3–4 weeks to achieve its major effect. It is important not to become anxious while waiting for the WBC count to start to drop, as increasing the busulfan dose does not cause it to start to fall sooner but steepens the rate of decline once an effect is achieved. Commonly used initial doses are 4 mg ($\sim$2.0 mg/m^2) and 8 mg ($\sim$4.0 mg/m^2) PO per day. Both doses are equally effective. In general, the dose of busulfan is cut in half each time the WBC count decreases by 50%. The busulfan is usually stopped when the WBC count reaches 20,000/µl; however, experienced clinicians may allow the WBC count to decrease to 15,000/µl when an initial dose of 4 mg is used. Because busulfan affects the stem cell, the WBC count continues to fall for 1–2 weeks after busulfan is discontinued. As a rule, it is best to err on the side of underdosing, as overaggressive use of busulfan may result in protracted (and potentially fatal) bone marrow suppression. In general, an initial dose of 4 mg/day is preferable because of the slower rate of decline of the WBC count and the lessened chance of producing overshoot marrow suppression. Because busulfan affects the stem cell it produces a "smoother," or more stable, effect on the WBCs than does hydroxyurea. Side effects of busulfan in addition to marrow suppression include pulmonary fibrosis, skin pigmentation, and an Addisonian-like wasting syndrome.

(2) **Hydroxyurea.** The recommended initial dose of hydroxyurea for CML is 0.5–1.5 gm/m^2 PO per day, although empiric initial doses of 500–2000 mg/day may be used. Hydroxyurea is given in a manner similar to that described for busulfan, except that the hydroxyurea is discontinued when the WBC count reaches 10,000–15,000/µl. Hydroxyurea may cause the WBC count to fall somewhat sooner than does busulfan. Because hydroxyurea is an enzyme inhibitor, it does

not have a prolonged effect on the stem cell, and a maintenance dose is often required. Hydroxyurea does not produce as "smooth" a decline in the WBC count as busulfan, which means that the dose of hydroxyurea frequently needs to be adjusted. Because of this feature, inexperienced physicians may complicate the problem by constantly altering the hydroxyurea dose based on modest fluctuations of the WBC count. Hydroxyurea is somewhat safer than busulfan, as unanticipated bone marrow suppression is usually not severe and is usually rapidly reversible.

b. Interferon-alpha (IFN-α). Although IFN-α has activity against CML, its exact role in the overall management of CML is unclear. The use of IFN-α for CML should still be considered experimental. IFN-α can control the leukocytosis of CML and when used aggressively can cause the disappearance of the Ph[1] chromosome. The drawbacks of IFN-α compared to busulfan and hydroxyurea are (1) IFN-α has not yet been shown to increase long-term survival or prevent the development of the aggressive phase of CML; (2) IFN-α is costly; (3) IFN-α has systemic side effects; and (4) neutropenia often develops at the doses used. Individuals with CML should be considered candidates for experimental protocols examining the role of IFN-α.

c. Leukapheresis. Individuals with CML may develop symptoms related to leukostasis when the WBC count approaches 600,000/μl. Leukapheresis may be of symptomatic benefit when combined with hydroxyurea administration in these individuals.

d. Birth control and pregnancy. CML is not uncommon in individuals during their reproductive years. Individuals receiving chemotherapy for chronic phase CML usually maintain their previous level of sexual activity. The advisability of pregnancy in a situation where one of the partners has a disease that is usually fatal within 3–4 years is a decision that can be made only by the affected couple. Given the potential teratogenic effects of chemotherapy, appropriate means of preventing conception need to be discussed. If conception is carefully planned, it may be possible to discontinue chemotherapy just prior to conception and for the first trimester. If conception is planned and it is not possible to interrupt chemotherapy, or if unplanned conception occurs while a patient is receiving hydroxyurea and a therapeutic abortion is not an option, it is recommended that busulfan be used during pregnancy, as busulfan appears to be associated with fewer teratogenic effects than hydroxyurea.

2. **Aggressive phase.** The aggressive phase of CML is often heralded by increasing cytopenia at doses of chemotherapy that have been well tolerated in the past. Management of the aggressive phase is usually unsatisfactory. Individuals treated initially with busulfan may respond to hydroxyurea; and those treated initially with hydroxyurea may respond to busulfan, although the neutropenia and thrombocytopenia produced tend to become dose-limiting. The use of aggressive multidrug regimens does not improve the overall outcome of the aggressive phase. The use of interferon during the aggressive phase has been disappointing. Individuals in the aggressive phase should be considered candidates for experimental protocols.

3. **Blast crisis.** The prognosis of a blast crisis remains dismal. The risks and benefits of further therapy must be weighed for each individual. In general, aggressive chemotherapy results in prolonged hospitalization. Remissions are difficult to induce and are short-lived. Supportive care often represents the best option unless the patient is young and "wants to go down swinging."

   a. **Lymphoblastic crisis** is characterized by blasts that are Tdt-positive. Lymphoblastic crisis may respond to vincristine and prednisone, with or without daunorubicin, as is used for de novo ALL.

   b. **Nonlymphoblastic crisis** responds poorly to therapy. No particular therapeutic regimen offers a significant advantage.

4. **Role of bone marrow transplantation (BMT).** BMT represents the only potentially curative therapy for CML. Allogeneic or syngeneic BMT should be considered the treatment of choice for individuals with CML in the chronic phase who are less than 40 years old. The timing of BMT during the chronic phase remains controversial. Although the relapse rate is high, BMT may produce long-term survival of selected individuals with aggressive phase CML and blastic crisis.

5. **Management of splenomegaly.** Splenomegaly usually responds to chemotherapy. Individuals with persistent symptomatic splenomegaly or excessive transfusion requirements due to splenic sequestration may respond to low-dose splenic irradiation. Although splenectomy is not advocated for routine use in CML, it may prove useful for select individuals whose splenic sequestration is unresponsive to other therapeutic modalities.

II. Chronic lymphoid leukemias

   A. **Definition.** The chronic lymphoid leukemias are a heterogeneous group of neoplastic lymphoproliferative disorders. Under current classifications they are grouped together because of their common stem cell and because they carry immunologic markers characteristic of "mature" rather than "immature" (blastic) lymphoid cells.

Despite the name "chronic," many have an aggressive clinical course.

B. Classification. The chronic lymphoid leukemias are categorized according to their cell of origin. Chronic lymphoid leukemias of B cell origin include B cell chronic lymphocytic leukemia, Waldenström's macroglobulinemia, leukemic phase of small cleaved follicular center cell lymphoma, prolymphocytic leukemia, and hairy-cell leukemia. Chronic lymphoid leukemias of T cell origin include T cell chronic lymphocytic leukemia, adult T cell leukemia/lymphoma syndrome, prolymphocytic leukemia, hairy-cell leukemia, and cutaneous T cell lymphoma. Given the scope of this chapter, only three are discussed in detail.

C. Chronic lymphocytic leukemia (CLL)

   1. Diagnosis and classification. CLL is a disorder seen in older adults (> 50 years). Its diagnosis is established by demonstrating a persistent accumulation of morphologically small, mature lymphocytes in the peripheral blood. In general, the presence of more than 5000–7500 lymphocytes/μl (normal 1500–3000/μl) over a 2- to 4-week period is compatible with a diagnosis of CLL. A bone marrow examination is done for prognosis rather than diagnosis, although the bone marrow in CLL should contain more than 30–40% small, mature lymphocytes. Approximately 95% of CLL is of B cell lineage [surface membrane immunoglobulin (IgM, IgD) present with monoclonal κ or λ light chains].

   2. Staging. Although CLL is a systemic disorder, it is one of the few leukemias where staging is of clinical importance, as management decisions are based on the stage of the disease. As originally described, the minimum absolute lymphocyte count was 15,000/μl for inclusion in both the Rai and International Workshop classifications.

   a. Rai classification. The Rai system has been the standard for staging CLL.

Stage	Criteria	Median Survival (years)
0	Blood and marrow lymphocytosis	> 12
I	Stage 0 plus palpable lymphadenopathy	8.5
II	Stage 0 plus splenomegaly or hepatomegaly	6
III	Stage 0 plus anemia (Hgb < 11 gm/dl)*	1.5
IV	Stage 0 plus thrombocytopenia (platelets <100,000/μl)*	1.5

*Autoimmune cytopenias may not be valid criteria for stages III and IV.

b. International Workshop classification. A more recent classification system is based on the extent of lymphoid organ involvement. In this system the body is divided into five anatomic lymphoid areas (cervical, axillary, and inguinal lymph nodes; spleen; and liver). Palpable lymphadenopathy or organomegaly are the criteria for clinical involvement. Unilateral and bilateral adenopathy both count for the involvement of one anatomic area only.

Stage	Criteria	Median Survival (years)
A	0–2 Anatomic areas	> 7
B	3–5 Anatomic areas*	< 5
C	Anemia or thrombocytopenia*	< 2

*Autoimmune cytopenias may not be valid criteria for stage C.

3. Approach to therapy. The therapy for CLL is palliative. Individuals with CLL are prone to life-threatening infections due to the neutropenia, hypogammaglobulinemia, and impaired cell mediated immunity that are part of the natural history of CLL. Because cytotoxic chemotherapy, prednisone, and splenic irradiation further immunosuppress these individuals, the potential risks and benefits must be weighed for each patient before initiating therapy.

Indications for initiating therapy include the following.

a. Advanced disease (stages III, IV, C) *or*

b. Disease of any stage with disfiguring or bulky adenopathy, adenopathy-producing neuropathy or organ dysfunction, symptomatic splenomegaly, systemic symptoms (fever, night sweats, weight loss) not due to occult infection or Richter's syndrome, and hyperlymphocytosis (usually > 500,000–800,000/μl) with symptomatic leukostasis.

c. In addition, individuals with early disease (stages I, II, A, B) with *diffuse marrow involvement* may benefit from chemotherapy. In general, the lymphocyte count per se is not used as a criterion for initiating therapy. Most times, however, a high or rising lymphocyte count is associated with indications for initiating therapy.

4. Chemotherapy. Single alkylating agents (with or without prednisone) are most commonly used for the initial treatment for CLL. The optimum duration of chemotherapy is unknown. Chemotherapy may be discontinued once the indication for therapy is under control or has disappeared. Maintenance therapy per se is not used; however, the prolonged use of chemotherapy may be necessary to keep the disease under control. Therapy is reinitiated as often as indications arise. Neither the initiation of cytotoxic chemotherapy during early stage asymptomatic disease nor the use of aggressive cytotoxic chemotherapy for advanced disease appear to offer a survival advantage to the usual individual with CLL. Combination chemotherapy may be of benefit to individuals who are not responsive to single-agent alkylator therapy.

a. Chlorambucil (CLB) ± prednisone. Although both chlorambucil and cyclophosphamide are probably equally efficacious, chlorambucil is used more commonly for the initial treatment of CLL. CLB may be given continuously or intermittently.

(1) Continuous CLB. The initial dose of CLB is 4–6 mg/m^2 or 0.1–0.2 mg/kg PO per day. The dose of chlorambucil should be decreased for the development of hematologic toxicity or as the disease responds. Lower initial doses may be employed initially in individuals who are severely neutropenic or thrombocytopenic or in whom hematologic toxicity develops (absolute neutrophil count = ANC).

Dose (%)	ANC/µl	Platelets/µl
100	> 1000	> 75,000
50	500–999	50,000–75,000
0	< 500	< 50,000

(2) Pulse CLB. Some investigators believe that there is decreased toxicity with pulse CLB. The initial dose is 20–30 mg/m^2 PO repeated every 2–4 weeks depending on the time to bone marrow recovery.

(3) Prednisone. The use of prednisone must be weighed carefully in the patient with CLL. Except when treating autoimmune phenomena (see below), prednisone is not used as a single agent for CLL. Because of its lympholytic (or other) effects, prednisone may make individuals with CLL feel dramatically better within a matter of days. At the same time, however, prednisone significantly increases the risk of bacterial and opportunistic infection. The addition of prednisone to CLB has not been shown to improve overall survival compared to CLB alone. In general, prednisone is considered standard therapy in individuals with advanced disease (stages III, IV, C). Because the main role for prednisone is symptomatic relief, its potential risks and benefits must be considered carefully for individuals with asymptomatic but poor-prognosis early stage disease. A commonly employed dose of prednisone is 20–40 mg/m^2/day for 1–3 weeks.

Prednisone may produce a transient lymphocytosis (prior to or concomitantly with objective signs of disease regression) in CLL. It is due to lymphocyte redistribution and should not be taken as a bad prognostic sign or as an indication to alter therapy.

b. **Cyclophosphamide (CTX).** CTX may be used initially instead of CLB. The usual dose of CTX is 80–120 mg/m² PO per day. Because daily oral CTX predisposes to hemorrhagic cystitis, it should be taken in a single dose in the morning; it should never be taken at bedtime. Oral hydration (2–3 liters/day) should be encouraged.

c. **Combination chemotherapy** is generally reserved for individuals who are unresponsive to single-agent alkylator therapy. Commonly employed combinations are CVP and low-dose CHOP.

(1) **CVP.** Courses of CVP are repeated every 3–4 weeks.

Cyclophosphamide 400 mg/m² PO on days 1–5 *and*
Vincristine 2 mg IV on day 1 *and*
Prednisone 100 mg/m² PO on days 1–5

(2) **"Low-dose" CHOP.** Courses are given every 4 weeks.

Cyclophosphamide 300 mg/m² PO on days 1–5 *and*
Vincristine 2 mg IV on day 1 *and*
Doxorubicin (Adriamycin) 25 mg/m² IV on day 1 *and*
Prednisone 40 mg/m² PO on days 1–5

d. **Experimental chemotherapy.** 2-Deoxycoformycin (pentostatin), fludarabine, and 2-chlorodeoxyadenosine are experimental agents that have been shown to be active against CLL. They are currently under investigation.

5. **Irradiation.** Low-dose irradiation may be of significant benefit for controlling localized disease. Indications include symptomatic local adenopathy and symptomatic splenomegaly. The use of radiation therapy for CLL should be considered in (1) individuals with early stage disease (stages I, II, A, or B) to spare them the effects of systemic chemotherapy, and (2) individuals refractory to systemic chemotherapy or who are unable to tolerate therapeutic doses of chemotherapy owing to marrow suppression.

6. **Immunoglobulin.** Approximately 40–70% of individuals with CLL develop hypogammaglobulinemia as a complication of their disease. Although the use of prophylactic IgG (400 mg/kg every 3 weeks for 1 year) has been shown to decrease the number of "moderately severe" bacterial infections (particu-

larly pneumonia) in individuals with CLL in a randomized prospective study, it did not decrease the number of "mild" or "life-threatening" bacterial infections, nor did it improve the overall survival of the cohort of individuals. In addition, cost–benefit analyses have not been performed comparing the significant yearly expense of prophylactic IgG versus the cost of saved days in the hospital. Thus the use of IgG outside of controlled, clinical trials cannot be recommended at this time.

7. **Autoimmune hemolytic anemia (AIHA) and immune thrombocytopenia** occur in approximately 20% of individuals with CLL. The initial approach to their management is similar to that of individuals with these disorders but without CLL. Although prednisone (40 mg/m²) is the usual initial treatment of choice, a full discussion of the management of AIHA and immune thrombocytopenia is beyond the scope of this chapter. For individuals with AIHA and immune thrombocytopenia who do not respond to initial prednisone therapy, a trial of cytotoxic chemotherapy may be warranted prior to recommending splenectomy.

8. **Ineffective therapy.** Ineffective therapies for advanced CLL include interferon, monoclonal antibodies, and interleukin-2.

D. **Hairy-cell leukemia (HCL)**

1. **Diagnosis.** HCL is an uncommon chronic lymphoproliferative disorder that "characteristically" presents as leukopenia (> 50% with pancytopenia), splenomegaly (often massive), and fever (due to infection until proved otherwise) in elderly men. HCL gets its name from the shaggy or "hairy" cytoplasmic projections seen on the affected lymphocytes. "Hairy" lymphocytes may be seen in the blood of individuals with leukopenia, but the diagnosis is usually made by bone marrow examination. Although not pathognomonic for HCL, hairy cells are characterized cytochemically by the presence of tartrate-resistant acid phosphatase. Most commonly, HCL is of B cell origin.

2. **Staging.** There is no formal staging system per se. Rather, clinical features and laboratory tests are used to predict the patient's clinical course and thus the need for therapy.

3. **Approach to therapy.** Although therapy for HCL is palliative rather than curative, HCL should be thought of as a highly treatable disorder with a long median survival (> 5 years in individuals treated with splenectomy alone). The goals of therapy are to improve the pancytopenia that is secondary to marrow infiltration and splenic sequestration, decrease the risk of infectious death, and decrease the symptoms of splenomegaly. In general, therapeutic decisions are based on the degree of splenomegaly and

the severity of the cytopenias. In the past, splenectomy has been the mainstay of therapy. More recently, IFN-α and 2-deoxycoformycin (pentostatin) have come to have established roles in the treatment of HCL.

4. **Treatment of early disease.** Approximately 10% of individuals have early disease as manifested by minimal splenomegaly (< 4 cm below costal margin), modest changes on the complete blood count (CBC: hemoglobin > 12 gm/dl, ANC > 1000/μl, platelets >100,000/μl), and no infections or fevers. These individuals are best managed by careful observation until there is evidence of disease progression.

5. **Treatment of advanced disease.** Individuals with clinically significant cytopenias (hematocrit <25%, ANC < 500/μl, platelets <50,000/μl), splenomegaly (> 4 cm below costal margin), tissue infiltration with hairy cells, or fever or recurrent infections are considered to have disease that requires therapeutic intervention. Splenectomy and IFN-α are palliative therapies, whereas 2-deoxycoformycin and 2-chlorodeoxyadenosine may ultimately represent curative therapies.

   a. **Splenectomy** is the classic treatment of choice for HCL, as it may dramatically reduce the tumor burden and improve the anemia and thrombocytopenia due to splenic sequestration. The CBC returns to normal after splenectomy in 50% of individuals. However, splenectomy may not greatly improve the degree of marrow infiltration or decrease the risk of infection. Splenectomy works best in individuals with significant splenomegaly (> 4 cm below costal margin), low bone marrow tumor burden (< 50–85% infiltration), and no infiltration of other organs. Most individuals ultimately require subsequent therapy.

   b. **Interferon (IFN)** represents the treatment of choice for individuals with modest splenomegaly (< 4 cm below costal margin), high bone marrow tumor burden (> 50–85% infiltration), tissue infiltration with hairy cells, leukemic phase disease, and transfusion-dependent anemia, as well as individuals with disease progression after splenectomy. It is also indicated in those who cannot medically tolerate splenectomy. Although the CBC returns to normal in 80% of individuals treated with IFN, in association with a decrease in the marrow tumor burden, only 10% have a true complete remission. In addition, IFN may decrease the risk of infection. Although IFN-induced responses may be short-lived once therapy is stopped, individuals may respond multiple times to it. IFN-α-2a and IFN-α-2b appear to be equally efficacious. Individuals in whom IFN therapy is contemplated should be considered candidates for experimental protocols designed to determine the optimum use of IFN.

    (1) IFN-α-2a (Roferon A) is given at a dose of 3 million units/day IM for up to 6 months until a complete or maximal partial response is attained. This phase is followed by a maintenance dose of 3 million units IM 3 times a week. The optimum duration of maintenance is unknown. Although individuals often relapse soon after maintenance is stopped, the prolonged use of IFN-α-2a has not yet been associated with improved survival.

    (2) IFN-α-2b (Intron A) is given at a dose of 2 million units/m^2 SQ 3 times a week for 6–12 months. As for IFN-α-2a, the optimum duration of therapy is unknown.

  c. 2-Deoxycoformycin (pentostatin), an inhibitor of adenosine deaminase, may become the treatment of choice for HCL. In phase II studies, 78% of 78 individuals (including IFN nonresponders) had a complete pathologic response to pentostatin. Drug-induced neutropenia is a significant complication that may increase the risk of infection. Pentostatin is currently an experimental agent available from the U.S. National Cancer Institute. Its use outside of clinical trials should be limited to individuals who have failed splenectomy (if indicated) and who have failed or been intolerant of IFN. Individuals with HCL should be considered candidates for experimental protocols examining the use of pentostatin as initial therapy for HCL.

  d. 2-Chlorodeoxyadenosine is an experimental deoxyadenosine analog. Initial studies suggest that 2-chlorodeoxyadenosine is at least as efficacious as pentostatin and may be associated with fewer side effects. Long-term responses have been seen.

 6. Immune phenomena including vasculitis of the skin and arthritis occur in patients with HCL. Short courses of prednisone may provide symptomatic relief, although these potential benefits must be weighed carefully against the increased risk of infection associated with prednisone use.

E. Adult (Japanese) T cell leukemia/lymphoma syndrome (ATCLL)

  1. Definition. ATCLL is a newly recognized syndrome. It is clinically and biologically significant because of its etiologic relation with the HTLV-1 retrovirus. It has been estimated that 4% of individuals in the United States who are HTLV-1 positive will ultimately develop ATCLL.

  2. Clinical features and diagnosis. The clinical features of ATCLL include hepatosplenomegaly, lymphadenopathy, and a skin rash. ATCLL is associated with hypercalcemia and lytic bone lesions similar to those seen with multiple myeloma. The hallmark of the disease is the presence of characteristic multilobated lymphocytes in the peripheral blood. Bone marrow involvement is minimal. The lymphocytes have the immunologic characteristics of mature T-helper cells [OKT3 (CD3)- and OKT4 (CD4)-positive and OKT8 (CD8)-negative]. The diagnosis of ATCLL is established by finding the above features in an individual who has serologic evidence of prior HTLV-1 infection.

   3. Therapy. Most individuals with ATCLL die within a year owing to opportunistic infection or hypercalcemia (median survival is approximately 5 months). In general, therapy is supportive, as the use of single-agent and combination chemotherapy has not dramatically improved survival. Individuals with ATCLL should be considered candidates for experimental protocols based on the biology of HTLV-1.

Selected Reading

Allan, N. C. Therapeutic options in chronic myeloid leukaemia. *Blood Rev.* 3:45, 1989.

Baccarani, M., et al. Staging of chronic lymphocytic leukemia. *Blood* 59:1191, 1982.

Berman, E., et al. Incidence of response and long-term follow-up in patients with hairy cell leukemia treated with recombinant interferon alfa-2a. *Blood* 75:839, 1990.

Cheson, B. D., and Martin, A. Clinical trials in hairy cell leukemia: current status and future directions. *Ann. Intern. Med.* 106:871, 1987.

Doane, L. L., Ratain, M. J., and Golomb, H. M. Hairy cell leukemia: current management. In *Hematology/Oncology Clinics of North America,* W. B. Saunders: Philadelphia 1990. Pp. 489–502.

Neely, S. M. Adult T-cell leukemia-lymphoma. *West. J. Med.* 150:557, 1989.

Piro, L. D., et al. Lasting remissions in hairy-cell leukemia induced by a single infusion of 2-chlorodeoxyadenosine. *N. Engl. J. Med.* 322:1117, 1990.

Rai, K. R., et al. Clinical staging of chronic lymphocytic leukemia. *Blood* 46:219, 1975.

Talpaz, M., et al. Therapy of chronic myelogenous leukemia: chemotherapy and interferons. *Semin. Hematol.* 25:62, 1988.

Thomas, E. D., and Clift, R. A. Indications for marrow transplantation in chronic myelogenous leukemia. *Blood* 73:861, 1989.

Myeloproliferative and Myelodysplastic Syndromes

Peter White

I. Myeloproliferative syndromes

The myeloproliferative syndromes are clonal disorders of the marrow stem cell characterized by autonomous and sustained overproduction of morphologically and functionally mature granulocytes, erythrocytes, or platelets. The diagnostic labels of the individual syndromes indicate the cellular element most strikingly increased, but it is not uncommon to have modest or even major elevations in other lineages (e.g., thrombocytosis and leukocytosis in polycythemia vera). Studies of marrow karyotypes such as the Philadelphia chromosome and isoenzyme patterns, e.g., glucose-6-phosphate dehydrogenase (G-6-PD) isotypes in heterozygous females, have verified the concept that the common, trilineage marrow stem cell is the neoplastic cell of origin for these disorders. Maturation is typically normal, and bone marrow aspirates and biopsies show hyperplasia without a shift toward immature precursor cells. Also, the progeny of the neoplastic stem cells function normally in most respects, though it is not unusual to have platelet dysfunction, which may contribute to bleeding. Chronic granulocytic leukemia is discussed in Chapter 22. The other myeloproliferative disorders are discussed in this chapter.

A. Polycythemia vera (P. vera)

1. **Diagnosis.** P. vera must be distinguished from pseudopolycythemia [normal red blood cell (RBC) mass, decreased plasma volume] and from secondary erythrocytosis (increased RBC mass due to hypoxia, carboxyhemoglobinemia, inappropriate erythropoietin syndromes with tumors or renal disease, and so on). P. vera is characterized by increased RBC mass (men > 36 ml/kg; women > 32 ml/kg), normal arterial oxygen saturation (> 92%), and a low serum erythropoietin level. The marrow shows panmyelosis. Splenomegaly, leukocytosis, and thrombocytosis are typically present; secondary gout is common.

2. **Aims of therapy.** Thrombosis—which may cause stroke, myocardial infarct, or venous thromboembolism—is a major cause of morbidity in P. vera due primarily to increased blood viscosity and stasis. Lowering the hematocrit to 40–45% markedly reduces the risk of thrombosis. High platelet counts may also pose a risk for thrombosis, and spontaneous platelet activation occasionally causes erythromelalgia (hot, red, painful digits). Elective surgery should not be undertaken without correcting a high hematocrit and assessing platelet function.

3. **Treatment regimens**

   a. **Phlebotomy.** Removal of 350–500 ml every other day (more slowly in the elderly or in patients with cardiac disease) is the standard initial approach. The usual goal is to lower the hematocrit to 40–45%, then repeat the complete blood count (CBC) monthly, and phlebotomize as needed to maintain the hematocrit under 45%.

b. Myelosuppressive agents. Persistent thrombocytosis, recurrent thrombosis, enlarging spleen, or similar problems despite adequate phlebotomy indicate the need for myelosuppressive therapy. Alkylating agents such as chlorambucil carry a high risk of producing leukemia and are no longer recommended. Currently recommended choices are as follows.

   (1) Hydroxyurea 600–800 mg/m^2 PO daily. This drug requires weekly blood counts initially and dosage adjustments to maintain the hematocrit at 40–45%, the platelet count at 100,000–500,000/μl, and the white blood cell (WBC) count at over 3000/μl.

   (2) Radioactive phosphorus (^{32}P) 2.3 mC/m^2 IV (5 mC maximum single dose). Repeat in 12 weeks if the response is inadequate (25% dose escalation optional). An inadequate response after a third dose mandates a switch to other forms of therapy. Use of ^{32}P entails an approximately 10% risk of leukemia, and it is best reserved for use in the elderly and in patients refractory to other modalities.

   Supplemental phlebotomies may be required for patients with satisfactory platelets and WBC counts but rising hematocrit.

c. Ancillary treatments. Allopurinol 300 mg daily is frequently needed to control hyperuricemia. It may be discontinued if and when the disease and hyperuricemia are controlled by myelosuppressive therapy. Pruritus is a frequent problem but usually abates with myelosuppressive therapy. Antihistamines, cyproheptadine, and cimetidine may help. Aspirin and similar antiplatelet agents are often helpful for erythromelalgia but do not protect against most thrombotic complications; they may cause bleeding.

4. Evolution and outcome. The median survival in P. vera is approximately 10 years. One-third of deaths are caused by thrombosis. The risk of leukemia is small in patients treated by phlebotomy alone. Approximately 10% of patients develop myelofibrosis with myeloid metaplasia (see **I.C,** below). Many patients progress to the "spent phase," with increasing splenomegaly and stable or falling hematocrit. Splenectomy or splenic irradiation may be indicated for massive splenomegaly in such patients.

B. Essential thrombocythemia

   1. Diagnosis. The diagnosis of essential thrombocytopenia is based on a persistent elevation of the platelet count to over 600,000/μl without known cause. It must be distinguished from secondary thrombocytosis (e.g., due to iron deficiency, malignancy, chronic inflammatory disease) and other myeloproliferative disorders (e.g., bled-out P. vera). The marrow shows hyperplasia of megakaryocytes and granulocytes. Moderate leukocytosis and splenomegaly are common. Platelet function studies may show either spontaneous aggregation or impaired response to agonists such as epinephrine. Pseudohyperkalemia is common and should be detected by comparing plasma to serum potassium levels. Microvascular occlusion may cause digital gangrene, transient ischemic attacks, visual complaints, and paresthesias. Large-vessel occlusion (myocardial infarct, cerebrovascular accident) and hemorrhagic manifestations due to platelet dysfunction are also seen.

2. **Treatment regimens.** Consensus is lacking on the need to treat the asymptomatic patient, and observation may be the best course. In patients with hemorrhagic or thrombotic symptoms, however, the platelet count should be lowered.

   a. **Hydroxyurea** 600–800 mg/m^2 PO daily, with dosage adjustments per weekly CBC, should achieve satisfactory response in 2–6 weeks.

   b. **^{32}P and alkylating agents** are effective but carry increased risk of secondary leukemia.

   c. **Plateletpheresis** may be indicated in emergent situations (e.g., cerebral ischemia), but the effect is usually short-lived.

   d. **Antiplatelet drugs,** such as aspirin 300 mg daily, may control erythromelalgia and similar vasoocclusive problems but are contraindicated in patients with a history of hemorrhagic symptoms or evidence of platelet dysfunction, e.g., prolonged bleeding time.

   e. **Investigational agents.** Anagrelide and interferon appear promising in lowering platelet counts but are still investigational.

3. **Evolution and outcome.** The course is often indolent, particularly in young patients. Median survival probably exceeds 10 years. A few patients transform to other myeloproliferative disorders or to acute leukemia.

C. **Agnogenic myeloid metaplasia (AMM)**

   1. **Diagnosis.** This disorder of the stem cell, also called idiopathic myelofibrosis, is marked by an intense reactive fibrosis of the marrow, ectopic hematopoiesis in the spleen and other organs, and the presence of immature granulocytes, nucleated RBCs, and teardrop RBCs in the peripheral blood. Other causes of secondary marrow fibrosis such as metastatic carcinoma, hairy-cell leukemia, and granulomatous infections, should be distinguished from AMM. Acute myelofibrosis is also distinct from AMM and may be identical or closely related to acute megakaryoblastic leukemia (see Chap. 21).

2. Treatment regimens. Median survival is approximately 5 years, but asymptomatic patients may do well without treatment for a number of years. Intervention is indicated for problems related to the following problems.

    a. Anemia. Androgens—e.g., testosterone enanthate (400 mg IM weekly) for men or danazol (600 mg PO daily) for women—or corticosteroids (prednisone 1 mg/kg PO daily) may be helpful to correct ineffective erythropoiesis or major hemolysis, respectively.

    b. Splenomegaly. Massive splenomegaly may lead to cytopenias, portal hypertension, variceal bleeding, abdominal pain, or compression of adjacent organs. Options for control include myelosuppressive therapy with hydroxyurea as for P. vera in **I.A.3.b,** above, or busulfan 2 mg daily in older patients; splenic irradiation (may cause a marked decrease in WBCs and platelets); and splenectomy (high risk of perioperative bleeding, postoperative thrombocytosis, or both).

    c. Marrow failure. Erythropoietin, other growth factors, and allogeneic marrow transplantation (for patients < 50 years) may prove useful. Antifibrosing agents such as penicillamine, vitamin D_3, and interferon are under investigation.

II. Myelodysplastic syndromes. These disorders, also referred to as "preleukemia" or "oligoblastic leukemia," represent clonal abnormalities of hematopoietic stem cells. In contrast to myeloproliferative syndromes, dysplastic morphologic features are prominent, reflecting impaired maturation; and functional abnormalities of granulocytes and platelets may lead to infection and bleeding despite normal WBC and platelet counts.

    A. Diagnosis. The bone marrow is normocellular or hypercellular, but hematopoiesis is ineffective, and anemia with or without other cytopenias is the rule. Reticulocyte counts are normal or low, despite erythroid hyperplasia. Diagnostic features include megaloblastoid changes in RBC precursors, ring sideroblasts, bilobed neutrophils (i.e., pseudo-Pelger-Huet anomaly), hypogranulation of neutrophils, monolobular or hypolobular megakaryocytes, and agranular platelets. Small numbers of blast cells may be found in the peripheral blood, as well as a variable number of myeloblasts in the marrow. Distinction from frank acute leukemia may be difficult, but most cases can be assigned to one of the following categories in the widely accepted FAB classification.

    1. Refractory anemia (<5% blasts in marrow)
    2. Refractory anemia with ring sideroblasts
    3. Refractory anemia with excess blasts (RAEB) (5–20% blasts in marrow)
    4. Refractory anemia with excess blasts "in transformation" (RAEBt) (20–30% blasts in marrow)

5. Chronic myelomonocytic leukemia (5–20% blasts in marrow)

Sideroblastic anemia may also be secondary to lead poisoning, severe alcoholism, and other toxic states. Dysplastic morphology is not uncommon in patients infected with human immunodeficiency virus (HIV). It is helpful to distinguish idiopathic or primary cases from those arising secondary to prior exposure to mutagenic agents, most commonly chemotherapy with alkylating drugs and therapeutic irradiation. Aneuploidy is demonstrable in approximately 50% of idiopathic cases and in a high percent of secondary cases, where deletions of chromosomes 5 and 7 are especially common.

B. Treatment regimens

    1. Supportive therapy. The following agents may improve anemia and other cytopenias in occasional patients, despite lack of efficacy in standardized trials.

        a. Pyridoxine 100 mg PO daily (for sideroblastic anemia)

        b. Folic acid 1–5 mg PO daily

        c. Androgens, e.g., oxymetholone 50 mg PO qid or danazol 600 mg PO daily (the latter particularly for thrombocytopenia)

        d. Corticosteroids, e.g., prednisone 30–80 mg PO daily

Transfusion support with RBCs is required for many patients and should follow standard guidelines. Transfusional hemochromatosis develops in a small percentage of patients.

    2. Cytotoxic chemotherapy. Patients having RAEB or RAEBt frequently progress to outright acute nonlymphoblastic leukemia (risk correlates with marrow blast count, circulating blast count, or both). Options for therapy prior to this progression include the following.

        a. Standard dose antileukemic therapy (e.g., cytarabine, daunorubicin) (see Chap. 21). It is appropriate to consider this therapy for young patients with clinically aggressive disease, but complete remission rates are lower and early therapy-related deaths are higher than with de novo primary acute nonlymphocytic leukemia. A prohibitive rate of early deaths mandates caution in the elderly.

        b. Low-dose cytosine arabinoside (10 mg/m^2 SQ q12h for 14–21 days) may improve cytopenias in a significant percentage of patients and complete remission in a small percentage of patients, but the impact on long-term survival is questionable. This regimen carries significant risk of morbidity due to neutropenia and thrombopenia, particularly in the elderly, and cannot be considered standard therapy.

        c. Allogeneic bone marrow transplantation is widely considered as the treatment of choice for a young patient with a high risk of progression to frank leukemia or life-threatening cytopenias and a suitable donor. The optimal pretransplant preparative regimen is not yet established. The potential cure rate may approximate that of de novo acute leukemia. Unfortunately, advanced age (median > 60 years at diagnosis) precludes marrow transplant for most patients with myelodysplasia.

d. **Hematopoietic growth factors.** Erythropoietin, granulocyte colony-stimulating factor (G-CSF), and granulocyte-monocyte-CSF (GM-CSF) are undergoing trials but do not yet have a defined role. The latter agents cause increased blast counts and progression to acute leukemia in significant numbers of patients.

e. **Differentiation agents.** Analogs of vitamin D and retinoic acid may enhance in vitro differentiation and maturation of precursor cells from patients with myelodysplasia, but they have not proved useful in clinical trials. Low-dose cytarabine has been touted as a differentiating agent, but the evidence for this mode of action is unconvincing.

C. **Evolution and outcome.** The median survival for patients with myelodysplastic syndromes is 1–2 years overall, but some patients (particularly those with refractory anemia or refractory anemia with ring sideroblasts) may do well for a number of years with occasional transfusions and supportive therapy. Adverse prognostic factors include advanced age, aneuploidy, thrombopenia, and a high percent of blasts in marrow. Conversion to acute leukemia is seen in 30% or more of patients with RAEBt but in 10% or less of patients without increased blasts. Many patients die from complications of bone marrow failure (infections, hemorrhage) without conversion to leukemia.

Selected Readings

Appelbaum, F. R., et al. Bone marrow transplantation for patients with myelodysplasia: pretreatment variables and outcome. *Ann. Intern. Med.* 112:590, 1990.

Bennett, J. M., et al. Proposals for the classification of the myelodysplastic syndromes. *Br. J. Haematol.* 51:189, 1982.

Brenner, B., et al. Splenectomy in agnogenic myeloid metaplasia and postpolycythemic myeloid metaplasia: a study of 34 cases. *Arch. Intern. Med.* 148:2501, 1988.

Cheson, B. D. The myelodysplastic syndromes: current approaches to therapy. *Ann. Intern. Med.* 112:932, 1990.

Murphy, S. Polycythemia vera. In W. J. Williams et al. (eds.), *Hematology* (4th ed.) New York: McGraw-Hill, 1990. Pp. 193.

Schafer, A. I. Bleeding and thrombosis in the myeloproliferative disorders. *Blood* 64:1, 1984.

Hodgkin's Disease and Malignant Lymphomas

Richard S. Stein

Hodgkin's disease and the non-Hodgkin's lymphomas constitute a diverse spectrum of lymphoproliferative malignancies that share a number of important clinical features. They commonly present as solitary or generalized adenopathy, and for both diseases accurate clinical staging is the base for rational therapeutic planning. Nevertheless, important clinical differences exist. With Hodgkin's disease contiguous spread of tumor from node to node is the rule, and most patients present with disease limited to the lymph nodes (or to the lymph nodes and spleen) and are therefore candidates for curative radiation therapy. In contrast, most patients with non-Hodgkin's lymphomas present with advanced disease. Furthermore, whereas Hodgkin's disease is curable regardless of stage (advanced Hodgkin's disease is curable by chemotherapy), only certain histologic types of non-Hodgkin's lymphoma are curable when disseminated. For this reason, Hodgkin's disease and the major histologic types of non-Hodgkin's lymphoma must be considered separately.

I. Hodgkin's disease

A. Incidence and histologic types.
Hodgkin's disease accounts for approximately 1% of newly diagnosed malignancies in the United States. The average age of new patients is 32 years, and the incidence curve is bimodal: One peak occurs near age 25 and another at age 55. Four major histologic types of Hodgkin's disease exist: lymphocyte predominance (10% of cases); nodular sclerosis (60% of cases); mixed cellularity (20% of cases); and lymphocyte depletion (10% of cases). Nodular sclerosis Hodgkin's disease is commonly seen in young adults and is frequently associated with a large mediastinal mass. Lymphocyte-depleted Hodgkin's disease is usually associated with symptomatic disease (see **I.B**) and frequent involvement of the bone marrow. Nevertheless, the critical variable with respect to the therapy of Hodgkin's disease is not the histologic type but the stage of disease.

B. Staging

1. **Modified Ann Arbor staging system.** The modified Ann Arbor staging system is used for patients with Hodgkin's disease. Clinically, patients are placed in one of four stages and are further classified as to the presence or absence of symptoms: A denotes that no symptoms are present; B denotes that any or all of the following are present: fever, night sweats, and unexplained weight loss of 10% or more of body weight. In addition, the subscript E (e.g., II_E) may be used to denote involvement of an extralymphatic site primarily or by direct extension, rather than by hematogenous spread, as in the case

of mediastinal mass extending to involve the lung. Stage III Hodgkin's disease is subdivided into stages III$_1$ and III$_2$ based on evidence that the clinical approaches to these two substages should be different. The modified Ann Arbor staging system is as follows.

Stage I—involvement of a single lymph node region.

Stage II—involvement of two or more lymph node regions on the same side of the diaphragm.

Stage III$_1$—involvement of lymph node regions on both sides of the diaphragm. Abdominal disease is limited to the upper abdomen: spleen, splenic hilar, celiac, or porta hepatis nodes.

Stage III$_2$—involvement of lymph node regions on both sides of the diaphragm. Abdominal disease includes paraaortic, mesenteric, iliac, or inguinal nodes, with or without disease in the upper abdomen.

Stage IV—diffuse or disseminated involvement of one or more extralymphatic tissues or organs, with or without associated lymph node involvement.

2. **Staging tests.** Staging must be performed with consideration of therapeutic options and not just to complete a "checklist." When performing staging tests, one should remember that Hodgkin's disease tends to spread in a contiguous manner. Considering that the thoracic duct makes the left supraclavicular area and the abdomen contiguous sites, it is not surprising that abdominal disease is found in 40% of patients with left supraclavicular presentations and in only 8% of patients with presentations in the right supraclavicular nodes. Procedures used for the staging of Hodgkin's disease are as follows.

   a. **History taking.** Symptoms to watch for are fever, night sweats, and weight loss.

   b. **Complete physical examination.** Attention must be paid to lymph nodes and spleen.

   c. **Laboratory tests.** Complete blood count (CBC), platelet count, erythrocyte sedimentation rate, serum alkaline phosphatase, and tests of liver and kidney function must be performed.

   d. **Chest x-ray film.** Chest computed tomography (CT) scans should be performed if the chest x-ray film is abnormal.

   e. **Lymphangiogram.** It is useful, as it can detect normal-sized nodes with disruption of internal architecture.

   f. **Liver and spleen isotope scan or abdominal CT scan.**

   g. **Bone marrow biopsy** may be omitted in patients who are in clinical stages IA or IIA after the above staging procedures have been performed.

   h. **Staging laparotomy** should be done in selected patients only. If performed, it should include inspection, splenectomy, liver biopsies (wedge biopsy of left lobe plus needle biopsy of both lobes), and lymph node biopsies of the splenic hilar, celiac, porta hepatis, mesenteric, paraaortic, and iliac nodes.

C. Therapy of Hodgkin's disease

1. **General considerations.** Therapy of Hodgkin's disease must be considered on a stage-by-stage basis. The incidence of the various stages of Hodgkin's disease is presented in Table 24-1 with an estimated cure rate for each stage. In general, limited stages of Hodgkin's disease are treated with radiation therapy (stages IA and IIA), and advanced stages (IVA and IVB) are treated with combination chemotherapy. The optimal therapy for the intermediate stages is controversial.

   Prior to initiating chemotherapy, patients should be placed on allopurinol 300 mg/day to avert the hyperuricemia that may follow tumor lysis. It may be discontinued after the first cycle of chemotherapy or after the first 2 weeks of radiotherapy.

2. **Radiotherapy.** With respect to radiation therapy, studies have shown that the optimal dose for local control is 36–40 Gy given over 3.5–4.0 weeks. With modern equipment, adequate radiation can be administered to involved areas while shielding adjacent tissues. Nevertheless, radiation injury such as radiation pneumonitis or pericarditis occurs infrequently. Similarly, inappropriate overlapping of radiation ports can result in damage to the overtreated area. If this damage involves radiation myelitis, the results can be disastrous owing to resultant paraplegia. Other potential side effects of irradiation include hypothyroidism (often subclinical) and sterility (unless the ovaries are moved at the time of staging laparotomy, prior to pelvic irradiation). See Figure 24-1 for standard radiation therapy ports.

3. **Stages IA and IIA.** Patients with stage IA disease are most commonly treated with mantle irradiation when the disease occurs above the diaphragm (as it

Table 24-1. Hodgkin's disease: incidence of stages and results of therapy

Stage	Incidence (%)	Potential cure rate (%)
IA	10	95
IIA	30	85
IB, IIB	10	70
III$_1$A	15	85
III$_2$A	10	65
III	15	60
IVA, IVB	10	60

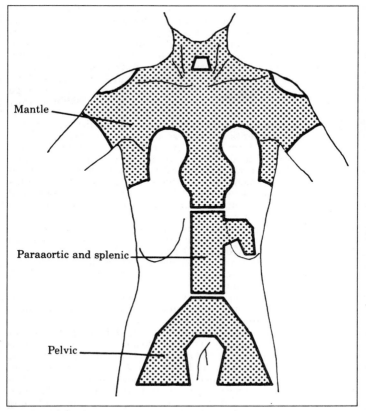

Fig. 24-1. Standard radiation therapy ports used for the treatment of Hodgkin's disease. For disease presenting above the diaphragm, the mantle plus paraaortic and splenic ports would be regarded as extended field therapy. The use of all three ports would be considered total nodal irradiation. (Reprinted by permission from J. R. Salzman and H. S. Kaplan. Effect of prior splenectomy on hematologic tolerance during total lymphoid radiotherapy of patients with Hodgkin's disease. *Cancer* 27:472, 1972.)

does in 90% of cases) or with pelvic radiotherapy when the disease presents in an inguinal node. Patients with stage IIA disease above the diaphragm are most commonly treated with mantle plus paraaortic-splenic radiotherapy. There is no firm evidence that adding chemotherapy or modifying the ports leads to either improved results or significantly decreased toxicity in these patients.

   4. **Stage IIE disease with bulky mediastinal mass.** Patients with bulky mediastinal masses (disease diameter 9 cm or more than one-third of the chest di-

ameter) present a special problem. When treated with radiotherapy alone, these patients have a risk of relapse approaching 50%. As a result, most clinicians treat patients having a bulky mediastinal mass with a combination of chemotherapy and radiotherapy. The optimal order of treatments and number of chemotherapy cycles is not firmly established. Six cycles of combination chemotherapy (as for stage IV disease) followed by involved field radiotherapy is a commonly used approach.

5. **Stages IB and IIB.** In view of the limited number of patients with these stages of disease, available data do not allow firm treatment recommendations to be made. These patients are most commonly treated with extended field radiotherapy or combined-modality therapy, i.e., radiation therapy plus 3–6 cycles of a combination regimen such as MOPP (outlined in **a–d** below). Dose adjustments appear in Table 24-2.

   a. Mechlorethamine 6 mg/m^2 IV on days 1 and 8 *and*

   b. Vincristine (Oncovin) 1.4 mg/m^2 (not to exceed 2.5 mg) IV on days 1 and 8 *and*

   c. Procarbazine 100 mg/m^2 PO on days 1–14 *and*

   d. Prednisone 40 mg/m^2 PO on days 1–14, cycles 1 and 4 only.

   Repeat the cycle every 4 weeks for 6 cycles, minimum. Complete remission should be documented prior to discontinuing therapy.

6. **Stage IIIA.** Therapy for stage IIIA is still a matter of controversy. The two options that are most commonly considered are total nodal radiotherapy alone or total nodal radiotherapy plus combination chemotherapy, such as mechlorethamine + vincristine + procarbazine + and prednisone (MOPP regimen). Although combined-modality therapy may appear to be optimal, it exposes all stage III patients to considerable toxicity—which may not be necessary in all patients. Also, studies have shown that combined-modality therapy is associated with an increased risk (about 4% at 7 years) of acute nonlym-

Table 24-2. Sliding scale of MOPP dose adjustment for myelotoxicity

Blood counts on day of treatment			Dose (%)			
WBC count/μl		Platelet count/μl	M	O	P	P
>4000	*and*	>100,000	100	100	100	100
3000–4000	*and*	>100,000	50	100	50	100
2000–3000	*or*	50,000–100,000	25	100	25	100
1000–2000	*and/or*	<50,000	25	50	25	100
<1000	*and*	<50,000	0	0	0	0

phocytic leukemia. Combined-modality therapy is best limited to patients in whom radiotherapy alone cannot produce adequate cure rates.

Studies suggest that the extent of abdominal disease may be a rational basis for determining therapy in patients with stage IIIA Hodgkin's disease. Patients with stage III_1A disease appear to achieve optimal results when treated with radiotherapy alone, leaving chemotherapy for salvage treatment at the time of relapse. For patients with stage III_2A, the results of radiotherapy alone are inadequate, and either radiotherapy with chemotherapy or chemotherapy alone appears to be appropriate. Because the use of radiotherapy plus chemotherapy requires evidence that these patients do not have stage IV disease, patients with clinical evidence of stage III_2 disease (e.g., positive lymphangiogram) are often treated with chemotherapy rather than being evaluated further by staging laparotomy.

7. **Stage IIIB, IVA, and IVB.** Therapy for these stages generally comprises combination chemotherapy. The demonstration that MOPP chemotherapy could cure advanced Hodgkin's disease was one of the major advances in modern cancer chemotherapy and has been one of the major rationales for the use of combination chemotherapy for other malignancies.

   a. **Dose and duration of the therapy.** The optimal chemotherapy regimen for use in Hodgkin's disease has not been established, and concerns about choosing the "best" regimen should not obscure the following principles. Drugs should be administered in accordance with prescribed schedules and not modified for toxicities such as nausea and vomiting (which should be controlled symptomatically with antiemetics). Vincristine should be decreased only in the presence of ileus, motor weakness, or numbness involving the entire fingers, not just the fingertips. Six cycles of chemotherapy represent the standard duration of therapy, but it is not an absolute, and the policy is to treat until a complete remission is documented (usually after four cycles), and then for two additional cycles. If tests are equivocal, it is better to treat with additional cycles and reevaluate than to prematurely discontinue therapy.

   b. **Response to MOPP chemotherapy.** When MOPP was administered in optimal fashion in one study, 81% of patients achieved a complete remission. Of these patients, 66% (representing 53% of the total series) remained in complete remission for 5 years, and an identical percentage remained in complete remission for 10 years. Thus 5-year disease-free survival is probably equivalent to cure. It should also be noted that the figure 53% is a minimal estimate for the cure of advanced Hodgkin's disease, as many patients who experience a complete remission and then relapse may still be cured with later salvage therapy.

c. **Alternatives to MOPP induction therapy.** Many efforts have been made to develop combination regimens that are more effective and less toxic than the standard MOPP regimen. Some of these regimens represent minor variations of the MOPP regimen, and others are combinations of non-cross-resistant drugs (Table 24-3). The latter regimens may be used for MOPP failures but may also be considered as initial therapy. Many regimens can produce remission rates similar to those achieved with MOPP therapy, but there are no data to indicate that the long-term results are superior to those achieved with MOPP. Of the regimens that are minimal variations of the MOPP regimen, only BVCPP (Table 24-3) has been shown to produce long-term results equivalent to those of MOPP.

Other alternatives to MOPP have also generated considerable interest. It is well known that patients with nodular sclerosing Hodgkin's disease, the most common type of Hodgkin's disease, tend to relapse at the site of prior nodal disease when treated with MOPP alone. For this reason,

Table 24-3. Alternatives to MOPP chemotherapy

Regimen	Dosage
BVCPP	Carmustine 100 mg/m^2 IV on day 1 Vinblastine 5 mg/m^2 IV on day 1 Cyclophosphamide 600 mg/m^2 PO on day 1 Procarbazine 100 mg/m^2 PO on days 1–10 Prednisone 60 mg/m^2 PO on days 1–10 Repeat every 28 days
ABVD	Doxorubicin (Adriamycin) 25 mg/m^2 IV on days 1 and 15 Bleomycin 10 units/m^2 IV on days 1 and 15 Vinblastine 6 mg/m^2 IV on days 1 and 15 Dacarbazine 150 mg/m^2 on days 1–5 Repeat every 28 days
BCAVe	Bleomycin 2.5 units/m^2 IV or IM on days 1, 28, 35 Lomustine (CCNU) 100 mg/m^2 PO on day 1 Doxorubicin (Adriamycin) 60 mg/m^2 IV on day 1 Vinblastine 5 mg/m^2 IV on day 1 Repeat every 42 days
ABDIC	Doxorubicin (Adriamycin) 45 mg/m^2 IV on day 1 Bleomycin 5 units/m^2 IV or IM on days 1 and 5 Dacarbazine 200 mg/m^2 IV on days 1–5 Lomustine (CCNU) 50 mg/m^2 PO on day 1 Prednisone 40 mg/m^2 PO on days 1–5 Repeat every 28 days

a number of programs combining MOPP or its variants with radiotherapy have been proposed for stage IV disease, and results of these approaches appear equivalent to, or slightly better than, MOPP alone.

8. **MOPP/ABV regimen.** Another approach to advanced disease is to use a hybrid regimen that integrates both the MOPP and ABV regimens (ABVD without dacarbazine) into the chemotherapy cycle. Based on the Goldie-Coldman model of development of tumor resistance, initial studies alternated 1 month of MOPP with 1 month of ABVD. More recent approaches involve giving the drugs included in MOPP on day 1 and giving ABV on day 8 (Table 24-4). Using supplemental radiotherapy to single areas of residual adenopathy, this regimen has been associated with complete remission rates of 97.5% and a 3-year relapse-free survival of 90.5%.

9. **Salvage therapy** for treatment failures. Relapse of Hodgkin's disease does not mean death, as salvage therapy is capable of producing cures. However, the chance of curing a patient with Hodgkin's disease who has relapsed is greater if the recurrence is nodal than if it is visceral. Also, the chance of salvaging a patient with Hodgkin's disease is greater when the initial stage of disease was limited than when it was relatively advanced.

For patients with limited nodal relapses following radiation therapy, additional irradiation may be considered. Alternatively, chemotherapy may be used in these patients and in those who relapse following chemotherapy. It has been appreciated that patients who relapse following initial radiotherapy may achieve a complete remission and may be potentially cured with combination chemotherapy. It has also been shown that patients who achieve a complete remission with MOPP therapy and who remain in remission for more than 1 year may have remission reinduced with MOPP therapy at the time of relapse and may be cured by this salvage therapy. In

Table 24-4. MOPP/ABV for Hodgkin's disease

Drug	Dose
Mechlorethamine	6 mg/m^2 IV on day 1
Vincristine (Oncovin)	1.4 mg/m^2 IV on day 1 (not to exceed 2 mg)
Procarbazine	100 mg/m^2 PO on days 1–7
Prednisone	40 mg/m^2 PO on days 1–14
Doxorubicin	35 mg/m^2 IV on day 8
Bleomycin	10 units/m^2 IV on day 8
Vinblastine	6 mg/m^2 IV on day 8
	Repeat every 28 days

past years, many of these patients, who were not truly MOPP-resistant, were treated with one of the regimens listed in Table 24-3 as salvage therapy. Inclusion of these relatively favorable patients in studies of such newer regimens as salvage therapy has led to overestimating the value of these regimens as salvage therapy in the patient who is truly MOPP-resistant.

Because of the heterogeneity of patient groups studied in reports of salvage therapy, it has not been established that any one salvage regimen is optimal. However, in patients truly resistant to primary treatment, the possibility of cure with salvage regimens such as ABVD or BCAVe is probably 15% or less. Furthermore, the use of regimens such as MOPP–ABV as primary therapy, by exposing patients to multiple agents, clearly decreases the possibility that they will respond to salvage therapy.

For this reason, using high-dose chemotherapy with or without radiotherapy in conjunction with reinfusion of autologous bone marrow has been investigated as either primary or secondary salvage therapy in patients with Hodgkin's disease. Although results are variable, because of differing criteria for selection of patients, studies suggest that as many as one-third of patients with advanced refractory disease may be salvaged by this approach.

II. Non-Hodgkin's lymphoma

A. Introduction. The non-Hodgkin's lymphomas (NHLs) are a group of malignancies that involve lymphocytes. The disorders included in NHLs differ in many basic characteristics. At the time of presentation some types of lymphoma, e.g., small cleaved cell lymphoma (poorly differentiated lymphocytic lymphoma), are almost always disseminated and have a high incidence of bone marrow and hepatic involvement. Other lymphomas, e.g., diffuse large noncleaved cell lymphoma (diffuse "histiocytic" lymphoma), may be limited to one or two lymph node areas in 30% of cases and involve the bone marrow at presentation in fewer than 20% of cases. In most adult lymphomas the malignant cell is a B lymphocyte. In a few cases the malignant cell is a T lymphocyte. Some types of lymphoma (primarily nodular lymphomas) have a slow, indolent course that initially responds to therapy but eventually progresses to a fatal outcome. Other types of lymphoma (mostly diffuse large cell lymphomas) have a rapidly fatal course in the absence of therapy but may be cured by combination chemotherapy.

In these circumstances, accurate classification of lymphomas is essential for scientific and clinical purposes. Ideally, one would want a classification system to divide lymphomas into entities that were both scientifically and clinically meaningful, i.e., a classification system that would define entities that were relatively homogeneous from a morphologic, immunologic, and clinical point of view. One would also want a classification system that could be widely used by pathologists so results could be compared from one institution to another, enabling clinicians to apply the results of studies to individual patients secure in the knowledge that the term used in the study meant the same thing to the academic pathologist writing the paper as to the local pathologist reviewing a particular case. Unfortunately, such an ideal classification system does not exist, and what is commonly used, the "New Working Formulation," is an attempt to use pathologic and immunologic principles to classify lymphomas into broad prognostic categories. The good news for clinicians is that this approach may facilitate treatment decisions. The bad news is that classification of lymphomas remains a suboptimal situation in which diverse disorders may be "lumped" together in the interests of simplifying care. Because the confusion over classification systems often prevents understanding the clinical state of the art with respect to lymphoma, a brief consideration of the classification of lymphomas is relevant prior to a discussion of therapy.

1. **Classification—historical perspective.** During the 1960s Rappaport divided lymphomas on the basis of whether the predominant cell was small (poorly differentiated lymphocytic lymphoma), large ("histiocytic" lymphoma), or a mixture of the two (mixed cell lymphoma). Lymphomas were also categorized as nodular or diffuse, although in many cases it was a continuum and not an absolute distinction. Entities such as diffuse "histiocytic" lymphoma were defined.

This system predated the understanding that there were B cells and T cells, and that most adult lymphomas involved the cells usually found in normal follicular centers. The Lukes-Collins classification system attempted to classify lymphomas on the basis of cell of origin and, by definition, define immunologically homogeneous entities. Several problems limited the adoption of this system. First, several systems considering immunologic features were simultaneously advocated by various hematopathologists, creating an atmosphere of confusion. Second, while attempting to define lymphomas by immune origin, as many as 25% of cases were "unclassified" in the "newer" Lukes-Collins system unless fresh tissue was available for the study of surface markers or until techniques to detect gene rearrangements were developed. Third, although the Rappaport system clearly had limitations, because of its widespread use by the mid-1970s there was concordance among pathologists regarding the classification of cases with respect to the Rappaport classification. Lacking a history of practical experience, none of the newer systems, including that of the Lukes-Collins system, had this level of agreement among pathologists with respect to cases. Fourth, although the Lukes-Collins system emphasized that a disorder such as "histiocytic" lymphoma was actually many disorders (i.e., large noncleaved cell lymphoma, large cleaved cell lymphoma, immunoblastic sarcoma of B cells, peripheral T cell lymphoma), there was no evidence that any or all of these hematopathologic distinctions were of clinical significance. Thus although the Lukes-Collins system appeared to be a scientific step forward, concerns over its practical application led to confusion.

2. **Classification—New Working Formulation.** In this context the National Cancer Institute created a working panel of hematopathologists who created the New Working Formulation. This classification system put the ideas of the Lukes-Collins system (and other immunologically oriented systems) into the mainstream; but instead of emphasizing the creation of many entities based on "cell of origin," the New Working Formulation defined broad categories of lymphoma based on general clinical prognosis, specifically low grade, intermediate grade, and high grade. The following is only a slight oversimplification.

Low grade lymphomas are indolent lymphomas, e.g., chronic lymphocytic lymphoma and follicular (nodular) small cleaved cell lymphoma. In asymptomatic patients, even with widespread disease, they may require no initial treatment. These disorders are associated with a high response rate, but after a prolonged clinical course (often 5 to 10 + years) they are invariably fatal. *Intermediate grade lymphomas* are more aggressive lymphomas that are associated with a fatal course within months (or occasionally a few years) in the absence of therapy but that have a high response rate and probably a cure rate approaching 50% with combination chemotherapy. This category includes diffuse small cleaved cell lymphoma and diffuse large noncleaved cell lymphoma, the most frequently seen subset of "histiocytic" lymphoma. *High grade lymphomas* are those lymphomas associated with a high growth fraction, rapidly progressive clinical course in the absence of effective therapy, and a response rate to most chemotherapy regimens generally lower than that seen with intermediate grade lymphomas. The New Working Formulation is presented in Table 24-5 and represents more of a framework for clinical trials and therapeutic decisions than a pathologic classification system.

B. **Staging**
1. **Limited versus advanced disease.** The Ann Arbor staging system for Hodgkin's disease (see **I.B**) is also used for NHLs. However, in contrast to Hodgkin's disease, which arises at an extranodal site in fewer than 1% of cases, approximately 10–20% of NHL cases arise at extranodal sites. Furthermore,

Table 24-5. New Working Formulation for non-Hodgkin's lymphoma

Low grade
　Small lymphocytic consistent with CLL or plasmacytoid cell
　Follicular, predominantly small cleaved cell
　　Diffuse areas
　　Sclerosis
　Follicular, mixed, small cleaved cell and large cell
　　Diffuse areas
　　Sclerosis

Intermediate grade
　Follicular, predominantly large cell
　　Diffuse areas
　　Sclerosis
　Diffuse small cleaved cell
　Diffuse mixed, small cleaved cell and large cell
　　Sclerosis
　　Epitheloid cell component
　Diffuse large cell
　　Cleaved cell
　　Noncleaved cell
　　Sclerosis

High grade
　Large cell, immunoblastic
　　Plasmacytoid
　　Clear-cell
　　Polymorphous
　　Epithelioid cell component
　Lymphoblastic
　　Convoluted cell
　　Nonconvoluted cell
　Small noncleaved cell
　　Burkitt's
　　Follicular areas

Miscellaneous
　Composite
　Mycosis fungoides
　Histiocytic
　Extramedullary plasmacytoma
　Unclassifiable
　Other

Source: Modified from the Non-Hodgkin's Lymphoma Pathologic Classification Project. National Cancer Institute-sponsored study of classification of non-Hogdkin's lymphomas: summary and description of a working formulation for clinical usage. *Cancer* 49:2112, 1982.

the clinical applicability of the four stages of Hodg-kin's disease to non-Hodgkin's lymphoma is lim-ited. For practical purposes there may be only two stages: limited disease (stage I) and advanced dis-ease (stages II, III, and IV). With the exception of low grade lymphomas, it is established that radiother-apy has no role in the curative therapy of stage II NHL and that chemotherapy is required in these pa-tients. (As noted below, even for stage I intermediate grade lymphoma, the role of radiotherapy has gen-erally been supplanted by chemotherapy.)

2. **Special considerations** apply to the staging of pa-tients with NHL.
   a. **When performing a physical examination** special care must be given to sites such as Wal-deyer's ring, epitrochlear nodes, femoral nodes, and popliteal nodes, which are rarely involved by Hodgkin's disease.
   b. **Bone marrow biopsy** is a key diagnostic proce-dure in NHLs owing to the high incidence of in-volvement, especially in small cleaved cell lym-phoma.
   c. **Abdominal CT** scanning is of greater value in NHLs than in Hodgkin's disease. In Hodgkin's disease involved abdominal nodes are small and may be missed by CT scanning, whereas lym-phangiography can detect small nodes in which the internal architecture is disrupted. With NHLs, retroperitoneal masses are often large and easily detected by CT scanning. In addition, whereas mesenteric nodes are rarely involved in Hodgkin's disease, they are involved in approxi-mately 70% of patients with nodular NHLs and may be detected by CT scanning but are not opa-cified by lymphangiography. As for Hodgkin's dis-ease, tests that are performed for purposes of staging establish a baseline so patients can be evaluated for a complete remission when therapy has been given with curative intent.

C. **Therapy of non-Hodgkin's lymphomas**
   1. **Radiation therapy; general considerations.** Be-cause most patients with NHLs have disseminated disease, radiotherapy plays a more limited role in NHLs than in Hodgkin's disease. However, the value of radiotherapy should not be overlooked. With most histologic types of nodular lymphoma, doses of 44 Gy can achieve control of local disease. Because disease occurs outside of treatment fields, e.g., bone marrow disease, irradiation is rarely curative. However, when patients with nodular lymphoma have large masses, local radiotherapy may be the most effective means of palliation. A dose-response curve for large cell lymphoma is less well established, although ra-diotherapy may play a role in palliating patients with large cell lymphoma who have become refrac-tory to chemotherapy. Although 30% of patients with

large cell lymphoma have stage I or II disease, the role of radiotherapy in these patients is not firmly established.

Radiotherapy has been associated with cure rates exceeding 80% in stage I large cell lymphomas *only* when patients have been staged by laparotomy. Rather than subject these patients to a laparotomy, the usual procedure is to treat stage I patients with chemotherapy with or without involved field irradiation. This approach is associated with cure rates exceeding 90%. It is not clear whether this approach should involve an aggressive chemotherapy regimen (e.g., ProMACE–MOPP) or a simpler regimen (e.g., CHOP) is adequate for these cases (Tables 24-6 and 24-7).

Prior to initiating intensive chemotherapy, patients should be placed on allopurinol 300 mg/day to avert the hyperuricemia that may follow tumor lysis.

2. **Low grade lymphoma** predominantly small cleaved cell lymphoma—nodular (SCC-N), also called poorly differentiated lymphocytic lymphoma—nodular). Patients with this type of lymphoma generally have widespread disease at presentation. Nevertheless, median survival of patients with SCC-N has ranged from 4 to 8 years in most series. Combination regimens such as those in Table 24-6 have produced com-

Table 24-6. Combination chemotherapy for the clinically indolent lymphomas

Regimen*	Dosage
CVP	Cyclophosphamide 400 mg/m² PO on days 1–5
	Vincristine (Oncovin) 1.4 mg/m² IV on day 1 (not to exceed 2.0 mg)
	Prednisone 100 mg/m² PO on days 1–5
	Repeat every 21 days
COPP	Cyclophosphamide 600 mg/m² IV on days 1 and 8
	Vincristine (Oncovin) 1.4 mg/m² IV on days 1 and 8 (not to exceed 2.5 mg)
	Procarbazine 100 mg/m² PO on days 1–10
	Prednisone 40 mg/m² on days 1–14
	Repeat every 28 days
CHOP	Cyclophosphamide 750 mg/m² IV on day 1
	Doxorubicin (Adriamycin) 50 mg/m² IV on day 1
	Vincristine (Oncovin) 1.4 mg/m² IV on day 1 (not to exceed 2.0 mg)
	Prednisone 100 mg PO on days 1–5
	Repeat every 21 days

*These regimens employ a sliding scale for myelotoxicity similar to that used for the MOPP regimen (Table 24-2). The alphabetic abbreviations used for these regimens consider doxorubicin (Adriamycin) as hydroxyldaunomycin. Mitoxantrone (Novantrone) 10 mg/m² may be substituted for doxorubicin to limit toxicity.

Table 24-7. Chemotherapy regimens for diffuse histiocytic lymphoma

Regimen	Dosage
BACOP	Bleomycin 5 units/m^2 IV on days 15 and 22
	Doxorubicin (Adriamycin) 25 mg/m^2 IV on days 1 and 8
	Cyclophosphamide 650 mg/m^2 IV on days 1 and 8
	Vincristine (Oncovin) 1.4 mg/m^2 IV on days 1 and 8 (not to exceed 2.0 mg)
	Prednisone 60 mg/m^2 PO on days 15–28
	Repeat every 28 days.
COMLA	Cyclophosphamide 1500 mg/m^2 IV on day 1
	Vincristine (Oncovin) 1.4 mg/m^2 IV on days 1, 8, 15 (not to exceed 2.5 mg)
	Methotrexate 120 mg/m^2 IV on days 22, 29, 36, 43, 50, 57, 64, 71
	Leucovorin 25 mg/m^2 PO q6h for 4 doses starting 24 hours after each methotrexate dose
	Cytarabine 300 mg/m^2 IV on days 22, 29, 36, 43, 50, 57, 64, 71
	Repeat every 91 days.
m-BACOD	Methotrexate 200 mg/m^2 IV on days 8 and 15
	Leucovorin 10 mg/m^2 PO q6h for 8 doses starting 24 hours after methotrexate
	Bleomycin 4 units/m^2 IV on day 1
	Doxorubicin (Adriamycin) 45 mg/m^2 IV on day 1
	Cyclophosphamide 600 mg/m^2 IV on day 1
	Vincristine (Oncovin) 1 mg/m^2 IV on day 1
	Dexamethasone 6 mg/m^2 PO on days 1–5
	Repeat every 21 days.
ProMACE/MOPP	Prednisone 60 mg/m^2 PO on days 1–14
	Methotrexate 1.5 gm/m^2 IV on day 14
	Leucovorin 50 mg/m^2 IV q6h for 5 doses starting 24 hours after methotrexate
	Doxorubicin (Adriamycin) 25 mg/m^2 IV on days 1 and 8
	Cyclophosphamide 650 mg/m^2 IV on days 1 and 8
	Etoposide 120 mg/m^2 IV on days 1 and 8
	Cycles are given every 28 days.
	ProMACE is given for a variable number of cycles based on tumor response; then MOPP therapy is given for approximately the same number of cycles.
MACOP-B	Methotrexate 400 mg/m^2 IV weeks 2, 6, and 10; one-fourth of dose as IV bolus, then three-fourths over 4 hours

Table 24-7 (continued)

Regimen	Dosage
	Leucovorin 15 mg PO q6h for 6 doses, starting 24 hours after each methotrexate dose
	Doxorubicin (Adriamycin) 50 mg/m^2 IV weeks 1, 3, 5, 7, 9, 11
	Cyclophosphamide 350 mg/m^2 IV weeks 1, 3, 5, 7, 9, 11
	Vincristine (Oncovin) 1.4 mg/m^2 IV weeks 2, 4, 6, 8, 10, 12
	Bleomycin 10 units/m^2 IV weeks 4, 8, 12
	Prednisone 75 mg/day PO for 12 weeks; taper to 0 during weeks 10–12
	Trimethoprim-sulfa 1 double-strength tablet PO bid × 12 weeks

plete remissions in up to 80% of patients. However, such remissions are not durable, and these regimens are associated with considerable toxicity (myelotoxicity, nausea, vomiting, alopecia, and neurotoxicity). Because therapy is palliative and there is no proof that survival is improved by the early use of combination chemotherapy, many clinicians use a policy of "watchful waiting," as might be employed for chronic lymphocytic leukemia. Nevertheless, it should be noted that some clinicians still advocate the early use of combination chemotherapy for these patients in the hope of having a favorable impact on individual cases.

Patients with minimal symptoms or moderate lymphadenopathy may be treated with chlorambucil, either 2–4 mg/m^2 PO daily or 30 mg/m^2 PO every 2 weeks, with or without prednisone. In patients with enlarging nodes or spleen, cytopenias, fever, sweats, weight loss, or visceral involvement other than bone marrow or microscopic liver involvement, one would generally initiate therapy with one of the simple chemotherapy regimens shown in Table 24–6. In many patients years elapse before such treatment is required.

Interferon-alpha (IFN-α) has also been shown to be effective against low grade lymphomas, often in patients refractory to chemotherapy. The optimal dose and schedule for use of interferon has not been established, nor has it been established if it should be incorporated into primary treatment programs.

Low grade lymphomas are slowly progressive by definition, although they eventually reach a phase where they are refractory to alkylating agents, prednisone, and anthracyclines. In some cases repeat biopsy reveals that this phase is associated with a pathologic change to large noncleaved cell lymphoma. In other cases it is associated with a biologic change and involvement of visceral sites or with total replacement of the bone marrow. Any of the regimens used as primary therapy (Table 24-7) or salvage therapy for intermediate or high grade lymphomas can be considered, but therapy of this clinical situation is generally unsatisfactory. Survival after pathologic transformation rarely exceeds 1 year.

3. **Intermediate grade lymphomas**

   a. **Small cleaved cell—diffuse.** The disease initially described by Rappaport as "poorly differentiated lymphocytic lymphoma diffuse" (PDL-D) has been shown to be composed of two disorders. One group of patients have a disease similar to small cleaved cell nodular lymphoma, which is indeed composed of small cleaved lymphocytes. This disease is similar to SCC-N but tends to be associated with a shorter survival. Although it is not known if initial chemotherapy produces results superior to "watchful waiting" in this group of patients, the general tendency is to treat at the time of diagnosis with either CHOP or a more aggressive regimen (Table 24-7). The other group of patients included in the Rappaport category PDL-D have a T cell lymphoma generally equivalent to T cell acute lymphocytic leukemia that is often associated with a large mediastinal mass. These patients clearly have a high grade lymphoma and require aggressive treatment programs.

   b. **Large cleaved cell lymphoma (LCCL) or "mixed cell" lymphoma.** These lymphomas, in which large cleaved cells are often the predominant cell, are generally mixtures of large cleaved cells and small cleaved cells. Large noncleaved cells are often present. Classification of these cases is also complicated by the fact that most of them have both a nodular and a diffuse pattern, rendering moot the New Working Formulation recommendation that nodular cases of large cleaved cell lymphoma should be regarded as low grade whereas diffuse cases are considered intermediate grade.

   When watchful waiting is employed in this group of patients, therapy is generally initiated within less than a year, so most clinicians treat these patients at the time of diagnosis. Nevertheless, there has not been a consistent demonstration that the patients have a curable disease when aggressive chemotherapy is employed. Optimal therapy for this group of patients is clearly undefined. Some clinicians prefer minimal therapy on the grounds that treatment is palliative, as in small cleaved cell lymphoma—nodular disease. Other clinicians believe that aggressive chemotherapy, e.g., MACOP-B, is indicated, as some of these lymphomas behave in an aggressive fashion and prospective identification of these cases is not possible.

There is less concordance among pathologists regarding classification of mixed cell lymphomas or large cleaved cell lymphomas than for any other NHL. Because these lymphomas are mixtures of cell types and are generally both nodular and diffuse, what is one pathologist's "large cleaved cell—nodular" or "mixed cell—nodular" lymphoma may be interpreted as "large noncleaved cell—diffuse by another. Fortunately, this confusing disorder represents only 5–10% of the cases of adult NHL.

c. **Large noncleaved (transformed) cell lymphoma, immunoblastic sarcoma of B cells, and peripheral T cell lymphoma.**

(1) **Immunologic and pathologic subtypes.** These disorders represent most of the cases previously considered "diffuse histiocytic" lymphoma and now entered into studies of "diffuse large cell lymphoma." Exact percentage breakdowns are not known, but T cell lymphomas comprise only 5–10% of cases of "large cell lymphoma," and approximately 10% of cases are immunoblastic sarcoma of B cells. Controversy still exists as to whether the immunologic subtype of "large cell" lymphoma is clinically important. Some studies have found immunologic subclassification to be clinically insignificant, whereas others have found that such subclassification is a major prognostic variable in this group of patients. These differences may reflect differences in the use of the pathologic classification systems, or an interaction between prognosis and therapy. At Vanderbilt University Medical Center, we have found that when one uses regimens such as CHOP, BACOP, or COMLA the prognosis is significantly worse for patients with peripheral T cell lymphoma compared to those with large noncleaved cell lymphoma (a B cell lymphoma). As therapy has become more aggressive (e.g., treatment with m-BACOD), immunologic subclassification has become clinically less significant.

(2) **Combination chemotherapy: historical perspective.** In the era of single-agent chemotherapy, the lymphomas classified as "diffuse histiocytic" were associated with a median survival of 6 months, with approximately 5–10% of patients surviving for 2 years. The demonstration that COPP che-

motherapy (Table 24-6) could produce complete remissions in approximately 40% of patients, with 35% of patients continuing as long-term relapse-free survivors, was a major clinical advance. Numerous regimens have replaced COPP since the early 1970s, but all of these regimens (see CHOP, Tables 24-6 and 24-7) can be interpreted relative to the COPP study.

(a) COPP showed that "histiocytic" lymphoma was curable. As noted above, there is suggestive evidence that certain subsets, e.g., large cleaved cell lymphoma (LCCL) and possibly peripheral T cell lymphoma (PTCL), are less curable than other subsets.

(b) The COPP study showed that approximately 80% of complete remissions are associated with cure. However, patients receiving CHOP appear to be more likely to relapse. Patients with LCCL and PTCL also appear to have higher rates of relapse after achieving a complete remission.

(c) The COPP study showed that 2-year relapse-free survival is a good estimate of cure. Late relapses occur but are rare. Because patients with large masses may have some residual mass (either fibrosis or residual disease) upon completion of therapy, the complete remission rate may be an overestimate of the cure rate based on "wishful thinking." The 2-year relapse-free survival rate is more meaningful because if the residual mass represents persistent disease it will be clinically evident within 2 years.

(d) The complete remission rate reported for newer regimens (Table 24-7) has increased from the 40% observed with COPP to $80 + \%$ with regimens such as MACOP-B. Although this development almost certainly represents a real clinical advance, the magnitude of true improvement is difficult to evaluate for several reasons. These lymphomas are a heterogeneous group clinically and immunologically, and the patients in different studies may not be comparable. First, as therapies have become more aggressive, the median age of the patients in the studies has decreased because older patients are excluded (reasonably so) as being too old to tolerate toxic therapies. Second, whereas chemotherapy studies initially included only patients with stage III and IV disease, patients with stage II disease are now routinely treated with chemotherapy. Because a lower tumor burden appears to be a favorable prognostic feature, these patients favorably bias results of clinical trials. Third, as noted above, the natural history of LCCL (mixed cell lymphoma) is not firmly established. These lymphomas tend to be both nodular and diffuse and may behave somewhat like indolent lymphomas. Inclusion of these patients in studies of large cell diffuse lymphoma may create a favorable bias, as these patients may have a high response rate and may relapse beyond the point at which one is looking for relapses in large cell diffuse lymphoma.

(3) **Combination chemotherapy: current recommendations.** Most clinicians favor the use of the more aggressive regimens shown in Table 24-7, e.g., MACOP-B, ProMACE/MOPP, or m-BACOD, and would regard CHOP as undertreatment for this group of lymphomas. However, there is no published evidence from controlled clinical trials that these regimens are superior to CHOP.

(4) **Salvage chemotherapy.** As primary therapies have become more aggressive and more effective, patients who fail such therapy represent a less and less favorable group of patients. As a result, it is not surprising that salvage chemotherapy of these lymphomas has not produced outstanding results. Some investigators have claimed response rates above 50% with salvage therapy; but complete response rates are generally in the 20–30% range, and long-term relapse-free survival has been observed in fewer than 5% of patients treated in most salvage studies. Salvage regimens generally include drugs such as cisplatin, high-dose cytosine arabinoside, etoposide, or ifosfamide. No regimen is standard, and for this reason no specific regimens are recommended in this chapter. In younger patients with refractory lymphoma, experimental high-dose chemotherapy in conjunction with autologous bone marrow transplantation is a viable option. However, successful results with this approach are generally limited to patients showing some responsiveness to standard chemotherapy.

Selected Reading

Armitage, J. O. Bone marrow transplantation in the treatment of patients with lymphoma. *Blood* 73:1749, 1989.

Bakemeier, R. F., et al. BCVPP chemotherapy for advanced Hodgkin's disease: evidence for greater duration of complete remission, greater survival, and less toxicity than with a MOPP regimen. *Ann. Intern. Med.* 101:447, 1984.

Connors, J. M. and Klimo, P. MACOP-B chemotherapy for malignant lymphomas and related conditions: 1987 update and additional observations. *Semin Hematol.* 25(suppl.2):41, 1988.

DeVita, V. T., et al. Curability of advanced Hodgkin's disease with chemotherapy. *Ann. Intern. Med.* 92:587, 1980.

Fisher, R. I., et al. Prolonged disease free survival in Hodgkin's disease with MOPP re-induction after first relapse. *Ann. Intern. Med.* 90:761, 1979.

Fisher, R. I., et al. Diffuse aggressive lymphomas: increased survival after alternating flexible sequences of ProMACE and MOPP chemotherapy. *Ann. Intern. Med.* 98:304, 1983.

Greer, J. P., et al. Peripheral T-cell lymphoma: a clinicopathologic study of 42 cases. *J. Clin. Oncol.* 2:788, 1984.

Harker, W. G., et al. Combination chemotherapy for advanced Hodgkin's disease after failure of MOPP, ABVD, and B-CAVe. *Ann. Intern. Med.* 101:440, 1984.

Klimo, P., and Connors, J. M. An update on the Vancouver experience in the management of advanced Hodgkin's disease treated with the MOPP/ABV hybrid program. *Semin. Hematol.* 25(suppl. 2):34, 1988.

Mauch, P., et al. Influence of mediastinal adenopathy on site and frequency of relapse in patients with Hodgkin's disease. *Cancer Treat. Rep.* 66:809, 1982.

Non-Hodgkin's Lymphoma Pathologic Classification Project. National Cancer Institute sponsored study of classification of non-Hodgkin's lymphomas: summary and description of a working formulation for clinical usage. *Cancer* 49:2112, 1982.

Portlock, C. S., et al. "Good risk" non-Hodgkin's lymphomas: approaches to management. *Semin. Hematol.* 20:25, 1983.

Prosnitz, L. R., et al. Combined modality therapy for advanced Hodgkin's disease: long-term follow-up data. *Cancer Treat. Rep.* 66:871, 1982.

Shipp, M. A., et al. Identification of major prognostic subgroups of patients with large cell lymphoma treated with m-BACOD or M-BACOD. *Ann. Intern. Med.* 104:757, 1986.

Stein, R. S., et al. Anatomic substages of stage III-A Hodgkin's disease: followup of a collaborative study. *Cancer Treat. Rep.* 66:733, 1982.

Sweet, D. L., et al. Hodgkin's disease: problems of staging. *Cancer* 42:957, 1978.

Multiple Myeloma and Other Plasma Cell Dyscrasias

Martin M. Oken

I. Introduction

A. Types of plasma cell dyscrasias. Plasma cell dyscrasias or plasma cell neoplasms are a group of conditions characterized by unbalanced proliferation of cells that normally synthesize and secrete immunoglobulins. They range from malignant neoplasms such as multiple myeloma to monoclonal gammopathy of undetermined significance, a usually benign condition that is sometimes termed benign monoclonal gammopathy. Associated with the abnormal cellular proliferation in nearly all instances is the production of homogeneous monoclonal immunoglobulin, referred to either as myeloma protein or M protein, or of excessive quantities of homogeneous polypeptide subunits of a monoclonal protein. The latter usually appear as monoclonal free light chains excreted into the urine. Frequently both whole immunoglobulin M protein and free light chains are produced. The plasma cell dyscrasias discussed in this chapter are multiple myeloma, macroglobulinemia (Waldenström's macroglobulinemia), heavy-chain diseases, amyloidosis, and monoclonal gammopathy of undetermined significance.

B. M protein. Unlike most neoplastic diseases, which are followed objectively by serial evaluation of palpable or radiographically measurable tumor masses, most plasma cell dyscrasias are best followed by serial measurements of the monoclonal protein (M protein) elaborated by the tumor. Effective use of this tumor marker is important for the proper evaluation of the disease course of most plasma cell dyscrasias and is usually essential to the determination of response to treatment. The basic immunoglobulin unit comprises two identical heavy chains with a molecular weight of 55,000 daltons linked to two identical light chains with molecular weights of 22,500 daltons. The heavy chains are either γ, α, μ, δ, or ε corresponding to IgG, IgA, IgM, IgD, and IgE, respectively. The light chains exist as either κ or λ subtypes. Serum M protein is a monoclonal whole immunoglobulin and therefore possesses only one heavy chain type and one light chain type. Urine M protein consists of free light chains or, in the case of some heavy chain diseases, free heavy chain fragments of single specificity. Serum M protein may be quantitatively evaluated by either serum protein electrophoresis or determining the concentration of the individual immunoglobulins (particularly IgG, IgA, and IgM) by radial immunodiffusion or nephelometry. Urinary M protein, usually in the form of free light chain, should be characterized by immunoelectrophoresis as monoclonal κ or λ light chain and then followed sequentially expressed as urinary light chain excretion in grams per 24 hours. This characterization requires determination of 24-hour urine protein excretion and scanning the urine protein electrophoresis to determine the percentage of urine protein present as free monoclonal immunoglobulin light chain.

II. Multiple myeloma
A. General considerations and aims of therapy

1. **Diagnosis.** Multiple myeloma is a neoplasm of malignant plasma cells invading bone and bone marrow, causing widespread skeletal destruction, bone marrow failure, and problems related to quantitatively abnormal serum or urinary M proteins. The diagnosis of multiple myeloma requires histologic documentation by the demonstration of increased numbers (usually > 10%) or abnormal, atypical, or immature plasma cells in the bone marrow in addition to finding serum or urinary M protein or characteristic osteolytic bone lesions. Some patients have multiple plasmacytomas of bone with intervening normal areas of bone marrow. In these patients a random bone marrow aspirate and biopsy may fail to reveal the tumor, and biopsy of specific bone lesions may be necessary to establish the diagnosis.

2. **Incidence.** The annual incidence of multiple myeloma is 3/100,000 population with a peak occurrence between ages 60 and 70. Although as many as 4% of patients with myeloma have indolent or smoldering disease at diagnosis, and an additional 5% have an isolated plasmacytoma of bone, most patients with multiple myeloma require chemotherapy of their disease soon after diagnosis.

3. **Effect of treatment.** The goal of therapy is to improve the duration of survival and to diminish or prevent the serious manifestations of this disease, such as bone pain, pathologic fractures, severe anemia, renal failure, or hypercalcemia. Treatment produces objective response in at least 50% of patients as determined by a sustained 50% decline in the levels of serum or urine M protein. Temporary, sometimes long-lasting, alleviation of symptoms occurs in nearly all patients exhibiting objective response to treatment and in some additional patients with lesser degrees of objective improvement. Median survival times usually reported for treated patients range from 2 to 3 years and are strongly influenced by response to treatment and by the initial tumor load.

4. **Prognostic factors.** Table 25-1 presents a clinical staging system developed to estimate myeloma tumor cell mass utilizing readily obtained clinical findings. Severe anemia, hypercalcemia, advanced osteolytic lesions, and extremely high M protein production rates are all associated with a high tumor burden and a poor survival prognosis. Renal failure,

Table 25-1. Myeloma clinical staging system

Stage	Criteria	Myeloma cell mass (cells/m^2)

I	All of the following
	1. Hemoglobin >10 gm/dl
	2. Serum calcium value normal (≤12 mg/dl)
	3. On x-ray film, normal bone structure or solitary bone plasmacytoma only
	4. Low M component production rates
	   a. IgG value <5 gm/dl
	   b. IgA value <3 gm/dl
	   c. Urine light chain M component on electrophoresis <4 gm/24 hours
		<0.6 × 10^{12} (low)

II	Fitting neither stage I nor III	0.6 × 10^{12} to 1.2 × 10^{12} (intermediate)

III	One or more of the following
	1. Hemoglobin <8.5 gm/dl
	2. Serum calcium value > 12 mg/dl
	3. Advanced lytic bone lesions
	4. High M-component production rates
	   a. IgG value >7 gm/dl
	   b. IgA value >5 gm/dl
	   c. Urine light chain M component on electrophoresis >12 gm/24 hours
		>1.2 × 10^{12} (high)

Subclass of any stage		
A	Serum creatinine <2 mg/dl	
B	Serum creatinine ≥2 mg/dl	

Source: Modified from Durie, B. G. M. and Salmon, S. E. A clinical staging system for multiple myeloma: correlation of measured myeloma cell mass with presenting clinical features, response to treatment and survival. *Cancer* 36:842, 1975.

although not well correlated with tumor burden, is associated with poor prognosis. Advanced age, poor performance status, and λ light chain disease have also been established as adverse prognostic signs.

The serum level of β_2-microglobulin correlates with the myeloma tumor burden but is of questionable value for serially monitoring patients with myeloma. Serum β_2-microglobulin usually falls during response to therapy and may increase during relapse, but it has been inconsistent in detecting fulminant progression in which the serum or urinary M proteins may fail to reflect the increasing tumor mass. Another prognostic factor is the plasma cell labeling index as a reflection of the proportion of myeloma cells that are synthesizing DNA. Patients with a labeling index higher than 3% who have a high cell mass have a particularly poor survival prognosis. A low labeling index has been associated with more indolent disease and particularly with a stable plateau phase during an objective response to therapy.

B. Initial treatment

1. **General measures.** Complications of myeloma, e.g., hypercalcemia and renal failure, may be present at the time of diagnosis (see **II.C**). These complications should be promptly identified and treated before the start of chemotherapy. The small percentage of patients who present with stable or indolent, asymptomatic stage IA disease may be followed with observation alone until evidence of progression appears. Most patients have more advanced or progressive disease at diagnosis and require chemotherapy. Patients should be maintained on allopurinol 300 mg/day PO through the first 2 months of chemotherapy to prevent urate nephropathy. A general supportive care regimen emphasizing ambulation and hydration should be maintained throughout the initial treatment.

2. **Standard induction chemotherapy** recommendations are based on an Eastern Cooperative Oncology Group (ECOG) prospective, randomized clinical trial comparing moderate (MP) therapy (see **b**, below) to a more intensive regimen (VBMCP) (see **a**, below). In that study VBMCP yielded an objective response rate of 72%, in contrast to 51% objective responses with MP. Median survival was similar for the two treatments at 28–30 months, but 26% of VBMCP patients survived 5 years compared with 19% five-year survival with MP.

   a. **Most patients** should receive VBMCP. With this regimen the prednisone schedule is frequently individualized so that slowly responding patients with persistent generalized bone pain or severe anemia may receive low-dose prednisone each day of the first two or three cycles in addition to the higher scheduled prednisone dose on days 1–

14. Furthermore, the second cycle may begin on day 29 if blood counts reflect complete recovery from the myelotoxic effects of the initial cycle of treatment.

The **VBMCP regimen** consists of the following.

Vincristine 1.2 mg/m^2 IV on day 1 (up to 2.0 mg) *and*

Carmustine (BCNU) 20 mg/m^2 IV on day 1 *and*

Melphalan 8 mg/m^2 PO on days 1–4 *and*

Cyclophosphamide 400 mg/m^2 IV on day 1 *and*

Prednisone 40 mg/m^2 PO on days 1–7 (all cycles), 20 mg/m^2 PO on days 8–14 (cycles 1–3 only)

Repeat cycle of VBMCP every 35 days for at least 1 year.

   b. **Patients over 70 years of age who have poor performance status,** defined as partially or completely bedridden (ECOG grade 2–4), do not tolerate VBMCP. These high-risk patients, who comprise 10–15% of myeloma patients, should instead be treated with MP according to the following schedule.

   Melphalan 8 mg/m^2 PO on days 1–4 *and*

   Prednisone 60 mg/m^2 PO on days 1–4

   Repeat cycle every 28 days for at least 1 year.

   Because of the similarity in median survival data between VBMCP and MP, the later regimen can also be considered an alternative to VBMCP even for some patients not in the above high-risk group if a less aggressive approach is required. Because of erratic absorption of melphalan in most patients, some investigators recommend cautiously escalating the dose of melphalan on subsequent cycles of chemotherapy until a dose is reached that produces moderate nadir leukocyte counts of 2000–3000 cells/µl. For reliable absorption, melphalan should be taken on an empty stomach.

3. **Alternative induction chemotherapy.** VBMCP + interferon-alpha (rIFN-α2) represents a promising alternative approach to induction therapy. With this regimen, two initial cycles of VBMCP are given followed by alternating 3-week cycles of rIFN-α2 with 3-week cycles of VBMCP. The rIFN-α is administered at 3×10^6 units/m^2 SQ 3 times a week for a total treatment duration of 2 years. A complete remission rate of 30% has been observed with this regimen, leading to the controlled comparison of VBMCP + rIFNα2 to VBMCP alone now being conducted by the ECOG.

4. **Duration of therapy and the role of maintenance therapy.** Although no study has conclusively demonstrated benefit by continuing chemotherapy beyond 1 year in responding patients, several investigators have noted prompt reemergence of active

myeloma shortly after cessation of therapy. Therefore one acceptable approach is to continue the induction regimen for a total duration of 2 years in responding patients but to decrease its frequency to every 6–8 weeks while continuing to follow M protein production carefully. It is probably safe to stop treatment at 1 year in those patients who started therapy with stage I disease and who maintain a 75% reduction in M protein production. These patients should be observed carefully, with reevaluation of serum and urine M protein at least once every 3 months.

A randomized study demonstrated that in patients with responding or stabilized disease after 12 months of chemotherapy, maintenance therapy with rIFNα2 3×10^6 units/m² SQ 3 times a week prolonged the response and survival when compared to no maintenance therapy. Confirmatory studies are in progress. There are no data as yet that establish whether interferon maintenance can prolong responses in patients who have received induction courses longer than 1 year.

5. **Role of radiotherapy.** Solitary plasmacytoma of bone is best treated by local radiation therapy and may not require chemotherapy for months to years. Radiotherapy is also useful as palliative therapy for patients with extraskeletal plasmacytomas, large lytic lesions threatening fracture of long bones, spinal cord or root compression by plasma cell tumor, and certain pathologic features. Repeated local irradiation should be avoided where possible in patients with disseminated myeloma, as chemotherapy is the only treatment demonstrated to improve survival while controlling systemic manifestations of the disease. Excessive use of radiation therapy can impair marrow reserves and render the patient less able to tolerate subsequent chemotherapy.

C. **Complications of disease or therapy.** Chemotherapy for multiple myeloma typically causes myelosuppression, and packed red blood cell transfusions are often required during the early weeks of treatment and the late refractory period. Toxicity of each chemotherapeutic agent is described in Chapter 8. In addition to these problems, several complications characteristic of multiple myeloma may occur.

1. **Hypercalcemia.** This common complication of multiple myeloma is believed to result from the liberation of bone calcium stimulated by osteoclast-activating factor released by the tumor cells. Presenting symptoms may include anorexia, nausea, vomiting, constipation, and polyuria progressing to lethargy, confusion, coma, and death. Dehydration and potentially reversible renal failure frequently occur during hypercalcemic crises. Control of hypercalcemic crises of multiple myeloma is usually accomplished with saline hydration (initially 200–300 ml/hour IV), furosemide (20–40 mg q4–6h), and prednisone (40–80

mg PO daily for 3–7 days). When hypercalcemia occurs in previously untreated patients, prompt initiation of chemotherapy of the myeloma, in addition to these measures, usually produces effective, durable control. In some patients oral inorganic phosphates, calcitonin, etidronate, or, more exceptionally, mithramycin may be needed and can be used on the following schedules.

   a. Inorganic phosphate, e.g., Neutra-Phos or Fleet Phospho-Soda, at a dose equivalent to 0.5 gm of phosphorus PO qid (diluted in water to reduce diarrhea).

   b. Calcitonin 100–300 units SQ q8–12h for up to 2–3 days. Calcitonin is usually given with prednisone 10–20 mg PO 2–3 times daily to prolong its effectiveness.

   c. Etidronate 7.5 mg/kg in 250 ml saline given as a daily 4 to 6-hour infusion for 3 days once the patient has been rehydrated.

   d. Mithramycin 1.0 mg/m^2 IV every 3–7 days. This agent is myelosuppressive and can cause hemostatic disorders and nausea. Its long-term or repeated use in myeloma patients should be avoided except refractory instances of hypercalcemia.

   e. Hemodialysis is effective but seldom needed for hypercalcemia.

2. Infection. Myeloma patients are highly susceptible to respiratory and urinary tract infections with common gram-positive and gram-negative bacterial pathogens. Deficiency of normal immunoglobulins, diminished bone marrow reserves, and immobilization due to skeletal disease are important predisposing factors. The weeks immediately following initiation of chemotherapy are a particularly high-risk period for infection. Prompt evaluation of fever or other manifestations of infection is essential. Antibiotic coverage for gram-positive and gram-negative organisms should be instituted while awaiting culture results from patients whose clinical pictures suggest infection. Infection prophylaxis with γ-globulin injections or antibiotics has not been proved of value, although the concept is reasonable and further evaluation is needed.

3. Hyperviscosity may present as central nervous system (CNS) impairment, congestive heart failure, ischemia, or bleeding tendency. It is more characteristic of Waldenström's macroglobulinemia than of multiple myeloma, but it may be seen in patients with extremely high IgG or IgA concentrations or in patients whose M protein tends to form aggregates. The treatment for symptomatic hyperviscosity is plasmapheresis.

4. Renal dysfunction may be caused by myeloma kidney, amyloidosis, pyelonephritis, hypercalcemia, hyperuricemia with urate nephropathy, hyperviscosity syndrome, plasma cell infiltration of both kidneys (rare), and renal tubular acidosis. Most of these problems are at least partially reversible if recognized and treated promptly. Hypercalcemia and hyperuricemia are especially common potential causes of reversible renal failure and should be ruled out at the onset of the evaluation of a patient with myeloma. In patients with severe renal failure, hemodialysis should be considered so long as chemotherapy offers the potential for a prolonged remission.

5. **Skeletal destruction** is a major cause of disability and immobilization in multiple myeloma. Radiation therapy or surgery, or both, may be needed to treat fractures or to prevent impending fractures of weight-bearing bones. The role of fluoride, calcium, and vitamin D in promoting skeletal repair during remission is under study.

6. **Leukemia.** Acute nonlymphocytic leukemia (ANLL) develops in about 4% of myeloma patients who receive chemotherapy. The incidence of ANLL is appreciably greater in patients surviving 4 years or more after the start of chemotherapy. Leukemia in this setting appears to be caused by the interaction of a carcinogenic drug with a predisposed host. ANLL complicating multiple myeloma is usually preceded by sideroblastic anemia as part of a myelodysplastic syndrome.

E. **Recurrence and treatment of refractory disease.** Objective responses to chemotherapy have a median duration of about 2 years. Response duration is influenced by the degree of reduction of tumor burden as reflected by the degree of reduction of myeloma proteins in the serum and urine. Eventually, virtually all patients develop recurrent or refractory disease. These patients pose a difficult clinical problem because of the small number of chemotherapeutic agents with proved activity in myeloma. Patients relapsing months or years after last receiving chemotherapy can frequently be reinduced with the original regimen.

1. **Treatment of patients refractory to melphalan.** Patients refractory to melphalan or melphalan + prednisone regimens may still respond to other alkylating agents. Two regimens that may be considered are as follows.

   a. **VBMCP** (see **II.B.2.a**)
   b. **BCP**

   Carmustine (BCNU) 75 mg/m^2 IV on day 1 *and*
   Cyclophosphamide 400 mg/m^2 IV on day 1 *and*
   Prednisone 75 mg PO on days 1–7
   Repeat every 4 weeks.

   Treatment with these alkylating agent-based regimens can be expected to yield objective responses in about 20% of patients refractory to prior MP therapy.

These regimens remain useful as conservative treatment choices for patients in their first relapse or for some patients who have failed initial MP therapy.

2. **Alternative regimens** not based on standard dose alkylating agents include the following.

   a. **VAD**

   Vincristine 0.4 mg/day as a continuous IV infusion on days 1–4 *and*

   Doxorubicin (Adriamycin) 9.0 mg/m^2/day as a continuous IV infusion on days 1–4 *and*

   Dexamethasone 40 mg PO on days 1–4, 9–12, 17–20

   Repeat cycle every 28–35 days until 4 cycles beyond occurrence of maximum reduction in myeloma protein. Maximum cumulative doxorubicin dose is 540 mg/m^2. To avoid problems related to adrenal steroid excess, the frequency of dexamethasone courses should be decreased once clinical response is reached.

   b. **High-dose cyclophosphamide.** Cyclophosphamide 600 mg/m^2 IV is given on days 1–4, with this dosage repeated in 1–2 months. This aggressive regimen effectively produces pain relief of more than 1 month's duration and yields short-term objective responses in more than 30% of patients refractory to prior treatments. Because the regimen is highly myelotoxic (it is employed without dose modification), its use should generally be limited to patients with active, markedly symptomatic refractory disease in institutions equipped to render intensive support, including platelet transfusion and infectious disease consultation. Simultaneous use of mithramycin should be avoided.

   c. **Interferon-alpha-2** (rIFNα2) 5 × 10^6 units/m^2 SQ 3 times a week. This regimen produces clinical benefit in 35% of patients by objective and symptomatic standards but full objective responses (50% decrease in serum myeloma protein) in only 10%.

   d. **Autologous bone marrow transplantation** has been employed after preparative regimens such as high-dose cyclophosphamide plus total body irradiation to induce good quality responses in some patients with refractory myeloma. There are issues related to marrow purge, the intensity of antitumor therapy, age range, expense, and the presence or absence of cure potential for this approach in myeloma.

III. **Waldenström's macroglobulinemia**

A. **General considerations and aims of therapy.** This neoplasm is characterized by the proliferation of plasmacytoid lymphocytes that elaborate a monoclonal IgM. In contrast to multiple myeloma, skeletal destruction does not occur, but hepatosplenomegaly and lymphadenopathy are common. The major problems are hyperviscosity syndrome, severe anemia, and occasionally pancytopenia. The median survival is only about 5 years from diagnosis partly owing to the advanced age of most affected patients (60–75 years old), as well as to the common association with second neoplasms (20% of patients) and chronic or recurrent infections (25% of patients). The primary aims of therapy are to control complications and to decrease their incidence. Although response to chemotherapy has, not surprisingly, been associated with a more favorable median survival, the actual role of chemotherapy in prolonging survival in this disease has not been fully defined.

B. Treatment

   1. Anemia. Most patients with macroglobulinemia are anemic; however, transfusions should generally be reserved for those with symptomatic anemia. Overtransfusion is dangerous because of the important contribution of red blood cells to whole blood viscosity.

   2. Hyperviscosity. Hyperviscosity syndrome requires plasmapheresis for acute management and chemotherapy with alkylating agents for long-term control.

   3. Chemotherapy. In general, chemotherapy is withheld until symptomatic disease or progressive cytopenias occur.

   a. Standard chemotherapy

   Chlorambucil 2–6 mg PO daily *or*
   Cyclophosphamide 50–100 mg PO daily
   (Prednisone 40–60 mg PO on days 1–4 every 4 weeks may be added.)

   b. Alternatively, a high-dose intermittent chlorambucil-prednisone regimen may be used every 2–3 weeks.

   Chlorambucil 30 mg/m^2 PO on day 1 *and*
   Prednisone 40 mg/m^2 PO on days 1–4

   c. VBMCP is described in **II.B.2.a.**

   4. Disease variants. Some patients with IgM monoclonal proteins have clinical chronic lymphocytic leukemia (CLL) or lymphoma and should have their treatment directed at that disease. Rare patients with macroglobulinemia have prominent skeletal disease, and their disease should be approached as IgM myeloma and treated similarly to other multiple myelomas.

IV. Heavy chain diseases comprise a group of rare plasma cell dyscrasias in which the abnormal clone of plasma cells or B lymphocytes elaborates an abnormal polypeptide consisting of anomalous γ, α, or μ heavy chains with deleted segments.

   A. Gamma heavy chain disease presents as a lymphoma usually with lymphadenopathy, hepatosplenomegaly and involvement of Waldeyer's ring. The latter may lead to characteristic palatal edema. Bone marrow involvement is the rule. Treatment by local radiotherapy or lymphoma-directed chemotherapy regimens is sometimes effective.

B. Alpha heavy chain disease appears to be the most common of the heavy chain diseases and occurs mainly in people under the age of 50. Its most common clinical presentation is in the enteric form with chronic diarrhea, malabsorption syndrome, and marked lymphoplasmacytic infiltration of the small bowel mucosa. Remissions have been reported using lymphoma chemotherapy regimens and occasionally antibiotics alone.

C. Mu heavy chain disease is rare, usually presenting as CLL, and it should be managed as such.

V. Amyloidosis. Only primary amyloidosis with or without associated plasma cell or lymphoid neoplasms is considered in this section. With these disorders the amyloid substance consists of fragments of immunoglobulin light chains and is therefore termed an *amyloid L chain protein* (AL-protein). This type of amyloid characteristically infiltrates the tongue, heart, skin, ligaments, and muscle and occasionally the kidney, liver, and spleen. In patients with documented lymphomas or plasma cell neoplasms, treatment is for the underlying neoplasm, but the decline in the amount of amyloid is often minimal. With primary amyloidosis without a demonstrable underlying neoplasm, treatment with MP has been shown to be of moderate benefit when tested in a randomized double-blind study, although the exact role of chemotherapy for this disease is not yet clear.

VI. Monoclonal gammopathy of undetermined significance has been found in up to 3% of persons over 70 years of age. It has been termed *benign monoclonal gammopathy*; however, because approximately 20% of patients with this finding progress to more severe plasma cell dyscrasias, the term *monoclonal gammopathy of undetermined significance* has been introduced as more appropriate. With this condition, patients usually have an M spike of less than 2.0 gm/dl, no bone lesions, no conclusive evidence of myeloma on bone marrow aspirate or biopsy, no anemia or bone marrow failure, and stability of the clinical picture and M protein studies over a period of follow-up. The serum β-2 microglobulin and the plasma cell labeling index are both low. Once initial stability has been demonstrated, these patients should be followed at yearly intervals with evaluation of hemoglobin levels and M protein status. No treatment is indicated unless progression to myeloma or symptomatic macroglobulinemia occurs.

Selected Reading

Barlogie, B., et al. Plasma cell myeloma: New biological insights and advances in therapy. *Blood* 73:865, 1989.

Barlogie, B., Smith, L., and Alexanian, R. Effective treatment of advanced multiple myeloma refractory to alkylating agents. *N. Engl. J. Med.* 310:1353, 1984.

Case, D. C., Lee, B. J., and Clarkson, B. D. Improved survival times in multiple myeloma treated with melphalan, prednisone, cyclophosphamide, vincristine and BCNU: M-2 protocol. *Am. J. Med.* 68:897, 1977.

Costanzi, J. J., et al. Phase II study of recombinant alpha-2 interferon in resistant multiple myeloma. *J. Clin. Oncol.* 3:654, 1985.

Durie, B. G. M., and Salmon, S. E. A clinical staging system for multiple myeloma: correlation of measured myeloma cell mass with presenting clinical features, response to treatment and survival. *Cancer* 36:842, 1975.

Durie, B. G. M., Salmon, S. E., and Moon, T. E. Pretreatment tumor mass, cell kinetics and prognosis in multiple myeloma. *Blood* 55:364, 1980.

Greipp, P. R., et al. Value of beta-2 microglobulin level and plasma cell labeling indices as prognostic factors in patients with newly diagnosed myeloma. *Blood* 72:219, 1988.

Kyle, R. A., and Lust, J. A. Monoclonal gammopathies of undetermined significance. *Semin. Hematol.* 26:176, 1989.

Lenhard, R. E., et al. High-dose cyclophosphamide: an effective treatment for advanced refractory multiple myeloma. *Cancer* 53:1456, 1984.

Mandelli, F., et al. Maintenance treatment with recombinant interferon alfa-2b in patients with multiple myeloma responding to conventional induction chemotherapy. *N. Engl. J. Med.* 322:1430, 1990.

Oken, M. M. Multiple myeloma. *Med. Clin. North Am.* 68:757, 1984.

Metastatic Cancer of Unknown Origin

Martin M. Oken

In approximately 5 percent of patients with newly diagnosed cancer (excluding nonmelanoma skin cancer), the primary site remains unknown despite a detailed history and
physical examination, routine blood chemistries, complete
blood count, urinalysis, chest x-ray film, and histologic
evaluation of the biopsy. The problem of metastatic cancer
of unknown origin raises difficult questions for both diagnosis and treatment. While the median survival of patients
with cancer of unknown origin is less than 6 months,
subgroups of patients have been defined who have a far better outlook with proper management. A major responsibility of the clinician is to identify those patients who might
benefit from active intervention while not consuming the
remaining days of the other patients with futile or unnecessary diagnostic procedures.

I. General considerations and aims of therapy
  A. Histology and presenting clinical manifestations.
     Adenocarcinoma and undifferentiated carcinoma each
     comprise up to 40% of all cancers of unknown origin.
     Fewer than 15% of cancers of unknown origin are squa-
     mous cell carcinomas, and only 2–5% are malignant mel-
     anoma. Other histologies that may present as cancer of
     unknown origin include lymphomas, germ cell tumors,
     and neuroendocrine carcinomas. These histologies are
     particularly important to identify because they repre-
     sent tumors that may be effectively managed with sys-
     temic chemotherapy. Nearly 50% of all patients with un-
     known primaries and well over 50% of those with
     adenocarcinoma present with hepatomegaly, abdominal
     mass, or other abdominal symptoms. Lymphadenopathy
     is the presenting clinical manifestation in 15–25% of pa-
     tients. Lower cervical or supraclavicular lymph nodes
     usually contain adenocarcinoma or undifferentiated
     carcinoma, and middle to high cervical adenopathy gen-
     erally represents squamous cell carcinoma (SCC).
     Between 10% and 20% of patients present with manifes-
     tations of bone, lung, or pleural involvement, whereas
     fewer than 10% present with evidence of central nervous
     system (CNS) disease. Most of the latter group are even-
     tually found to have either lung or gastrointestinal tract
     primaries.

     Two presentations of advanced carcinoma of unknown
     primary site have been recognized as more treatable
     than others: (1) poorly differentiated carcinoma with
     predominant sites of involvement in the mediastinum,
     retroperitoneum, lymph nodes, or lungs; and (2) adeno-
     carcinoma in women predominantly involving the peri-
     toneal surfaces. In these instances, platinum-based che-
     motherapy regimens designed for germ cell or ovarian

cancers, respectively, have produced many useful objective responses and occasional long-term disease-free survival.

B. Sites of origin. It is sometimes possible to predict the most likely primary sites from the histology and location of the metastatic lesion of unknown origin. Pancreas and lung are the most common ultimately determined sites of origin. Together they represent over 40% of the adenocarcinomas of unknown origin. Colorectal, gastric, and hepatobiliary carcinoma each represents about 10% of the cancers of unknown origin.

In general, adenocarcinomas or undifferentiated carcinomas presenting with hepatic metastases or left supraclavicular adenopathy are eventually demonstrated to be of gastrointestinal origin. SCCs that present in the supraclavicular or low cervical lymph nodes are usually from lung primaries, whereas similar lesions of higher cervical nodes are more likely to have originated from occult primary lesions in the head and neck region.

The pattern of metastatic involvement associated with occult primary tumors differs from that associated with overt primaries. For example, occult lung cancer rarely involves bone, a common site of metastasis from overt lung cancer; however, bone metastases appear to be more common in patients with gastrointestinal cancer who have occult primaries than in those who have overt primaries.

C. Aims of diagnostic evaluation. The first objective in the management of a patient newly diagnosed with cancer of unknown origin is to plan the appropriate diagnostic evaluation. There are three chief aims of this evaluation.

1. Identify a tumor in which cure or effective disease control is possible
2. Determine if the tumor is regionally confined or widely metastatic
3. Identify any complication for which immediate local therapy is indicated

D. Goal of treatment. In patients with tumors for which effective systemic therapy is available and in patients with disease regionally confined to peripheral lymph nodes alone, active management with the goal of prolongation of life through extended disease control or cure should be considered. These patients represent about 25% of patients with occult primaries. For the remaining patients, the chance of prolonging life is unlikely, and treatment should be directed toward palliation of symptoms and preservation of the best possible quality of life. Whether to employ systemic therapy depends largely on the patient's general condition and desire for active therapy.

II. Diagnostic evaluation

A. Analysis of the biopsy specimen. If possible, the pathologist should receive fresh, unfixed material to allow electron microscopy, histochemistry, immunohistology, and hormone receptor studies to be done, if needed, after routine examination. Careful review of the biopsy material should be undertaken to classify the tumor conclusively as SCC, adenocarcinoma, or other identifiable histology. Up to 40% of cancers of unknown origin are undifferentiated or poorly differentiated tumors based on evaluation of hematoxylin and eosin-stained material. Electron microscopy may be useful for the further classification of these tumors through the identification of desmosomes and intercellular bridges (SCC), tight junctions, microvilli, and acinar spaces (adenocarcinoma), premelanosomes (amelanotic melanoma), neurosecretory granules (small cell or neuroendocrine carcinoma), and absence of junctions (lymphoma). Immunohistochemical studies on the tumor may be used to demonstrate the presence of prostatic acid phosphatase or prostate-specific antigen (prostate carcinoma), human chorionic gonadotropin (β-hCG: germ cell tumors), α-fetoprotein (germ cell tumors or hepatocellular carcinoma), or monoclonal immunoglobulin (lymphoma, plasmacytoma). Immunoglobulin or T cell receptor gene rearrangements may be helpful for identifying tumors of lymphoid origin. Undifferentiated carcinomas or adenocarcinomas in women should be evaluated for estrogen and progesterone receptors. Mucin positivity is helpful for eliminating the possibility of renal cell carcinoma.

Clearly, the use of many of these specialized studies must be balanced against their expense. If judiciously applied, they can aid in the identification of some of the undifferentiated or poorly differentiated tumors of unknown origin and help to focus their subsequent diagnostic evaluation and management.

One exception to the policy of seeking a definitive histologic diagnosis as the first step in evaluating a tumor of unknown origin is when the patient presents with a potentially resectable neck mass (other than supraclavicular adenopathy) and no other apparent lesion. In these patients, a head and neck primary should be sought by detailed head and neck examination, x-ray films of the sinuses, and, if necessary, panendoscopy under general anesthesia to include laryngoscopy, bronchoscopy, esophagoscopy, and nasopharyngoscopy with blind biopsy of the base of the tongue, piriform sinuses, nasopharynx, and tonsillary fossae if no gross primary is found. A computed tomography (CT) scan of the head and neck may also be of value. If this workup is negative, biopsy of the neck mass is undertaken. This order of evaluation is chosen so that if a resectable squamous cell head and neck cancer is found, the neck mass can be removed as part of the curative procedure.

B. **Squamous cell carcinoma.** For SCCs with apparent involvement of only one lymph node group, the possibility of long-term survival exists if proper treatment is carried out. The diagnostic evaluation depends on the lymph node region involved. The most common lymph node presentation for SCCs of unknown origin is in the cervical or supraclavicular region. Cervical lymph node metastases above the supraclavicular region usually originate from head and neck primary lesions. The diagnostic approach to these lesions is discussed in **II.A.** Because surgery or irradiation, or both, with curative intent is employed if disease is localized to this region, distant metastases should be ruled out with a bone scan, a chest x-ray film, and in some instances a chest CT scan. SCC of supraclavicular lymph nodes is usually of lung or esophageal origin and seldom represents regionally confined disease. Evaluation is the same as that discussed in the last paragraph in **II.B** for disease that extends beyond regional lymph nodes.

Squamous cell carcinoma in axillary or inguinal lymph nodes is rarely associated with an occult primary. Regional skin and lung should be examined as possible primary sites with axillary disease, whereas the skin, anus, and genitalia should be carefully examined when the presentation is SCC in inguinal nodes.

Squamous cell carcinoma with generalized lymphadenopathy or, more commonly, with disease that extends beyond lymph nodes represents disease that cannot be satisfactorily controlled by present-day techniques. The search for the primary lesions should consist mainly in a chest x-ray film and careful physical examination of the appropriate organs. Serum chemistries including the calcium level should be determined. Further diagnostic studies are needed only if indicated by signs, symptoms, or abnormalities on the initial studies.

C. **Adenocarcinoma and undifferentiated carcinoma.** Women with adenocarcinoma or undifferentiated carcinoma of unknown origin should undergo mammography, careful pelvic examination, and hormone receptor evaluation of the tumor. In men, serum acid phosphatase, prostate-specific antigen, β-hCG, and α-fetoprotein should be determined to help rule out prostate and germ cell tumors, respectively. All patients should have stools and urine examined for occult blood, and the serum should be tested for abnormalities in the liver chemistries, creatinine, and electrolytes. With disease apparently confined to axillary lymph nodes, mammography is particularly important in women and should be considered in some men as well. Undifferentiated carcinoma found only in mid to high cervical lymph nodes should be evaluated in the same manner as described in **II.B** for cervical SCC.

Traditional contrast studies, such as intravenous pyelogram, barium enema, and upper gastrointestinal series, are not indicated unless specifically suggested by signs or symptoms (e.g., occult blood in the stool). Abdominal CT scan with intravenous contrast is a reasonable option in view of the frequency with which it detects carcinoma of the pancreas or hepatobiliary cancer in this setting.

D. **Malignant melanoma.** The finding of malignant melanoma confined to a single lymph node group and without a detectable primary lesion represents stage II disease and is associated with a 30% five-year survival following lymphadenectomy. Evaluation to exclude more extensive disease should include a history, physical examination (emphasizing skin and ophthalmoscopic examination), chest x-ray film, liver chemistries, liver scan, and brain CT scan.

III. Treatment

A. General strategy. The importance of identifying tumors that may be treated effectively, such as lymphomas, germ cell tumors, trophoblastic tumors, and breast, prostate, ovarian, and neuroendocrine carcinomas, is readily apparent. Once identified, these lesions should be treated as described in their respective chapters. In patients whose primary lesion remains obscure, a therapeutic distinction must be made between those with disease confined to one lymph node region and those with more widespread disease or involvement of visceral organs. In the former, some may be treated with curative intent, whereas in the latter the aims of treatment are palliative.

B. Squamous cell carcinoma. Patients with SCC confined to cervical lymph nodes above the supraclavicular region should receive full-course radiotherapy to fields extending from the base of the skull to the clavicles. Alternatively, they may be treated with radical lymph node dissection followed by radiation therapy. In either case, the irradiation is designed to include any possible head and neck primary carcinoma. Survival of patients so treated is at least as good as that for patients with known head and neck primaries. More limited lymph node dissection or regional irradiation may also be indicated for SCC confined to axillary or inguinal nodes.

More widespread SCCs of unknown origin are treated with palliative intent. No treatment except for local radiotherapy to symptomatic lesions is the standard approach. In patients who are symptomatic or who have progressive disease and desire chemotherapy, regimens designed mainly for head and neck cancer should be considered.

1. MBP

Methotrexate 40 mg/m^2 IM on days 1 and 15 *and*
Bleomycin 10 units IM on days 1, 8, 15 *and*
Cisplatin 50 mg/m^2 IV on day 4
Repeat every 3 weeks.

2. DF

Cisplatin 100 mg/m^2 IV on day 1 *and*
Fluorouracil 1000 mg/m^2 as a continuous 24-hour IV
   infusion for 4 days (days 1–4)
Repeat every 3 weeks.

Do not use these regimens if the serum creatinine level is more than 1.5 mg/dl. Bleomycin cumulative dose should not exceed 300 units. Use proper hydration with cisplatin as described in Chapter 8, section III.

C. **Adenocarcinoma and undifferentiated carcinoma.** In women, if these carcinomas are confined to unilateral axillary lymph nodes, they should be considered possible breast cancer and treated accordingly as stage II disease (see Chap. 13). A woman with adenocarcinoma or poorly differentiated carcinoma predominantly confined to the peritoneal surface should be considered for a cisplatin-based ovarian cancer regimen. Undifferentiated carcinoma confined to middle or high cervical lymph nodes should be treated actively as SCC (see **III.B**). Patients with more advanced adenocarcinoma or undifferentiated carcinoma in whom the evaluation previously described in **II.C** does not suggest breast, prostate, or other highly treatable primary should be managed palliatively with local radiotherapy given as needed for symptomatic lesions. For patients in whom symptomatic or progressive disease suggests the need for systemic chemotherapy, the DM regimen may produce partial responses in about one-third of patients.

Doxorubicin (Adriamycin) 50 mg/m^2 IV on days 1 and 22
and
Mitomycin 20 mg/m^2 IV on day 1
Repeat every 42 days.

This regimen is worthy of consideration in patients with good performance status, as occasional durable responses have occurred. Responding patients show improvement within two cycles, and chemotherapy should be stopped after two cycles if no improvement is seen. Do not exceed a cumulative doxorubicin dosage of 540 mg/m^2.

Patients with poorly differentiated or undifferentiated tumors predominantly of lymph nodes or midline structures (e.g., mediastinum, retroperitoneum, or lung) may benefit from chemotherapy with a cisplatin-containing germ cell regimen as described in Chapter 15. Complete responses in more than 20% and long-term disease-free survival in 13% have been described.

Women with adenocarcinoma predominantly involving the peritoneal surface should be considered for treatment with a cisplatin-based ovarian cancer regimen.

D. **Malignant melanoma.** For disease confined to a single lymph node group, radical lymph node dissection yields long-term survival in 30% of treated patients. Treatment of disseminated melanoma is discussed in Chapter 17.

Selected Reading

Altman, E., and Cadman, E. An analysis of 1539 patients with cancer of unknown primary site. *Cancer* 57:120, 1986.

Greco, F. A., Vaughn, W. K., and Hainsworth, J. D. Advanced poorly differentiated carcinoma of unknown primary site: recognition of a treatable syndrome. *Ann. Intern. Med.* 104:547, 1986.

Hainsworth, J. D., Dial, T. W., and Greco, F. A. Curative combination chemotherapy for patients with advanced poorly differentiated carcinoma of unknown primary site. *Am. J. Clin. Oncol.* 11:138, 1988.

Levine, M. N., Drummond, M. F., and Labelle, R. J. Cost effectiveness in the diagnosis and treatment of carcinoma of unknown primary origin. *Can. Med. Assoc. J.* 133:977, 1985.

McMillan, J. H., Levine, E., and Stephens, R. H. Computer tomography in the evaluation of metastatic adenocarcinoma from an unknown primary site. *Radiology* 143:143, 1982.

Moertel, C. G. Adenocarcinoma of unknown origin. *Ann. Intern. Med.* 91:646, 1979.

Neumann, K. H., and Nystrom, J. S. Metastatic cancer of unknown origin: nonsquamous cell type. *Semin. Oncol.* 9:427, 1982.

Silverman, C., and Marks, J. E. Metastatic cancer of unknown origin: epidermoid and undifferentiated carcinomas. *Semin. Oncol.* 9:435, 1982.

Stewart, J. F., et al. Unknown primary adenocarcinoma: incidence of overinvestigation and natural history. *Br. Med. J.* 1:1530, 1979.

Strnad, C. M., et al. Peritoneal carcinomatosis of unknown primary site in women: a distinctive subset of adenocarcinoma. *Ann. Intern. Med.* 111:213, 1989.

Woods, R. L., et al. Metastatic adenocarcinomas of unknown primary site: a randomized study of two combination chemotherapy regimens. *N. Engl. J. Med.* 303:87, 1980.

Acquired Immunodeficiency Syndrome and Related Malignancies

Bahu S. Shaikh

Acquired immunodeficiency syndrome (AIDS) was first recognized in 1981 when the Centers for Disease Control (CDC) reported five cases of *Pneumocystis carinii* pneumonia and 26 cases of Kaposi sarcoma in previously healthy homosexual men. Since then there has been a virtual explosion of knowledge and an epidemic of this disease in the United States. By September 1985 there were more than 13,000 cases of AIDS reported to the CDC; and in 1989 a total of 35,238 new cases of AIDS were reported (14.1/ 100,000 population), a 9% increase from the 32,196 new cases reported in 1988.

The etiologic agents for AIDS is a human T lymphocyte-tropic retrovirus initially named *human T cell lymphotropic virus III (HTLV III)* by Gallo et al. in the United States and lymphadenopathy-associated virus (LAV) by Montagnier et al. in France. This infectious agent is now known by its official designation *human immunodeficiency virus (HIV),* which more closely reflects its associated clinical disorders.

I. **Immunodeficiency and cancer.** A long-standing history of association between immunodeficiency states and human cancer has been noted. "Histiocytic" (large cell) lymphoma is seen in association with certain congenital immunodeficiency states, e.g., Wiskott-Aldrich syndrome. Kaposi sarcoma has been described in patients on immunosuppressive drugs following renal transplantation. There is a characteristic temporal sequence of cancers after transplant. Kaposi sarcoma occurs on the average at 16 months, non-Hodgkin's lymphoma at 30 months, and epithelial cancers at about 5 years. In immunodeficient states, as in the normal host, individual susceptibility to cancer is variable, is poorly defined, and may be related to a complex interplay of factors such as age, sex, genetic factors, diet, hormonal status, immunologic status, preexisting diseases, use of tobacco and alcohol, exposure to radiation or sunlight, occupational exposure, and treatment with carcinogenic drugs or radiotherapy.

The Cincinnati Tumor Registry has analyzed the types of tumor that occur in immunosuppressed transplant patients. The 10 most frequent cancers were skin and lip carcinomas, lymphomas, uterine carcinomas, lung cancer, colorectal cancer, Kaposi sarcoma, breast cancer, kidney cancer, leukemia, and tumors from unknown primary sites.

Nontransplant immunosuppressed patients are also susceptible to the development of certain cancers. In patients who were taking drugs such as cyclophosphamide, azathioprine, and chlorambucil, non-Hodgkin's lymphoma, small cell lung cancer, bladder cancer, liver cancer, and leukemia were seen. The dose and duration of therapy may determine the kind of cancer that may develop in these patients.

AIDS is one of the most crippling diseases that affects the human immune system. Qualitative and quantitative abnormalities of helper/inducer T cells are seen. Functional abnormalities are widespread and involve virtually all limbs of the immune system. As with other immunodeficient states, selected cancers appear with increased frequency in AIDS patients and present special management problems.

II. **AIDS-associated malignancies.** There is a high prevalence of viral infections in patients with AIDS, and many of these viruses are known to be associated with cancers in humans. For example, Epstein-Barr virus (EBV) infects B cells, causing polyclonal B cell proliferation. Normally, this situation is controlled by cytotoxic T cells, viral antibodies, and natural killer cells. In the immunodeficient patient with AIDS, this proliferation remains unchecked. A second cytogenic event may result in a monoclonal growth of these cells leading to a B cell malignancy. Whether any virus leads directly to malignancy in patients with AIDS, however, is unknown. The most common malignancies in patients with AIDS are Kaposi sarcoma and non-Hodgkin's lymphoma.

A. **Kaposi sarcoma associated with AIDS**

1. **Background.** Kaposi sarcoma (KS) was described in 1872 by Moritz Kaposi as an "idiopathic multiple pigmented sarcoma." It was considered a rare dermatologic entity until the discovery of an endemic form of the disease in tropical Africa during the 1960s and its association with immunosuppression following renal transplantation. It has now occurred epidemically in the United States in association with the viral infection that causes a state of immunodeficiency in AIDS patients.

2. **The natural history** of KS associated with AIDS is highly variable. It may remain localized (stage I or II) and indolent for months. Individuals with AIDS-related KS may therefore be asymptomatic for a period of time. It is often aggressive, however, and may disseminate to involve viscera and nodes. Gastrointestinal involvement is fairly common and occurs in about 50% of patients. AIDS-related KS can involve almost any organ in the body. Patients usually succumb to opportunistic infections caused by the worsening underlying immunologic dysfunction.

3. **Classification.** AIDS-related KS has been variously classified. Groopman and Mitsuyasu have proposed the staging criteria shown in Table 27-1.

4. **Association of cytomegalovirus and KS.** There is highly suggestive evidence that cytomegalovirus (CMV) plays an important role in the pathogenesis of KS in patients with AIDS. CMV gene products have been shown in KS; CMV nuclear antigens are present in nuclei of KS cells; and CMV DNA and viral particles are present in KS tumor. It is possible

Table 27-1. Staging classification of Kaposi's sarcoma associated with AIDS

Stage/subtype	Criteria
Stage	
I	Limited cutaneous
II	Disseminated cutaneous
III	Visceral or nodal
IV	Cutaneous plus visceral
Subtype	
A	No symptoms
B	Fevers, night sweats, weight loss, or unexplained diarrhea
C	Opportunistic infection

that CMV reactivation occurs after tumor inception. However, there is further evidence linking CMV to KS in AIDS, including the observations that KS resembles murine sarcoma, which has a viral etiology; CMV infections are common in AIDS and transplant patients; CMV causes profound immunosuppression and is capable of transforming human cell in vitro; and epidemiologic, serologic, and virologic studies link CMV to KS in AIDS.

5. **Treatment of superficial AIDS-related KS.** There is no uniform agreement as to the treatment of choice for early-stage cutaneous AIDS-related KS. Some choose to watch the lesions and treat only when they become symptomatic or have serious cosmetic effect. When treatment is deemed desirable, it may consist in simple excisional surgery or electron beam radiotherapy. This modality is not effective in deep dermal lesions, for which standard supervoltage photon radiotherapy should be chosen because of its deeper penetration. A small number of patients who have failed routine radiotherapy have been treated with hemibody radiotherapy with good regression of lesions and minor hematologic, hepatic, or pulmonary toxicities.

6. **Chemotherapy of late-stage KS associated with AIDS.** Patients with uncontrolled cutaneous AIDS-related KS or those with systemic spread of the disease (stages III and IV) have been treated with chemotherapy consisting in single agents or combination chemotherapy.

Local therapy should be used for patients with limited disease and chemotherapy reserved for those with widespread involvement. Patients with slowly progressive disease are usually treated with single agents, whereas those with advanced or rapidly progressive disease are treated with combination chemotherapy.

7. **Single-agent chemotherapy.** Drugs with activity in AIDS-related KS include vincristine, vinblastine, etoposide (VP-16), cisplatin, bleomycin, and doxorubicin. The single agents of choice in AIDS-related KS are vincristine, vinblastine, and etoposide.

   a. **Vincristine** 2 mg IV weekly for 2–5 weeks is associated with a response rate of 61% and with a 4-month or more median duration of response. Vincristine is preferred in patients who are thrombocytopenic, especially if the thrombocytopenia is of the immune type, as such patients stand a good chance of responding with a significant increase in their platelet counts as well.

   b. **Vinblastine** 4–8 mg IV weekly is more myelosuppressive than vincristine; therefore its dose should be adjusted according to the white blood cell (WBC) count. It occasionally produces a complete response; however, 30% of patients with AIDS-related KS experience a partial remission, and 50% have stabilization of their disease. Patients with anemia, elevated erythrocyte sedimentation rate, or symptoms such as fever, night sweats, or weight loss are less likely to respond. Median duration of response is 3 months or more.

   c. **Etoposide (VP-16)** 150 mg/m^2 IV daily for 3 days every 28 days is active against AIDS-related KS. Complete response rates of up to 30% and partial responses of 46% have been reported. Because etoposide is also myelosuppressive, opportunistic infections may complicate therapy.

8. **Combination chemotherapy.** The preferred regimen for combination chemotherapy is ABV, which consists of doxorubicin (Adriamycin), bleomycin, and vinblastine.

   Doxorubicin 40 mg/m^2 IV on day 1 *and*
   Bleomycin 15 units IV on days 1 and 15 *and*
   Vinblastine 6 mg/m^2 IV on day 1
   This cycle is repeated every 28 days.

   ABV has been reported to produce an overall response rate of 84% (23% complete response and 61% partial response, with a median duration of 8 months). The toxicity of the regimen is higher than with single-agent chemotherapy. The risk of acquiring an opportunistic infection with ABV is 50% versus 12–27% for patients treated with single-agent chemotherapy. This regimen, however, can also be used with success in patients who have failed single-agent chemotherapy. Because of the increased risk of opportunistic infections, other approaches, e.g., correction of the underlying immune dysfunction by the use of immunoregulators and modifiers, have received much attention.

9. **Immunotherapy of KS associated with AIDS.** Immunotherapy of AIDS-related KS is intellectually appealing, as the main underlying derangement of AIDS is itself immunologic.

   a. **Interferon-alpha (IFN-α).** Interest in immunotherapy of AIDS-related KS has centered primarily on the interferons. Various doses and schedules of interferon have been used in the treatment of KS, varying from 1 to 50 × 10^6 units/m^2 daily for 5 days on alternate weeks. Both IM and IV therapy has been used. Overall response rates range from 40% to 66%. Remission is more likely to occur in those patients who have baseline CD4 counts above 200/μl. About 30% of patients with AIDS-related KS experience a complete remission that may last more than 29 weeks. There are few objective data that can be used to recommend one regimen over another, although it has been suggested that a combination of IFN-α and zidovudine may be more effective in producing longer lasting remissions than interferon alone. Patients ought to be entered on study protocols whenever possible.

      (1) **Recommended regimen.** The best responses for interferon alone have been reported with a dose schedule of 20 million units/m^2 IM daily for 4–8 weeks, followed by a maintenance dose of 20 million units/m^2 IM three times a week.

      (2) **Toxicity** is significant and includes chills, fever, fatigue, and asthenia, any of which may be debilitating. Hematologic toxicity consists mainly in moderate leukopenia and thrombocytopenia. Patients experience improved performance status, and the treatment is not associated with an exacerbation of opportunistic infections as is seen with chemotherapy of AIDS-related KS. Immunologic dysfunction, however, is not fully corrected even though partial restoration of some aspects of cell-mediated immune function has been reported.

B. **Non-Hodgkin's lymphoma and AIDS**
   1. **Clinical features.** The non-Hodgkin's lymphoma (NHL) associated with AIDS has some unusual clinical features. It is the second most common malignancy after KS in these patients. It may present with fever, weight loss, or central nervous system (CNS) symptoms; it frequently is found to involve extranodal sites; and histologically it is likely to be a high-grade B cell neoplasm. Primary CNS involvement is common; and the prognosis, even with aggressive therapy, is poor.

   The median age at diagnosis occurs during the late thirties, and more than 60% have a high grade histology. The median survival of patients with high grade lymphomas is about 6 months, whereas those with low grade lymphomas have a median survival of more than 30 months.

The extranodal sites are commonly the CNS, skin, mucous membranes, bowel, lung, liver, and kidney. In patients with CNS presentation, multicentricity is demonstrated in most cases. Clinical and radiologic features are thought to be nonspecific; therefore histologic confirmation is essential. Although such tumors are radiosensitive, the ultimate prognosis is poor.

2. **Therapy of NHL associated with AIDS.** Various regional, intrathecal, and systemic treatment regimens have been used in patients with AIDS-associated NHL. The standard combination therapy with cyclophosphamide, doxorubicin, vincristine, and prednisone (CHOP) has commonly been used, but results have been suboptimal. The rate of durable remissions has not been as good as that seen in patients with *de novo* NHL. Therefore CHOP is not considered the regimen of choice for AIDS-associated high grade NHL. The use of aggressive cytoreductive regimens (including prophylactic craniospinal treatment in patients with high-grade NHL) coupled with immune reconstruction by biologic response modifiers and reversal of cytopenias with the use of hematopoietic growth factors offers some hope of improved survival. Because therapy of AIDS-associated lymphoreticular diseases is still evolving, such patients should be entered in ongoing clinical trials whenever possible.

Overall response rates of 50–70% with 25–65% complete remissions have been reported in various series. Patients given more aggressive therapy have higher response rates than those treated with less aggressive regimens, although complications are great. Patients achieving complete remission have a median survival of 11–20 months depending on the histology. The presence of opportunistic infections, Kaposi sarcoma, or both have a negative impact on the ability to induce a complete remission. Current therapies are not effective in patients with *P. carinii* pneumonia with or without Kaposi sarcoma, as high death rates are seen in such patients. The survival of patients with large noncleaved NHL is better than that of the immunoblastic type of NHL.

C. **Hodgkin's disease and AIDS** is a recognized association. The mean age of such patients is 38 years, and the most common histologic types are nodular sclerosis and mixed cell type. Most patients present with a late stage of the disease. Extranodal sites of presentation are common and the CD4/CD8 ratio is less than 1:1. Patients have been treated with standard combination chemotherapy using MOPP or ABVD. Complete remissions are possible, but most patients die of opportunistic infections.

D. Other cancers in patients with AIDS. Cancers of the mouth, rectum and anus, and hepatomas are also seen in patients with AIDS. The median age of these patients is 25 years younger than non-AIDS patients with such cancers. The cancers may be related to viral infection at these sites. Inflammatory lesions here can be difficult to distinguish from carcinomas; therefore biopsy of all suspicious lesions is recommended.

Selected Reading

Bermudez, M. A., et al. Non-Hodgkin's lymphoma in a population with or at risk for acquired immunodeficiency syndrome: indications for intensive chemotherapy. *Am. J. Med.* 86:71, 1989.

Biggar, R. J. Cancer in acquired immunodeficiency syndrome: an epidemiological assessment. *Semin. Oncol.* 17:251–260, 1990.

Gelmann, E. P., et al. Human lymphoblastoid interferon treatment of Kaposi's sarcoma in the acquired immune deficiency syndrome. *Am. J. Med.* 78:737, 1985.

Groopman, J. E., and Mitsuyasu, R. T. Biology and therapy of Kaposi's sarcoma. *Semin. Oncol.* 11:53, 1984.

Knowles, D. M., et al. Lymphoid neoplasia associated with the acquired immunodeficiency syndrome (AIDS): the New York University Medical Center experience with 105 patients (1981–1986). *Ann. Intern. Med.* 108:744, 1988.

Krown, S. E., et al. Interferon-α with zidovudine: safety, tolerance, and clinical and virologic effects in patients with Kaposi sarcoma associated with the acquired immunodeficiency syndrome (AIDS). *Ann. Intern. Med.* 112:812, 1990.

Lane, C. H., et al. Qualitative analysis of immune function in patients with the acquired immunodeficiency syndrome. *N. Engl. J. Med.* 313:79, 1985.

Laubenstein, L. J., et al. Treatment of epidemic Kaposi's sarcoma with etoposide or a combination of doxorubicin, bleomycin, and vinblastine. *J. Clin. Oncol.* 2:1115, 1984.

Levine, A. M. Non-Hodgkin's lymphomas and other malignancies in the acquired immune deficiency syndrome. *Semin. Oncol.* 14:(suppl. 3):2, 1987.

Penn, I. The occurrence of malignant tumors in immunosuppressed states. *Prog. Allergy* 37:259, 1986.

Rios, A., et al. Treatment of acquired immunodeficiency syndrome-related Kaposi's sarcoma with lymphoblastoid interferon. *J. Clin. Oncol.* 3:506, 1985.

Volberding, P. Therapy of Kaposi's sarcoma in AIDS. *Semin. Oncol.* 11:60, 1984.

Ziegler, J. L., et al. Non-Hodgkin's lymphoma in 90 homosexual men: relation to generalized lymphadenopathy and the acquired immunodeficiency syndrome. *N. Engl. J. Med.* 311:565, 1984.

Selected Aspects of Supportive Care of Patients with Cancer

Endocrine Syndromes

Roberto Franco-Saenz

I. General considerations. The occurrence of endocrine syndromes secondary to the ectopic production of hormones by nonendocrine tumors has been recognized with increasing frequency. Recognition of an endocrine or metabolic manifestation of cancer is most important, as in some patients the effects of the endocrine syndrome are more deleterious to the patient than the neoplasm itself. Study of the responsible hormones and related products has further significance, as it is possible that they have the potential to be used clinically as tumor markers for early detection of tumors, an indication of the response to therapy, or an indication of tumor recurrence.

A. Hormone production and clinical expression. Production of hormone precursors is a common occurrence in malignancy, but the clinical expression of an endocrine syndrome is less common, as it appears to depend on the capability of the neoplasm to release the active hormone from its precursor. Malignant tumors may also produce subunits of the parent hormone that under normal circumstances are not released by themselves. For example, the precursors of adrenocorticotropic hormone (ACTH), calcitonin, and other peptide hormones and their subunits are usually present in all lung tumors regardless of histologic type. However, only a few patients develop clinical or biochemical abnormalities related to ectopic hormone production. The so-called oncofetal proteins, e.g., α-fetoprotein and carcinoembryonic antigen, and the oncoplacental proteins represent another major category of ectopic production of proteins; and although they do not cause specific endocrine syndromes, their production by tumors probably has similar pathogenetic significance.

B. Ectopic hormone production by nonendocrine tumors has been documented by several lines of evidence.

1. Arteriovenous differences in the hormone concentration across a tumor bed
2. High concentrations of hormone precursors in tumor extract
3. Incorporation of radiolabeled amino acid into the hormone by tumors
4. Production of the hormone by tumors grown in tissue culture

Furthermore, correction of the endocrine syndrome has followed total excision of the tumor and recurrence of the syndrome when metastases developed.

C. Mechanism of ectopic hormone production. Data indicate that most normal nonendocrine tissues synthesize and store small quantities of a variety of peptide hormones and their precursors. Moreover, when cancer develops in these tissues, they continue to produce the hormones, often in increased amounts, leading to various humoral syndromes. Therefore the term "ectopic hormone production" may not be accurate.

II. Ectopic Cushing's syndrome (ectopic ACTH/β-LPH)

A. Production of hormones. ACTH-producing tumors have been shown to synthesize and release ACTH, β-lipotropin hormone (β-LPH), and β-endorphin, which are known to originate from a common precursor molecule, *proopiomelanocortin*; γ-LPH, α- and β-melanocyte-stimulating hormone, and corticotropin-like intermediate lobe peptide have also been found in some tumors causing the ectopic ACTH syndrome. In view of these findings, the term *ectopic ACTH/β-LPH* is being used with increasing frequency. Simultaneous production of other unrelated peptide hormones, e.g., vasopressin [antidiuretic hormone (ADH)] and calcitonin, has been reported. Furthermore, production of corticotropin-releasing factor has been documented in several of these neoplasms.

The following tumors are most commonly associated with ectopic Cushing's syndrome.

1. Small cell anaplastic (oat-cell) carcinoma of the lung
2. Thymoma
3. Pancreatic carcinoma (including carcinoid and islet cell tumors)
4. Medullary thyroid carcinoma
5. Pheochromocytoma, neuroblastoma, ganglioma, and paraganglioma
6. Bronchial adenoma and bronchial carcinoid
7. Melanoma
8. Prostatic carcinoma

B. Symptoms and signs. The ectopic ACTH syndrome is more common in men and has a higher frequency in patients over 50 years of age, probably because oat-cell carcinoma of the lung, which is the most common cause of the syndrome, is 10 times more common in men of this age group. Most patients with ectopic ACTH syndrome do not have the characteristic clinical appearance of Cushing's syndrome. The absence of this clinical picture is probably due to the catabolic effects of the neoplasm as well as to the sudden onset and rapidly deteriorating clinical course of patients with these malignant neoplasms. However, when the syndrome is caused by a less malignant or a benign tumor, such as bronchial carcinoid, classic cushingoid features may be found. Anorexia and weight loss, rather than obesity, are common. Hypertension and hyperpigmentation are more common than with other causes of Cushing's syndrome. Severe muscular weakness is one of the most common manifestations of the syndrome. Edema, polyuria, and polydipsia are often seen. The course of patients with ectopic ACTH syndrome is usually more rapid and the prognosis is worse than in patients with similar tumors without the ectopic ACTH syndrome. However, cures have been reported after successful removal of the bronchial carcinoids causing the ectopic ACTH syndrome.

C. **Laboratory findings**
1. **Hypokalemic alkalosis.** Severe, unexplained hypokalemia—with serum potassium levels usually below 3 mEq/liter and metabolic alkalosis with venous bicarbonate frequently more than 30 mEq/liter—is one of the most common findings. *Hypokalemic alkalosis in a patient with cancer in the absence of diuretics should alert the physician to the possibility of ectopic ACTH syndrome.* Severe muscle weakness, hyporeflexia, paresthesias, and muscle paralysis may occur. Cardiac arrhythmias, electrocardiographic (ECG) findings of hypokalemia, and increased sensitivity to the effects of digitalis glycoside may occur.
2. **Hyperglycemia** or abnormal glucose tolerance is common.
3. **Hormone abnormalities.** Plasma cortisol is usually greatly elevated (>40 µg/dl) and lacks diurnal variation. The plasma ACTH level is also high. Free urinary cortisol, 17-hydroxysteroids, and 17-ketosteroids are markedly increased. Typically, patients with ectopic ACTH syndrome caused by bronchogenic carcinoma show lack of suppression of plasma cortisol, plasma ACTH, and urinary free cortisol with high-dose dexamethasone (2 mg dexamethasone q6h for 2 days). In contrast, 20–50% of the patients with this syndrome due to bronchial carcinoids show consistent suppression with 2 mg of dexamethasone.

D. **Treatment**
1. **Primary Tumor.** The therapy of choice for ectopic ACTH syndrome is treatment of the primary tumor by surgery, radiotherapy, or chemotherapy. Unfortunately, as the most common cause of the syndrome is small cell anaplastic carcinoma of the lung, complete removal or permanent eradication of this tumor is seldom possible. Complete removal of less aggressive tumors, e.g., bronchial carcinoids, may result in total cure of the syndrome.
2. **Correction of hypokalemia**
   a. **Oral therapy.** Because of the concomitant alkalosis and hypochloremia, *only potassium chloride supplements should be employed.* The severe potassium depletion may require that potassium 40–100 mEq/day be given. Potassium chloride preparations are available in liquid, powder, and tablet forms. Liquid preparations of potassium chloride are available as 5%, 10%, and 20% solutions that contain 10, 20, and 40 mEq/15 ml (tablespoon), respectively. Nausea, vomiting, and gastrointestinal irritation may be important deterrents for the use of oral potassium supplementation, especially in patients who may be receiving simultaneous chemotherapy. To minimize

this irritation, each 20 mEq of potassium chloride solution should be diluted with at least 2 ounces of water or fruit juice and taken after meals. The powder form of potassium chloride should be diluted in at least 4 ounces of water and taken after meals. The slow-release tablet forms of potassium chloride cause less irritation of the gastrointestinal tract. However, some patients develop intestinal or gastric ulcerations and bleeding. Furthermore, the concentration of potassium chloride in the tablets is too low for it to be an effective treatment.

b. **IV administration.** IV therapy is necessary for severe hypokalemia (serum potassium < 2 mEq/liter), if the patient cannot tolerate oral potassium or when cardiac arrhythmias, extreme muscle weakness, or paralysis is present. Under these conditions, the potassium chloride solution should be dissolved *only* in *normal saline or 0.5 N saline solutions*—not in glucose-containing solutions, as the availability of glucose in nondiabetic patients may cause an intracellular shift of potassium and may aggravate hypokalemia. Potassium chloride solutions at concentrations of no more than 60 mEq/liter should be used, and the rate of IV administration should never exceed 40 mEq/hour. However, if hypokalemia is not severe, more dilute solutions are advisable (20–30 mEq/liter), and slower infusion rates (10–20 mEq/hour) are recommended. The total daily dosage of potassium chloride should not exceed 200 mEq/day. IV potassium therapy should be monitored by frequent determinations of serum potassium, venous bicarbonate, and pH. Also at high infusion rates (30–40 mEq/hour), *continuous monitoring of the ECG is necessary.* Potassium chloride therapy should not be given to anuric or severely oliguric patients. In some patients with tumors producing multiple hormones, e.g., ACTH and antidiuretic hormone (ADH), correction of the hypokalemia may restore ADH sensitivity, and hyponatremia and water intoxication may develop.

c. **Spironolactone** (Aldactone) is a specific pharmacologic antagonist of aldosterone that acts primarily through competitive binding of the mineralocorticoid receptors at the sodium-potassium exchange sites of the distal tubules. Doses of 100–400 mg/day may be necessary to correct hypokalemia. Spironolactone should not be used in conjunction with potassium supplements or other potassium-sparing drugs, as severe hyperkalemia may develop. Spironolactone does not always effectively prevent hypokalemia and metabolic alkalosis in patients with ectopic Cushing's syndrome, but it may be used temporarily until more effective measures are established. Spironolactone should not be used in the presence of severe impairment of renal function or oliguria. The most common side effects include gynecomastia, abdominal cramping, diarrhea, dizziness, lethargy, and confusion.

3. Management of sodium and water retention. In patients with severe hypertension and edema, moderate sodium restriction and diuretics are indicated.

   a. Thiazides are the most commonly used drugs for the treatment of sodium retention and hypertension in patients with ectopic Cushing's syndrome. Hydrochlorothiazide 50 mg bid or long-acting diuretics such as chlorthalidone 50–100 mg/day or metolazone (Zaroxolyn) 2.5–5.0 mg/day are equally effective.

   b. Other diuretics. When severe hypertension with fluid overload and pulmonary congestion is present, more potent diuretics such as furosemide and ethacrynic acid are useful. Furosemide 20–80 mg PO may be used. If a good diuretic response is obtained, the dose may be repeated 6 hours later. If there is no significant response, the dosage of furosemide may be increased by 20–40 mg q6h until the desired diuretic effect has been obtained. Furosemide is the diuretic of choice in patients with renal insufficiency. For more critical situations of pulmonary edema, furosemide should be administered IV (20–40 mg over 1–2 minutes); if necessary, increments of 20 mg can be given q2h. The maximum dosage of furosemide should not exceed 600 mg/24 hours. Caution must be exerted with the use of diuretics for ectopic Cushing's syndrome, as hypokalemia may be aggravated by their use. Careful monitoring of serum potassium and adequate potassium supplementation can prevent this complication.

4. Treatment of metabolic alkalosis. Metabolic alkalosis is the chloride-resistant type and is caused by excess mineralocorticoids. This excess causes intracellular shifts of hydrogen ions and increased hydrogen ion secretion by the renal tubule, and it results in severe alkalosis. Characteristically, urinary chloride levels are less than 15 mEq/liter. Treatment consists in potassium chloride supplement, spironolactone, and, more importantly, correction of the mineralocorticoid excess by the use of inhibitors of adrenal steroid synthesis.

5. Adrenal enzyme inhibitors

   a. Metyrapone (Metopirone)

      (1) Mechanism of action. Metyrapone is a synthetic compound that inhibits adrenal 11β-hydroxylase, causing a rapid reduction of cortisol production.

      (2) Therapeutic use. When used for therapeutic purposes, metyrapone can be used at a dosage of 500 mg PO q4–6h (2–3 gm/day); and according to the clinical response, the dosage may be lowered.

(3) **Effects of therapy.** Although metyrapone rapidly lowers plasma cortisol levels, it does not lower the levels of deoxycorticosterone, which is a powerful mineralocorticoid. In patients with the ectopic ACTH syndrome, the plasma deoxycorticosterone levels are usually 9- to 12-fold higher than normal. Therefore rapid relief of symptoms caused by the excess cortisol is expected after metyrapone treatment, but hypokalemia and metabolic alkalosis may not improve after treatment with metyrapone alone. The most common adverse reactions have been nausea, abdominal discomfort, dizziness, headache, sedation, and allergic reactions.

b. **Aminoglutethimide (Cytadren)** is derived from the hypnotic drug glutethimide, which was formerly used for the treatment of epilepsy. Approximately two-thirds of the patients with ectopic ACTH syndrome treated with aminoglutethimide show clinical as well as biochemical evidence of improvement.

(1) **Mechanism of action.** Aminoglutethimide is a competitive inhibitor of the mitochondrial enzyme cholesterol side-chain-cleaving enzyme, and its primary effect is to inhibit the conversion of cholesterol to pregnenolone. By blocking the conversion of cholesterol to pregnenolone, aminoglutethimide causes a reversible medical adrenalectomy, with marked reduction in the production of adrenal glucocorticoids, mineralocorticoids, androgens, and estrogens.

(2) **Dosage and administration.** The recommended dosage of aminoglutethimide for the treatment of Cushing's syndrome is 1 gm/day in four divided doses. In some patients dosages of 1.5–2.0 gm/day may be necessary.

(3) **Prevention of adrenal insufficiency.** To prevent the development of adrenal insufficiency, glucocorticoids and mineralocorticoid should be replaced. Aminoglutethimide increases the rate of metabolism of hydrocortisone and dexamethasone, and it is necessary to use larger doses of dexamethasone or hydrocortisone than those required for physiologic replacement. Adrenal replacement therapy can be done with one of the following agents.

(a) **Hydrocortisone** 40–60 mg/day (10 mg at 8 A.M., 10 mg at 5 P.M., and 20 mg hs).

(b) **Dexamethasone,** 0.50–0.75 mg qid (2–3 mg/day).

In patients receiving hydrocortisone replacement, the response to aminoglutethimide therapy should be monitored by the plasma levels of dehydroepiandrosterone sulfate. In patients receiving dexamethasone replacement, response to therapy can be monitored by the levels of plasma or urinary cortisol, or both. If hypotension or hyperkalemia develops, the patient should also receive mineralocorticoid replacement therapy with fludrocortisone (Florinef) 0.05–0.10 mg/day. Development of hyponatremia may be another indication of mineralocorticoid deficiency, but the possibility of concomitant production of ADH by the tumor has to be considered.

(4) Side effects. The most common side effects are related to central nervous system (CNS) toxicity and include lethargy, sedation, dizziness, blurred vision, and depression. Morbilliform skin rashes with or without fever may also be seen 9–14 days after the initiation of aminoglutethimide therapy. These rashes may disappear spontaneously with continuation of therapy. CNS symptoms are usually transient and dose-related, and they rarely occur in patients receiving 1 gm/ day. Gastrointestinal symptoms such as anorexia, nausea, and vomiting may also occur.

c. Mitotane (Lysodren, *o,p'*-DDD)

(1) Mechanism of action. Mitotane is an oral chemotherapeutic agent best known by its trivial name *o,p'*-DDD. Mitotane is an adrenal cytotoxic agent, although it can also cause inhibition of steroidogenesis without cellular destruction.

(2) Dosage and administration. Treatment with mitotane should be instituted in the hospital until a stable dosage regimen is achieved. *Signs and symptoms of adrenal insufficiency may develop in patients receiving mitotane.* Therefore adrenal steroid replacement should be started [see **II.D.5.b.(3)**] together with the mitotane, although the effect of the drug on adrenal steroidogenesis is not immediate. Mitotane should be started at dosages of 4–8 gm/day in divided doses either qid or tid. If severe side effects appear, the dosage should be reduced until the maximum tolerated dosage is achieved. If the patient can tolerate higher dosages and if there is a possibility of further clinical improvement, the dosage should be increased until adverse reactions interfere. Maximum tolerated dosages vary from 2 to 16 gm/day. Treatment should be continued as long as clinical benefits are observed. If no clinical benefits are observed after 3 months at the maximum tolerated dose, the drug should be discontinued. Dosages as low as 4 gm/day, when combined with metyrapone (500 mg q4h), have been reported to cause complete remission of hypercorticism in patients with the ectopic ACTH syndrome.

(3) **Side effects.** A high percentage of patients treated with mitotane manifest at least one side effect. Approximately 80% of the patients develop gastrointestinal disturbances, e.g., anorexia, nausea, vomiting, and diarrhea. CNS side effects occur in approximately 40% of patients and consist primarily of depression, lethargy, and less frequently dizziness or vertigo. Dermatologic toxicity occurs in about 15% of patients, but the symptoms usually subside with continuation of treatment. A variety of other side effects have been reported but seem to occur only rarely. The combined administration of metyrapone, aminoglutethimide, and mitotane has been reported to be effective in some patients with ectopic Cushing's syndrome.

d. Ketoconazole (Nizoral)

(1) **Mechanism of action.** Ketoconazole is an imidazole derivative antifungal agent that has been shown to inhibit the production of androgens and adrenal glucocorticoids. Ketoconazole has been used successfully for treatment of patients with Cushing's syndrome of different etiologies including the ectopic Cushing's. Ketoconazole blocks steroidogenesis by inhibiting 11β-hydroxylase as well as both cytochrome P450-dependent mitochondrial enzymes, which function at the site of side chain cleavage. In addition, there is evidence that ketoconazole binds to glucocorticoid receptors acting as a peripheral glucocorticoid antagonist. Ketoconazole has been shown to block the cortisol response to ACTH in healthy men. Furthermore, ketoconazole blocks androgen synthesis by inhibiting the C_{17-20} lyase enzyme.

In several reported cases the drug causes rapid correction of hypercortisolism and in high doses may lead to hypoadrenalism requiring supplemental doses of glucocorticoids.

(2) **Dosage and administration.** Ketoconazole has not been approved for treatment of Cushing's syndrome. The doses employed for treatment of Cushing's syndrome varies

from 200 mg PO twice daily to a total of 1 gm/day in divided doses.

(3) Prevention of adrenal insufficiency. Ketoconazole in high doses may cause adrenal insufficiency, so careful monitoring of the patient for clinical and laboratory signs of adrenal insufficiency is required. To prevent adrenal insufficiency some use hydrocortisone replacement in a schedule similar to that recommended for patients treated with aminoglutethimide. Alternatively, patients may be treated with dexamethasone 1 mg daily PO.

(4) Side effects. Although the drug is well tolerated by most patients, severe hepatotoxicity has been reported in some, including a few fatalities. Therefore patients should be instructed to report any signs or symptoms suggestive of liver disease so that appropriate liver function tests can be obtained. In rare cases anaphylactic reactions have been reported after the first dose. Doses of 800–1600 mg/day cause testosterone deficiency and adrenal insufficiency.

e. RU 486. This experimental drug is a 19-nor-steroid glucocorticoid antagonist. RU 486 has high affinity for the glucocorticoid receptor and no agonistic effects. This medication has been used successfully to treat a patient with Cushing's syndrome secondary to ectopic ACTH secretion. Treatment with this drug produced clinical and biochemical remission of hypercortisolism despite persistently elevated levels of cortisol. The drug was well tolerated, and no side effects were reported; however at high doses it may cause glucocorticoid insufficiency, which may be difficult to recognize as cortisol levels remain elevated or even increase. Lower cost and future increased availability make this drug a promising therapy for the ectopic ACTH syndrome.

III. Hyponatremia and cancer

A. Syndrome of inappropriate secretion of antidiuretic hormone (SIADH) and water intoxication. Another endocrine syndrome that is frequently associated with cancer is *hyponatremia*. Hyponatremia in patients with cancer can be caused by either inappropriate secretion of ADH of central origin or ectopic production of ADH by the tumor. Also, hyponatremia can be caused by several drugs, including some drugs frequently used for cancer chemotherapy. A variety of tumors have been associated with ectopic production of ADH. The material synthesized by neoplasms has been characterized by bioassay, immunoassay, and chromatography and appears to be arginine vasopressin (AVP). Ectopic production of ADH has been reported in approximately 40% of the patients with carcinoma of the lung and carcinoma of the colon without clinical evidence of this syndrome. The most common tumors associated with SIADH are as follows.

1. Small cell anaplastic (oat-cell) and occasionally non-small-cell carcinomas of the lung
2. Carcinoid tumors
3. Pancreatic carcinoma
4. Esophageal carcinoma
5. Prostatic carcinoma
6. Adrenocortical carcinoma
7. Bladder carcinoma
8. Hodgkin's disease
9. Acute myelogenous leukemia

B. Other causes of SIADH and hyponatremia. It is important to distinguish between ectopic production of ADH and other causes of SIADH. Also it is important to eliminate the possibility that the syndrome is caused by drugs that can affect water metabolism. The most common drugs that impair water metabolism and that are associated with hyponatremia are listed in Table 28-1.

C. Spurious hyponatremia and hyperglycemia. It must be recognized that lower than normal levels of serum sodium not always imply hypoosmolarity.

　1. Spurious or artifactual hyponatremia can occur

Table 28-1. Drugs associated with hyponatremia

Drugs	Potentiates renal action of AVP	Potentiates release of AVP
Chlorpropamide (Diabinese)	x	x
Tolbutamide (Orinase)	x	
Clofibrate (Atromid-S)		x
Carbamazepine (Tegretol)		x
Vincristine (Oncovin)		x
Vinblastine (Velban)		x
Cyclophosphamide (Cytoxan)		x
Opiates		x
Histamine		x
Phenformin	x	
Thiazides		x(?)
Nicotine		x
Barbiturates		x(?)
Isoproterenol		x
Thioridazine (Mellaril)*		

Key: AVP = arginine vasopressin.
*Increases thirst

in patients with marked elevation of *serum lipids* or *serum proteins*.

2. **Severe hyperglycemia** is another common situation that can lead to hyponatremia without hypoosmolarity. With this condition the increased osmolarity due to hyperglycemia causes water to be drawn from cells and results in dilution of plasma sodium.

D. **Diagnosis of SIADH.** In the absence of direct and clinically applicable measurements of ADH, the important criteria for the diagnosis of SIADH are the following.

1. Hyponatremia with hypoosmolarity of the serum
2. Inappropriate antidiuresis (urine osmolarity that is higher than that expected for the degree of hyponatremia and hypoosmolarity of the serum)
3. Normal renal, adrenal, thyroid, and pituitary function
4. Evidence of sodium wasting in the urine (urine sodium commonly > 20–40 mEq/liter)
5. Absence of clinical signs of hypovolemia and dehydration
6. Absence of generalized edema or ascites
7. Correction of the hyponatremia and hypoosmolarity of the plasma by severe fluid restriction

Patients with mild SIADH may be asymptomatic. However, when the serum sodium levels fall to the range of 120–125 mEq/liter, loss of memory, apathy, and impairment of abstract thought may occur. When serum sodium levels fall below 115 mEq/liter, extrapyramidal signs, asterixis, convulsions, and coma may occur. Serum sodium levels below 115 mEq/liter indicate severe water intoxication and constitute a medical emergency.

E. **Treatment of SIADH.** Successful treatment of the tumor usually corrects SIADH, and reappearance of the syndrome is seen with recurrence of the tumor.

1. **Fluid restriction.** For mildly symptomatic patients or patients whose serum sodium has fallen below 125 mEq/liter, fluid restriction is necessary. In these patients the major source of water loss is insensible. Therefore to effectively raise the serum sodium concentration, fluid restriction to 500 ml/day or less is necessary in some patients. Once the serum sodium returns to normal, fluid administration should be increased to replace sensible and insensible losses plus the urine output. Unfortunately, because of the continuous production of ADH by tumors, this approach alone is often impractical and unsuccessful.

2. **Demeclocycline (Declomycin)** antagonizes the renal actions of AVP and therefore causes a reversible, dose-dependent nephrogenic diabetes insipidus. Demeclocycline, in divided doses of 600–1200 mg/day and combined with moderate water restriction, has been highly successful in treating chronic SIADH associated with tumors. The most common side effects of this drug have been anorexia, nausea, and vomiting. Skin rashes and hypersensitivity to

ultraviolet light are also common. Because of the antianabolic effect of the tetracyclines, this drug may cause a rise in blood urea nitrogen (BUN). Also, when combined with fluid restriction, it may lead to sodium depletion and dehydration.

3. **Lithium carbonate** has also been used for the treatment of chronic tumor-associated SIADH, but it is more toxic and inferior to demeclocycline.

4. **Phenytoin** inhibits the release of ADH from the pituitary gland. At dosages of 100 mg tid, phenytoin has been successful in the treatment of SIADH of CNS origin. However, this drug is not effective for the treatment of SIADH caused by ectopic production of ADH by tumors.

5. **Hypertonic sodium chloride.** For the treatment of severe hyponatremia and water intoxication (serum sodium < 115 mEq/liter associated with confusion, stupor, convulsions, and muscle twitching), therapy should be aimed at reversing the flow of water into the cells. Such therapy may require the administration of small amounts of hypertonic sodium chloride: 3% sodium chloride (513 mEq/liter) or 5% sodium chloride (855 mEq/liter). The quantity of hypertonic sodium chloride should not exceed the amount required to raise the concentration of serum sodium one-half the distance to normality within 8 hours. It is unnecessary to correct serum sodium to normal levels within the initial 12–24 hours. The amount of sodium necessary to accomplish the desired correction can be estimated by the following formula.

Sodium for replacement (mEq) = [desired serum sodium (mEq/liter) − observed serum sodium (mEq/liter)] × body weight (kg) × 0.6

Use of hypertonic sodium chloride is potentially dangerous and may result in fluid and circulatory overload, especially in elderly patients. To prevent these complications, IV furosemide can be added to the regimen. Alternatively, furosemide (1 mg/kg IV) as initial therapy followed by hourly replacement of the urinary losses of sodium and potassium with 3% sodium chloride with potassium chloride added to it can correct severe hyponatremia within 6–8 hours. This approach requires careful monitoring of fluid and electrolyte balance and ready access to the laboratory, as hourly measurements of sodium and potassium in the urine are required. *Rapid correction of hyponatremia may lead to neurologic damage due to central pontine myelinolysis and should therefore be avoided.*

IV. **Hypercalcemia**

A. **Causes** of tumor hypercalcemia are in Table 28-2.

1. **Associated tumors.** Hypercalcemia is relatively common in patients with malignancy. In fact, in one study it was shown that the most common cause of hypercalcemia in hospitalized patients is malignancy. Hypercalcemia of malignancy can be associ-

Table 28-2. Factors responsible for hypercalcemia of malignancy

Direct resorption of bone by tumor cells

Production of PTH-related peptide (PTHrP)

Production of osteoclast-activating factors (OAFs)
Interleukin 1
Tumor necrosis factor (TNF-α)
Lymphotoxin (TNF-β)
Colony stimulating factor
Interferon-γ

Production of 1,25-dihydroxyvitamin D

Production of prostaglandins (PGE_2)

Production of transforming growth factors (TGF)
TGF-α
TGF-β

Coexistence of tumor with primary hyperparathyroidism or
other cause of hypercalcemia (e.g., vitamin D intoxication,
sarcoidosis)

ated with bone metastasis, or it may occur in the absence of any direct bone involvement by the tumor. Based on the findings of a study on 433 patients with hypercalcemia of cancer, 86% of the patients had identifiable bone metastasis. More than one-half ($n = 225$) of the cases were accounted for by patients with breast carcinoma, and cancer of the lung and kidneys accounted for a smaller proportion. Patients with hematologic malignancies accounted for approximately 15% of the cases. These patients usually had hypercalcemia in the presence of diffuse tumor involvement of bone, although in a small percentage there was no evidence of bone involvement.

2. **Humoral mediators.** In approximately 10% of the cases of malignancy, hypercalcemia develops in the absence of radiographic or scintigraphic evidence of bone involvement. In this group of patients, the pathogenesis of hypercalcemia appears to be secondary to humoral mediators.

Although for years it was thought that humoral hypercalcemia of malignancy was associated with increased production of parathyroid hormone (PTH), it has been shown that PTH levels are normal or low in patients with hypercalcemia of malignancy and that nonendocrine tumors associated with hypercalcemia do not contain PTH mRNA. On the other hand, a PTH-related peptide (PTHrP) has been extracted and purified from a large number of nonparathyroid tumors associated with the syndrome of humoral hypercalcemia of cancer.

a. **PTHrP.** In 1987 a parathyroid-like humoral factor was isolated from lung and renal carcinomas. The gene for PTHrP is located on the short arm of chromosome 12, and the cDNA has been cloned and sequenced. The amino-terminal region of the PTHrP shares a similar amino acid sequence (8 of 13 amino acids) with PTH. Beyond amino acid 13, the sequence of the two peptides is completely different. Alternative splicing of the gene leads to three related peptides with lengths of 139, 141, and 173 amino acids, respectively.

The biologic activity of the molecule resides in the initial N-terminal 34 amino acids. The peptide interacts with the PTH receptor and stimulates cyclic adenosine monophosphate (cAMP) production and bone resorption, and when injected into animals it causes hypercalcemia.

The peptide has been measured by radioimmunoassay using two antibodies directed against the N-terminal 1-70 and the C-terminal 109-138 regions. These studies suggest that the PTHrP does not circulate in its intact form in the plasma, and that the C-terminal 109-139 fragment circulates as a separate peptide. Normal individuals have low or undetectable levels of the N-terminal fragment and undetectable C-terminal peptide. In 30 patients with humoral hypercalcemia of cancer, the plasma levels of the two fragments of PTHrP were 10-fold higher than normal. In some patients the concentration decreased after the tumor was resected. Patients with renal failure have marked elevations of the C-terminal peptide but normal N-terminal peptide. Patients with hyperparathyroidism and hypercalcemia from other causes had normal levels of PTHrP. The peptide has been found in a number of normal tissues, including skin keratinocytes, CNS tissue, placenta, and lactating mammary tissue, and is present in high concentrations in human milk (10,000 times higher than normal plasma), suggesting that the peptide may have a still unknown physiologic role in calcium homeostasis.

b. **Osteoclast activating factors.** A number of cytokines with potent bone-resorbing activities have been identified. These cytokines may account for the previously designated osteoclast-activating factor (OAF). Interleukin-1 (IL-1) produced by monocytes has potent bone-resorbing activity in vitro. Tumor necrosis factor (TNF-α) also produced by monocytes, and lymphotoxin or tumor necrosis factor-beta (TNF-β), produced by lymphocytes, have potent bone-resorbing properties. Lymphotoxin plays an important role in the pathogenesis of bone destruction and hypercalcemia of multiple myeloma. Adult T cell lymphomas are frequently associated with hypercalcemia, and this tumor produces several bone resorbing factors, including lymphotoxin, colony stimulating factor, and interferon-gamma.

    c. Production of 1,25-dihydroxyvitamin D. Hypercalcemia with increased serum calcitriol (1,25-dihydroxyvitamin D) levels in patients with malignant lymphomas was first reported in 1984. Since then this observation has been confirmed, and elevated levels of 1,25-dihydroxyvitamin D have been reported in patients with other tumors associated with hypercalcemia such as leiomyoblastomas, Hodgkin's disease, and a large plasma cell granuloma.

    d. Production of prostaglandins (PGs). There is convincing experimental and clinical evidence indicating that PGs play a role in the hypercalcemia of malignancy. PGs are potent stimulators of bone resorption. There are some reports of metastatic renal cell carcinomas in which high concentrations of PGE_2 have been found in the tumor or its metastases and in which hypercalcemia responded to indomethacin. Also, the urinary metabolite of PGE_2 has been found to be elevated in a number of patients with hypercalcemia associated with solid tumors, primarily bronchogenic carcinoma, and suppression of the PGE_2 metabolite levels and normalization of the serum calcium have been seen after treatment with indomethacin or aspirin in some patients. However, the prostaglandin metabolite has weak bone-resorbing activity, and the concentrations found in the blood are insufficient to account for the hypercalcemia. Therefore it appears that prostaglandins may play a role, primarily as local mediators in the pathogenesis of hypercalcemia of cancer.

    e. Transforming growth factors. Transforming growth factors are small peptides characterized by their ability to stimulate cell growth and replication. Transforming growth factor-alpha (TGF-α) is a 5000-dalton peptide, and transforming growth factor-beta (TGF-β) is a homodimer protein with a molecular weight of 24,000 daltons. Both peptides have in vitro bone-resorbing activities more potent than those of PTH. These peptides are produced by many solid tumors and have been implicated in the humoral hypercalcemia of malignancy.

B. Symptoms, signs, and laboratory findings. Hypercalcemia often produces symptoms in patients with cancer and, in fact, may be the patients' major problem. Polyuria and nocturia, resulting from the impaired ability of the kidneys to concentrate the urine, occur early. Anorexia, nausea, constipation, muscle weakness, and fatigue are common. As the hypercalcemia progresses, severe dehydration, azotemia, mental obtundation, coma, and cardiovascular collapse may appear. In addition to hypercalcemia, the laboratory studies may reveal hypokalemia and increased BUN and creatinine levels.

Patients with hypercalcemia of malignancy frequently have hypochloremic metabolic alkalosis, whereas with primary hyperparathyroidism metabolic acidosis is more common. The concentration of serum phosphorus is variable. PTH levels may be normal, low, or high; but marked elevations are rarely seen. Bone involvement is best evaluated by a bone scan, which is often positive in the absence of radiographic evidence of bone involvement.

C. **Treatment.** The management of hypercalcemia of malignancy has two objectives: (1) reducing elevated levels of serum calcium; and (2) treating the underlying cause. When hypercalcemia is mild to moderate (serum calcium < 12–13 mg/dl) and the patient is not symptomatic, adequate hydration and measures directed against the tumor (e.g., surgery, chemotherapy, or radiation therapy) may suffice. Severe hypercalcemia, on the other hand, is a life-threatening condition that requires emergency treatment. Therefore for more severe degrees of hypercalcemia other measures must be taken, including enhancement of calcium excretion by the kidney in patients with adequate renal function.

1. **Saline diuresis.** Sodium competitively inhibits the tubular resorption of calcium. Therefore IV infusion of saline causes a significant increase in calcium clearance. Because of the large amounts of saline that may be required to correct hypercalcemia, it is advisable to monitor the central venous pressure continuously. The infusion of normal saline (0.9% sodium chloride) at a rate of 250–500 ml/hour, accompanied by IV administration of furosemide 20–80 mg q2–4h, results in significant calcium diuresis and lowering of the serum calcium in most patients. This type of therapy requires *strict* monitoring of cardiopulmonary status to avoid fluid overload and electrolyte imbalance. Also, it requires ready access to the laboratory, as the urinary losses of sodium, potassium, magnesium, and water must be replaced to maintain metabolic balance. In many cases, saline infusions at rates of 125–150 ml/hour plus the addition of furosemide 40–80 mg IV once or twice a day may significantly reduce the serum calcium until other measures aimed at inhibiting bone resorption take effect.

2. **Glucocorticoids.** Large initial doses of hydrocortisone 250–500 mg IV q8h (or its equivalent) can be effective in the treatment of hypercalcemia associated with lymphoproliferative diseases, e.g., non-Hodgkin's lymphoma and multiple myeloma, and in patients with breast cancer metastatic to bone. It may take several days for glucocorticoids to lower the serum calcium level. Maintenance therapy should be started with prednisone 10–30 mg/day PO. The mechanisms by which glucocorticoids lower the serum calcium are multiple.

1. Inhibition of OAFs
2. Inhibition of phospholipase A_2, thereby blocking PG synthesis
3. Reduction of the rate of bone turnover
4. Reduction of the rate of intestinal absorption of calcium
5. Reduction of the rate of renal tubular resorption of calcium

3. Calcitonin (Calcimar) is a peptide hormone that inhibits osteocytic and osteoclastic bone resorption. Salmon calcitonin, when given by infusion, causes a modest reduction of serum calcium levels, usually by 1–3 mg/dl, which commonly reverses after discontinuation of therapy. To avoid anaphylactic reactions, skin testing should be performed prior to the administration of calcitonin. To avoid inconsistencies in the response, it is recommended that albumin (approximately 5 gm) be added to the infusion to coat the infusion set and prevent absorption of the peptides to the walls of the set. The usual initial dose of calcitonin is 50–100 International Units (I.U.) IV followed by 4–8 I.U./kg SQ or IM q12–24h according to the serum calcium levels. In patients who develop resistance to salmon calcitonin, human calcitonin may be tried.

Nausea with or without vomiting has been noted in approximately 10% of the patients treated with calcitonin. It is more common at the beginning of the treatment and usually subsides with continuous administration. Local inflammatory reactions at the site of SQ or IM injections have been reported in about 10% of the patients. Skin rashes and flushing occur occasionally.

4. Disodium etidronate (Didronel)
   a. Mechanism of action. Didronel is the only diphosphonate available for clinical use in the United States. The diphosphonates or bisphosphonates are analogs of pyrophosphate in which the oxygen in the backbone of pyrophosphate (P–O–P) is replaced by a carbon (P–C–P), rendering the molecule resistant to degradation by phosphatases. The diphosphonates are potent inhibitors of normal and abnormal bone resorption and inhibit bone formation. They bind to the surface of calcium phosphate crystals and inhibit crystal growth and dissolution. In addition, they may directly inhibit osteoclast resorptive activity. Oral etidronate has been used for the treatment of Paget's disease of bone for many years. However, the intravenous preparation was only recently made available for treatment of hypercalcemia of malignancy. In several clinical studies intravenous Didronel therapy has been shown to be effective and well tolerated for the treatment of hypercalcemia of malignancy. In one clinical study with 26

patients with hypercalcemia of malignancy, intravenous Didronel had a beneficial effect in more than 90% of the patients, and complete normalization of serum calcium was seen in 19 patients (73%). Also, in a large multicenter double-blind placebo-controlled trial sponsored by the manufacturer, normalization of serum calcium was attained within 1 week in 72 of 114 Didronel-treated patients (63%) compared with only 14 of 43 patients (33%) in the placebo group. Intravenous etidronate at a dose of 7.5 mg/kg for 3–7 days usually leads to normalization of the serum calcium after 4–7 days. The serum calcium level may continue to fall for several days after discontinuation of therapy and may remain normal for up to 2 weeks. Oral etidronate has been reported to maintain the hypocalcemic response and to prevent recurrence of hypercalcemia in some trials but not in others.

Second generation bisphosphonates, in particular 3-amino-1,hydroxypropylidene-1,1-bisphosphonic acid (AHP,BP), are more potent inhibitors of bone resorption and are the most effective agents for the treatment of hypercalcemia of malignancy. AHP,BP is currently undergoing clinical trials in the United States. Administration of 30–60 mg IV or 1200 mg PO for 6 days causes normalization of the serum calcium in most patients after 4–9 days. The drug appears to be well tolerated and, when clinically available, probably will become the treatment of choice for hypercalcemia of malignancy.

A potentially important use of diphosphonates is for preventing bone metastasis. Experimental evidence shows that etidronate prevented bone metastases after intraarterial inoculation of tumor into rats. Also there is preliminary clinical evidence suggesting a decrease in bone metastasis in breast cancer patients treated with bisphosphonates.

b. **Dosage and administration.** The recommended dose of didronel is 7.5 mg/kg body weight diluted in at least 250 ml of normal saline and administered IV over a period of at least 2 hours every day. It is of great importance that the infusion be given slowly to minimize complications. The usual course of treatment is one infusion a day for 3 days, but some patients have been treated for up to 7 days. However, hypocalcemia may occur after prolonged treatment.

c. **Side effects.** Loss of taste or a metallic taste has been reported that usually disappears within hours. In approximately 10% of patients transient, mild elevations of the BUN and creatinine may be observed. In the presence of preexistent renal impairment, the dose should be reduced and renal function monitored frequently.

5. **Mithramycin (Mithracin)** is a potent antineoplastic agent that was formerly used for the treatment of some malignant tumors of the testes. Mithramycin inhibits bone resorption and causes hypocalcemia. Mithramycin at dosages of $0.6-1.0$ mg/m^2 given by IV push as a single bolus usually causes a significant fall in serum calcium within 12 hours, and the effect may last $3-7$ days. Additional doses may be administered at intervals of $3-4$ days to maintain the serum calcium below $12-13$ mg/dl. Mithramycin should generally be used only for the treatment of hypercalcemia of malignancy that has been refractory to other modalities of therapy.

The most common side effects reported with the use of mithramycin are gastrointestinal symptoms of anorexia, nausea, vomiting, diarrhea, and stomatitis. Other less frequent side effects include fever, drowsiness, weakness, lethargy, malaise, facial flushing, and skin rash. The most important form of toxicity associated with the use of mithramycin consists in a bleeding syndrome that usually begins with an episode of epistaxis. This syndrome appears to be dose-related and is rarely seen at the dosages used for the treatment of hypercalcemia.

6. **Oral phosphate supplements (Neutra-Phos or Fleet Phospho-Soda).** Oral phosphate therapy is a useful adjunct for the treatment of hypercalcemia of malignancy. Oral phosphate decreases the intestinal absorption of calcium and enhances the deposition of insoluble calcium salts in bone and tissue. Oral phosphate supplements at dosages of $1.5-3.0$ gm of elemental phosphorus per day can result in lowering of the serum calcium levels as well as a reduction in urinary calcium excretion. Diarrhea usually limits the amount of phosphate that can be given. Phosphate supplements should *never* be given to patients with renal failure or when hyperphosphatemia is present, as soft tissue calcification may occur. Monitoring the calcium and phosphorus levels as well as the calcium $\times$ phosphorus ion product is important to prevent metastatic calcifications.

7. **PG inhibitors.** Nonsteroidal anti-inflammatory agents inhibit cyclooxygenase and thereby block PG synthesis. Inhibitors of PG synthesis have been clearly effective in selected cases of metastatic renal cell carcinoma and squamous cell carcinoma of the lung. Indomethacin 50 mg tid is the most potent inhibitor of PG synthesis. Aspirin 1 gm tid has also been shown to be effective in selected cases.

8. **Gallium nitrate.** Gallium nitrate has been shown to inhibit bone resorption and cause hypocalcemia in patients in whom the drug has been used as an experimental antitumor agent. The drug appears to in-

hibit bone resorption by reducing the solubility of bone crystals. In one study, gallium nitrate was more than twice as effective as calcitonin in reducing serum calcium to normal in patients with hypercalcemia of malignancy. Moreover, normocalcemia was maintained for a longer period in the gallium nitrate-treated group. Gallium nitrate has been associated with nephrotoxicity, and there is little information regarding its long-term efficacy or toxicity.

9. **WR-2721.** WR-2721 is an agent used in patients with cancer undergoing radio- or chemotherapy to protect noncancerous tissues from the effects of ionizing radiation and chemotherapy. WR-2721 was shown to cause hypocalcemia in normocalcemic patients with cancer undergoing chemotherapy. The hypocalcemia was associated with low PTH levels.

WR-2721 affects calcium metabolism at several levels. It inhibits PTH secretion, decreases bone resorption, and decreases the renal tubular reabsorption of calcium. Unfortunately, there are no reports of clinical trials in patients with hypercalcemia, and therefore the overall efficacy of the agent for the treatment of humoral hypercalcemia of cancer is unknown.

V. **Hypoglycemia and cancer.** A wide variety of non-islet-cell tumors may be associated with hypoglycemia. Hypoglycemia may occur months or even years before recognition of the tumor; it may be present at the time of diagnosis, or it may develop after the diagnosis of malignancy has been well established.

A. **Most of the neoplasms associated with hypoglycemia** are large and may present as masses in the mediastinum or retroperitoneal space. The most common non-beta-cell tumors associated with hypoglycemia are as follows.

1. Mesenchymal or mesodermal: fibrosarcomas, mesotheliomas, neurofibromas, neurofibrosarcoma, spindle cell sarcoma, rhabdomyosarcomas, and leiomyosarcomas
2. Hepatocellular carcinoma
3. Adrenocortical carcinoma
4. Pancreatic and bile duct carcinomas
5. Lymphomas and leukemias
6. Miscellaneous: lung, ovary, neuroblastoma, Wilms' tumor, and hemangiopericytoma

B. **Pathogenesis of hypoglycemia** in patients with malignancy is not clear. The possible causes of hypoglycemia are as follows.

1. Production and secretion of insulin
2. Production of nonsuppressible insulinlike protein (NSILA-p)
3. Production of insulinlike growth factor II (IGF-II)
4. Proliferation of insulin receptors
5. Increased glucose utilization by the tumor

6. Production of metabolites that interfere with gluconeogenesis
7. Inhibition of glycogen breakdown
8. Suppression of counterregulatory hormones
9. Destruction of liver by tumor

Secretion of insulin by tumors is rare. In only a few cases has an increased insulin concentration in the blood or in the tumors been reported. Such tumors are teratoma of the mediastinum containing beta cells, bronchial carcinoid, carcinoma of the cervix, retroperitoneal fibrosarcoma, and bronchogenic metastasis.

At present, the best documented mechanisms are (1) production of the high molecular weight protein NSILA-p, whose action is not suppressed by insulin antibodies; (2) production of a biologically active but not immunoreactive insulinlike growth factor II; and (3) increased glucose utilization due to proliferation of insulin receptors in liver and muscle induced by an unknown humoral substance. There is also evidence for a high rate of glycolysis of these large tumors associated with hypoglycemia, and this glycolysis could possibly contribute to excessive glucose utilization. It is likely that a variety of mechanisms may be responsible for the hypoglycemia in different tumors. In patients with hematologic malignancies and markedly elevated white blood cell counts, artifactual hypoglycemia may be seen owing to increased in vitro glucose utilization by glycolysis. In such patients plasma glucose should be measured in freshly obtained specimens to avoid possible confusion.

C. **Symptoms, signs, and laboratory findings.** The hypoglycemia that occurs with non-beta-cell tumors usually occurs during fasting in the early morning or late afternoon, and its onset is generally insidious. In most patients symptoms of neuroglycopenia predominate. They usually develop when the plasma glucose falls below 45–50 mg/dl, at which point the patients may experience symptoms and signs that resemble a variety of neurologic or psychiatric disturbances. When the hypoglycemia is severe and protracted, generalized convulsions and coma may occur. Typically, the symptoms of hypoglycemia are relieved by ingestion of food. The hypoglycemia caused by non-islet-cell tumors cannot be differentiated clinically from that caused by insulinomas, but they can be differentiated by measuring the fasting plasma insulin and glucose levels. Whereas patients with insulinomas have fasting hyperinsulinemia in the presence of hypoglycemia, patients with non-islet-cell tumors have hypoglycemia with low levels of insulin.

D. **Treatment.** Therapy of hypoglycemia associated with non-islet-cell tumors is difficult because no specific agents are available. Amelioration of hypoglycemia may result from partial or complete resection of the tumor or by control of the tumor by chemotherapy or radiation therapy.

1. **Diet.** The primary form of therapy is dietary. Frequent feedings between meals, at bedtime, and throughout the night may decrease the frequency of hypoglycemic attacks. In severe cases it may be necessary to place an ileostomy tube to facilitate continuous feeding, especially during the night. In some patients, it is also necessary to administer continuous infusions of 10–20% glucose.

2. **Hyperglycemic hormones.** High doses of glucocorticoids (prednisone 20–80 mg or dexamethasone 10–15 mg/day) may be used in patients who do not respond to dietary therapy. Also, patients may benefit from the use of long-acting glucagon (zinc glucagon) and human growth hormone. In most cases, however, the effect of these agents is only temporary.

3. **Diazoxide (Hyperstat)** is a nondiuretic derivative of the benzothiadiazine group that inhibits insulin secretion and thereby causes hyperglycemia. Diazoxide has been effective for the treatment of hypoglycemia associated with malignant insulinomas at dosages of 300–600 mg/day IV given in conjunction with hydrochlorothiazide 100 mg/day PO. However, in patients with hypoglycemia due to non-islet-cell tumors, diazoxide is frequently ineffective.

   Hypotension occasionally results from the IV administration of diazoxide. Infrequently, severe hypotension and shock may be seen. Sodium and water retention after repeated injections is common but may be obviated by the simultaneous use of hydrochlorothiazide or other diuretics.

4. **Phenytoin and somatostatin** are usually ineffective in patients with hypoglycemia due to non-insulin-producing tumors.

5. **Streptozotocin and chlorozotocin,** which may be effective in insulinomas, can be tried in refractory cases, but the results have been disappointing in non-islet-cell tumors.

VI. **Acromegaly and cancer.** The association of acromegaly with bronchial carcinoid tumors has been known since the 1970s. Reversibility of growth hormone hypersecretion and cure from acromegaly have been reported in several patients after removal of bronchial carcinoid tumors. In most of these patients no therapy was directed against the pituitary, suggesting that the carcinoid tumor was the cause of the acromegaly. Production of growth hormone-releasing hormone has been documented in eight patients with clinical evidence of growth hormone hypersecretion. Most of these patients had carcinoid tumor, pancreatic islet cell tumor, or small cell carcinoma of the lung. A 40- to 44-amino-acid peptide has been isolated from these tumors. This peptide appears to be similar, if not identical, to the hypothalamic growth hormone-releasing factor.

Ectopic production of growth hormone has also been reported by bronchogenic, gastric, ovarian, and breast cancer. However, clinical evidence of acromegaly has been lacking in these patients. Squamous cell tumors of the lung are commonly associated with *hypertrophic pulmonary osteoar-thropathy,* a subperiosteal bone deposition along the shaft of the tibia, fibula, radius, ulna, and phalanges. This new bone growth resembles that observed in acromegaly and may regress after removal of the tumor. Although growth hormone excess has been suggested as a possible cause of this abnormality, there is no clinical or laboratory evidence to support this hypothesis.

VII. Ectopic production of gonadotropins

   A. Causes and clinical observations. Ectopic production of gonadotropin can result in gynecomastia in adults and precocious puberty in children. Gynecomastia has been associated with carcinoma of the lung and is sometimes accompanied by hypertrophic pulmonary osteoarthropathy. Increased estrogen production has been reported in several patients with carcinoma of the lung and has been attributed to the production of gonadotropins by the tumor. Arteriovenous differences in follicle-stimulating hormone (FSH) concentration have been found across the tumor from adenocarcinoma of the lung, providing substantial evidence of hormone production by the tumor. Also, increased luteinizing hormone (LH) activity has been found in a hepatoblastoma from a patient with precocious puberty. In addition to carcinoma of the lung and hepatoblastoma, tumors of the testes, ovaries, pineal gland, mediastinum, adrenals, breast, bladder, and melanomas may be associated with gonadotropin production. Assays not only for FSH, LH, and human chorionic gonadotropin (hCG) but also for the α- and β-subunits of these hormones have been developed and are used primarily for screening as tumor markers. hCG is closely related biochemically and biologically to LH and is generally produced by tumors that have trophoblastic characteristics. However, there is no specific syndrome that can be attributed to the ectopic production of hCG.

   B. Treatment. There is no specific treatment for the ectopic production of gonadotropins other than therapy of the primary tumor. Symptomatic gynecomastia in men can be controlled by radiotherapy to the breast area.

VIII. Ectopic thyrotropin secretion

   A. Causes. Hyperthyroidism has been described primarily in patients with trophoblastic tumors, although a similar syndrome has been reported with epidermoid cancers of the lung and mesothelioma. The hyperthyroidism in these patients is usually mild, although severe cases have been reported in association with choriocarcinomas. The nature of the thyroid stimulator in chorionic tumors has been named *molar thyroid-stimulating hormone* (molar TSH), and evidence suggests that thyrotropic activity cannot be distinguished from that of hCG.

   B. Treatment. In patients with hydatidiform mole and hyperthyroidism, surgical removal is the treatment of choice and should be performed as soon as possible. If the hyperthyroidism is severe, administration of sodium iodide effectively reduces the concentrations of triiodothyronine (T_3) and thyroxine (T_4) in the plasma. Propranolol 40–160 mg/day may be used for control of the tachycardia. In patients with choriocarcinoma, symptomatic hyperthyroidism can be treated with propylthiouracil or methimazole as well as propranolol. Effective chemotherapy of the tumor reduces the hCG levels, thereby providing definitive treatment of the hyperthyroidism.

IX. **Osteomalacia and hypophosphatemia associated with tumors**

  A. **Clinical observations.** There are approximately 30 reports of patients displaying profound hypophosphatemia and osteomalacia associated with tumors. This condition has been called *oncogenic osteomalacia* and has been associated with a variety of mesenchymal tumors, including mesenchymomas, pleomorphic sarcomas, neurofibromas, sclerosing and cavernous hemangiomas, and hemangiopericytomas. Clinically, the patients may have profound muscle weakness and frequent fractures. Laboratory examinations reveal severe hypophosphatemia and phosphaturia. PTH levels are usually normal, and 1,25-dihydroxycholecalciferol levels are usually low. The pathogenesis of the syndrome appears to be abnormal vitamin D metabolism. It is thought that the tumor secretes a substance that inhibits the 25-hydroxycholecalciferol-1-hydroxylase activity, resulting in decreased synthesis of 1,25-dihydroxycholecalciferol, which causes the osteomalacia and the attendant biochemical abnormalities.

  B. **Treatment.** Successful surgical removal of the tumor causes healing of the osteomalacia and restores the levels of serum phosphorus and 1,25-dihydroxycholecalciferol to normal. Treatment with 1,25-dihydroxycholecalciferol (Rocaltrol) 3 μg/day for 2 weeks, has been shown to correct the biochemical abnormalities and cause healing of the bone lesions. Oral phosphate supplements (Neutra-Phos or Fleet Phospho-Soda) may be used for severe hypophosphatemia (see **IV.C.6**).

X. **Erythrocytosis and tumors.** Erythrocytosis has been seen in association with a number of benign and malignant tumors. Because erythropoietin is normally produced in the kidney, the most common tumors associated with erythrocytosis are hypernephroma and Wilms' tumor. Other tumors associated with this syndrome are uterine fibromas, cerebellar hemangioblastomas, hepatocellular carcinoma, pheochromocytoma, and ovarian carcinoma. In contrast to patients with polycythemia vera, the plasma and urinary levels of erythropoietin are elevated, and there is no splenomegaly. Patients with tumoral erythrocytosis have an elevated hemoglobin, hematocrit, red blood cell count, and red blood cell mass. Remissions are usually seen after complete removal of the tumor. For inoperable cases, periodic phlebotomies may reduce the incidence of thromboembolism and hemorrhage.

XI. **Hyperreninism and cancer.** Excess renin production has been reported in a number of renal and extrarenal neoplasms. Tumoral hyperrenism is usually associated with severe hypertension, secondary aldosteronism, and hypokalemia. Plasma renin activity and plasma aldosterone are markedly elevated and usually do not respond to position or blood volume changes. The levels of prorenin or inactive renin are also markedly elevated. The most common tumors associated with this syndrome are juxtaglomerular tumors of the kidney (renal hemangiopericytoma), Wilms' tumors, adenocarcinoma of the kidney, adenocarcinoma of the pancreas, adenocarcinoma, small cell carcinoma of the lung, ovarian carcinoma, adrenocortical adenoma, and angioid hyperplasia with eosinophilia, which is a benign tumorlike lesion of the subcutaneous tissue. Medical therapy with angiotensin-converting enzyme (ACE) inhibitors has a variable response. Remission of the syndrome has been seen after successful therapy of the tumor.

Selected Reading

Baylin, S. B., and De Bustros, A. Hormone synthesis and secretion by cancer. In K. L. Becker (ed.), *Principles and Practice of Endocrinology and Metabolism.* Philadelphia: Lippincott, 1990. Pp. 1626–1629.

Becker, K. L., and Silva, O. L. Paraneoplastic endocrine syndromes. In K. L. Becker (ed.), *Principles and Practice of Endocrinology and Metabolism.* Philadelphia: Lippincott, 1990. Pp. 1629–1638.

Odell, W. D. Paraendocrine syndromes of cancer. *Adv. Intern. Med.* 34:325, 1989.

Ectopic Acth Syndrome

Farwell, A. P., Devlin, J. T., and Stewart, J. A. Total suppression of cortisol excretion by ketoconazole in the therapy of the ectopic adrenocorticotropic hormone syndrome. *Am. J. Med.* 84:1063, 1988.

Nieman, K. L., et al. Successful treatment of Cushing's syndrome with the glucocorticoid antagonist RU 486. *J. Clin. Endocrinol. Metab.* 61:536, 1985.

Hypercalcemia and Cancer

Attie, M. F. Treatment of hypercalcemia. *Endocrinol. Metab. Clin. North Am.* 18:807, 1989.

Bockman, R. S., et al. Gallium nitrate inhibits bone resorption, increases bone calcium content and crystallite perfection of hydroxyapatite. *Calcif. Tissue Int.* 39:376, 1986.

Breslau, N. A., et al. Hypercalcemia associated with increased serum calcitriol levels in three patients with lymphoma. *Ann. Intern. Med.* 100:1, 1984.

Burtis, W. J., et al. Immunochemical characterization of circulating parathyroid hormone-related protein in patients with humoral hypercalcemia of cancer. *N. Engl. J. Med.* 322:1106, 1990.

Elomaa, A., et al. Diphosphonates for osteolytic metastases. *Lancet* 1:1155, 1985.

Ryzen, E., et al. Intravenous etidronate in the management of malignant hypercalcemia. *Arch. Intern. Med.* 145:449, 1985.

Simpson, E. L., et al. Absence of parathyroid hormone mRNA in nonparathyroid tumors associated with hypercalcemia. *N. Engl. J. Med.* 309:325, 1983.

Van Holten-Verzantvoort, A. T., et al. Reduced morbidity from skeletal metastases in breast cancer patients during long-term bisphosphonate (APD) treatment. *Lancet* 2:983, 1987.

Warrell, R.P., Jr., et al. Gallium nitrate for acute treatment of cancer-related hypercalcemia: a randomized double-blind comparison to calcitonin. *Ann. Intern. Med.* 108:669, 1988.

Hypoglycemia and Cancer

Li, T. C., et al. Surgical cure of hypoglycemia associated with cystosarcoma phylloides and elevated nonsuppressible insulin-like protein. *Am. J. Med.* 74:1080, 1983.

Stuart, C. A., et al. Insulin receptor proliferation: a mechanism for tumor associated hypoglycemia. *J. Clin. Endocrinol. Metab.* 63:879, 1986.

Bony Metastases

Gerald W. Marsa

Second in importance to maximizing a patient's chances for cure, perhaps, is the challenge the physician faces in minimizing the potential complications of cancer, which can markedly diminish the quality of remaining life for a patient with incurable disease. Metastatic involvement of the skeleton is the most commonly encountered problem. It has the potential to drastically change a patient's ability to continue living a relatively normal life. It is imperative that physicians and others caring for patients with cancer be continually alert to the possibility of skeletal metastases so the devastating end result of pathologic fracture may be avoided. Accurate assessment of the patient's future course by knowledge of a tumor's natural history and realistic appraisal of chances for success of remaining therapy programs assists the team of primary physician, orthopedic surgeon, radiation oncologist, and medical oncologist in deciding the correct approach to managing each patient with bony metastases.

I. Clinical presentation

A. Pain.

Bony metastases manifest by producing pain or limiting function. Pain from skeletal metastases is usually of two coexisting types. Patients with bone pain frequently complain first of constant gnawing pain in the affected bone, which usually is worse at night and may awaken the patient from sleep. This pain is attributable to pressure erosion of bone by an expanding metastatic deposit within the bone. A second component of pain, usually sharp in quality, is noticed by patients when stress (e.g., weight bearing) is applied to the affected bone; classically, this component is more prominent during the day while a patient is active and is relieved by resting. While the constant ache caused by bony erosion is frequently relieved within a few days of initiating radiotherapy or effective chemotherapy, the pain caused by structural weakening persists until additional support is provided by external devices (brace, cast), internal orthopedic support (e.g., intramedullary rod, compression plate, methylmethacrylate cement), or adequate bone reconstitution by the normal reparative process.

B. Radiologic studies

1. Bone scans and radiography.

Radiographic evidence of bony metastasis may be lacking despite great pain, as nearly one-half of the bone structure must be destroyed before the destruction is apparent on a routine bone x-ray film. Isotope bone scanning is much more sensitive and usually shows the increased bone turnover at a much earlier stage. It must be remembered, however, that the scan identifies an area of increased osteoblastic activity that can be the result of a variety of processes. Radiographs of abnormal areas are a prerequisite to ensure against a benign cause of the abnormality.

2. Types of lesions. Metastatic involvement may appear radiographically as a pure osteoblastic process (prostate carcinoma, osteosarcoma), a pure osteolytic process (multiple myeloma, oat-cell carcinoma of lung), or a mixed process with varying amounts of each type (breast carcinoma, lung carcinoma, and most other malignancies, including those that can present as a pure process). Because bone scanning identifies areas of increased osteoblastic activity, lesions that are purely osteolytic may appear silent on bone scan in the presence of a large defect on the x-ray film.

3. Site of metastasis. Malignancies that frequently metastasize to a solitary skeletal site include hypernephroma and gastrointestinal carcinomas. Breast carcinoma, lung cancer, and prostatic carcinoma nearly always involve several bones on initial metastasis. For this reason, a systematic search for other, as yet asymptomatic, lesions should be undertaken as part of the overall reevaluation, including a bone scan and x-ray films of the pelvis, proximal femurs, and any bones identified as abnormal on scan. Most metastases involve the axial skeleton and proximal extremities, but skull involvement is common with multiple myeloma and breast carcinoma. Metastasis to distal extremity bones, although rare, is most frequently seen with hypernephroma, lung cancer, and neuroblastoma.

II. Surgical therapy
A. Pathologic fractures

1. Long bones and ribs. Because rapid return of the patient to as normal a life as possible is an overriding concern when treating patients with metastatic disease, surgical stabilization is most often the initial step in treating pathologic fractures of the long bones. If the fracture is the initial manifestation of tumor relapse, biopsy confirmation can also be obtained. Whereas fractures at sites of significant residual bony architecture can be satisfactorily stabilized with an intramedullary rod or pin, marked lytic destruction may necessitate additional structural support such as methylmethacrylate cement to fill the intramedullary canal and cortical defects. Casts are infrequently utilized owing to the long interval until restoration of normal bone strength through the healing process. In addition, a cast's bulkiness interferes with restoration of normal ambulation and makes administration of adjuvant irradiation difficult. Pathologic fractures of non-weight-bearing bones can be managed by splinting (ribs) or sling immobilization (humerus or clavicle) while delivering radiotherapy to promote healing. Fixation may also be used in the upper extremities to speed recovery of function, particularly of the humerus.

2. **Compression fractures.** Compression fractures of the spine not only are a source of severe pain but also are a potential source of spinal cord or nerve root compression. Adequate support to the weakened vertebral body can be provided with external supportive devices, ranging from a tight girdle in the least severe cases to a rigid spine brace in the most severe. In this manner, weight from the upper body can be partially transferred to the pelvic bones by way of the ribs and soft tissues, preventing further deformity by reducing stress on the affected vertebral body. In many cases this support must be maintained a number of months until adequate healing has occurred following intervening radiotherapy or systemic chemotherapy. In some circumstances, surgical stabilization of the spine is required. Anterior and posterior stabilization procedures may be done, depending on the nature of the bony deficit. Although such procedures are technically difficult and require an orthopedic/neurosurgical team experienced in these techniques, the relief of pain and improvement of mobility may be dramatic. If the patient has an anticipated survival of more than 3 months, serious consideration of surgical stabilization of the spine is recommended.

3. **Prostheses.** Occasionally, severe destruction of the femoral head or acetabulum makes restoration to an ambulatory state impossible unless the bone is replaced by a prosthesis. Replacement is warranted when the prognosis suggests a reasonable life expectancy of 3 months or more with continued stability of health following the procedure. An appropriate example of a situation in which such replacement might be used is breast carcinoma in a patient without prior exposure to combination chemotherapy (of which several systemic therapy programs exist with high probability of response). A prosthetic device is less often appropriate in patients with lung carcinoma, a disease for which survival is short following the diagnosis of systemic metastasis and responses to chemotherapy are less frequent and of shorter duration. With careful selection, total hip arthroplasty can give excellent palliation with marked improvement in the quality of life for the affected patient.

B. **Impending fractures.** Weight-bearing bones with marked cortical destruction are at high risk for subsequent fracture during the course of palliative radiotherapy or, after irradiation, while awaiting restoration of adequate bone structure. Rather than consigning a patient to a prolonged interval of non-weight-bearing on the affected extremity with continued high risk of fracture with passive movement, better management is immediate "prophylactic" stabilization with an intramedullary rod or pin. Following stabilization, radiotherapy can be initiated without high risk of fracture and with the patient significantly more active. Prophylactic nailing is easy to perform and is associated with less morbidity than fracture fixation.

III. Radiation therapy

A. Indications. Irradiation of weight-bearing bones with metastatic involvement is indicated early in the disease process before pathologic fracture can occur. Surgical stabilization does not obviate the need for irradiation to prevent further bony destruction by residual tumor. Symptomatic metastases to non-weight-bearing bones are also an indication for palliative irradiation. Relatively low doses of irradiation (15–20 Gy) are frequently sufficient to afford dramatic pain relief, and 80–90% of patients with pain secondary to bone metastases show significant improvement with intermediate doses (30–40 Gy).

B. Treatment schedules. Treatment is structured to give therapy as rapidly as possible to afford relief of pain and promote bone healing for the remainder of the patient's life while minimizing any concurrent radiation symptoms. In a patient in the terminal stage of illness with a life expectancy of a few weeks, a single fraction of 10 Gy if the portal is small or 15–20 Gy in three to five fractions gives the desired effect. Conversely, an occasional patient has the potential for prolonged survival (i.e., early metastatic breast carcinoma), in which instance one might use high doses for longer control of disease and a large number of fractions to minimize late normal tissue effects (i.e., 50 Gy in 25 fractions). Most patients receive optimal results from courses of 30 Gy in 10 fractions (2 weeks) or 40 Gy in 15 fractions (3 weeks). Should recurrent symptoms develop owing to reactivation of treated disease, a repeat course of radiotherapy can be undertaken with excellent prospects for another response, as patients with relapsing metastatic disease seldom survive long enough to develop the late radiation consequences of multiple radiotherapy courses.

C. Treatment fields. Radiotherapy fields should include the evident bone involvement, as shown on x-ray film and bone scan, with a sufficient extension to prevent relapse at the portal margin. It is seldom necessary to treat the entire bone unless the entire bone is involved, as encroachment on marrow reserve may compromise any systemic chemotherapy that may also be indicated. Supervoltage radiotherapy (cobalt or linear accelerator) is always preferable to minimize acute skin reactions and late soft tissue fibrosis as a source of patient morbidity and to maximize the capacity to re-treat the patient at a late date if required.

D. Hemibody irradiation

1. Indications. Experience has shown that sequential hemibody irradiation for palliation of widespread symptomatic bony metastases is an effective modality. It is indicated only in patients with diffuse symptomatic bony involvement for whom no effective systemic chemotherapy remains, as significant marrow depression can be expected.

2. **Technique.** The more symptomatic half of the body, divided at the umbilicus, is irradiated as a single large field through anterior and posterior portals, usually giving a single fraction of 10 Gy to the lower half-body or 7 Gy to the upper half-body. The other half is treated approximately 1 month later, after marrow recovery within the irradiated field.

3. **Side effects.** Despite the following side effects, because of the excellent transient responses that can be achieved, hemibody irradiation should be considered for patients with diffuse symptoms who have exhausted conventional systemic therapies.

   a. **Nausea and vomiting** during the first 12 hours after treatment is usually controlled with sedation and antiemetics.

   b. **Blood count depression** at 7–10 days after treatment, which rarely requires transfusion support, occurs in the patient heavily pretreated with chemotherapy.

   c. **Hypotension** may be seen during the first 24 hours after upper hemibody irradiation in patients not pretreated with steroids.

   d. **Acute radiation pneumonitis** may occur 4–6 weeks after upper hemibody irradiation, especially if the patient has had prior thoracic radiotherapy.

IV. **Systemic therapy.** Patients developing bone metastasis have obvious need for effective systemic therapy of their disease if therapy is available. For disease such as lymphoma or breast carcinoma, there is a high probability of response to chemotherapy, and institution of systemic treatment alone can induce healing of the metastatic bony lesions. Even in such favorable instances, the physician must evaluate any involved weight-bearing bones regarding the potential for pathologic fracture and maintain this close vigilance throughout the course of therapy. Any evidence of progressive bony involvement, especially in the proximal femurs, warrants immediate radiotherapy to reduce the risk of pathologic fracture and prevent the need for surgical stabilization. Many neoplasms, e.g., gastrointestinal malignancies and non-oat-cell carcinomas of the lung, have a low probability of response to chemotherapeutic regimens; and in these patients local irradiation to affected weight-bearing bones should be considered part of the initial systemic program. With closely coordinated care among the primary physician, medical oncologist, and radiotherapist, concurrent or sequential therapies can be given to minimize the risks of orthopedic catastrophe without compromising the systemic chemotherapy.

Selected Reading

Blitzer, P. Reanalysis of the ROTG study of the palliation of symptomatic osseous metastasis. *Cancer* 55:1468, 1985.

Malawer, M., and Delaney, T. Treatment of metastatic cancer

to bone. In V.T. DeVita (ed.), *Cancer Principles and Practice of Oncology* (3rd ed.). Philadelphia: Lippincott, 1989. Pp. 2298–2317.

Montague, E., and Delclos, L. Palliative radiotherapy in the management of metastatic disease. In G. H. Fletcher (ed.), *Textbook of Radiotherapy* (3rd ed.). Philadelphia: Lea & Febiger, 1980. Pp. 943–948.

Turek, S. Secondary tumors of bones. In *Orthopaedics: Principles and Their Application* (4th ed.). Philadelphia: Lippincott, 1984. Pp. 664–677.

Superior Vena Cava Syndrome and Other Obstructive Syndromes

Gerald W. Marsa

Obstruction of blood vessels and other tubular passages is a common problem of untreated cancer, occurring as a presenting sign of localized tumor as well as a late manifestation of widespread disease. Irrespective of the extent of tumor involvement, it is a process that requires prompt recognition and appropriate treatment to avoid loss of organ function and to reduce the risk of abscess or other infection. Superior vena cava obstruction is among the most common of the obstructive syndromes encountered, although a variety of sites can become obstructed by neoplastic growths. Prompt treatment is important to relieve the patient's symptoms and reduce the likelihood of serious consequences.

I. **Superior vena cava (SVC) syndrome**
   A. **Clinical presentation.** Symptoms of SVC obstruction include edema and cyanosis of the face, neck, and upper extremities (usually worse on arising in the morning and lessening during daytime activities), headache, dyspnea, and changes in sensorium. Examination reveals venous distention and elevated venous pressure in the neck and upper extremities, normal venous pressure of the lower extremities, and frequently visible superficial collateral circulation on the trunk with venous flow toward the groin.
   B. **Etiology**
      1. **Malignant tumors.** The high incidence of lung carcinoma today has made SVC obstruction increasingly common. SVC obstruction is nonetheless frequently overlooked in its early stages because of an insidious presentation. Although most SVC obstructions are caused by bronchogenic carcinoma (usually metastatic to mediastinal lymph nodes), any neoplasm involving the upper right mediastinum in the vicinity of the SVC can obstruct this vein. Other neoplasms frequently associated with SVC syndrome include undifferentiated carcinoma of the thyroid, diffuse non-Hodgkin's lymphomas, and mediastinal germinomas.
      2. **Nonmalignant disorders.** The flagrant symptoms associated with SVC syndrome in cancer are caused by the rapid occlusion of the vena cava that occurs before sufficient collateral venous circulation can develop. The slow growth of benign mediastinal tumors allows more collaterals to develop and thus explains the much lower frequency of these symptoms with complete SVC compression by benign neoplasms. SVC syndrome due to nonneoplastic conditions is un-

common, and it is generally appropriate to presume that the obstruction is caused by a malignant neoplasm.

3. Intrinsic luminal occlusion. Although obstruction usually is due to extrinsic compression, intrinsic venous involvement by tumor can also be seen. The syndrome can also develop from intraluminal thrombosis in the absence of neoplastic involvement.

C. Diagnosis. Superior venacavography using radionuclide or radiocontrast techniques can be useful for defining the site and extent of vena cava involvement. Because of the high risk of bleeding due to elevated venous pressure, other invasive diagnostic studies (e.g., mediastinotomy) are frequently delayed until treatment has been initiated and signs of obstruction have subsided. If biopsy is contemplated, careful thought must be given to the relative risks and benefits of pretreatment biopsy in the face of veins engorged by increased venous pressure. Although biopsy carries an increased risk for bleeding, biopsy specimens may be obtained from areas in which hemostasis can be reasonably ensured. As a rule, bronchoscopy (with washings, brushings, and biopsy) or supraclavicular node biopsy may be safely undertaken. Mediastinoscopic biopsy is more hazardous but may be undertaken by a skilled surgeon provided meticulous hemostatic dissection is used. If the risk of biopsy is deemed too great, radiotherapy can be initiated and the biopsy undertaken within 2–3 days after there has been initial relief of signs and symptoms. Before taking this approach, it must be recognized that even a short course of radiotherapy may make an accurate histologic diagnosis difficult or impossible.

D. Treatment

1. General measures. Because some tissue edema is usually associated with tumor obstruction, diuretics and high doses of corticosteroids can provide initial relief of symptoms and should be promptly prescribed. Dexamethasone 8–16 mg daily in divided doses or prednisone 30–60 mg daily frequently gives a partial response within 24 hours; additionally, either helps avoid further exacerbation of signs and symptoms at the initiation of antineoplastic therapy. Furosemide 40 mg PO is an effective diuretic with rapid action and can be used repeatedly as symptoms require, provided cardiac output remains adequate.

2. Surgery. Because SVC obstruction is prima facie evidence of mediastinal involvement, surgical therapy is contraindicated because of tumor unresectability and the high risks of excessive bleeding.

3. Radiotherapy. Prompt irradiation of the site of vena cava obstruction is indicated as soon as SVC syndrome is recognized. Treatment need not be withheld pending histologic confirmation of malignancy, as benign conditions are so rare and the danger of waiting is high. Several daily high-dose fractions (4

Gy daily for 2 or 3 days) is usually sufficient to provide temporary relief of symptoms. Additional diagnostic and staging procedures then can safely be undertaken to determine the overall plan of therapy. For non-oat-cell lung carcinomas and other mediastinal neoplasms without evidence of systemic dissemination, definitive radiotherapy with high total radiation doses is indicated. Emergency irradiation should be interrupted as soon as the desired response is seen in order to avoid compromising definitive diagnosis and treatment.

4. **Chemotherapy.** In patients with previously diagnosed neoplasms that are highly responsive to systemic chemotherapy (e.g., lymphomas, small cell undifferentiated lung carcinoma), chemotherapy can be initiated as primary treatment. Obviously, subsequent staging studies will be compromised after a course of systemic therapy; hence local irradiation is still preferred for new patients presenting with cancer. Chemotherapy cannot be relied on to provide the desired rapid relief of SVC obstructive symptoms for neoplasms with low response rates to drug therapy and neoplasms for which the chemotherapy response is achieved only after a prolonged interval. In these situations, local irradiation should precede planned chemotherapy.

II. Bronchial and tracheal obstruction

A. Bronchial obstruction: etiology and diagnosis. One of the most common complications of uncontrolled bronchogenic carcinoma is loss of respiratory function secondary to airway obstruction. Symptoms can develop suddenly with increased dyspnea; or if obstruction is gradual, they can manifest as fevers caused by distal pneumonitis or abscess. Because obstruction can develop owing to causes other than neoplastic growth (especially mucous plugging), bronchoscopy should be performed if the etiology is uncertain. Bronchoscopy can be therapeutic if the obstruction is due to nonneoplastic sources. Other neoplastic causes of bronchial obstruction include the lymphomas and a rare endobronchial metastasis from another site, such as breast or gastrointestinal carcinoma.

B. Surgery. In cases in which only segmental atelectasis is present, a curative surgical resection is indicated if the neoplasm is localized and if the patient's medical condition can tolerate pulmonary resection. In cases that are otherwise nonsurgical, palliative surgical resection may be necessary if significant localized pulmonary destruction owing to infection has occurred and can be resected to remove the nidus of an otherwise chronic infection.

C. Radiotherapy

1. **General considerations.** The most common therapy for major bronchial obstruction is localized irradiation. Lung tissue is sensitive to x rays, with the risk of acute radiation pneumonitis and late pulmo-

nary fibrosis rising rapidly at doses above 15 Gy. It
is thus important to achieve reexpansion of the collapsed normal lung as rapidly as possible to shield
uninvolved lung from higher doses of irradiation. Intermittent positive-pressure breathing should be
employed regularly during radiotherapy until reexpansion is achieved.

2. **Potentially curative treatment.** For newly diagnosed neoplasms with which there is evidence of only
localized or regional involvement, irradiation should
be carried out with curative intent, delivering doses
of 50 Gy or more for attempted long-term control of
the tumor.

3. **Palliative treatment.** More commonly, local obstruction due to lung carcinoma is only a local manifestation of generalized disease; nevertheless, local
irradiation is necessary to palliate what is or may
progress to a devastating complication of cancer—respiratory insufficiency. In such cases, a rapid course
of lower total doses of radiation can be undertaken
to be delivered to the local area of tumor involvement
in order to provide relief of obstructive symptoms or
at least to prevent further progression of lung collapse.

4. **Prophylactic treatment.** Anticipation of major
bronchial obstruction with prophylactic treatment
prior to onset of symptoms can be of marked value in
maintaining a high quality of life in the patient with
incurable disease, as it is often easier to avoid obstruction than to reverse the process once atelectasis
has developed.

D. **Chemotherapy.** Systemic therapy should usually be reserved for the secondary management of disseminated
carcinoma once the local problem of bronchial obstruction has been treated with local irradiation. Lymphomas
and small cell undifferentiated carcinoma of the lung
have high response rates when treated with combination
chemotherapy, and frequently bronchial obstruction can
be relived with systemic drug therapy alone. Even in
these instances, the response is seldom as rapid and may
not be as complete as when local irradiation is also delivered.

E. **Endoscopic laser therapy.** A new treatment modality
for palliation of obstructing or bleeding bronchial tumors is the neodymium-yttrium-aluminum-garnet (Nd-
YAG) laser. This laser produces a powerful, highly fo-
cused beam of light in the near-infrared range that can
be transmitted through a flexible fiberoptic endoscope to
the tumor site by means of a separate fiber in the biopsy
channel. The Nd-YAG laser is suitable for lesions of the
larger airways that can be reached by means of a flexible
bronchoscope. Patients in poor condition are at increased risk of developing acute respiratory distress and
cardiac decompensation during the laser therapy. Usually several treatment sessions are preferred in order to
avoid injury to large blood vessels. Necrotic debris can

also be removed by means of the bronchoscope prior to each treatment.

F. **Photodynamic therapy (PDT).** Light-absorbing chemicals have been used to cause photoreactions in living tissues. The most prominent example involves psoralen and ultraviolet light (PUVA) for the treatment of psoriasis. Porphyrins given IV to patients with malignancies result in (1) concentration of the porphyrins in the neoplastic tissues; (2) visible fluorescence when illuminated with violet light (a possible method of visually detecting small malignant deposits); and (3) cellular damage when the site of porphyrin concentration is exposed to light. Porphyrin also concentrates in the reticuloendothelial system of normal liver, spleen, kidneys, lymph nodes, and skin. Patients are cautioned to avoid sun exposure for 1 month following treatment to avoid skin photosensitization.

Increasing use of PDT for treating human cancers of skin, lung, esophagus, head and neck, bladder, cervix, and vagina is being reported. Two porphyrin mixtures have been used: hematoporphyrin derivative (HPD) and dihematoporphyrin ethers (DHE). To treat a tumor the patient receives an intravenous injection of the drug a few days prior to exposure of the tumor to laser light, usually red light of 630 nm wavelength. The laser penetrates tissue for several millimeters and in combination with porphyrins can cause tissue necrosis up to 1 cm deep. For definitive treatment it is effective only for small early lesions, where limitations of light penetration in tissues are minimized. It is also useful for palliation in patients with advanced lesions where surgery, radiotherapy, and chemotherapy have failed. Research is under way on delivering light by interstitially implanted optic fibers to treat large tumors and on combining PDT with hyperthermia.

G. **Tracheal obstruction.** Airway obstruction within the trachea is obviously acutely life-threatening. Tracheal obstruction is caused most frequently by extrinsic compression by a mediastinal neoplasm. Because temporizing measures, e.g., tracheostomy, are impossible, recognition and treatment of pending obstruction before its development is vital.

1. **Endotracheal neoplasms** are rare. They are usually managed with corticosteroids and bronchoscopic resection to temporarily enlarge the airway followed by irradiation to the tracheal neoplasm and regional lymphatics. Tracheal resection with reanastomosis can seldom be accomplished, and utilization of prosthetic tracheal replacements has thus far proved unsatisfactory. Experience has also shown the Nd-YAG laser via the bronchoscope to be of value for maintaining a patent airway, and early work suggests that photodynamic therapy may also be effective.

2. **Extrinsic tracheal obstruction,** which is more common, can be anticipated because tracheal narrowing can be observed on the chest x-ray film prior

to development of obstruction. Because the trachea is composed of U-shaped rings of cartilage, it can withstand significant pressure before collapse, usually complete, develops suddenly after the integral strength of the cartilage is exceeded. Emergency endotracheal intubation can be life-sparing, but it is seldom successful. It is therefore important that tracheal narrowing be noted early, be recognized for the potentially fatal complication it is, and be treated promptly with radiotherapy.

II. Biliary tract obstruction

A. Etiology and diagnosis. Obstruction of the biliary tract can develop owing to (1) intrinsic blockade by a primary neoplasm or biliary stones, or (2) extrinsic compression by lymphadenopathy secondary to metastatic carcinoma. Identification of the site and probable cause of obstructive jaundice has been made easier with the advent of computed tomography (CT) body scanning; but other studies, including transhepatic cholangiography and endoscopic retrograde cholangiopancreatography (ERCP), may also be of benefit. Relief of obstructive jaundice is a legitimate goal even in patients with limited survival.

B. General measures. Fever due to a retrograde infection is a frequent symptom of biliary tract obstruction, and broad-spectrum antibiotics that cover enteric organisms, including anaerobes and enteric gram-negative bacteria, are often required. Pruritus can be relieved in patients with partial biliary tract obstruction by cholestyramine resin (4 gm in water tid before meals), which chelates bile salts in the gut. Pruritus can also be lessened by such medicines as trimeprazine (Temaril) 2.5 mg PO qid. Percutaneous biliary drainage through transhepatic catheter placement into the dilated proximal ducts can be utilized in instances in which the obstruction is not amenable to surgical bypass procedures or in a patient whose medical condition makes surgery risky. Hypoprothrombinemia should be corrected with vitamin K 5–10 mg IM or SQ.

C. Surgery

1. Curative resection. Radical resection can provide relief of obstructive symptoms and an opportunity for cure in some cases of ampullary carcinoma, an occasional carcinoma of the head of the pancreas, and rarely carcinoma of the distal common biliary duct with radical pancreaticoduodenectomy (Whipple's operation).

2. Palliative treatment. The remaining cases either have evidence of metastasis or involve proximal biliary tracts not amenable to surgical resection for cure. In those patients with unresectable disease caused by intrahepatic or proximal obstruction, a permanent internal biliary drainage catheter can sometimes be passed through the obstructing tumor to act as a drain into the duodenum. In unresectable cases with more distal obstruction, bypass can be accomplished through choledochojejunostomy or external drainage by way of a T-tube from the dilated ducts proximal to the obstruction.

D. Radiotherapy

1. **Highly responsive tumors.** In patients with biliary blockage due to highly radioresponsive neoplasms such as lymphomas or oat-cell carcinoma of the lung, local irradiation to the porta hepatis can provide rapid relief.

2. **Moderately responsive tumors.** Although radiotherapy eventually causes sufficient tumor regression to reduce jaundice in patients with most other neoplasms where only moderate radiosensitivity exists, the process may require several weeks or more; therefore for best results radiotherapy should be combined with a biliary drainage procedure whenever possible. Irradiation following operative bypass or percutaneous transhepatic cholangial drainage not only can provide improved biliary drainage as the initial obstruction improves but can also prevent reobstruction caused by progressive tumor growth. Palliative doses of irradiation (20–40 Gy in 1–3 weeks depending on portal size) are indicated in cases of metastatic disease.

3. **Tumors with potential for long-term control.** In cases of primary carcinomas of the pancreas and biliary ducts without evidence of hepatic or distant spread, radical irradiation should be undertaken following surgical delineation of tumor extent and biliary bypass procedure. Radiation doses of 60 Gy or more over 6–7 weeks, utilizing multiply-shaped portals to minimize injury to surrounding normal tissues, can provide better local tumor control and occasionally improve long-term survival.

E. Chemotherapy. Because response rates and regression intervals are poor in most tumors causing biliary tract obstruction, chemotherapy plays a secondary role of maintaining surgical and radiotherapeutic responses by preventing tumor extension with biliary tract obstruction.

IV. Alimentary tract obstruction

A. Clinical presentation and rationale of treatment. Nausea, vomiting, and abdominal pain are common symptoms experienced by the patient with cancer. Obstruction of the gastrointestinal tract must be constantly differentiated from other causes of these symptoms. Treatment of this complication is nearly always indicated, even in the patient with terminal disease, to relieve the undesirable alternatives of persistent symptoms or continued suctioning of the alimentary tract. Even obstruction of the esophagus, which is not associated with the same symptoms, is best palliated by relief of the obstruction because of the unpleasantness associated with an inability to handle salivary secretions.

B. General measures. Significant nutritional deficiencies are nearly always associated with gastrointestinal obstruction because of the long-standing condition that had existed subclinically before diagnosis of the blockage. Restoration of positive nutritional balance is vital to a good result. Usually nutritional balance should be initiated by IV hyperalimentation as a temporary supportive measure until gastrointestinal tract integrity can be restored. With proximal obstructions (esophagus and stomach), feeding gastrostomy or jejunostomy can provide similar support and is preferred because of diminished expense and potential complications. Also, continued hospitalization can be avoided. Intestinal dilatation associated with obstruction must be decompressed by nasogastric suction while preparing for surgery. Nonneoplastic causes of intestinal obstruction are occasionally resolved by decompression of intestinal dilatation and subsidence of tissue edema.

C. **Surgery.** With few exceptions, surgical correction of gastrointestinal obstruction is the treatment of choice.

    1. **Tumors not helped by surgical resection** include carcinoma of the proximal esophagus and extensive carcinomas of the distal esophagus and stomach. In these cases the morbidity of the procedure overwhelms the palliative results. Feeding gastrostomy or jejunostomy can temporarily circumvent the obstruction while awaiting the results of radiotherapy. Placement of a semirigid plastic tube through an obstructive esophageal neoplasm into the proximal stomach can also be useful, although late displacement of the tube is common and local irradiation postoperatively is still indicated.

    2. **Curative resections.** Resection is indicated for other localized gastrointestinal carcinomas causing obstruction, although it is often accomplished as a staged procedure following colostomy for colonic obstruction to reduce the risk of infection and anastomotic leak.

    3. **Palliative resection** is indicated in cases in which metastases are evident and whenever the procedure can be accomplished without high risk. Palliative resection decreases the tumor burden for subsequent chemotherapy and removes the most likely site of future symptoms from the cancer. The recommendation for palliative resection includes obstructing rectal carcinomas with metastasis, in which abdominal perineal resection can prevent future pelvic and perineal pain, rectal bleeding and drainage, and rectal tenesmus. When an obstructing neoplasm cannot safely be removed, bypass of the obstructed viscus with side-to-side anastomosis should be performed.

D. **Radiotherapy**

    1. **Potentially curative treatment.** Esophageal carcinoma is the only gastrointestinal tract carcinoma commonly treated definitively with irradiation. In the absence of evident systemic spread, radical irradiation is warranted to attempt long-term control of the local and regional disease, despite the dismal

cure rates. Doses in the range of 60–70 Gy are required, necessitating careful radiotherapy planning and multiple portals to avoid injury to the lungs, spinal cord, and heart. Vigorous nutritional support is required during the treatment course.

   2. Palliative treatment. Palliative irradiation of an unresectable gastrointestinal neoplasm usually requires doses of 40–50 Gy over 3–5 weeks. Restoration of esophageal and gastric patency can be accomplished in more than one-half of patients with significant improvement in quality of life. Irradiation of unresected intestinal and rectal neoplasms following bypass or colostomy is frequently indicated to relieve pain and perineal discharge of bladder dysfunction.

E. Chemotherapy. Primary gastrointestinal carcinomas have low response rates to chemotherapeutic agents, which should be considered only as an adjunct to surgery or radiotherapy in relieving obstructive symptoms. Responsive neoplasms such as lymphomas may be treated with drugs primarily in cases of incomplete obstruction, but usually they are best managed by relieving the obstruction surgically in order to improve nutrition before chemotherapy is begun. Experience shows that combining systemic chemotherapy with radiotherapy for squamous cell carcinomas of the esophagus promises more rapid and complete tumor regression.

F. Endoscopic Nd-YAG laser. Obstructing neoplasms of the esophagus can be palliated by a series of laser treatments that progressively reestablish a lumen through the tumor mass. Care must be taken to avoid excessive tumor destruction at one setting that could lead to esophageal perforation. Necrotic tissue from prior laser treatments is removed by means of an endoscope before each successive treatment. In some studies, patients with esophageal cancer treated with laser therapy combined with radiotherapy survived longer than those treated with radiotherapy. Obstructing neoplasms of the stomach and large bowel have been similarly treated for palliation.

G. Photodynamic therapy. See **II.F.**

V. Ureteral obstruction

A. Etiology and diagnosis. Because of the long abdominal and pelvic course of the ureter, it is subject to obstruction due to pressure or invasion by a variety of cancers. The upper ureter can be compressed or invaded by carcinomas of the kidney or pancreas. The pelvic segment is most commonly compressed by extensive retroperitoneal lymph node metastases from carcinomas of the urinary bladder, prostate, uterus, cervix, or rectum. Intraluminal obstruction by urothelial carcinoma must be distinguished from obstruction caused by clot or stone. Obstruction secondary to retroperitoneal fibrosis caused by previous surgery, previous radiation therapy, or primary disease should also be considered. Symptoms can be nonexistent until uremia develops, or they can develop acutely with flank pain, fever, or hematuria. Assessment of the site and extent of ureteral obstruction can be accomplished with an excretory urogram, cystoscopy with retrograde pyelography, and CT body scanning.

B. **General measures.** Preservation of remaining renal function requires prompt relief of ureteral back-pressure. Indwelling retrograde catheters can be left in place until obstruction has been relieved or corrective surgery is undertaken. Ureteral stents can be utilized with lower obstructions to avoid the need for indwelling catheters. When bilateral ureteral obstruction has occurred owing to uncontrolled neoplasm, one must assess the quality of remaining life before undertaking relief of ureteral obstruction. Because renal failure is one of the easiest modes of demise for patients with terminal cancer, it is inappropriate to prevent it in the patient with cancer who has significant pain and a minimal probability of future treatment response.

C. **Surgery.** In patients with localized recurrence of pelvic tumor following irradiation, exenterative surgery with ureteral implantation into an ileal or colonic conduit should be considered for possible salvage cure. If tumor resection is impossible, conduit diversion may still be the best palliation. Other diverting procedures such as ureterosigmoidostomy are less desirable. Occasionally, ureteral reimplantation into an unirradiated tumor-free bladder can be accomplished with excellent prognosis for success. Nephrectomy should be considered in the relatively healthy patient with unilateral nonfunctioning kidney caused by ureteral obstruction because of the high risk of future infection.

D. **Radiotherapy.** Ureteral obstruction caused by retroperitoneal lymphadenopathy or pelvic neoplasms not previously irradiated are usually best treated with radiotherapy. In instances of widespread metastases, palliative doses of 30–40 Gy over 2–3 weeks are usually adequate (in conjunction with anticipated postirradiation systemic therapy). The objective response may take several weeks or more to be maximal. In cases of only localized or regional tumor involvement, higher doses are indicated in anticipation of longer potential survival or even cure.

E. **Chemotherapy.** With the exception of lymphomas, most neoplasms causing ureteral obstruction have low chemotherapy response rates. However, cisplatin alone or in combination may produce a satisfactory response by sensitive tumors. Nephrotoxicity is markedly enhanced by poor renal function, so chemotherapy with cisplatin is best withheld until ureteral obstruction has been relieved by surgery or irradiation. Ureteral obstruction due to disseminated lymphomas can be treated with combination chemotherapy in lieu of localized irradiation, but it should be recognized that the local response rate is higher and the time to response shorter for patients undergoing irradiation.

VI. Lymphatic obstruction. Lymphedema of an extremity in the patient with cancer can be discomforting and disabling. It can result from uncontrolled tumor growth within nodes blocking lymphatic pathways or from successful cancer therapy with surgery or irradiation. Determination of the etiology of the edema in each patient, including distinguishing lymphatic from venous obstruction, maximizes the chances for successful therapy.

A. General measures. Reduction in total body fluids by salt restriction and diuretic therapy can somewhat reduce extremity lymphedema. Elevation of the affected extremity when possible and avoidance of strenuous muscular activities can also be of limited benefit. A fitted elastic stocking, encompassing the affected extremity and worn while nonrecumbent, can alleviate some of the aching and heaviness associated with this complication. A trial of intermittent elevated extremity pressures using a pneumatic pump occasionally enhances the development of collateral lymphatic channels.

B. Surgery. Patients without evidence of neoplasm and with lower extremity lymphedema owing to fibrotic obliteration of the lymphatic system have, on occasion, improved following placement of an omental graft across the area of prior high-dose irradiation to reestablish a lush lymphatic pathway.

C. Radiotherapy. Lymphatic blockage with distal lymphedema caused by metastatic lymphadenopathy usually responds best to local irradiation, although the probability of totally reversing the process is less than 50% except in highly radiosensitive tumors, such as the lymphomas. Because the local tumor burden is obviously great, relatively high doses of irradiation are required. High-dose irradiation carries with it high risks of late radiation fibrosis and reexacerbation of initial symptoms should the patient survive several years. The optimal radiation dose in the patient with reasonable life expectancy and regional metastatic carcinoma is 60–65 Gy over 6–7 weeks. Patients with poor prognosis can be treated with 30–40 Gy over 2–3 weeks for optimal results.

D. Chemotherapy. Because lymphedema is not an emergency, systemic therapy with drugs or hormones can also be utilized in lieu of local irradiation for attempted relief of symptoms. Breast and prostate carcinomas and the lymphomas are associated with higher expectations of response than many other neoplasms, for which a lower probability of remission exists. In the latter cases, combined-modality therapy with local irradiation and systemic therapy can provide maximal benefit.

Selected Reading

Ahmann, F. R. A reassessment of the clinical implications of the superior vena caval syndrome. *J. Clin. Oncol.* 2:961, 1984.

Davenport, D., et al. Radiation therapy in the treatment of superior vena caval obstruction. *Cancer* 42:2600, 1978.

Dougherty, T. J. Photodynamic therapy. *Clin. Chest Med.* 6:219, 1985.

Dougherty, T. J. Photodynamic therapy of malignant tumors. *CRC Crit. Rev. Oncol. Hematol.* 2:83, 1984.

Fair, W. Urologic emergencies. In V. T. DeVita (ed.), *Cancer Principles and Practice of Oncology* (3rd ed.). Philadelphia: Lippincott, 1989. Pp. 2016–2028.

Fielding, L. P., Stewart-Brown, S., and Blesovsky, L. Large bowel obstruction caused by cancer: a prospective study. *Br. Med. J.* 2:515, 1979.

Kanji, A., et al. Extrinsic compression of superior vena cava: an analysis of 41 patients. *Int. J. Radiat. Oncol. Biol. Phys.* 6:213, 1980.

Kessel, D. Hematoporphyria and HPD: photophysics, photochemistry, and phototherapy. *Photochem. Photobiol.* 39:851, 1984.

MacCarthy, R. Nonsurgical management of obstructive jaundice in the patient with advanced cancer. *J.A.M.A.* 244:1976, 1980.

McNamara, T. E., and Butkus, D. E. Nephrostomy in patients with ureteral obstruction secondary to nonurologic malignancies. *Arch. Intern. Med.* 140:494, 1980.

Mellow, M., and Pinkos, H. Endoscopic therapy for esophageal carcinoma with Nd-YAG laser: prospective evaluation of efficacy, complications, and survival. *Gastrointest. Endosc.* 30:334, 1984.

Meyer, J. E. Palliative urinary diversion in patients with advanced pelvic malignancy. *Cancer* 45:2698, 1980.

Montague, E., and Delclos, L. Palliative radiotherapy in the management of metastatic disease. In G. H. Fletcher (ed.), *Textbook of Radiotherapy* (3rd ed.). Philadelphia: Lea & Febiger, 1980. Pp. 943–948.

Oho, K., et al. Indications for endoscopic Nd-YAG laser surgery in the trachea and bronchus. *Endoscopy* 15:302, 1983.

Osteen, R. T., et al. Malignant intestinal obstruction. *Surgery* 87:611, 1980.

Scarantino, C., et al. The optimum radiation schedule in treatment of superior vena caval obstruction: importance of ^{99m}Tc scintiangiograms. *Int. J. Radiat. Oncol. Biol. Phys.* 5:1987, 1979.

Shapshay, S. Laser therapy for the cancer patient. In V. T. DeVita (ed.), *Cancer Principles and Practice of Oncology* (2nd ed.). Philadelphia: Lippincott, 1985. Pp. 2326–2331.

Sharer, W., et al. Palliative urinary diversion for malignant ureteral obstruction. *J. Urol.* 120:162, 1978.

Singh, B., et al. Stent versus nephrostomy: is there a choice? *J. Urol.* 121:268, 1979.

Sise, J. G., and Crichlow, R. W. Obstruction due to malignant tumors. *Semin. Oncol.* 5:213, 1978.

Wilson, R. Surgical emergencies: obstructive disease. In V. T. DeVita (ed.), *Cancer Principles and Practice of Oncology* (3rd ed.). Philadelphia: Lippincott, 1989. Pp. 2008–2012.

Yahalom, J. Superior vena cava syndrome. In V. T. DeVita (ed.), *Cancer Principles and Practice of Oncology* (3rd ed.). Philadelphia: Lippincott, 1989. Pp. 1971–1978.

Malignant Pleural, Peritoneal, and Pericardial Effusions and Meningeal Infiltrates

Walter D. Y. Quan and Roland T. Skeel

Malignant pleural, peritoneal, and pericardial effusions and malignant meningeal infiltrates are uncommon early in the course of the malignancy. They occur more frequently with disseminated disease and often herald a poor prognosis. Although pleural and peritoneal effusions may initially have little adverse effect on quality of life, when progressive they (as well as pericardial effusions and meningeal infiltrates) can result in incapacitating disability and death. It is therefore necessary for the clinician to have a high index of suspicion for these problems and to be prepared to take appropriate action and deliver palliative treatment promptly.

I. Pleural effusions

A. Causes. Malignant pleural effusions arise in association with malignant cells lining the pleura, exuded into the pleural space, or blocking veins or lymphatics. The most common malignancy associated with pleural effusions in women is carcinoma of the breast, whereas in men it is carcinoma of the lung. Other causes of malignant pleural effusions include lymphoma, mesothelioma, and carcinomas of the ovary, gastrointestinal tract, urinary tract, and uterus. Malignancy is not the only cause of effusions even in patients with known neoplastic disease, and therefore it is important to attempt to rule out other possible causes such as congestive heart failure, infection, and pulmonary infarction.

B. Diagnosis

1. **Clinical diagnosis.** Effusions may be asymptomatic or may be suspected because of respiratory symptoms, such as shortness of breath with exertion or at rest, orthopnea, paroxysmal nocturnal dyspnea, or occasionally chest pressure or cough. The patient may feel more comfortable when lying on one side when the effusion is unilateral. On physical examination dullness to percussion, decreased tactile fremitus, diminished breath sounds, and egophony are typical signs over the area of the effusion.

2. **A chest x-ray film** should be obtained to confirm the clinical impression. If fluid appears to be present, a lateral decubitus film must be obtained to help estimate the volume of the effusion and how free it is within the pleural space.

3. **Diagnostic thoracentesis** should be performed. Ultrasonographic guidance is helpful if loculation is present. Fluid should be obtained for bacterial and fungal cultures, cytologic examination, protein concentration (> 3.0 gm/dl in most exudates), and cell

count. The cytologic examination is important because if it is positive, as in 50–70% of cases with malignant effusion, the diagnosis is established. Other studies of the pleural fluid that may be helpful in establishing that the fluid is an exudate and not a transudate include a specific gravity of more than 1.015, protein concentration that is more than 0.5 times the serum protein concentration, lactic dehydrogenase (LDH) level more than 0.6 times the serum LDH level, and low glucose level. A cytologic examination of fluid from a newly discovered pleural effusion is wise, regardless of whether the patient is known to have malignancy, because for nearly one-half of all malignant effusions this finding is the first sign of malignancy. The role of analyzing the pleural fluid for tumor markers such as carcinoembryonic antigen (CEA) and human chorionic gonadotropin (β-hCG) has yet to be determined. Likewise, the utility of monoclonal antibodies and gene rearrangement studies in patients with lymphomas to distinguish reactive mesothelial or lymphocytic cells from malignant cells is under investigation but has not been established as clinically useful.

4. **Pleural biopsy** may be helpful in establishing the diagnosis in up to 20% of cases in which the pleural fluid cytology is negative.

5. **Thoracotomy and open biopsy** may be done in patients who have negative cytology and pleural biopsy but about whom there is still high suspicion of malignancy.

C. **Treatment.** As malignant pleural effusions are generally a sign of systemic rather than localized disease, the best therapy is treatment that effectively treats the malignancy systemically. Unfortunately, effective systemic treatment is often not possible, particularly when the malignancy is commonly refractory to systemic treatment (e.g., in non-small-cell carcinoma of the lung) or in patients who have previously been heavily treated and systemic therapy is no longer effective. In these circumstances, local-regional therapy is required for palliation of the patient's symptoms.

1. **Drainage.** Most malignant pleural effusions recur within 1–3 days after simple thoracentesis; about 97% recur within 1 month. Chest tube drainage (closed tube thoracotomy) allows the pleural surfaces to oppose each other and, if maintained for several days, may result in obliteration of the space and improvement in the effusion for several weeks to months. It does not appear to be as effective when used alone as when a cytotoxic or sclerosing agent is added, and therefore one of these agents is commonly instilled into the space while the chest tube is in place.

2. **Cytotoxic and sclerosing agents.** A wide variety of agents, including radioactive isotopes (gold, phos-

phorus, yttrium), talc, tetracycline, quinacrine, mechlorethamine, thiotepa, fluorouracil, bleomycin, and *Corynebacterium parvum* have been used to treat pleural effusions. All are of similar effectiveness but vary in toxicity and ease of administration. All require the pleural fluid to be drained as completely as possible prior to instillation for maximal effectiveness.

    a. Method of administration. The drug to be used is diluted in 50–100 ml of saline and instilled through the thoracostomy tube into the chest cavity after the effusion has been drained for at least 24 hours and the rate of collection is less than 100 ml/24 hours. Throughout the procedure, care must be taken to avoid any air leak. The thoracostomy tube is clamped, and the patient is successively repositioned on his or her front, back, and sides for 15-minute periods over the next 2–6 hours. The tube is then reconnected to gravity drainage or suction for at least 18 hours to ensure that the pleural surfaces remain opposed and to prevent the rapid accumulation of any fluid in reaction to the instillation. Some clinicians repeat the instillation daily for a total of 2–3 days, although the value of this practice is not certain. If the drainage is less than 40–50 ml over the previous 12 hours, the tube may be removed and a chest x-ray film obtained to be certain that pneumothorax has not occurred during removal of the tube. If the thoracostomy tube continues to drain more than 100 ml/24 hours after the last instillation, it may be necessary to leave it in place for an additional 48–72 hours to ensure that a maximum amount of adhesion between the pleural surfaces has taken place.

  b. Recommended agents

    (1) Bleomycin 1 mg/kg or 40 mg/m^2, has relatively little myelosuppressive effect and is highly effective.

    (2) Tetracycline 500–1000 mg also has the advantage of being nonmyelosuppressive. [An injection of 10 ml of 1% lidocaine (100 mg) through the chest tube prior to tetracycline often reduces the pleuritic pain associated with the agent.]

  c. Alternative agents

    (1) Mechlorethamine (nitrogen mustard) 8–16 mg/m^2. Systemic effects, including nausea, vomiting, and myelosuppression, are seen. Mechlorethamine may have an advantage because it is locally cytotoxic, particularly in the lymphomas.

    (2) Thiotepa 20–30 mg/m^2 causes less intense inflammation and therefore less pain than mechlorethamine. It also causes less nausea.

> > (3) **Fluorouracil** 500 mg/m^2, may have a theoretical advantage in sensitive carcinomas, but whether that advantage is significant is not yet established.
> >
> > (4) *Corynebacterium parvum* 7 mg in 20 ml saline may cause nausea, chest pain, and higher fever than the other agents.
>
> > d. **Responses.** A combination of chest tube drainage and instillation of one of the agents discussed in **I.C.2.b,c** controls pleural effusions more than 75% of the time. The durations of response are short, with a median between 3 and 6 months unless the patient's systemic disease comes under adequate control. In that circumstance the effusion may not recur for years or at least until the systemic disease once more emerges.
> >
> > e. **Side effects** common to most agents include chest pain, fever, and occasional hypotension. These effects are usually not severe and may be controlled by standard symptomatic management.
>
> 3. **Thoracotomy and pleural stripping** may be tried subsequently for effusions refractory to medical treatment.

II. Peritoneal Effusions

> A. **Causes.** Malignant peritoneal effusions usually occur in association with diffuse seeding of the peritoneal surface with small malignant deposits. The impairment of subphrenic lymphatic or portal venous flow may result in peritoneal effusions. Alternatively, it has been postulated that a "capillary leak" phenomenon mediated by tumor cells or immune effector cells could be a contributing factor. Carcinoma of the ovary is the most commonly associated malignancy in women, whereas in men gastrointestinal carcinomas are most common. Other neoplasms that may cause peritoneal effusions include lymphoma, mesothelioma, and carcinomas of the uterus and breast. Liver metastasis by itself, unless it is far advanced, is not usually associated with symptomatic peritoneal effusions.
>
> B. **Diagnosis**
>
> > 1. **Symptoms and signs.** Patients may be completely asymptomatic or have so much fluid that they have severe abdominal distension, abdominal pain, and respiratory distress. In the presence of peritoneal metastases, there may be abnormal bowel motility that at times resembles a paralytic ileus and may result in loss of appetite, early satiety, nausea, and vomiting. On examination, the lower abdomen and flanks bulge when the patient is supine. Confirmatory signs include shifting dullness, a fluid wave, diminished bowel sounds, or the "puddle sign" (periumbilical dullness when the patient rests on knees and elbows).
> >
> > 2. **Radiographic studies.** Ascites may be suggested on a recumbent film of the abdomen, although x-ray

films are less sensitive than computed tomography (CT) for detecting fluid. CT is also helpful for defining whether there are enlarged retroperitoneal nodes, tumor masses in the abdomen or pelvis, or liver metastases in association with the ascites.

3. **Paracentesis** is used to distinguish malignancy from other causes of peritoneal effusions, including congestive heart failure, hepatic cirrhosis, and peritonitis. Malignant cells are found in about one-half of patients in whom the effusion is due to malignancy. Other tests are less reliable, and treatment decisions must often be based on incomplete data. Elevated lactate dehydrogenase (LDH) and protein along with a negative Gram's stain and cultures are supportive but nonspecific for malignancy. The use of monoclonal antibodies to identify tumor cells is still experimental.

C. **Therapy.** As with malignant pleural effusions, malignant peritoneal effusions as a rule are optimally treated with effective systemic therapy. (The possible exception to this is peritoneal effusions from carcinoma of the ovary. In this circumstance, there may be advantage to intraperitoneal therapy because most systemic disease is on the peritoneal surface.) If the patient is resistant to all further systemic treatment, regional treatment should be tried, but the likelihood of success is less and the complications are greater with peritoneal effusions than with pleural effusions. Success probably is less because of the greater likelihood of loculations to areas inaccessible to therapy and the impossibility of obliterating the peritoneal space in the same way that the pleural space can be obliterated. Complications are greater because of the increase in adhesions caused by instillation therapy and the resultant increase in obstructive bowel problems.

1. **Paracentesis** may be helpful in acutely relieving intraabdominal pressure. If the ascites has caused impairment of respiration, paracentesis may thus give temporary relief. Rapid withdrawal of large volumes of fluid (> 1 liter) can result in hypotension and shock, however; and if frequent paracenteses are performed, severe hypoalbuminemia and electrolyte imbalance may result. Repeated procedures could also subject the patient to increased risk for peritonitis or bowel injury. This procedure thus results in only temporary benefit.

2. **Bed rest and dietary salt restriction,** although helpful in the treatment of various nonmalignant causes of ascites, is of less benefit in malignant ascites.

3. **Diuretics** may be helpful in reducing ascites, but care must be taken not to be too vigorous in attempts at diuresis because of the possibility of dehydration and hypotension. A reasonable choice of diuretic is a combination of hydrochlorothiazide 50–100 mg daily and spironolactone 50–100 mg daily.

4. **Intracavitary therapy.** Radioisotopes, cytotoxic drugs, and sclerosing agents have been used with some benefit for treating malignant ascites; but, overall, probably fewer than one-half of patients have a satisfactory response. The utility of these agents has less to do with direct tumor cytotoxicity and more with the induction of a local inflammatory response with subsequent sclerosis. The radioactive isotopes ^{198}Au and ^{32}P should be used only by those with experience and appropriate certification. Cytotoxic agents such as thiotepa are associated with less risk to the person administering the therapy.

a. **Method.** The peritoneal fluid should be drained slowly through a Tenckhoff catheter over a 24 to 36-hour period. The potential distribution of the therapeutic agent can be determined by instilling ^{99}Tc glucoheptonate macroaggregated albumin in 50 ml of saline and obtaining an abdominal scintigram. Two liters of warmed 1.5% peritoneal dialysis solution is instilled, allowed to remain for 2 hours, and then drained. The chemotherapeutic agent is next mixed with 2 liters of fresh 1.5% dialysate solution containing 1000 units of heparin/liter. After warming, this solution is instilled through the Tenckhoff catheter. For some agents draining after 4 hours is recommended, but for others it is not.

b. **Agents**

(1) **Bleomycin** 150 units. Drainage is recommended. The dose is repeated weekly for 3 weeks.

(2) **Thiotepa** 20–30 mg/m². Drainage is optional. Thiotepa is likely to cause myelosuppression, and so the dose should not be repeated until blood counts have returned to normal, and then only if there has been objective improvement in the ascites.

(3) **Cisplatin** 50–100 mg/m² (for carcinoma of the ovary). Drainage is optional. Saline diuresis is recommended. Dosages higher than 100 mg/m² should not be used without protection by intravenous sodium thiosulfate. The dose is repeated every 3 weeks. Systemic toxicity is to be expected.

(4) **Other agents** used intraperitoneally include nitrogen mustard, cytosine arabinoside, fluorouracil, methotrexate, and doxorubicin. These days are not recommended at this time for routine use. Monoclonal antibodies conjugated to radioactive isotopes such as ^{131}I and ^{90}Y are undergoing clinical trials.

III. **Pericardial effusions.** Although 5–10% of patients dying with disseminated malignancy have cardiac or pericardial metastases, far fewer have symptomatic pericardial effusion. However, although malignant pericardial effusions are not particularly common, they are of great importance because of their potential to cause acute cardiac tamponade and death.

A. Causes. The most common neoplasms causing pericardial effusions are carcinomas of the lung and breast, leukemias, lymphomas, and melanoma.

B. Diagnosis

1. **Clinical diagnosis.** Patients with developing cardiac tamponade may exhibit a variety of grave symptoms, including extreme anxiety, dyspnea, orthopnea, precordial chest pain, cough, and hoarseness. On examination, they are likely to have engorged neck veins, generalized edema, tachycardia, distant heart tones, lateral displacement of the cardiac apex, a low systolic blood pressure and low pulse pressure, and a paradoxical pulse. They may also have tachypnea and a pericardial friction rub.

2. **Electrocardiogram** (ECG) may show nonspecific low voltage, T wave abnormalities, elevation of ST segments, and ventricular alterans or the more specific total electrical alterans.

3. **Chest x-ray film** typically shows an enlarged cardiac silhouette, often with a bulging appearance suggestive of an effusion. There is frequently an associated pleural effusion.

4. **Echocardiography** can confirm the diagnosis and provide important information on the location of the effusion within the pericardium.

5. **Pericardiocentesis** reveals neoplastic cells on cytologic examination in more than 75% of patients.

C. Treatment

1. **Volume expansion and vasopressor support** is applied (if necessary) to maintain blood pressure. Adequate oxygenation must be maintained.

2. **Pericardiocentesis** under ECG and blood pressure monitoring should be done in emergent circumstances. If the patient can be stabilized or in cases of pericardial effusion without tamponade, pericardiocentesis under two-dimensional echocardiography is preferable as it significantly reduces the incidence of cardiac laceration, arrhythmia, and tension pneumothorax as a complication of the procedure.

3. **Instillation of chemotherapeutic or sclerosing agents.** Because pain may be associated with the intrapericardial therapy, xylocaine 100 mg may be administered intrapericardially as a local anesthetic. (Check with the cardiologist on the safety for each patient.) After the cytotoxic or sclerosing agent is instilled, the pericardial catheter is clamped for 1–2 hours and then allowed to drain. One of the following agents may be used.

   a. **Tetracycline** 500–1000 mg in 10 ml of normal saline. The dose may be repeated every 2–3 days until the pericardial drainage has slowed to less than 25 ml during the preceding 24 hours.

      b. Fluorouracil 500–1000 mg in aqueous solution as supplied commercially. This dose is generally not repeated.

      c. Thiotepa 25 mg/m^2 in 10 ml of normal saline may be preferred in tumor deemed sensitive to alkylating agents. Myelosuppression may occur. The dose is usually not repeated.

    Complications of intrapericardial therapy include arrhythmias, pain, and fever.

  4. Radiotherapy with radioisotopes or 2000–4000 cGy external beam therapy may help control effusions.

  5. Systemic chemotherapy (with standard regimens) following pericardiocentesis is a possible alternative for newly diagnosed, potentially responsive malignancies such as leukemias and selected lymphomas. Chemotherapy, intrapericardial or systemic, or radiotherapy controls the effusion for at least 30 days in 60–70% of patients. If they are ineffective, surgical intervention to create a pericardial window may be necessary and can be effective for several months. It is not recommended, however, unless simpler measures fail.

IV. Malignant subarachnoid infiltrates

  A. Causes. Leptomeningeal involvement with non-central-nervous-system (CNS) cancer is an uncommon complication of most neoplasms, although in children with acute lymphocytic leukemia who have not received prophylactic treatment the incidence approaches 50%. Of the nonleukemic diseases, breast carcinoma and lymphomas account for about 30% each in cases of malignant subarachnoid infiltrates. Carcinoma of the lung and melanoma account for 10–12% each.

  B. Diagnosis

    1. Clinical diagnosis. Patients commonly present with headache, change in mental status, cranial nerve dysfunction, or spinal root-derived pain, paresthesia, or weakness. Any onset of change in neurologic status, particularly of cerebral, cranial nerve, or spinal root origin, should alert the clinician to the possibility of subarachnoid infiltrates.

    2. Radiologic studies

      a. Myelography may be helpful for finding large infiltrates that may cause cord compression and for identifying areas that may benefit from radiotherapy.

      b. CT or magnetic resonance imaging (MRI) can demonstrate tumor masses in the brain parenchyma or meninges, hydrocephalus, and evidence of increased intracranial pressure.

  C. Treatment. Malignant subarachnoid infiltrates may be treated with radiotherapy, intrathecal chemotherapy, or a combination of the two.

    1. Radiotherapy. The radiation field is usually limited to the most involved field (frequently the brain), and intrathecal chemotherapy is used to control the infiltrates elsewhere. This technique is used even though the entire neuraxis is usually involved because total craniospinal irradiation causes severe myelosuppression, which limits the patient's tolerance to concurrent or subsequent cytotoxic chemotherapy.

2. **Chemotherapy** may be administered by lumbar puncture or preferably into a surgically implanted (Ommaya) reservoir that communicates with the lateral ventricle. The latter has the advantages of being easily accessible in patients who require repeated treatments and of giving a better distribution of drug than can be obtained via lumbar puncture. When the Ommaya reservoir is used, a volume of cerebrospinal fluid (CSF) equal to that to be injected (6–10 ml) should be removed through the reservoir with a small-caliber needle. The chemotherapy should then be given as a slow injection. When the chemotherapy is given via lumbar puncture, the volume of injection (usually 7–10 ml) should be greater than that of the CSF withdrawn in order to have a higher closing than opening pressure. This method facilitates distribution of the drug and minimizes postlumbar puncture headache. The most commonly used drugs are the following.

   a. **Methotrexate** 12 mg/m^2 (maximum 15 mg) twice weekly until the CSF clears of malignant cells, then monthly.

   b. **Cytarabine** 30 mg/m^2 twice weekly until the CSF clears of malignant cells, then monthly.

   c. **Thiotepa** 2–10 mg/m^2 twice weekly until the CSF clears of malignant cells, then monthly.

   Each of the agents is given in preservative-free saline or, if available, buffered preservative-free diluent similar to Elliot's B solution. Any subsequent flush solution should be of similar composition. Other drugs used to treat effusions, e.g., fluorouracil, mechlorethamine, or radioisotopes, *must not* be used to treat meningeal disease.

3. **Immunotherapy with intrathecal interleukin-2** has been described, but experience concerning response and toxicity is currently insufficient.

D. **Response to treatment.** Most patients with meningeal leukemia or lymphoma respond to a combination of radiotherapy and intrathecal chemotherapy. Carcinomas are less likely to improve, but mild to moderate improvement may be seen in up to 50% of patients.

E. **Complications.** Aseptic meningitis or arachnoiditis, seizures, acute encephalopathy, myelopathy, leukoencephalopathy, and radicular neuropathy may result from intrathecal chemotherapy with or without radiotherapy.

Bone marrow suppression is not usually severe unless the patient undergoes spinal irradiation or systemic chemotherapy as well. Oral leucovorin can be given after the intrathecal methotrexate (10 mg leucovorin PO q6h × 6–8 doses, starting 24 hours after the methotrexate) to prevent marrow toxicity. Serious complications are infrequent, however, and in patients with advanced metastatic disease they usually are not a major problem.

Selected Reading

Pleural Effusions

Bayly, D. D., et al. Tetracycline and quinacrine in the control of malignant pleural effusions: a randomized trial. *Cancer* 41:118, 1978.

Chernow, B., and Sahn, S. A. Carcinomatous involvement of the pleura: an analysis of 96 patients. *Am. J. Med.* 63:695, 1977.

Friedman, M. A., and Slater, E. Malignant pleural effusions. *Cancer Treat. Rev.* 5:49, 1978.

Hausheer, F. H. and Yarbro, J. W. Diagnosis and treatment of malignant pleural effusions. *Cancer Metastasis Rev.* 6:23, 1987.

Johnson, W. W. The malignant pleural effusion: a review of cytopathologic diagnoses of 584 specimens from 472 consecutive patients. *Cancer* 56:905, 1985.

Ostrowski, M. J. Intracavitary therapy with bleomycin for the treatment of malignant pleural effusions. *J. Surg. Oncol. (suppl. 1):*7, 1989.

Ostrowski, M. J., and Halsall, G. M. Intracavitary bleomycin in the management of malignant effusions: a multicenter study. *Cancer Treat. Rep.* 66:1903, 1982.

Pavesi, F., et al. Detection of malignant pleural effusions by tumor marker evaluation. *Eur. J. Cancer Clin. Oncol.* 24:1005, 1988.

Tamura, S., et al. Tumor markers in pleural effusion diagnosis. *Cancer* 61:198, 1988.

Van Hoff, D. D., and LiVolsi, V. Diagnostic reliability of needle biopsy of the parietal pleura: a review of 272 biopsies. *Am. J. Clin. Pathol.* 64:200, 1975.

Peritoneal Effusions

Baker, A. R. Treatment of malignant ascites. In V. I. DeVita, S. Hellman, and S. A. Rosenberg (eds.), *Cancer: Principles and Practice of Oncology* (3rd ed.). Philadelphia: Lippincott, 1989. P. 2317.

Bitran, J. D. Intraperitoneal bleomycin: pharmacokinetics and results of a phase II trial. *Cancer* 56:2420, 1985.

Lacy, J. H., et al. Management of malignant ascites. *Surg. Gynecol. Obstet.* 159:397, 1984.

Papac, R. J. Treatment of malignant disease in closed spaces. In F. F. Baker (ed.), *Cancer, A Comprehensive Treatise* (Vol. 5). New York: Plenum, 1977.

Pericardial Effusions

Buzaid, A. C., et al. Managing malignant pericardial effusion. *West. J. Med.* 150:174, 1989.

Callahan, J. A., et al. Two-dimensional echocardiographically guided pericardiocentesis: experience in 117 consecutive patients. *Am. J. Cardiol.* 55:476, 1985.

Helms, S. R., and Carlson, M. D. Cardiovascular emergencies. *Semin. Oncol.* 16:463, 1989.

Shepherd, F. A., et al. Tetracycline sclerosis in the management of pericardial effusion. *J. Clin. Oncol.* 3:1678, 1985.

Theologides, A. Neoplastic cardiac tamponade. *Semin. Oncol.* 5:181, 1978.

Malignant Subarachnoid Infiltrates

Gutin, P. H., et al. Treatment of malignant meningeal disease with intrathecal thiotepa: a phase II study. *Cancer Treat. Rep.* 61:885, 1977.

Hubbard, S. M., et al. Administration of cancer treatments: practical guide for physicians and oncology nurses. In V. T. DeVita, S. Hellman, and S. A. Rosenberg (eds.), *Cancer: Principles and Practice of Oncology* (3rd ed.). Philadelphia: Lippincott, 1989. P. 2384.

Mitchell, M. S. Relapse in the central nervous system in melanoma patients successfully treated with biomodulators. *J. Clin. Oncol.* 7:1701, 1989.

Olson, M. E., et al. Infiltration of the leptomeninges by systemic cancer. *Arch. Neurol.* 30:122, 1974.

Infections: Etiology, Treatment, and Prevention

Rodger D. MacArthur

I. **Overview.** Infection is a major source of morbidity and mortality among patients with cancer, despite advances in prevention and treatment. In many series, infection is the most frequent cause of death, exceeding all other causes combined. Granulocytopenia, cellular immune dysfunction, humoral immune dysfunction, and splenectomy can predispose patients to certain types of infection. In addition, mucosal or integumentary damage, prolonged hospitalization, lack of ambulation, malnutrition, neurologic dysfunction, and local tumor effect contribute to the risk of infection.

Most bacterial and fungal infections in patients with cancer arise from their own flora. Environmental reservoirs also contribute to infection in certain circumstances. Prolonged hospitalization and antibiotic use tend to favor the acquisition of resistant strains of organisms. Careful hand washing by health care workers is the most important means of reducing the occurrence of infection. Reverse isolation of patients can be justified only rarely. The prompt initiation of therapy with broad-spectrum antibiotics in documented and suspected bacterial infections is essential. The addition of antifungal therapy should be considered in patients who do not respond within a reasonable period to antibiotics. Daily reevaluation of all patients is critical.

II. **Reasons for infection**
   A. **Granulocytopenia**
   1. **General comments.** Acute leukemias or lymphomas after chemotherapy are prototypical malignancies in which infection resulting from granulocytopenia is seen. An increase in the incidence of infection can be expected when the granulocyte count is less than $500/\mu l$. A substantial increase in the incidence and severity of infection occurs when there are fewer than 100 granulocytes/μl. Infection early in the course of granulocytopenia typically is caused by relatively nonresistant endogenous bacteria. Fungal infections and infection with resistant bacteria most often occur during prolonged periods of granulocytopenia.
   2. **Sites of infection.** Damage to skin and mucosal membranes (e.g., from venipuncture or chemotherapy) greatly increases the risk of infection in granulocytopenic patients. The integument, periodontium, oropharynx, colon, and perianal area are common foci from which organisms can seed the bloodstream and disseminate. Pneumonia typically is caused by bacteria that have colonized the oropharynx.
   3. **Microbiology**
      a. **Gram-negative bacteria.** *Escherichia coli, Klebsiella pneumoniae,* and *Pseudomonas aeruginosa*

predominate. *Enterobacter cloacae, Acinetobacter anitratum, Serratia marcescens, Pseudomonas cepacia,* and *Xanthomonas maltophilia* are less common, but still important, pathogens.

b. Gram-positive bacteria. Infection with either *Staphylococcus epidermidis* or *Staphylococcus aureus* is now almost as common as infection with gram-negative bacteria. The increase in gram-positive infections is probably due to the increase in the use of central venous catheters. *Corynebacterium* JK occasionally is found in association with catheter infections.

c. Fungi. *Candida* and *Aspergillus* species and the agents of mucormycosis are the important pathogens. *Pseudallescheria boydii* is seen less frequently.

B. Cellular immune dysfunction

1. General comments. Cellular immune dysfunction and its associated infections can result from the underlying disease or from antineoplastic agents and corticosteroids. Hodgkin's disease or acute lymphocytic leukemia (ALL) in long-term remission are characteristic malignancies in which cellular immune dysfunction-related infection is encountered.

2. Microbiology

a. Bacteria. *Legionella pneumophila* is of special concern, as are the *Nocardia* species. Nocardiosis typically presents with one or more lesions in the lung, skin, and brain. Infections caused by *Salmonella* species and *Listeria monocytogenes* are considerably less frequent.

b. Mycobacteria. *Mycobacterium avium/Mycobacterium intracellulare* is being seen with increasing frequency in patients with non-Hodgkin's lymphomas receiving intensive cytotoxic therapy. The incidence of infection with *Mycobacterium kansasii* is increased in patients with hairy-cell leukemia. *Mycobacterium tuberculosis* is surprisingly unusual in patients with cancer with altered cell-mediated immunity.

c. Fungi. *Cryptococcus neoformans* is seen frequently. Meningitis is the most common presentation, but pulmonary and cutaneous infections also occur.

d. Viruses. Herpes zoster virus, causing either varicella or zoster, is particularly common in this group of patients. Varicella can be life-threatening in children with ALL, causing pneumonitis, purpura fulminans, and encephalitis. Oropharyngeal or esophageal lesions due to herpes simplex virus can predispose to infection with bacterial or fungal pathogens. Cytomegalovirus (CMV) is seen most often in patients undergoing bone marrow transplantation.

e. Protozoa and parasites. *Pneumocystis carinii* is a frequent cause of pneumonia, especially in children with ALL. Infection with *Toxoplasmosis gondii* presents as either chorioretinitis or cerebral abscesses. *Strongyloides stercoralis* can cause diarrhea or life-threatening disseminated infections. Diffuse pulmonary infiltrates, shock, and sepsis due to enteric gram-negative bacilli are the typical features of disseminated strongyloidiasis.

C. Humoral immune dysfunction

1. **General comments.** Agammaglobulinemic or hypogammaglobulinemic patients are susceptible to infections because they often lack opsonizing antibodies to the common encapsulated pyogenic bacteria. Many of these patients also have deficient functional complement activity. Multiple myeloma or chronic lymphocytic leukemia are prototypical neoplasms with humoral immune dysfunction.

2. **Microbiology.** *Streptococcus pneumoniae* predominates. In addition, decreased complement activity increases the risk of infection by *Hemophilus influenzae, Neisseria meningitidis,* and *Escherichia coli.*

D. Splenectomy

1. **General comments.** The spleen is the organ most efficient at removing nonopsonized bacteria. Specific opsonizing antibodies are required for effective killing of the encapsulated bacteria. Thus splenectomized patients are at risk of overwhelming sepsis when infected with a strain of encapsulated bacteria against which they have never had an opportunity to make antibodies.

2. **Microbiology.** Infections are usually caused by *Streptococcus pneumoniae* and, to a lesser extent, *Hemophilus influenzae* and *Neisseria meningitidis.*

E. Other factors

1. **Indwelling vascular catheters** increase the risk of bacterial and fungal infections. The risk increases with the length of time they have been in place. Concurrent granulocytopenia magnifies the infection risk.

2. **Nonambulation and length of stay** have been identified as independent risk factors for infection in most studies. Other factors, e.g., previous antibiotic use and the presence of a Foley catheter, are correlated with nonambulation and length of stay but are not themselves independent risk factors for infection.

3. **Malnutrition and neurologic dysfunction.** Whether malnutrition is an independent risk factor for immunosuppression is controversial. On the other hand, malnourished patients who require enteral feedings are certainly at increased risk for aspiration. Loss of the gag reflex also increases the risk of aspiration. Loss of sensation facilitates the development of cutaneous ulcers.

4. **Local tumor effect.** Complete or partial obstruction by tumor may lead to infection behind the ob-

struction. Postobstructive pneumonia in a patient with bronchogenic cancer and ascending cholangitis in a patient with an intraabdominal lymphoma are two examples of this phenomenon.

III. Diagnosis of infection

A. Clinical findings that suggest the diagnosis of infection

1. **Symptoms**
   a. **General.** Malaise, fatigue, confusion, or other nonspecific or subtle symptoms may be the first indication of infection. Any unexplained change in the patient's condition should be evaluated clinically and microbiologically.
   b. **Localizing.** Symptoms referable to a particular organ system are particularly worrisome and demand an immediate and thorough evaluation.

2. **Signs**
   a. **Fever** is the single most important indicator of infection in cancer patients. Often it is the only abnormal finding. Never assume that an unexplained fever is due to the underlying malignancy. Similarly, never rely exclusively on fever to diagnose infection: Debilitated or elderly patients occasionally are afebrile in the presence of infection.
   b. **Hypotension and shock** occur with a variety of infections; they are not specific for infections caused by gram-negative bacteria.
   c. **Tachycardia,** especially if new or unexplained, also suggests infection.
   d. **Inflammation,** if present, suggests underlying infection. Note, however, that granulocytopenic patients often fail to show a normal inflammatory response to infection. Consequently, bacterial pneumonia can present without an identifiable infiltrate on chest x-ray film or even without significant sputum production. Similarly, abscess formation is often minimal or absent despite significant local or systemic infection.

3. **Leukocytosis,** especially when accompanied by an increase in neutrophils or band-form neutrophils, suggests infection. Of course, patients who are leukopenic owing to chemotherapy do not have this response. Toxic granulation of neutrophils also suggests infection.

B. Evaluation of patients with suspected infection

1. **General.** A thorough, daily evaluation of all patients with cancer is necessary to properly diagnose and treat infections. Areas that should not be overlooked include the retinae, ears and sinuses, mouth, skin, catheter sites, axillae, perineum, perianal region, and extremities.

2. **Cultures**
   a. **General approach.** Samples for cultures need to be obtained from multiple sites whenever infection is suspected. All culture material must be

delivered promptly to the microbiology laboratory.

b. Blood

    (1) Technique. At least two sets of blood (in aerobic and anaerobic bottles) should be obtained, each set being from a different site. At least 5 ml of blood is injected into each culture bottle.

    (2) Central venous catheters. If these indwelling devices are present, it is important to obtain additional cultures through each port of the device, as well as to obtain peripheral specimens in the usual manner.

    (3) Resin bottles. Culture bottles containing an antibiotic-binding resin or other antibiotic binding substance should be included with each culture set for patients who are receiving antibiotics at the time of evaluation.

c. Urine. Clean-catch or straight-catheterization specimens are preferred. Urine that has been present in a closed collection system for more than an hour should not be sent for culture. If necessary, urine can be obtained from the catheter tubing using a syringe and a small-gauge needle.

d. Sputum

    (1) Spontaneously expectorated. A good specimen should have fewer than 10 squamous epithelial cells per low-power ($100 \times$) field.

    (2) Induced. The yield on culture can be increased by using 3% saline delivered through an ultrasonic nebulizer. Three percent saline can cause significant bronchospasm and should be administered cautiously only by trained personnel.

    (3) Transtracheal aspiration. This procedure is used rarely. More commonly, patients are bronchoscoped or undergo open lung biopsy if pulmonary pathology is suspected and the first two techniques fail to provide an answer.

e. Cerebrospinal fluid (CSF)

    (1) Criteria. A lumbar puncture should be performed on any patient who has an abnormal or a changed neurologic examination without other apparent cause for these findings. It should be strongly considered in any patient in whom no other source can be found to explain the suspected infection.

    (2) Studies. CSF should always be sent for a Gram's stain, bacterial cultures, cell count with differential, and glucose and protein determinations. A cryptococcal antigen titer or India ink preparation should be performed if there are reasons to suspect cellular immune dysfunction. Acid-fast bacillus

(AFB) stains and cultures probably are not indicated routinely.

f. Stool

(1) ***Clostridium difficile.*** This toxin-producing anaerobic bacterium is a common cause of diarrhea in patients who have been on antibiotics. A mild-to-moderate leukocytosis and a fever to 38.5°C typically are part of the syndrome. All patients with diarrhea who are at risk should have stool sent for a cytotoxic assay for *C. difficile* toxin. Rapid antigen detection tests are unreliable.

(2) Bacterial cultures. A stool culture should be sent to the microbiology laboratory from patients in whom the diagnosis of infectious diarrhea is suspected. Occasionally, *Salmonella* species and *Listeria monocytogenes* are causes of nosocomial diarrhea and sepsis.

(3) Fecal leukocytes. The presence of white blood cells in the stool suggests an invasive inflammatory process of the colon. Fecal leukocytes are seen with *Shigella* species, *Campylobacter* species, invasive *Escherichia coli*, and, variably, *Salmonella* species and *C. difficile*. A methylene blue stain of the stool should be requested routinely along with the culture.

(4) Ova and parasites. Diarrhea that develops more than 3 days after hospitalization is almost never caused by a parasite. Routine performance of this test is therefore discouraged. The important exception is in geographic regions in which *Strongyloides stercoralis* is endemic (e.g., southeastern United States).

g. Viral cultures

(1) Herpes simplex virus (HSV) and varicella zoster virus (VZV). Suspicious vesicular lesions must be cultured for HSV or VZV. Fluid-filled lesions should be carefully unroofed. A swab is then rubbed on the base of the lesion and sent in viral transport medium to the laboratory within 30 minutes. These specimens must be promptly inoculated into tissue culture or stored at 4–9°C for no more than 18 hours.

(2) Cytomegalovirus. Bone marrow transplant patients who are suspected of being infected with CMV should have blood (in a dark blue sodium heparin tube) and urine sent to the virology laboratory. When appropriate, induced sputum or bronchoalveolar lavage fluid also should be sent. No special transport medium is required for any of these specimens, but they should be handled as noted above.

    h. Other. Cultures of biopsy or aspirate specimens from any accessible suspected site of infection should be obtained as soon as possible. The risk of complications from such procedures (e.g., infection, bleeding) must be weighed against the possible gains.

3. Imaging studies

    a. Radiographs. A chest x-ray film should be obtained routinely on any patient suspected of having an infection. Sinus films are also frequently important.

    b. Computed tomography (CT). CT scans of the chest, abdomen, brain, head and neck, spine, and other areas can add considerable information to the diagnostic workup. Ordering of these tests must be individualized to the specific clinical situation.

    c. Ultrasonography. An echocardiogram should be obtained when endocarditis is suspected. Ultrasonography is also helpful for detecting ascites and biliary, hepatic, and pancreatic pathology. A portable (bedside) ultrasonography machine can be useful in critically ill patients who are too sick to be transported to the radiology department.

    d. Nuclear medicine. Unfortunately, radionuclide scanning using indium-labeled granulocytes or gallium is not sufficiently sensitive or specific to be diagnostically helpful. False-positive and false-negative results occur too frequently to recommend these tests on a routine basis.

4. Invasive studies

    a. Bronchoscopy. Bronchoalveolar lavage for fungi, CMV, and *Pneumocystis carinii* should be considered for patients at risk for one of these organisms. The adequacy of the specimen can be ascertained by noting the presence of alveolar macrophages on subsequent stains. Specimens also should be sent for Gram's stain, AFB stain and culture, and bacterial culture.

    b. Skin biopsy. Suspicious dermatologic lesions should be biopsied and sent for culture and silver (fungal) staining.

    c. Open lung biopsy. A persistent unexplained infiltrate on chest x-ray film often is evaluated best with this approach. Morbidity is low in patients with adequate platelets and normal coagulation indices.

    d. Bone marrow biopsy. Specimens should be sent for AFB stains and culture.

    e. Percutaneous liver biopsy. Occasionally this procedure is helpful if abnormalities referable to this organ are suspected based on imaging studies or serum chemistries.

    f. Exploratory laparotomy. Even multiple imaging studies sometimes fail to reveal intraabdominal abscesses. A positive blood culture and abdominal tenderness are clues to this diagnosis. Exploratory laparotomy may be required if symptoms persist. Alternatively, surgery may be considered if intraabdominal abnormalities detected by other studies fail to resolve with therapy.

5. Miscellaneous studies

    a. Complete blood count with differential should be performed on every patient suspected of having an infection.

    b. Liver function tests are often abnormal in the presence of generalized sepsis or infections involving the organ itself.

    c. Urinalysis can help differentiate infection from contamination: the absence of white blood cells (WBCs) suggests the latter diagnosis. Note, however, that WBCs may be absent in neutropenic patients.

    d. Erythrocyte sedimentation rate. This nonspecific test is rarely useful and is seldom indicated for diagnosing infection.

IV. Therapy of Infection

  A. Empiric therapy

    1. Timing. Two or three instances of oral temperature elevation above 38°C, or one elevation above 38.5°C, suggests infection. Patients with fewer than 500 neutrophils/μl should be started on antibiotics at this time. Nonneutropenic patients also may require antibiotics, but that decision should be individualized based on other findings.

    2. Neutropenic coverage. Prompt initiation of empiric antibiotic therapy has been shown to reduce mortality. Despite some success with monotherapy, the use of combination therapy remains the standard of care for neutropenic patients.

      a. Recommended regimens. Two antipseudomonal antibiotics should be included. Current popular combinations are piperacillin + tobramycin or ceftazidime + amikacin. Other regimens are possible; the one that is chosen should reflect local sensitivity patterns.

        (1) Aminoglycoside dosing. A loading dose of tobramycin 2 mg/kg or amikacin 7.5 mg/kg should be given initially. High peak serum levels (e.g., tobramycin 7–8 μg/ml) have been shown to be beneficial in treating infections in neutropenic patients. To avoid unacceptably high trough levels (>2 μg/ml), it often is necessary to decrease the dosing frequency and increase the amount given with each dose. A reasonable approach is to give slightly less than a loading dose (e.g., tobramycin 1.7–2.0 mg/kg) with each dose, and adjust only the dosing interval by monitoring peak and trough levels.

        (2) Piperacillin is given at a dose of 3 gm q6h.

    b. Double β-lactam combinations. These regimens have the potential advantage of avoiding aminoglycoside nephrotoxicity and ototoxicity. Unfortunately, cross-resistance to all β-lactams occurs commonly with many gram-negative organisms. Resistance has been much slower to develop to the aminoglycosides, especially tobramycin and amikacin.

    c. Duration. Antibiotics should be continued for a full 14-day course in patients who remain neutropenic, even if the patient becomes afebrile during therapy. In patients whose granulocyte counts recover to more than 500/μl the antibiotics can be discontinued after the patient is afebrile for at least 72 hours.

    d. Antifungal therapy. Amphotericin B, at a dose of 0.5 mg/kg/day, should be started if neutropenic patients remain febrile despite broad-spectrum antibiotic coverage for more than 5–7 days. Although the optimal duration of therapy is unknown, it is prudent to continue antifungal therapy at least as long as neutropenia exists. The imidazole derivatives ketoconazole and fluconazole show promise but cannot be recommended in place of amphotericin B at this time.

3. Gram-positive coverage. The addition of an antistaphylococcal antibiotic to the initial empiric regimen should be considered in patients with indwelling vascular catheters. Vancomycin is preferred because of its efficacy against methicillin-resistant *Staphylococcus aureus, Staphylococcus epidermidis,* and *Corynebacterium* JK. Patients with integumentary damage from any cause also should receive an antistaphylococcal antibiotic.

4. Additional coverage. Patients at risk for pneumonia caused by *Pneumocystis carinii* or the *Legionella* species should have trimethoprim/sulfamethoxasole and erythromycin, respectively, included in their antibiotic regimens, if evidence for pulmonary infection exists. Anaerobic coverage (e.g., metronidazole or clindamycin) should be considered for patients with necrotizing gingivitis or perianal tenderness.

B. Definitive therapy

  1. Antibiotics

    a. General. Reevaluation of the empiric antibiotic regimen is mandatory when the identity and sensitivity pattern of an isolated pathogen become available.

    b. Gram-negative infections. Neutropenic patients should be treated with two antibiotics, each effective against the isolated organism. Nonneutropenic patients with *Pseudomonas aeruginosa* pneumonia also should be treated with two antibiotics, at least initially.

    c. Gram-positive infections. One antibiotic is sufficient, but coverage against gram-negative organisms should be continued in neutropenic patients, as discussed previously.

2. **Specific infections**

a. **Catheter-related sepsis.** Staphylococcal infections predominate. Removal of infected indwelling intravascular devices is optimal but not always possible. Eradication of infection often can be accomplished with long-term antibiotics alone. There is an approximately 70–80% chance of curing a gram-positive infection with 3–4 weeks of antibiotics administered through each port of the device. The chance of success drops to 30–50% for gram-negative infections. Fungal infections require immediate removal of the catheter. Tunnel infections also generally require catheter removal.

b. ***Candida* infections**

(1) **Significance.** Isolation of *Candida* species from sputum, urine, stool, or drainage fluid is not necessarily synonymous with infection. On the other hand, isolation of *Candida* species from three or more nonblood sites has been shown to correlate with disseminated candidiasis in neutropenic patients. Isolation of this organism from the blood is always significant. The presence of macronodular skin lesions shown on biopsy to be consistent with candidal infection is synonymous with dissemination.

(2) **Therapy.** Amphotericin B remains the treatment of choice. Although the optimum dose and length of administration are unknown, especially in patients who remain neutropenic, a dose of 0.5 mg/kg/day for the duration of the neutropenia or a minimum of 300 mg is recommended. Treatment may be less for patients with only superficial infection. The addition of 5-fluorocytosine (flucytosine) is often synergistic and may increase response rates. This agent is potentially bone marrow-suppressive, and serum levels should be monitored. Liposome-encapsulated amphotericin B may prove to be better tolerated than conventional amphotericin B.

(3) **Dissemination.** Candidemia or other evidence of dissemination should prompt a search for deep organ involvement. Weekly funduscopic examinations are essential in such circumstances. Surgery, when feasible, may improve survival in selected cases of deep organ involvement.

c. ***Aspergillus* infections.** Even a single positive culture for one of the *Aspergillus* species warrants initiation of therapy. Pulmonary involvement is the most common disease manifestation, but thrombosis of major blood vessels and widespread dissemination occur in neutropenic patients. Aggressive therapy is necessary to reduce mortality: early initiation of amphotericin B at doses of 1.0–1.5 mg/kg/day is recommended. A total course of 2 gm is typical.

d. HSV and VZV infections. Early initiation of therapy helps to prevent dissemination. The dose of acyclovir for herpes simplex infections in immunocompromised patients with normal renal function is 6.25 mg/kg IV q8h. Varicella zoster infections require acyclovir 12.5 mg/kg q8h. Serum levels following an oral dose average about 25% of levels obtained after an intravenous dose; for this reason, oral acyclovir typically is not used for acute HSV or VZV infections in cancer patients. High-dose oral regimens (800 mg 5 times daily) have been tried with some success, but gastrointestinal distress is a common side effect.

e. *Nocardia* infections. Altered cell-mediated immunity, whether intrinsic or corticosteroid-induced, is the main risk factor for infection with these organisms. The treatment of choice remains oral sulfadiazine 6–8 gm/day. Therapy should be continued for at least 3 months, and regimens of 6–12 months are not uncommon. Trimethoprim–sulfamethoxazole (IV or PO), sulfisoxazole, and triple sulfonamide combinations are likely to be as efficacious as sulfadiazine. Minocycline is an alternative for patients with sulfa allergies, and imipenem has shown impressive *in vitro* activity.

3. Biologic response modifiers

a. Granulocyte transfusions. Beneficial results have not been seen consistently in controlled trials. Transfusion reactions, allosensitization to HLA antigens, and transfusion-associated CMV infection occur frequently and further limit the usefulness of this approach. An increased incidence of severe pulmonary reactions, especially when transfusions are given to patients receiving amphotericin B, has also been noted.

b. Granuloycyte and granulocyte-macrophage colony-stimulating factors (G-CSF, GM-CSF). Controlled trials have shown an acceleration of myeloid recovery in patients who were neutropenic secondary to high-dose chemotherapy.

c. Passive immunization

(1) Monoclonal antibodies. Immunization with high-titer antibody directed against the core glycolipid of gram-negative organisms (J-5 antisera) appears to reduce mortality due to infection, presumably by neutralizing endotoxin. Preparation of the antisera is difficult and expensive, and the technique remains primarily a research tool at this time. Immunization with a "cocktail" of antibodies directed against different antigenic determinants of gram-negative bacilli is the newest approach utilizing monoclonal antibody technology.

   (2) Pooled immunoglobulin preparations. These preparations contain antibodies to many potential pathogens. Results of early controlled trials have been disappointing.

   (3) Tumor necrosis factor (TNF) antiserum. TNF has been shown to be a mediator of endotoxic shock. However, antibody to TNF does not appear to reduce mortality. More recent data suggest that TNF might even have a beneficial effect on host defenses as an activator of macrophages.

   d. Interleukins and interferon. Activation of monocytes and neutrophils by these substances might be expected to reduce mortality from certain kinds of infections. Unfortunately, systemic side effects might limit the usefulness of this approach.

V. Prevention of infection
A. Environmental manipulations
   1. Hand washing. Numerous studies have confirmed that scrupulous adherence to good hand washing technique reduces infections. Patients should be told to remind their physicians to wash their hands before allowing them to proceed with the examination. In addition, hand washing signs should be placed outside the rooms of neutropenic patients as a reminder to all personnel.

   2. Protective isolation
   a. Definition. The concept of a "total protected environment" includes the use of laminar airflow rooms; sterilization of all objects placed in those rooms; gowning, masking, and gloving of personnel before entering the rooms; decontamination of the skin and gut with antimicrobial agents; and special food preparation to reduce the number of microorganisms present on the food.

   b. Disadvantages. This approach is expensive and cumbersome for patients, their families, and hospital personnel; and it decreases the perceived quality of life. It also is difficult to justify, as studies have not shown a significant advantage of protective isolation when compared with other preventive techniques.

   3. Reservoir recognition and removal
   a. Foods. Fresh fruits, vegetables, and nonprocessed dairy products are frequently contaminated with gram-negative bacteria, especially *Pseudomonas aeruginosa, Escherichia coli,* and *Klebsiella pneumoniae.* Adherence to a cooked

diet during periods of neutropenia helps to reduce the risk of infection with these organisms.

  b. Objects. Faucet aerators, sinks, shower heads, and flowers are known to harbor bacteria. However, most epidemiologic studies have not found these objects to be significant causes of infection. No special precautions, except for good hand washing technique, are necessary.

  c. Construction. The incidence of infections caused by *Aspergillus* species is increased in areas of construction. Patients at risk should be moved to other areas of the hospital during periods of renovation.

B. Surveillance cultures. Routine bacterial surveillance cultures are rarely of benefit. In centers where *Aspergillus* is a significant problem, periodic fungal cultures of the nares for this fungus might be useful for early detection.

C. Prophylaxis

 1. Antibiotics

   a. Nonabsorbable agents

    (1) Rationale. Oral vancomycin, gentamicin, and nystatin have been used in attempts to suppress gut flora and lessen the importance of this reservoir of infection.

    (2) Disadvantages. The combination of antibiotics is poorly tolerated by patients. Increased bacterial resistance develops, especially to gentamicin. The regimens do not provide protection against bacteria originating from other body sites. Some controlled studies have failed to demonstrate decreased infection rates.

    (3) Recommendations. These oral nonabsorbable antibiotics should not be utilized at this time.

   b. Quinolones

    (1) Efficacy. Norfloxacin and ciprofloxacin have been shown to reduce the incidence of infection (but not mortality) in neutropenic cancer patients.

    (2) Mechanism of action. The quinolones suppress gram-negative and gram-positive aerobic gut flora. They achieve therapeutic serum and tissue levels against many bacteria.

    (3) Recommendations. Side effects have been minimal, and resistance has been slow to develop. Some cancer centers now routinely place patients on a regimen of 400 mg of norfloxacin twice daily prior to beginning chemotherapy. The quinolones are not approved for use in children.

   c. Trimethoprim–sulfamethoxasole. The use of this agent has fallen out of favor for bacterial prophylaxis because of its potential for bone marrow suppression and other side effects. Increased bacterial resistance and breakthrough infections have been observed.

2. **Antifungals drugs.** Prophylaxis, usually against *Candida* species, has been attempted with a number of antifungal agents. Disadvantages include the potential for emergence of resistant strains and the lack of correlation between decreased colonization rates and the rate of invasive fungal disease. Consequently, the routine use of antifungal prophylaxis is not recommended.

3. **Antiviral drugs.** Intravenous (6.25 mg/kg bid) and oral (200–400 mg 3–5 times daily) acyclovir can prevent recurrences of herpes simplex infections. Acyclovir is ineffective for treatment of CMV infections; high-dose IV acyclovir therapy (12.5 mg/kg tid) for 1 month following bone marrow transplantation may reduce the incidence of subsequent CMV infections. Gancyclovir and foscarnet are two new antivirals with activity against all herpes-group viruses (including CMV). The efficacy of prophylactic regimens utilizing these two drugs is being investigated.

4. **Antiparasitic drugs**
   a. ***Pneumocystis carinii.*** Trimethoprim–sulfamethoxazole (1 double-strength tablet given twice daily on 2 or 3 consecutive days) is effective prophylaxis against this organism. Monthly aerosolized pentamidine may also be of value.
   b. ***Strongyloides stercoralis.*** Patients living in endemic areas should have stool cultures evaluated and treatment initiated (if necessary) before beginning immunosuppressive therapy.

D. **Immunization**
1. **Vaccines.** Live attenuated viral vaccines should not be used in immunocompromised patients. The efficacy of vaccines against *Streptococcus pneumoniae* and *Hemophilus influenzae* in immunocompromised patients is suspect. Nevertheless, many authorities recommend their use prior to immunosuppressive therapy.

   Note: Vaccination against *Streptococcus pneumoniae* is recommended prior to splenectomy in patients who have this operation as an elective procedure as part of staging or therapy for lymphoproliferative or myeloproliferative disorders.

2. **Biologic response modifiers**
   a. **Pooled immunoglobulin.** These preparations, given IV at doses of 0.1–0.2 gm/kg body weight at monthly intervals, have been used in patients with chronic lymphocytic leukemia, multiple myeloma, and other malignancies. Controlled trials seem to indicate some reduction in bacterial infections, but the preparations are expensive, and lifelong therapy is required.
   b. **Monoclonal antibodies**. Prophylactic administration of antibodies directed against virulence

determinants of gram-negative bacteria (e.g., J-5 antisera) may be of value in reducing the incidence of infection. However, mortality has been unaltered in early clinical trials.

   3. Varicella zoster immune globulin (1 vial/10 kg body weight to a maximum of 5 vials) effectively reduces morbidity and mortality in seronegative immunocompromised patients exposed to varicella. The product should be given IM within 96 hours of exposure.

E. Miscellaneous. IV catheters (nonsurgically placed) should be changed at least every 72 hours. Rectal temperatures, rectal suppositories, and unnecessary rectal examinations should be avoided in neutropenic patients.

Selected Readings

Berkman, S. A., Lee, M. L., and Gale, R. P. Clinical uses of intravenous immunoglobulins. *Ann. Intern. Med.* 112:278, 1990.

EORTC International Antimicrobial Therapy Cooperative Group. Ceftazidime combined with a short or long course of amikacin for empirical therapy of gram-negative bacteremia in cancer patients with gram-negative bacteremia in cancer patients with granulocytopenia. *N. Engl. J. Med.* 317:1692, 1987.

Hawkins, C., and Armstrong, D. Fungal infections in the immunocompromised host. *Clin. Haematol.* 13:599, 1984.

Hughes, W. T., *et al.* From the Infectious Diseases Society of America: guidelines for the use of antimicrobial agents in neutropenic patients with unexplained fever. *J. Infect. Dis.* 161:381, 1990.

Karp, J. E., Merz, W. G., and Hendricksen, C. Oral norfloxacin for prevention of gram negative bacterial infections in patients with acute leukemia and granulocytopenia. *Ann. Intern. Med.* 106:1, 1987.

Klastersky, J., *et al.* Empiric antimicrobial therapy for febrile granulocytopenic cancer patients: lessons from four EORTC trials. *Eur. J. Cancer Clin. Oncol.* 24(suppl. 1):S35, 1988.

Newman, K. A., *et al.* Venous access devices utilized in association with intensive cancer chemotherapy. *Eur. J. Cancer Clin. Oncol.* 25:1375, 1989.

Pizzo, P. Considerations for the prevention of infectious complications in patients with cancer. *Rev. Infect. Dis.* 11(suppl. 7):S1551, 1989.

Schimpff, S. C. Dilemmas and choices in infection management of the cancer patient. *Eur. J. Cancer Clin. Oncol.* 25:1351, 1989.

Disorders of Hemostasis and Transfusion Therapy

Mary R. Smith

Disorders of the hemostatic mechanisms are common in patients with malignancy. Disorders associated with thromboembolic events cause significantly more morbidity and mortality than disorders leading to hemorrhage.

I. Thromboembolism in cancer

A. Etiology.
The thromboembolic risk associated with neoplasia reflects an imbalance among platelet numbers and function, levels of coagulation factors, levels of inhibitors of hemostasis, and fibrinolytic activity. Thrombosis may be minor and localized or widespread and associated with multiple organ damage. There may also be hemorrhage of varying degrees of severity in association with the thromboembolic events.

1. Factors that may affect the risk of thromboembolism

1. Specific type of tumor
2. Nutritional status of the tumor
3. Type of chemotherapy
4. Effect of chemotherapy
5. Liver and renal function
6. Patient immobility and venous stasis

2. Factors that may initiate thrombus formation

1. Circulating tumor cells adhere to the vascular endothelium and form a nidus for clot formation.
2. Tumors may penetrate the vessel, destroying the endothelium and promoting clot formation.
3. Neovascularization associated with many tumors may stimulate clotting.
4. Arterial thrombosis associated with tumors may be due to vasospasm.

B. Disseminated intravascular coagulation (DIC).
DIC is a syndrome with many signs, symptoms, and laboratory abnormalities. As many as 90% of patients with neoplasms have some manifestation of DIC, but only a fraction of these patients suffer morbidity due to it. The initiation factor for DIC varies from one tumor to another.

1. Thromboplastic substances in granules from promyelocytes of acute promyelocytic leukemia (DIC may worsen with therapy). There is a significant secondary fibrinolysis in many cases.
2. Sialic acid from mucin produced by adenocarcinomas of the lung or gastrointestinal tract.
3. Trypsin released from pancreatic cancer.
4. Impaired fibrinolysis associated with hepatocellular carcinoma.

C. Fibrinolysis. Many tumors are associated with activation of fibrinolysis. Although fibrinolysis is primarily due to urokinase released from normal and malignant prostate tissue, it may develop secondary to DIC with many malignant disorders.

D. Lupus anticoagulant in neoplastic disease. The lupus anticoagulant is an antiphospholipid antibody—either immunoglobulin G (IgG) or IgM. Antiphospholipid antibodies are reported to be associated with a number of malignant disorders, most commonly leukemia or lymphoma. The lupus anticoagulant leads to a prolonged activated partial thromboplastin time but is paradoxically associated with an increased risk of thrombosis.

E. Platelet abnormalities associated with an increased risk of thromboembolism

1. Thrombocytosis
2. Increased platelet adhesion and aggregation.

Tumors may produce substances that cause increased platelet aggregation with subsequent release of platelet factor 3 and ensuing acceleration of coagulation.

F. Clinical syndromes associated with "the hypercoagulable state" of malignancy
1. **Migratory thrombophlebitis.** Suspect the possibility of neoplasia when:
    a. An unexplained thromboembolic event occurs after the age of 40 *or*
    b. Thromboses occur in unusual sites.
2. **Thrombotic neurologic syndromes** are present.
3. **Thrombotic events occur after surgery** associated with tumors of the lung, ovary, pancreas, or stomach.
4. **Nonbacterial thrombotic endocarditis** may be found in association with carcinoma of the lung. These thrombi are formed from accumulations of platelets and fibrin. The mitral valve is the most frequent site of origin of these thrombi, which frequently embolize.
5. **Thrombotic thrombocytopenic purpura (TTP).** TTP is a poorly understood syndrome characterized by thrombocytopenia, acute hemolysis, fever, fluctuating neurologic signs and symptoms, and acute renal failure. The prognosis for TTP is poor, and its therapy has been varied. At the present time, plasmapheresis and transfusion with fresh frozen plasma appear to be the best modalities of therapy.
6. **Thromboembolism associated with chemotherapy**
    a. The use of central arterial or venous catheters has markedly facilitated the delivery of chemotherapy, but all such catheters are associated with a significant risk of vascular thrombosis.
    b. Many chemotherapy agents cause significant chemical phlebitis. The most common offending

agents are mechlorethamine (nitrogen mustard), anthracyclines, nitrosoureas, mitomycin, fluorouracil, and dacarbazine.

   c. L-Asparaginase may be associated with an increase in risk of thromboembolism. It interferes with the synthesis of proteins, including coagulation proteins; therefore clotting events, bleeding, or both may occur.

   d. Estrogens may increase the risk of thromboembolism. The exact mechanism for this increased risk of thrombosis is unclear.

   e. Thrombotic microangiopathy may be associated with some chemotherapy agents. The most common agents are mitomycin, cisplatin, bleomycin, vinca alkaloids, doxorubicin, and dacarbazine. This thrombotic microangiopathy is associated with thrombi in small blood vessels. The therapy is similar to that for TTP, i.e., plasmapheresis and fresh frozen plasma transfusions. The prognosis is poor, with up to 50% mortality.

G. Principles of therapy for thrombosis associated with neoplasia

   1. Discrete vascular thrombosis

   a. Therapy should be directed at controlling the neoplasm. As an anticoagulant, heparin is superior to coumadin in these patients. Coumadin and antiplatelet drugs have been used with varying degrees of success in some patients with thromboembolism associated with tumors.

   b. Vascular interruption procedures such as Greenfield filters may be used in patients who cannot tolerate anticoagulant therapy or who have embolism while on adequate therapy.

   2. DIC. Therapy for DIC includes the following.

   a. Urgently correct shock.

   b. Treat the underlying disease process.

   c. Replace depleted blood components, e.g., platelets and fresh frozen plasma.

   d. Consider the use of heparin only in patients with acute promyelocytic leukemia or when there is evidence of ongoing organ damage to the brain, lungs, or kidneys due to DIC in a patient who has been resuscitated from shock. There is no evidence that chronic warfarin therapy is of value for treating the chronic DIC seen in some patients with neoplasia.

II. Bleeding in patients with cancer

   A. Tumor invasion. It is well recognized that bleeding may be a warning sign of cancer: Bloody sputum may indicate carcinoma of the lung, blood in the urine may be a sign of carcinoma of the bladder or kidney, blood in the stool may be due to carcinoma of the alimentary tract, and postmenopausal vaginal bleeding may be caused by endometrial carcinoma. In each of these instances, bleeding can be directly related to the invasive properties of cancer and disruption of normal tissue integrity.

B. Hematologic abnormalities. Often bleeding in patients with cancer is not due to direct effects of the neoplasm but to indirect effects of the cancer or its therapy on one of the components of the hematologic system. Because of the frequency and the special management problems caused by abnormalities in the hematologic system in patients with cancer and the frequency with which these problems occur, it is important to consider the possible causes and corrective measures in detail.

  1. **Increased vascular fragility** may be due to chronic corticosteroid therapy, chronic malnutrition, or "senile purpura." Bleeding is usually not severe, but bruising, particularly around IV infusion sites, is common.
  2. **Thrombocytopenia** may occur for a variety of reasons, each of which must be considered whenever the platelet count is low.
      a. **Chemotherapy and radiotherapy** regularly cause depression of platelets, and regular blood counts must be obtained while patients are being treated.
      b. **Bone marrow invasion or replacement** is common only with leukemias or lymphomas, and it may cause thrombocytopenia.
      c. **Splenomegaly** with splenic sequestration is most common with leukemia or lymphoma.
      d. **Poor nutrition causing folate deficiency and decreased platelet production** is common in patients with cancer because of poor appetites. Dietary history should provide the clues to the diagnosis.
  3. **Abnormalities of platelet function.** Most cases are secondary to drug effects, including nonsteroidal anti-inflammatory agents (e.g., aspirin), antibiotics (e.g., carbenicillin), antidepressants (tricyclic drugs), tranquilizers, and alcohol. Consider any drug that the patient is taking as a possible offender until proved otherwise.
  4. **Coagulation factor deficiencies** may develop in patients with malignancy for several reasons.
      a. **DIC** depletes most clotting factors but to variable degrees.
      b. **Liver failure** causes deficiency of all clotting factors except factor VIII.
      c. **Malnutrition** leads to deficiency of factors II, VII, IX, and X (the vitamin K-dependent factors).
      d. **Circulating anticoagulants,** if present, are most commonly fibrin-fibrinogen split products. Specific anticoagulants may also be seen but are not common.
      e. **Functionally abnormal clotting factors** are occasionally seen. The most commonly diagnosed abnormality is dysfibrinogenemia.

III. Laboratory evaluation of hemostasis in patients with malignancy. Up to 90% of patients with malignancy demonstrate some abnormality of tests of hemostasis.

  A. Screening tests for bleeding. The following tests provide an adequate screening battery.

1. Platelet count
2. Bleeding time
3. Prothrombin time (PT)
4. Activated partial thromboplastin time (APTT)
5. Thrombin time
6. Fibrinogen level

  B. Interpretation of screening laboratory studies. Abnormal results of the screening tests reflect hematologic problems caused by blood vessels, platelets, or coagulation factors. The following list provides clues to the interpretation of the screening tests that help determine the most likely cause or causes of the patient's bleeding.

1. Platelet count
  a. Normal is 150,000–450,000/μl.
  b. If thrombocytopenia is less than 100,000/μl, consider the following.
    (1) Bone marrow failure
    (2) Increased consumption of platelets
    (3) Splenic pooling of platelets
  c. Thrombocytosis with a platelet count of more than 500,000/μl.
    (1) Common in patients with neoplasms.
    (2) Sometimes seen in association with iron-deficiency states.
    (3) Usually poses no risk for arterial thrombosis unless the patient has a primary marrow disorder.

2. Bleeding time
  a. Normal bleeding time requires both adequate platelet number and function and adequate blood vessel function.
  b. Prolonged bleeding time may be due to thrombocytopenia, abnormal platelet function, or rarely inadequate vessel wall function.

3. Prolonged PT is seen in the presence of the following.
  a. Deficiency of one or more of the following clotting factors: VII, X, V, II (prothrombin), or I (fibrinogen). (Oral anticoagulant therapy leads to a deficiency of factors II, VII, IX, and X.)
  b. Circulating anticoagulant(s) against factor VII, X, V, or II.

4. Prolonged APTT
  a. Deficiency of any of the following clotting factors: XII, XI, IX, VIII, X, V, II, I. Factor XII deficiency is not associated with bleeding. Fletcher and Fitzgerald factor deficiencies (both rare) may also prolong the APTT.
  b. Circulating anticoagulants against factor XII, XI, IX, VIII, X, V, or II.

    c. Anticoagulant therapy with:

      (1) Heparin.

      (2) Oral anticoagulants.

  5. Prolonged thrombin time. Prolongation of the thrombin time may be due to the following.

    1. Hypofibrinogenemia

    2. Some forms of dysfibrinogenemia

    3. Fibrin-fibrinogen split products

    4. Heparin therapy

    If the thrombin time is prolonged, further studies to clarify the cause may be required.

  6. Low fibrinogen level. When evaluating the results of a fibrinogen assay, one must be familiar with the assay method used. Many laboratories use immunologic assays, which measure both functionally normal and abnormal fibrinogens. If such an assay is in use, the thrombin time can be used to evaluate the functional integrity of the fibrinogen. A low functional fibrinogen level means that production is decreased or that consumption is increased.

C. Laboratory findings in patients with DIC. Acute DIC is often associated with significant hemorrhage, whereas chronic DIC may have few signs or symptoms. Screening and confirmatory laboratory tests are shown in Table 33-1.

D. Additional laboratory studies. The tests listed in Table 32-2 show abnormalities that may occur in cancer patients with few or no indications of hemostatic derangements.

Table 33-1. Laboratory diagnosis of DIC

Tests	Acute DIC	Chronic DIC
Screening tests		
PT, APTT	Usually prolonged	Normal
Platelets	Usually decreased	Normal or slightly decreased
Fibrinogen	Usually decreased but may be normal	Usually normal
Confirmatory tests		
Fibrin monomer	Positive	Positive
FDP	Strongly positive	Positive
D-Dimer	Positive	Positive
Thrombin time	Normal or abnormal	Usually normal
Factor assays	Decreased factors V and VIII	Normal factors V and VIII
Antithrombin III	May be reduced	Usually normal

Table 33-2. Laboratory tests of coagulation tests in patients with cancer that may be abnormal without clinical bleeding or thrombosis

Test	Common result in patients with malignancy
Antithrombin III	Decreased
β-Thromboglobulin	Increased
Cryofibrinogen	Present
D-Dimer	Increased
Factor VIIIC	Increased
Fibronectin	Decreased
Fibrin monomer (soluble)	Present
Fibrinogen	Increased
Fibrin(ogen) degradation products	Present
Fibrinopeptide A	Increased
Fibrinopeptide B	Increased
Plasmin	Increased
Plasminogen	Decreased
Platelet count	Increased or decreased
Platelet factor 4	Increased
Protein C	Decreased

IV. Transfusion therapy

A. General guidelines

1. Use the specific blood component needed by the patient.
2. Minimize complications of transfusion by using:
   a. Only the amount and type of blood product indicated for the patient in the specific clinical setting.
   b. Special filters or irradiated blood when indicated.

B. Blood component therapy

1. **Platelet transfusions**
   a. **Available forms of platelets** for transfusion
      (1) **Random-donor platelets.** Six to ten units are usually given in rapid sequence each day they are needed.
      (2) **Single-donor platelets.** They come as a single pack but represent the platelets from 3–4 liters of blood.
      (3) **HLA-matched platelets.** They come as a single pack but represent the platelets from 3–4 liters of blood.
      The latter two forms are reserved for use in patients who fail to respond to random-donor platelets or who may be candidates for bone marrow transplantation or in patients expected to need many platelet transfusions.
   b. **Check platelet count** 4 and 24 hours after platelet transfusion to estimate survival of plate-

lets in the patient. An ideal increment at 4 hours would be 7000–10,000/μl for each unit transfused.

c. **Criteria for transfusing platelets**

(1) **Prophylactic platelet transfusion** should be considered when the platelet count is 10,000/μl or less. A higher threshold (20,000/μl) should be used if the patient is infected, bleeding, or febrile or experiences a rapid fall in the platelet count. This point is particularly important in patients with acute leukemia. Patients with immune thrombocytopenia (e.g., ITP) are not likely to benefit from platelet transfusions,

(2) **If surgery is contemplated** (with the exception of intracranial surgery), the platelet count should be increased to 60,000/μl. (Check the bleeding time before surgery; results should be within 2 minutes of the upper limits of normal.)

(3) **For intracranial surgery** transfuse to a platelet count of 100,000/μl (bleeding time must be checked before surgery and must be normal).

d. **Management of patients** who become refractory to platelet transfusions.

(1) Patients who become refractory to random donor platelets may well respond to HLA-matched or cross-matched platelets.

(2) All such patients should be evaluated for alloimmunization.

(3) Evaluate the patient for other causes of poor response to platelet transfusions, e.g., fever, DIC, or splenomegaly.

2. **Coagulation factor support**

a. **Fresh frozen plasma (FFP)** contains all clotting factors (but not platelets) and should be used for multiple coagulation factor deficiencies. FFP requires 20–30 minutes to thaw, as it must be thawed at 37°C or lower.

b. **Cryoprecipitated factor VIII ("cryo")** is a source of factor VIII, fibrinogen, and factor XIII. Each bag of cryo contains the factor VIII and fibrinogen harvested from 1 unit of fresh whole blood. Cryoprecipitate is stored in a frozen state and has the advantage of concentrating the clotting factors in a small volume (≤ 10 ml/unit). About 10–20 units are usually given, and the patient is evaluated to determine if the laboratory abnormalities have been corrected.

c. **Factor IX concentrates** contain factors II, VII, IX, and X. Several precautions are worth noting.

(1) This concentrate is made from pooled plasma; therefore the risk of hepatitis is high, and the risk of contamination with HIV is significant. The dose depends on the preparation

to be used. The goal is to bring the factor to more than 50% of normal.

    (2) There is a small risk of DIC resulting from the use of factor IX concentrates. Patients with liver dysfunction and newborns are at increased risk.

    (3) Factor IX concentrates are stored in the lyophilized state. Do not shake when reconstituting.

  d. DDAVP (Desmopression) 0.4 μg/kg IV over 15–30 minutes every 8–12 hours for 2–4 days may be used to elevate factor VIII and von Willebrand factor levels. Tachyphylaxis may occur if therapy is continued for longer periods. Because DDAVP also activates fibrinolysis, ε-Aminocaproic acid (EACA) or tranexamic acid may need to be given as well to prevent bleeding from this cause. Intranasal DDAVP 0.25 ml bid using a solution containing 1.3 mg/ml has been given for minor bleeding episodes.

C. Leukocyte filters. Filters designed to remove leukocytes from cellular blood products are now readily available. The following should be considered as a guideline for the use of such filters: Patients not previously transfused, particularly with platelets, in whom a need for long-term platelet support is anticipated should receive all cellular blood products via filters to remove leukocytes. These filters are not useful for preventing febrile transfusion reactions but may be expected to delay white blood cell alloimmunization.

D. Cytomegalovirus (CMV)-negative blood. Only patients known to be anti-CMV-negative with impaired immunity should be considered for the use of CMV-negative blood. This group comprises children for the most part. The use of CMV-negative blood seriously restricts the potential donor pool for these patients.

    Frozen-deglycerolized blood is considered free of CMV contamination. White blood cell depletion filters also remove CMV virus; however, irradiation of blood products does not appear to render them CMV-free.

E. Irradiated blood products. The use of irradiated blood products should be limited to those patients with one of the following indications.

    1. Immunocompromised host
    2. Premature babies
    3. Bone marrow transplant patients
    4. Directed blood donations to first-degree relatives
    5. Transfusion of patients with Hodgkin's disease (a relative indication)

Selected Reading

Bauer, K., et al. Tumor necrosis factor infusions have a procoagulant effect on the hemostatic mechanisms in humans. *Blood* 74:165, 1989.

Bick, R. L. Alterations of hemostasis associated with malignancy: etiology, pathophysiology, diagnosis and management. *Semin. Thromb. Hemost.* 5:1, 1978.

Esparaz, B., Kies, M., and Kwaan, H. Thromboembolism in cancer. *Clinical Thrombosis.* Boca Raton: CRC Press, 1989. Pp. 317–333.

Griffin, M., et al. Deep venous thrombosis and pulmonary embolism, risk of subsequent malignant neoplasms. *Arch. Intern. Med.* 147:1907, 1987.

Leitman, S. F., and Holland, P. V. Irradiation of blood products: indications and guidelines. *Transfusion* 25:293, 1985.

Mannucci, D. M. Desmopressin: a non-transfusional form of treatment for congenital and acquired bleeding disorders. *Blood* 72:1449, 1988.

Mollison, P. L., Engelfried, C. P., and Contreras, C. *Blood Transfusion in Clinical Medicine* (8th ed.). Boston: Blackwell Scientific Publications, 1987.

Murgo, A. Thrombotic microangiopathy in the cancer patient including those induced by chemotherapy agents. *Semin. Hematol.* 24:161, 1987.

Schafer, A. The hypercoagulable state. *Ann. Intern. Med.* 102:814, 1985.

Emotional and Psychiatric Problems in Patients with Cancer

Kathy S. N. Franco

I. **General principles.** Clinical psychiatric disorders occur in up to 50% of patients with cancer at some point during their treatment. Delirium, depression, and anxiety are those most frequently seen and may coexist in the same patient. Careful monitoring for the early symptoms of psychiatric distress is important to the care of these patients. The clinician should inquire regularly about symptoms in the affective and cognitive domains. Symptom clusters help differentiate anxiety, depression, and organic brain syndromes from other psychiatric disorders. Once an accurate diagnosis is made, appropriate treatment that may include medication can be planned for the target symptoms. More than one psychiatric diagnosis may be present requiring a hierarchical approach. For example, if both delirium and depression are present, the etiology of the delirium should be determined and treated before starting antidepressant therapy (which could worsen the delirium). Once organicity has improved, treatment for the depression can be considered. When major depression and an anxiety disorder coexist, treatment for the depression is started first and may adequately manage both disorders.

II. **Acute confusional states**

A. **Precepts.** Psychiatrists are often asked to assist in the care of "agitated" patients. The initial request may be for medication advice, but prescribing psychotropic drugs without understanding the cause of the patient's distress can have serious consequences. Delirium is characterized by fluctuating levels of alertness/consciousness, shortened attention and concentration, rapidly changing moods, irregular sleep–wake cycles, garbled or slurred speech, hypervigilance, and behavior not consistent with good judgment. The delirious patient may also have delusional ideas or hallucinations. Visual, auditory, tactile, and occasionally olfactory hallucinations can be present. The more sensory modalities that are involved in the hallucinations, the greater is the likelihood the patient is experiencing an acute confusional state.

B. **Etiologies**

1. **Medications** remain the most common reason for acute confusional states. The most frequently identified medications to cause delirium are sedatives, narcotics, analgesics, anxiolytics, anticholinergic drugs, and corticosteroids.

2. **Metabolic causes** are often seen in patients with cancer and include hyper- and hyponatremia, hyper- and hypothyroidism, poorly controlled diabetes mellitus, and hypercalcemia.

459

3. **Infections** of the respiratory, urinary, central nervous and other systems are common, especially in immunosuppressed patients.

4. **Chemical withdrawal** from benzodiazepines, alcohol, and others can induce delirium.

5. **Vitamin deficiencies** (B_{12}, folate, thiamine), tumors, cardiac arrhythmias, congestive heart failure, liver disease, trauma, strokes, renal failure, and a variety of other conditions can cause acute changes in mental status.

C. **Therapeutic approach.** Once an acute confusional state is identified, the primary therapeutic approach is to treat the cause. Antipsychotic medications may be helpful for managing symptoms such as hallucinations, delusions, and extreme agitation, but they do not treat the cause of the delirium.

1. **Orientation** aids in the reduction of confusion.

   a. It is helpful to frequently orient the patient to place, time, and why they are at the hospital, and to give current explanations of procedures. This routine should be done once or more per shift when the delirious patient is awake. Because patients' attention, concentration, and recent memory are often impaired, they often do not recall instructions given to them earlier. Leaving a large, legibly written note card with the patient's name, date, hospital name, and so on is beneficial in some instances.

   b. A large calendar, a clock, and family pictures or mementos can assist the patients in feeling less estranged from their environment.

   c. Some patients are reassured by a small night light in their room, which cuts down on illusions or misinterpretations. Individuals with compromised vision or hearing are particularly distraught when they are even less able to discern what is happening around them.

2. **Medication** helps to control hallucinations, delusions, and psychotic agitation. The lowest dose to control symptoms is usually preferable.

   a. **Haloperidol** (Haldol) (Table 34-1) is a butyrophenone, antipsychotic agent with potent dopamine blocking action. It is less likely to produce cardiovascular, respiratory, gastrointestinal, and general anticholinergic side effects than many of the other antipsychotic medications. However, moderate doses may cause extrapyramidal symptoms. The starting dose in a patient with an acute confusional state is 0.25–2.00 mg PO or IM, on an "as needed" or regular dosing schedule every 4–6 hours. A marked advantage of haloperidol is that sedation is minimized while controlling agitation. There are exceptions to the usually preferred low doses of antipsychotic medications. For example, if patients tolerate higher doses with few side ef-

Table 34-1. Antipsychotic medications: dosage for patients with cancer and prominent characteristics

Agent	Starting dose (mg)*	Characteristics
Phenothiazines		
Chlorpromazine (Thorazine)	10–25	Significant hypotension risk, lowers seizure threshold, highly sedating, anticholinergic
Thioridazine (Mellaril)	10–25	Similar to chlorpromazine but more likely to alter ECG; not available IM
Mesoridazine (Serentil)	10–25	Similar to chlorpromazine and thioridazine
Perphenazine (Trilafon)	4	Moderate sedation and hypotension
Trifluoperazine (Stelazine)	2	High frequency of extrapyramidal side effects
Fluphenazine (Prolixin)	2	High frequency of extrapyramidal side effects
Prochlorperazine (Compazine)	5–10	Weak antipsychotic; used more as an antiemetic
Others		
Haloperidol (Haldol)	0.5–2.0	High frequency of extrapyramidal side effects
Thiothixene (Navane)	1–2	High frequency of extrapyramidal side effects
Loxapine (Loxitane)	10	Moderate in most side effects noted above
Molindone (Moban)	5–10	Less weight gain
Clozapine (Clozaril)	Little experience with the physically ill patient	Recommended for patients who have chronic schizophrenia or evidence of tardive dyskinesia

*Dose generally can be repeated every 4–6 hours, either on an as-needed or a regular schedule (e.g., qid).

fects, they may benefit by having improved pain control.

b. Additional **high-potency, low-sedation options** include thiothixene (Navane), trifluoperazine (Stelazine), and fluphenazine (Prolixin).

c. **A delirious patient** with vision or hearing impairment is likely to hallucinate during periods of excessive sedation.

d. If the patient demonstrates a **predictable period of confusion,** e.g., early evening ("sundowning") when there is less environmental activity, a once-a-day dose at that time may be adequate.

e. **When increasing the dose of antipsychotic drugs,** muscle spasms, restlessness, or pseudoparkinsonian symptoms may occur. Adding a small amount of trihexyphenidyl (Artane) 1–2 mg bid, benztropine (Cogentin) 1 mg bid, or diphenhydramine (Benadryl) 25 mg bid can often reduce the side effects. However, increasing the level of anticholinergic activity with these choices may cause an atropiniclike psychosis. Constipation, urinary retention, dry mouth, tachycardia, and increasing confusion are warnings of this potential problem, especially when multiple anticholinergic medications (e.g., antiemetics, analgesics) are being prescribed. Therefore antiparkinsonian drugs are not prescribed prophylactically but only if clearly indicated.

f. **Intravenous haloperidol** has not been approved by the U.S. Food and Drug Administration (FDA), although it is commonly used in the seriously agitated patient. Half the oral dosing is prescribed when the medication is given IV.

g. **Benzodiazepines,** e.g., lorazepam (Ativan) 0.5–2.0 mg q8h, are sometimes given in small doses to a patient who needs some sedation without added anticholinergic activity or whose cardiac status is at risk (i.e., heart block) if the antipsychotic medication is increased. Using both benzodiazepines and antipsychotics is sometimes helpful. One pattern might be 0.5–2.0 mg haloperidol at 4 P.M., 1–2 mg of lorazepam at 8 P.M., and so forth if the patient is agitated.

h. **Increasing delerium.** Too much medication may have been given if the patient's level of agitation increases with higher doses.

i. **Hypotension.** Avoid adding other antipsychotics, e.g., thorazine, as they predispose to hypotension and shock. If the blood pressure does drop significantly, norepinephrine bitartrate (Levophed) or a similar choice may be necessary because the antipsychotic medications block the action of dopamine. The half-life of the antipsychotic is generally 24–48 hours.

III. Depression. Patients with cancer have various emotional responses to their diagnoses. The mourning period for some is brief, does not inhibit their ability to interact with family and friends, and does not hinder participation in their own treatment. Support from others, acceptance of their feelings, and time may be all that is necessary for them to continue the emotional work ahead. However, approximately one-fourth of patients with cancer develop longer, more severe depressions. There are many variables that influence this process, including emotional conflicts with loved ones, disproportionate guilt, previous losses that were never resolved, long-standing debilitating illness, some personality characteristics such as dependency, and inadequate support systems. Any of these factors, along with a family history of depression, are warnings for the doctor to heed.

  A. Therapeutic approach

  1. Emotional support at frequent intervals from the physician is generally needed. Some patients explore old emotional conflicts, whereas others just need a safe person to whom they can express their feelings. It is important for patients to be able to hold on to hope. A degree of "denial" is acceptable, normal, and upheld. Only when this denial makes it impossible for a patient to make informed treatment decisions is it necessary to probe into the denial.

  Psychotherapy of a supportive nature is often provided by the primary care physician, oncologist, psychiatrist, clergy, nurse, family, or friend individually or in any combination. For patients who wish to explore ambivalence, a professional psychotherapist trained in psychodynamic or interpersonal therapy is a good option. Cognitive therapy is helpful in letting go of detrimental interpretations while increasing one's ability to deal with emotional pain.

  2. Psychiatric care may be particularly instrumental when the patient's other physicians are struggling with how much of the patient's preexisting personality style is interfering with treatment. Anniversary responses to previous losses, important family events, or past hospitalizations may have a great impact on the presentation of the depression and deserve exploration by a psychotherapist if a pattern is found. If there is a designated psychiatric consultant, this individual must work closely with the rest of the oncology team, communicating in a helpful way to the patient, family, and staff.

  If a patient has felt depressed, distressed, or irritable for some time or describes a loss of pleasure from formerly enjoyable relationships or activities, inquiry about the following symptoms is necessary: insomnia or hypersomnia, alteration in appetite with expected weight change, reduced interest in family, sexuality, work, or hobbies, increased guilt, low energy level, poor concentration, thoughts of death or suicide, frequent crying episodes, and psy-

Table 34-2. Commonly used antidepressants and side effect profiles

Antidepressant	Sedation*	Anticholinergic actions†	Other characteristics
Amitriptyline (Elavil, Endep)	+ 4 to + 5‡	+ 4 to + 5	Also available IM
Amoxapine (Asendin)	+ 2-3	+ 2 to + 3	Blocks dopamine (has antipsychosis effect but can cause extrapyramidal symptoms including tardive dyskinesia)
Buproprion (Wellbutrin)	+ 1	+ 1	Increases seizure risk especially if organic brain pathology or eating disorder is present; more activating; less weight gain
Clomipramine (Anafranil)	+ 3	+ 3	Recommended for obsessive-compulsive disorders
Desipramine (Norpramin)	+ 1 to + 2	+ 1 to + 2	Less TCA seizure risk alteration
Doxepin (Sinequan, Adapin)	+ 4	+ 3	Less TCA seizure risk alteration; highest appetite increase

Fluoxetine (Prozac)	+1	+1	May cause restlessness and GI upset; more activating; less weight gain; safe in patients with renal disease but not in those with liver disease
Imipramine (Tofranil)	+3	+3	Also available IM
Maprotiline (Ludiomil)	+2	+2	Lowers seizure threshold significantly
Nortriptyline (Pamelor, Aventyl)	+3	+3	Less likely to cause orthostasis than other TCAs
Protriptyline (Vivactyl)	+1	+3 to +4	More activating; less pulmonary suppression
Trazodone (Desyrel)	+4	+1	Least anticholinergic of sedating options; priapism rate increased
Trimipramine (Surmontil)	+4	+4	

Key: TCA = tricyclic antidepressant.
*Associated with histaminergic blockade; appetite increase follows somewhat similar trends.
†Constipation, dry mouth, urinary retention, and so on.
‡Scale of 1–5, where 1 is least and 5 is most.

chomotor hypo- or hyperactivity. These symptoms are characteristic of a major depressive disorder for which antidepressant medication in addition to psychotherapy is recommended.

3. **Medications.** Patients with cancer are often undertreated for major depression that has been mistaken for simple grief. Evidence is beginning to accumulate that psychosocial adjustment and improved life adaptation, in general, occur when patients with cancer and major depression are treated with antidepressant medications.

   a. **Selection of agents and their side effects.** An antidepressant medication should be selected on the basis of its tendency to sedate or activate, cause orthostatic changes, or produce anticholinergic effects. Medication selection should also be tailored to the patient's symptom cluster, such as the need for sedation or weight gain versus the need for activation (Table 34-2). Route of metabolism and elimination may also figure into a choice as well as the medication's tendency to cause seizures.

   Highly anticholinergic medications frequently produce dry mouth, blurred vision, tachycardia, and constipation. They can also produce urinary retention, ileus, and acute confusion. Those drugs that are also antihistaminergic can increase sedation, appetite, and hypotension. Medications that produce adrenergic receptor blockade are associated with increased orthostatic hypotension, dizziness, and reflex tachycardia.

   b. **Dosages** (Table 34-3). Weak, debilitated, or elderly patients need protection from many of these side effects. Starting out with small doses and gradually increasing the dose is prudent. Splitting doses may also be helpful for minimizing side effects and maximizing pain relief from these medications.

   If a patient has a personal history, family history, or previous drug response that reflects mania or hypomania, it is necessary to proceed carefully, perhaps with lithium alone (Table 34-4).

   c. **Monoamine oxidase inhibitors (MAOI)** (Table 34-5) may be used to treat major depression or panic disorder but are somewhat inconvenient in that tyramine dietary restrictions and medication interactions require much attention. They are often tried as an alternative when other choices have failed if the depression is accompanied by phobic and histrionic features or if the individual was effectively treated with an MAOI for an earlier depression.

IV. **Anxiety**

A. **Approach to the problem.** As grieving is described as normal, so is anxiety in patients with cancer. However, this anxiety varies in its etiology, severity, and treat-

Table 34-3. Dosages for antidepressant therapy

Drug	Starting dose (mg)	Average daily dose for patient with cancer (mg)
Amitriptyline	10–25	75–150
Amoxapine	25	75–150
Buproprion	75–150	300
Clomipramine	25	75–150
Desipramine	25	75–150 (tid)
Doxepin	25	75–150
Fluoxetine	20	20
Imipramine	10–25	75–150
Maprotiline	25	75
Nortriptyline	10–25	50–100
Protriptyline	5–10 qam	20 (10 mg A.M. & noon)
Trazodone	50	150–300
Trimipramine	10–25	75–150

ment. A detailed history of the onset, characteristics, and length of distress is important. Knowledge of the patient's previous symptoms, current and past physical illness, and chemical and medication usage is essential to the evaluation process. Antianxiety agents may be helpful for alleviating patients' distress and helping them to cope with other problems associated with their cancer (Table 34-6).

- **B. Problems that present as anxiety.** The duration of the symptom is one of the first factors to assess in the anxious patient.
    - **1. Suspect an adjustment disorder** when maladaptive anxious symptoms have persisted (less than 6 months) and apparently represent an adjustment to learning the diagnosis or reactions to the treatment. This kind of anxiety may benefit from supportive therapy, relaxation therapy, or benzodiazepines.
    - **2. Generalized anxiety.** If the anxiety has been present for more than 6 months, continuing no matter what environmental alterations occur, and is accompanied by signs of physical tension or poor attention to conversation or other daily activities, the patient is likely to have generalized anxiety. Supportive therapy, relaxation tapes, biofeedback, buspirone, and benzodiazepines are useful.
    - **3. Brief, isolated episodes of anxiety** that come and go lead the examiner to consider other diagnoses.
        - **a. Panic attacks.** If the patient has repeated "attacks" that have a rapid onset and last 20 minutes to a few hours, and if they are accompanied by tachycardia, palpitations, hyperventilation, sweating, dizziness, and the wish to flee without

Table 34-4. Other medications used to treat affective disorders

Drug	Starting dose	Average dose for cancer patients	Treatment	Pretreatment workup	Follow-up studies	Comment
Stimulants*						
Methylphenidate (Ritalin)	2.5–5.0 mg qA.M.	5–20 mg qA.M. + noon	Medically ill patient with depression	CBC	R-CBC	
Pemoline (Cylert)	18.75 mg qA.M.	37.5 mg qA.M. + noon	Medically ill patient with depression	Liver function tests	Liver function tests	
Dextroamphetamine (Dexedrine)†	2.5 mg qA.M.	5–20 mg qA.M. + noon	Medically ill patient with depression			
Lithium carbonate (Eskalith, Eskalith-CR, Lithobid)	300 mg qhs	300 mg tid	Depression‡ (may need to add an antidepressant) Mania‡ (may need to add clonazepam or an antipsychotic)	ECG, electrolytes, UA, BUN/ creat., thyroid (T₄, TSH, CBC (esp. WBC & platelets)	Lithium level initially 2 ×/wk. Gradually lengthen to q3mo. Thryoid studies q6mo or earlier if indicated. UA/BUN/creatinine, CBC if infection	Monitor blood level 12 hr after evening dose. 0.8–1.0 mEq/ liter *is* most effective. Watch for hypothyroidism, diabetes insipidus, nephropathy, dehydration.

Anticonvulsants						
Carbamazepine (Tegretol)	100 mg bid	200 mg tid	Depression or mania	CBC (including platelets, reticulocytes, & serum iron), liver function tests, UA, BUN	CBC, thyroid studies, blood level	Watch for leukopenia, hepatotoxicity.
Valproic acid (Depakene, Depakote)	15 mg/kg/day	500–750 mg/day (divided into tid doses)	Mania	Liver function tests, CBC	Liver function tests, CBC, blood level	Watch for hepatotoxicity, especially in young children.
Benzodiazepines						
Clonazepam (Clonopin, Klonopin)	0.5 mg qhs	2 mg or higher	Mania	CBC, liver function tests	CBC, liver function tests	Do not withdraw rapidly. Impaired renal function and respiratory distress require extremely cautious use.
Alprazolam (Xanax)	0.5 mg qhs	1 mg tid or higher	Depression			Do not withdraw rapidly (reduce daily dose by 0.25 mg weekly). Use cautiously if respiratory impairment.

*Checks on weight, pulse, and blood pressure. Tolerance may develop, and doses may require adjustment.
†Caution required because of multiple drug interactions.
‡Natural or corticosteroid-induced.

Table 34-5. Antidepressants: monoamine oxidase inhibitors

	Starting dose (mg bid)	Average dose (mg)	Characteristic
Tranylcypromine (Parnate)	10	20–60	More activating
Phenelzine (Nardil)	15	30–90	More sedating
Isocarboxazid (Marplan)	10	20–40	Greater risk of hepatotoxicity

Avoid

Foods: Tyramine-containing foods: aged cheeses, flat, broad beans, sausage, pickled herring, chianti wine

Drugs: Meperidine, phenylethylamine compounds including stimulants, appetite suppressants, decongestants, bronchodilators, large doses of aspartame sweeteners

a physical or chemical explanation, they are most likely panic attacks that often preexisted. They are best treated with antidepressants such as tricyclics and MAOIs. β-blockers to block autonomic symptoms may be tried if performance anxiety around specific activities is identified.

   b. Organic etiologies are often responsible for the anxiety.

   (1) Hypoxia. Repeating episodes of anxiety accompanied by alterations in intellectual functioning, poor orientation, reduced judgment, shortened attention, a rapidly fluctuating mood, and difficulty with memory suggest hypoxia. When anxiety is induced by hypoxia, it is wise to reduce central nervous system (CNS) depressant medications and give small doses of an antipsychotic drug if the anxiety is accompanied by delirium. Antipsychotic medications, however, often produce akathisia, an extrapyramidal restlessness that anxiety mimics. Alternating the antipsychotic drug with small doses of a short-half-life benzodiazepine or antihistamine is one option for organically induced anxiety—if respiratory status or arterial blood gases (ABGs) measurements do not worsen.

   (2) Liver disease and other physical disorders. If anxiety is associated with liver disease, start by reducing CNS depressant medications. When needed, small, infrequent doses of a short-acting benzodiazepine that

Table 34-6. Antianxiety agents and nighttime sedatives

Agent	Half-life (hours)	Onset	Starting dose (mg)
Benzodiazepines			
Triazolam (Halcion)	1.5–3.5	Rapid	0.125 (qhs)
Oxazepam (Serax)	8–20	Moderate	10 (tid)
Lorazepam (Ativan)	10–20	Rapid	0.5 (tid)
Temazepam (Restoril)	12–24	Rapid	15 (qhs)
Alprazolam (Xanax)	12–24	Moderate	0.25 (tid)
Chlordiazepam (Libriuim)	12–48	Moderate	10 (bid or tid)
Clonazepam (Klonopin)	20–30	Rapid	0.5 (bid)
Diazepam (Valium)	20–90	Rapid	2–5 (bid)
Clorazepate (Tranxene)	20–100	Rapid	7.5 (bid)
Flurazepam (Dalmane)	20–100	Rapid	15 (qhs)

Antidepressants (for panic disorder)
See Tables 34-2, 34-3, 34-4, 34-5. May use lower doses than for depression; i.e., an imipramine starting dose of 10 mg tid.

β-Blockers (for autonomic symptom control)
Propranolol (Inderal) 10–20 mg tid.

Antipsychotics (for anxiety associated with delirium)
See Table 34-1.

Antihistamines
May be safer in some cases when respiratory impairment is a complication; also used for insomnia.

Diphenhydramine (Benadryl) 25 mg; starting doses bid or tid
Hydroxyzine (Vistaril) 50 mg; starting doses tid or qid

Note: Elderly or extremely debilitated patients should be given lower doses. Caution should be taken when prescribing long-acting sedating medications, as they have been associated with a high incidence of falls and hip fracture.

requires conjugation but not oxidation in the liver are prescribed. Many other physical disorders can also produce anxious symptoms, including various brain tumors, pheochromocytoma, carcinoid, hyperthyroidism, cardiac arrhythmias, drug or alcohol withdrawal, and hyperparathyroidism.

   (3) **Medications** such as theophylline, corticosteroids, antidepressants, and antipsychotic drugs can produce anxiety.
C. **Precipitants** can be identified in patients with cancer that initiate the previously discussed adjustment disorder lasting generally no longer than 6 months. Posttraumatic stress disorder, less often seen in patients with

cancer, follows a distressing event outside the range of usual human experience. More frequently observed, however, are individuals who describe intense fears of needles, radiotherapy rooms, or confined-space scanning devices. Often the history unfolds to describe previously existing phobias. These patients, like those with anticipatory anxiety about procedures or chemotherapy, may be assisted with relaxation or desensitization techniques, imagery, antianxiety medications, and reassurance. If patients begin to experience procedures, treatments, or interpersonal situations as being particularly stressful, anticipatory anxiety intensifies the requirement for larger doses of as-needed medication to attain some relief. Therefore regular scheduling of antianxiety medication similarly to that of pain medication is in order.

V. Insomnia

A. Principles.
An inability to fall asleep may be associated with anxiety, whereas awakening in the middle of the night is generally more closely related to depression. In addition, there are a variety of physical disorders that cause sleeping irregularities. The sleep–wake cycle is almost always disturbed in a delirious patient, no matter what the etiology. Pain often awakens a patient with cancer. Medications can awaken some patients directly (e.g., fluoxetine) or indirectly (e.g., diuretics). Aside from sorting out these influences, the physician must take into account the environment. Is the patient too hot or cold? Is the ward too brightly lit or too noisy? Do the patients awaken each time they are checked by the night staff? When any or several of these concerns are corrected, sleeping medication may not be necessary, although the need for sedatives remains in some patients.

B. Benzodiazepines
(Table 34-6). This class of drugs is most often prescribed if a patient needs nighttime sedation. The shorter half-life benzodiazepines (i.e., triazolam or temazepam) with a rapid onset produce less daytime grogginess than those with a longer half-life. Short-acting ones tend to accumulate less and are safer for patients with liver disease. On the other hand, longer half-life drugs (i.e., diazepam or flurazepam) with a rapid onset produce less rebound insomnia or unwanted awakening during the very early morning.

C. Antihistamines
(Table 34-6). These medications may be chosen if physicians are hesitant to prescribe benzodiazepines, e.g., for patients with respiratory disease. A disadvantage may be the higher anticholinergic potential of these drugs compared to the benzodiazepine family.

D. Others.
Chloral hydrate (500–1000 mg), an old standby hypnotic, can still be used so long as patients are free of gastrointestinal or liver disease. Barbiturates, e.g., sodium amytal, are occasionally used to treat some refractory sleeping disturbances for a short time but are not routinely used because they induce respiratory depression and have addictive potential.

Selected Reading

Adams, F., Fernandez, F., and Anderson, B. Emergency pharmacotherapy of delirium in the critically ill cancer patient. *Psychosomatics* 27(suppl. 1):33, 1986.

Anderson, B., Adams, F., and McCredie, K. High-dose neuroleptics for acute brain failure after intensive chemotherapy for acute leukemia. *Acta Psychiatr. Scand.* 70:193, 1984.

Bernstein, J. G. *Handbook of Drug Therapy in Psychiatry* (2nd ed.). Littleton, MA: PSG Publishing, 1988.

Cassileth, B., et al. Psychosocial correlates of survival in advanced malignant disease. *N. Engl. J. Med.* 312:1551, 1985.

Evans, D. L., et al. Treatment of depression in cancer patients is associated with better life adaptation: a pilot study. *Psychosom. Med.* 50:72, 1988.

Holland, J. C., and Rowland, J. H. (ed.). *Handbook of Psychooncology.* New York: Oxford University Press, 1989.

Maguire, P., and Faulkner, A. How to improve the counseling skills of doctors and nurses in cancer care. *Br. Med. J.* 297:847, 1988.

Massie, M. J., and Holland, J. C. Depression and the cancer patient. *J. Clin. Psychiatry* 51(suppl. 7):12, 1990.

Perry, P., Alexander, B., and Liskow, B. *Psychotropic Drug Handbook* (4th ed.) Cincinnati: Harvey Whitney Books, 1985.

Spiegel, D., et al. Effect of psychosocial treatment of patients with metastatic breast cancer. *Lancet* 2:1447, 1989.

Zonderman, D. B., Costa, P. T., and McCrae, P. R. Depression as a risk for cancer morbidity and mortality in a nationally representative sample. *J.A.M.A.* 262:1191, 1989.

Cancer Pain

Michael Weintraub and Ana Rubio

I. Goals and approach to therapy for cancer pain

A. Definition and significance. Pain may be defined as an unpleasant sensory and emotional experience associated with actual or potential tissue damage; or it may be described in terms of such damage. The sensory and emotional aspects of pain are particularly important for the patient with cancer. Whether or not specific therapy is available for the cancer, physicians always have the responsibility to attempt to achieve adequate analgesia for their patients. Cancer pain is not conceptually different from other chronic pain syndromes, but the emotional overtones of the pain of cancer make it even more important that it be adequately treated. Initially, pain may be a signal for reassessment and diagnostic procedures. If specific therapy is possible, it should be undertaken as soon as the etiology of the pain has been discovered. However, physicians must prescribe analgesic drugs while attempting to establish the etiology of the pain and while waiting to begin specific treatment.

Pain is most often associated with solid tumors or multiple myeloma. It is less common with the lymphomas and leukemias. Almost three-fourths of patients with cancer have severe pain that is controllable in most cases. Common reasons for inadequate pain control include incorrect narcotic dosing (dose size, interval), incorrect switching from one narcotic medication or one route of administration to another without paying attention to individual patient characteristics and intrinsic medication properties, "noncompliance," and incorrect choice of medication.

Cancer pathophysiology can interfere with the oral administration of medication, narrow the patient's therapeutic window for analgesic drugs, limit the effectiveness of psychologic pain therapies, and complicate or preclude invasive pain-relieving procedures. Cancer therapy can interfere with pain therapy by causing pain or producing other adverse effects. However, cancer therapy may also enhance analgesia by reducing the extent of cancer, acting as a "coanalgesic," and providing intravenous access for parenteral drug administration to patients who require it. Pain therapy can interfere with treatment of the cancer by increasing or complicating the adverse effects of the cancer therapy.

B. Goals of therapy. Recognizing that patients with advanced cancer often equate their symptoms with their disease is an important psychologic adjustment for both the doctor and the patient. It helps avoid a "nothing more can be done" syndrome. The overall goal of analgesic therapy is to allow the patient to have as comfortable a life as possible at the highest level of daily activity commensurate with his or her physical status. The patient must be able to rest comfortably, eat, and perform self-care activities. Analgesic therapy should aim to enable the patient with cancer to maintain meaningful interaction with family members. Other ancillary goals are to allow the patient to maintain independent living at home and to be cared for in as normal a situation as possible. Some pain in patients with cancer is not amenable to specific therapy. Nonetheless, analgesia should always be attempted.

C. **General guidelines for analgesic use.** There are a number of general guidelines for analgesic use in patients with cancer. With the goal of therapy established and kept firmly in mind, the physician must next choose the agent and the modality.

1. **Choice of agent.** The choice of analgesic should be based not only on the analgesic goal and pain severity but on a variety of other factors as well: the etiology of the pain, the anatomic location of the pain, and the characteristics of the pain (e.g., sharp, paroxysmal pain or dull, constant pain). Selection of analgesic modalities is, in part, related to the type and location of the tumor; e.g., pain in the bones can be successfully treated with peripherally acting analgesics such as nonsteroidal anti-inflammatory agents (NSAIDs). On the other hand, pain from some cancers, e.g., primary pancreatic or perianal tumors, requires local measures. Neuritic pain may respond best to tricyclic antidepressants.

2. **Dosage and schedule.** Once the agent has been chosen, the proper dose and dosing interval needed to achieve the therapeutic goal must be selected. This decision is not the end of the therapeutic process, however. The physician must continually assess the response to the analgesic selected and modify the dose or the dose schedule based on the patient's response. In general, it is most often efficacious to begin treatment with high doses when the pain is severe and taper medication as pain control is achieved. Regularly scheduled dosing is often more effective than "as needed" dosing. It is important to prevent recurrent "breakthroughs." Thus blocking the pain and erasing its memory in order to obtain continued, uninterrupted relief may be an appropriate goal of analgesia.

   When a previously effective chronic pain analgesic regimen fails, physicians should look for correctable new pain causes, such as infection, pathologic fractures, tumor extension, or neuritic pain due to radiation therapy or direct tumor extension.

3. **Adjunctive therapy.** Nonanalgesic adjunctive therapy such as muscle relaxants, sedatives, liniments, antiemetics, heat, cold, braces, and other appliances as well as other symptomatic therapy for cough, itching, or nausea can enhance the patient's response to analgesic medication and improve the overall quality of his or her life.

4. **Combinations of analgesics.** Often rational combinations of analgesics are beneficial for patients with cancer pain. Such combinations may provide improved pain relief, delay the appearance of tolerance to narcotic medications, and avoid side effects from the medications in the combination. In some cases combinations of narcotic analgesics and stimulants, e.g., amphetamines, may enhance narcotic effects, as is discussed in **IV.C.4.**

5. **Pain and suffering.** Physicians must always remember that chronic pain does not inure patients to pain; in fact, it makes them more sensitive to pain. Additionally, physicians and patients may share the puritanical belief that suffering builds character. Undertreatment with analgesic drugs may occur based on complicity between the patient and physician, nurse, or other health professional. Physicians may not prescribe enough analgesic treatment, a weak drug may be chosen, too low a dose may be given, or too long a dose interval may be utilized. Alternatively, patients may not ask for prescribed analgesics and suffer needlessly.

Often analgesic therapy fails owing to the use of an "as needed" policy and smaller daily doses than suggested by the literature. Undertherapy with narcotics may occur because of exaggeration of the risk of tolerance and addiction by both patients and medical personnel. Patients suffering from severe pain may benefit from a pain-free period of intensive treatment allowing sleep and freedom from discomfort. Such a respite often restores the response to previously ineffective analgesics. The need for a pain-free period may occur whenever patients have escaped from previous analgesic therapy or if a new pain problem has arisen.

Physicians should not be reluctant to prescribe narcotics. Lack of knowledge may intimidate physicians and keep them from prescribing rationally. For example, Hill indicated that prescribing very large doses and ordering an adequate quantity of a drug to have at home for a reasonable period of time, as is often required for the control of severe pain, may be perceived as an invitation for investigation of the physician. However, the evidence is clear that drug abuse is not a problem among cancer patients with pain.

II. **Cancer pain type and etiology.** Pain associated with cancer may result from tumor infiltration of pain-sensitive structures, injury to nerves, bone, and soft tissue resulting from chemotherapy, radiotherapy, surgery, or vascular occlusion by tumor. Less commonly, it is unrelated to cancer or cancer treatment.

A. **Visceral pain.** Cancer pain may arise from the pressure caused by the tumor growth in a tight tissue compartment. Occasionally, cancers impede venous return, causing engorgement and resulting in pain. Ischemia resulting from partial or complete arterial blockage causes severe pain. A hollow viscus may become obstructed as a consequence of tumor growth or surgical intervention. Pain arising in solid or hollow organs related to these etiologies is often called visceral pain. Patients may describe the character of visceral pain as dull, deep, constant or colicky, and aching. It can be referred to cutaneous areas that may even become tender. Except in the case of hollow viscus obstruction, visceral pain is often diffuse and poorly defined, with radiation that may not be in the pattern usually associated with classic descriptions of somatic dermatomes. Visceral pain often responds best to narcotic and narcotic antagonist analgesics, particularly when it is severe.

B. **Inflammatory and somatic pain.** Cancer pain may also arise from tissue damage, such as that caused by necrosis, infection, or inflammation in pain-sensitive structures. Patients with cancer may complain of bone or musculoskeletal pain, which may arise from periosteal irritation, fractures, or other causes. This pain is typically well localized, usually constant, and described as aching or gnawing. Metastases to bone cause the most common pain syndrome in patients with cancer. Pain from tissue damage, musculoskeletal pain, and dental and integumental pain respond best to antipyretic or anti-inflammatory analgesics such as aspirin, acetaminophen, or the NSAIDs.

C. **Neuritic, neuropathic, and atypical pain.** Neuritic pain arises from infiltration of nerves or nerve roots, as a distant effect caused by cancer, from extrinsic pressure on the nerves, or from postherpetic neuralgia. Patients may complain of a constant, dull, squeezing, aching sensation with superimposed paroxysms of burning, sharp, or "electric-shocklike" sensations. Patients may complain of unpleasant distortions in their perception of normal stimuli. There may also be changes in autonomic function, such as blood flow changes or sweating. Neuropathic pain occurs when the nervous system is damaged or degeneration occurs in the part of the nervous system that normally transmits information about painful stimuli. Neuropathic pain may be caused by direct irritation, metabolic problems, immunologic effects on the nervous system, or late effects of radiation therapy, surgery, or chemotherapy. Neuritic and neuropathic pain often responds poorly to both narcotic analgesics and to antipyretic, anti-inflammatory analgesics, but it may respond well to so-called nonanalgesic analgesics, e.g., tricyclic antidepressants, antiepileptic agents, and phenothiazines. Neuritic pain may be the most difficult to control, particularly if not treated early and aggressively.

III. **Drug groups**

A. **Narcotic and narcotic antagonist (partial agonist) analgesics.** Examples of drugs in this class of analgesic agents include the narcotic agonists morphine, methadone (Dolophine), and meperidine (Demerol), and the narcotic antagonist or partial agonist analgesics penta-zocine (Talwin), butorphanol (Stadol), and nalbuphine (Nubain). These drugs are most helpful for treating visceral pain (as described in **II.A**) and should be used for severe pain of any type arising from any structure.

1. **Mode of action.** Narcotic and narcotic antagonist medications are also called centrally acting analgesics. They work by interacting with specific receptors located in neuronal membranes and have their major effect within the central nervous system (CNS). These receptors are thought to be the same ones normally acted on by the "endogenous opioids"—primarily endorphins and enkephalins. The narcotic drugs presumably mimic the actions of these endogenous compounds. In addition to decreasing the patient's response to or processing of the pain stimulus at a central level, narcotic agonist and partial agonist analgesics also directly decrease the severity of the pain.

2. **Adverse effects.** CNS side effects ranging from sedation to hallucinations may be a problem when using narcotic analgesics and narcotic antagonist analgesics. Other adverse effects, e.g., bradycardia and hypotension, may be seen with some of the agents in this class. Respiratory depression occurs with the narcotic agonists. Nausea and vomiting may develop. Patients often need laxative treatment (or prophylaxis) for narcotic-induced constipation.

    Tolerance (the need to increase the dose to achieve the same therapeutic effect) and *physical dependence* (manifested by a characteristic withdrawal syndrome) have been described with the use of narcotic agonist and partial agonists; however, with appropriate adjustment of dose, patients can continue to obtain pain relief. True addiction (preoccupation with drug procurement and use) arising from the medical use of narcotic analgesics is a rare phenomenon. Psychologic and physical dependence may develop more or less rapidly based on various medication and patient characteristics. The medications that cause rapid psychologic and physical dependence are those that cross the blood-brain barrier quickly. Other effects of the medication, e.g., as anticholinergic and euphoriant effects, increase drug abuse liability. Large, frequent doses of medication speed the development of tolerance. It has been said that tolerance and physical dependence may develop over a 48 to 72-hour period when narcotic medications are administered in continuous IV infusions at a relatively high dose. Oral administration is less likely to lead to tolerance. The patient and the underlying physical problem also affect the rapidity and development of tolerance and physical dependence. Some patients do not develop this syndrome, whereas others develop it quickly.

3. **Effect of dose and route administration.** There is a ceiling effect for some of the weak narcotic analgesic agents, e.g., codeine and propoxyphene (Darvon). Thus increasing the dose of codeine above 120 mg PO q4h may do nothing but increase the adverse effects without a concomitant increase in analgesia. However, morphine does not exhibit the ceiling effect; and in fact open-heart surgery has been conducted using morphine as the sole anesthetic agent. Initial morphine doses are 5–10 mg parenterally every 4 hours. Physicians should increase the dose according to the pain reported by the patient. One suggested method utilizes steps of 5, 10, 15, 20, 30, 45, 60, 90, 120, 160, and 180 mg parenterally every 4 hours until the pain is controlled.

Many of the narcotic analgesics maintain some activity when administered orally. Morphine is almost completely absorbed after oral administration but has poor bioavailability (30–40%) due to extensive first pass metabolism in the gut and liver. The relative oral to parenteral potency ratio of morphine is 1:6. This potency improves to 1:2 or 1:3 following repeated dosage owing to (1) dose-dependent presystemic metabolism; (2) contribution of the metabolite morphine-6-glucuronide to the analgesic effect; and (3) enterohepatic circulation of morphine and metabolites. Initially, giving the same amount of drug orally as is given parenterally results in serious undertreatment with most narcotic analgesics. For example, an adequate IM dose of meperidine for an adult is 75–100 mg, whereas as much as 200–300 mg PO may be necessary to achieve the same analgesic response. However, oral narcotic doses may be reduced once pain control is achieved.

Several narcotic analgesics are not completely metabolized in the gut wall or by hepatic cells, and they reach the systemic circulation with a good PO/IM potency ratio. These drugs include levorphanol (Levo-Dromoran), methadone, and oxycodone. Codeine, although less active, also has a good PO/IM potency ratio. The starting doses of narcotic analgesics and narcotic antagonist-agonist analgesics are given in Table 35-1.

4. **Duration of action.** Most narcotic analgesics have a duration of action of at least 3 hours. Medications found at this lower end of the scale include hydromorphone (Dilaudid), oxycodone, pentazocine, and heroin (not available for medical use in the United States). Although heroin has been advocated as a superior therapeutic agent for use in terminal illnesses, it is difficult to make a judgment with the available data. It is 15 times more potent than morphine when given orally and 2–4 times more potent than morphine administered parenterally. When the potency difference is accounted for, the pharmaco-

Table 35-1. Starting doses and duration of action of narcotic analgesics and narcotic antagonist-agonist analgesics

Drug	Initial dose (mg)	Frequency	Duration of action (hr)
Parenteral narcotics			
Morphine	8–10	q3–6h	⁻4
Oxymorphone (Numorphan)	1	q3–6h	⁻4
Hydromorphone (Dilaudid)	1–2	q4–6h	⁻5
Levorphanol (Levo-Dromoran)	2–3	q4–6h	⁻5
Methadone (Dolophine)	8–10	q5–8h	6
Meperidine (Demerol)	75–100	q3–4h	2–4
Parenteral narcotic antagonist agonists			
Pentazocine (Talwin)	40–60	q3–6h	4–5
Butorphanol (Stadol)	2–4	q3–4h	3–4
Nalbuphine (Nubain)	10	q3–4h	3–4
Buprenorphine (Buprenex)	0.3	q6h	⁻6
Oral narcotics			
Meperidine (Demerol)	200–300	q4–6h	4–5
Codeine	30–60	q4–6h	4–5
Propoxyphene (Darvon)	130	q4–6h	4–5
Oxycodone (in mixtures)	20–30	q3–4h	⁻4
Methadone (Dolophine)	10–20	q6–8h	⁻6
Levorphanol (Levo-Dromoran)	2–4	q4–6h	⁻5
Hydromorphone (Dilaudid)	4–6	q3–5	3–4
Morphine, Sustained Release (MS Contin)	30–60	q8–12h	12
Morphine (tablets or liquid)	10–20	q4h	⁻4
Oral narcotic antagonist-agonist			
Pentazocine (Talwin)	50–100	q3–5h	3–4
Hydrocodone	2.5–5.0	q4–6h	5
Phenothiazines (parenteral)			
Methotrimeprazine (Levoprome)	10–20	q6–8h	⁻6

logic effects of heroin do not differ appreciably from those of morphine. Methadone has a longer duration of action (up to 6 hours), particularly after chronic dosing, owing to drug accumulation. Individual variation in the duration of action of methadone and its pharmacokinetics may lead to accumulation and a consequent need for careful monitoring. Buprenorphine, a mixed narcotic agonist-antagonist seems to have a longer duration of action than others in this class. Meperidine and morphine are intermediate-acting, with durations of action of approximately 4 hours. Physicians frequently overestimate the duration of action of narcotic analgesics, which may result in undertreatment. Morphine and other narcotics may accumulate in patients with decreased renal function. Thus naloxone (Narcan) reversal of excessive effects may be needed for long periods.

5. **Formulation.** Some patients prefer liquid oral formulations. These formulations are easy to take, have various flavors (limited only by the pharmacist's imagination), and are flexible in terms of dose titration. However, interest in liquid combination analgesics is not supported by objective data. Other patients find tablets or capsules more convenient. Suppositories may also be useful for patients who have swallowing difficulties or significant nausea. Patients must insert the suppository above the anal sphincter but not much further. This position allows the absorbed drug to bypass the portal system and enter the systemic circulation as the inferior and middle hemorrhoidal veins enter the inferior vena cava system. Occasionally, rectal administration of analgesics irritates the mucosa, or absorption may be irregular and slow. Patients also may not wish to use the suppositories. New formulations are continually being developed (see **III.A.6.c**), and most analgesics can be found in many formulations. The physician should prescribe one that the patient finds acceptable and at the same time accomplishes the therapeutic goal.

6. **New developments**

   a. **Epidural narcotic analgesics.** An important development in the use of opiate analgesics is the administration of these drugs into the extradural spaces, although studies find the improvement over oral analgesia questionable. Potential advantages of this route of administration include lower drug doses than those used for systemic therapy and analgesia without autonomic changes, loss of motor power, or impairment of sensation other than pain reduction. Various medications with differing durations of action and routes of elimination have been utilized for peridural or epidural analgesia. This method seems relatively safe, even if the material is inadvertently injected into the subarachnoid space. If the medication is accidentally given IV or intrathecally, respiratory depression and other adverse effects can easily be antagonized by naloxone, a specific, safe, pure opiate antagonist. The use of epidural narcotic analgesics is based on the existence of spinal opiate receptors in the substantia gelatinosa. Studies involving large numbers of patients have concluded that the use of indwelling epidural catheters for narcotic analgesic administration has resulted in few adverse effects, rare development of tolerance (even over a 3-week period), the need for low daily doses, and excellent analgesia. Respiratory depression may still follow epidural morphine use, however. There is no significant analgesic cross-tolerance to epidural morphine, but clear evidence exists for cross-tolerance regarding morphine's respiratory depressant action. The duration of the previous morphine therapy seems to exert a greater influence on the development of ventilatory cross-tolerance than the dose.

Concomitant administration of methylprednisolone can increase both analgesia and its duration, decreasing the chance of morphine-induced side effects.

Absorption from the epidural space into the blood varies depending on the agent used. Some data indicate that buprenorphine causes more respiratory depression than morphine, probably because of its greater systemic absorption. Nevertheless, the risk of delayed respiratory depression appears to be less after buprenorphine than after morphine.

b. Enkephalin derivatives. Several enkephalin derivatives are currently under study as analgesic medications. Further understanding of the endogenous opiate system may result in clinically useful medications. However, development remains slow.

c. New formulations. Several manufacturers have produced controlled, delayed, and sustained-release formulations of morphine. Controlled-release morphine sulfate tablets allow only two administrations per day. Analgesia nearly identical to oral aqueous morphine solution occurs. Controlled-release morphine offers an additional method of providing prolonged control with an associated overall improvement in quality of life. A review describing the European experience indicates that controlled-release morphine (MST) is effective in patients with opioid-responsive pain, that for almost all patients twice-daily administration is sufficient, that the potency ratio compared with standard (immediate release) oral morphine formulations is 1:1 and that the side effect profile is similar. MST is not recommended for titration when frequent dose adjustments may be required. However, once patients have been stabilized, MST is much more convenient and simpler to use.

For a particular patient new methods for administering morphine orally may avoid injections, thereby enabling patients to remain at home. A new combination of narcotic antagonist analgesic and acetaminophen has also been marketed. The combination of oral pentazocine and naloxone is a valuable formulation. The effect of naloxone is not present when ingested orally. However, if a drug abuser attempts to dissolve the preparation and inject it parenterally, naloxone blocks the psychic effects of pentazocine. Narcotic analgesics have also been formulated in so-called high-potency or concentrated solutions, so patients with decreased muscle mass can receive full narcotic doses easily. Morphine administered in a continuous subcutaneous infusion has been helpful in both children and adults with serious cancer pain. A new experimental approach is the administration of morphine intranasally or through tablets that dissolve against the buccal mucosa. Transdermal delivery of narcotics provides an option whose effectiveness is still under investigation.

B. Antipyretic, anti-inflammatory analgesics. The classic example of drugs in this class is aspirin. Acetaminophen is antipyretic, but only weakly, if at all, anti-inflammatory. Nonetheless, it remains a valuable analgesic to replace aspirin in patients who cannot tolerate the gastrointestinal or platelet inhibitory side effects of aspirin. Acetaminophen does not affect uric acid excretion. The doses used for aspirin as an analgesic agent are less than those required for full anti-inflammatory effect. Thus 650 mg (2 common tablets) of aspirin provide analgesia for 2–4 hours. Other examples of the antipyretic, anti-inflammatory analgesics include indomethacin and other NSAIDs, such as ibuprofen, fenoprofen, naproxen, sulindac, and tolmetin sodium. They seem to have a specific effect on pain caused by bone metastases by interfering with the production of prostaglandins. This point is doubly important, as this type of pain responds poorly to opioids.

1. Use and mode of action. These drugs work peripherally rather than centrally. They are most effective in the treatment of musculoskeletal, dental, or integumental pain of mild to moderate severity. They may also decrease inflammation. Data on the precise mechanism of action of the antipyretic, anti-inflammatory medications in decreasing pain are controversial. However, by blocking production of prostaglandins, NSAIDs may decrease sensitization of nociceptors (a receptor preferentially sensitive to a noxious or potentially noxious stimulus).

Newer members of this analgesic class may also block other mediators of the inflammatory process. Sedation, of course, is not a problem with peripherally acting antipyretic, anti-inflammatory analgesics. Acetylsalicylic acid has been successfully used intrathecally for the treatment of chronic refractory pain in cancer patients.

2. **Adverse effects** are usually related to the gastrointestinal tract, kidneys, and bone marrow. Cardiovascular effects, respiratory depression, tolerance, and dependence do not accompany therapy with these agents. They do have a ceiling effect, however. All of these agents except ketorolac, given orally, are effective with a usual duration of action of approximately 4 hours. The rationale for the development of the newer NSAIDs has been to achieve anti-inflammatory and analgesic effects similar to those of aspirin but with fewer side effects. Therefore the possibility of using these agents in patients who cannot tolerate the necessary doses of aspirin or acetaminophen always exists. (Table 35-2 lists common starting doses of the NSAIDs). Antipyretic, anti-inflammatory analgesics often form a logical component of rational combination analgesics either as manufactured by the pharmaceutical industry or as prepared individually for each patient by physicians.

One NSAID may be more effective for a specific patient than others. Trying one at a time is appropriate in order to select the most effective. The trial and error method is useful, as responses and side effects of the various NSAIDs vary.

C. **Nonanalgesic analgesics** (phenothiazines, tricyclic antidepressants, and antiepileptic agents). Sleep disorders and mood disturbances are related to the experience of pain. Anxiety and depression, which may be associated with cancer, can influence the pain experience and can be managed symptomatically with psychotropic drugs. In addition, some psychotropic drugs have analgesic properties or may be used to reduce some side effects of narcotics. They can be useful adjuvant analgesic agents for the management of cancer pain.

1. **Agents and their use.** Examples of this class of medications include the standard analgesic drug methotrimeprazine (Levoprome). This agent is a phenothiazine drug used in parts of the world other than the United States as an antipsychotic agent. It produces analgesia equivalent to that of morphine when given parenterally. The problems of its use include sedation (particularly after the first few doses) and postural hypotension. Tolerance and respiratory depression do not develop with methotrimeprazine.

Amitriptyline (Elavil and others) given with or

Table 35-2. Starting doses and dose ranges of some nonsteroidal analgesic agents

Drug	Starting dose (mg)	Frequency	Dose range (mg)
Salicylates			
Aspirin	650	q4–6h	Up to 1300 (q6h)
Choline salicylate	870	q4h	
Choline-magnesium salicylate	500	q6h	Up to 1000
Diflunisal	1000 (loading dose)	q8h	500–1000
Magnesium salicylate	545	q6–8h	Up to 600
Salsalate	1000	q8h	Up to 1500
Sodium salicylate	650	q4h	Up to 975
Phenylacetic acids			
Diclofenac	50	q8h	Up to 75
Ketorolac (IM only)	30 (loading dose)	q6h	15–60
Fenamates			
Mefenamic acid	250	q6h	Up to 375 (q6h)
Meclofenamate	50	q6–8h	Up to 100
Indoleacetic acids			
Indomethacin	50	q6–8h	Up to 100 (q6–8h)
Sulindac	150	q12h	Up to 200
Tolmetin	400	q8h	Up to 600
Propionic acids			
Ibuprofen	400	q4–6h	Up to 2400 (daily)
Fenoprofen	600	q6h	Up to 3200 (daily)
Flurbiprofen	50	q6–8h	Up to 75
Ketoprofen	50	q8h	Up to 100
Naproxen	250	q8–12h	Up to 1250 (daily)
Naproxen sodium	550	First dose	
	275	q6–8h	Up to 1375 (daily)
Oxicams			
Piroxicam	10	q12–24h	Up to 20

without a phenothiazine such as perphenazine (Trilafon) has been used for the treatment of atypical pain and a variety of painful syndromes involving nerves. Tricyclic antidepressants may have a specific analgesic action linked to a direct activity on the structure of the CNS. In addition, when administered concomitantly with morphine, amitriptyline produces a significant increase in the plasma availability of morphine with an increase in the half-life of this drug. Postherpetic neuralgia, phantom-limb pain, and other types of neuritic pain may respond dramatically and rapidly to tricyclic and other psychotherapeutic medications.

Amitriptyline plus perphenazine as well as other psychotropic drugs have been used with success for the treatment of serious postherpetic neuralgia pain and neuritic pain caused by direct or distant effects of cancer. Common starting doses include 50 mg of amitriptyline with 4 mg of perphenazine given before bedtime, followed by 25 mg of amitriptyline and 2 mg of perphenazine given in the morning. Patients with postherpetic neuralgia may report dramatic improvement in their pain after 1–2 days of such doses.

Carbamazepine (Tegretol) has been used for the treatment of tic douloureux. It is, of course, an important antiepileptic agent. Levodopa has been used to treat pain arising from bone metastases in patients with breast and other cancers. Along with a peripheral dopa-decarboxylase inhibitor, levodopa has also been successful in decreasing acute herpes zoster pain and perhaps preventing postherpetic neuralgia. The mechanism of levodopa's pain-decreasing effects is unclear.

These nonanalgesic analgesics may have both central and peripheral sites of action. Neuritic and atypical shooting paroxysmal pain responds best to these drugs. In fact, ablative neurosurgical procedures may be avoided by the appropriate use of these agents. They are efficacious against moderate to severe pain. Of course, methotrimeprazine may be used for any type of pain, particularly in bedridden patients or those needing the pain-free period previously discussed.

2. **Side effects.** Sedation may occur with amitriptyline and phenothiazine, but it is rarely a problem if these drugs are prescribed on an appropriate schedule, such as before sleep. Postural hypotension occurs with methotrimeprazine and less often with the amitriptyline plus perphenazine combination. However, patients rapidly become tolerant to this effect without loss of analgesic effect. Respiratory depression, the need for dose escalation, and physical dependence do not occur. Except for methotrimeprazine, the useful psychotropic medications are orally active and have relatively long half-lives.

D. Others

1. **Capsaicin.** Capsaicin is an extract of red pepper that may be helpful against neuritic pain. It is available over the counter in a cream formulation. Onset of effect may be delayed. Local burning is the primary adverse effect.

2. **Corticosteroids** seem to help pain caused by the destruction of nerves. Its psychostimulating, anti-anorexic, and strength-improving actions are beneficial in cancer patients.

E. Combination analgesics. Rational combinations of antipyretic, anti-inflammatory agents with mild narcotics, e.g., codeine, propoxyphene, or in some cases the more euphoria-inducing agent oxycodone, are valuable therapeutic approaches to the treatment of cancer pain. The addition of NSAIDs to a narcotic regimen may delay the appearance of tolerance to the narcotic while maintaining adequate pain control. Naloxone–pentazocine combinations have been marketed; and as noted in **III.A.6.c,** such a formulation decreases abuse potential. In the past, the pharmaceutic industry has altered the formulas of many of the combination analgesics. Therefore it is important that each physician keep up-to-date information and learn the exact ingredients of every combination drug. One important change has been to eliminate phenacetin from analgesic combinations. However, other ingredients have also been removed from some of the pharmaceutically produced analgesic combinations. Combination analgesics may, in the long run, save the patient money and produce the desired therapeutic effect more efficaciously than combinations created by the physician. Another valuable feature of pharmaceutically produced combination analgesics is ensurance of compatibility of both active ingredients and the excipients. Pharmacists may charge separate fees for filling each of two prescriptions, thereby increasing the cost of physician-created combinations. If physicians wish to create their own combinations, the names of the components not requiring a prescription should be given to the patient on a separate paper and bought over the counter. To reduce drug costs, only the prescription medications should be written on a prescription blank.

IV. Analgesics: additional considerations of rational pain management

A. Cost of therapy. Physicians must consider the cost of therapy, but they should not depend on price lists taken from wholesale catalogs, even with a standard markup added. The pharmacist, whose importance is often forgotten, represents one of the major components of drug price. Many studies have shown that prices for the same amount of the same medication vary enormously among pharmacies and even within the same pharmacies over time. Prescriptions written generically to allow substitution usually do save patients some money. However, generic drugs occasionally cost more than the brand-name product, depending on the pharmacy. Simplistic dependence on the prices in the "Red Book" often misleads prescribers. To achieve savings, patients must comparison-shop. Of course, the physician must prescribe the most effective medication for the patient, as the medicine achieving the therapeutic goal ultimately represents the least expensive treatment.

B. Escalation of analgesic requirement

   1. Increase in symptoms may connote a change in disease status. If a patient who has been previously well controlled on a therapeutic regimen of analgesics suddenly has increasingly severe pain, a diagnostic workup and perhaps new therapeutic approaches are required. Frequently the cause of the change in pain is a new disease process, which may be related to or unrelated to the cancer. The search for correctable causes, e.g., infections, pathologic fractures, and new metastases (which may be sensitive to localized irradiation or alterations in chemotherapy), should be carried out immediately. If the etiology of the pain is extension of the disease process (e.g., a new tumor mass) or the therapy form (e.g., late effects of radiation therapy or surgery) this etiology must be diagnosed and treated appropriately.

   2. Increase in symptoms may mean insufficient medication or tolerance. Another cause for the development of ineffective analgesia is that the patients have "fallen behind" in their therapy. Constant around-the-clock analgesic therapy is more effective than on-demand or as-needed therapy. Patients may omit analgesic doses either because they wish to avoid addiction or because they believe that the physician, nurse, and pharmacist may attribute their use of drugs to a weakness of character.

   The development of tolerance to narcotic analgesics is another potential etiology for ineffective analgesia. As tolerance develops, the patient first notices a decrease in the duration of action of the narcotic analgesics. Later the peak effect decreases, and finally the onset of effect is delayed. Simply increasing the dose of medication can overcome this problem. Addition of NSAIDs, stimulants, or other psychoactive medications may also help delay or overcome the development of tolerance.

C. Stepwise use of analgesic agents. If the need arises for the initiation of analgesics or for therapeutic escalation to more powerful analgesics for cancer pain, a stepwise approach is often valuable. This approach assumes that nondrug therapy and other adjunctive therapies have been attempted. Beginning with oral medication is a good idea unless the patient needs either a pain-free period or high analgesic doses to achieve initial pain control. The first step is to begin with a mild drug, later working toward combinations of mild drugs, and finally adding the more powerful agents.

1. **Mild drugs.** In step 1, the use of nonnarcotic oral analgesics, e.g., antipyretic, anti-inflammatory agents, is often helpful. Acetaminophen has less gastrointestinal toxicity than aspirin, although it may cause hepatic toxicity in overdose and in poorly nourished patients. It does not have anti-inflammatory effects, however. Aspirin is a good alternative that has not only analgesic effects but also anti-inflammatory effects. The NSAIDs, including indomethacin, the propionic acid derivatives, and newer agents, may also be useful as first-step agents, particularly if the pain is mild or if it involves either the musculoskeletal system or the integument. Depending on the etiology of their pain and its severity, some patients respond to a mild narcotic given alone. Mild narcotics include codeine and propoxyphene, either as the hydrochloride or the napsylate salt (Darvon-N). One of the mild, mixed agonist-antagonist analgesics (e.g., pentazocine) could also be used. Oxycodone, which is found mostly in combination drugs, may have a higher abuse potential than some of the other agents. Propoxyphene and its metabolite norpropoxyphene, at least in high doses, may be associated with cardiac toxicity. There is also some problem with abuse of propoxyphene.

2. **Adding mild narcotics to nonnarcotic analgesics.** Step 1A involves the combination of a nonnarcotic oral antipyretic, anti-inflammatory analgesic with a mild narcotic. In manufactured combinations, they frequently include the mild stimulant caffeine and, more rarely, barbiturates. Other combinations can be created by the physician.

3. **Using a stronger narcotic.** Step 2 involves the use of orally active, stronger narcotics. An example is hydromorphone: A dose of 8 mg PO is equivalent to 10 mg of parenteral morphine, but lower doses may be used for less severe pain. Hydromorphone is short-acting and should be given approximately q3–4h. Other examples are levorphanol, 4 mg of which is equivalent to 10 mg of morphine, and oxymorphone (Numorphan), which can be given as a suppository in patients who are nauseated. Approximately 6 mg of oxymorphone PO is equivalent to 10 mg of morphine. Methadone is the most useful of these orally active strong narcotics because of its long half-life and its tendency to accumulate with chronic dosing. A 20-mg dose of methadone has been said to be equal to 10 mg of parenteral morphine; patients frequently respond well to methadone in repeated doses of 10 mg PO. In fact, after several days, many patients are able to tolerate a reduction in their dose of methadone with maintained pain relief.

4. **Combining strong narcotics and NSAIDs or stimulants.** Step 2A involves combining the strong narcotics and the NSAIDs. In some institutions, strong narcotics have been used in combination

with stimulant drugs, e.g., amphetamine and, more rarely, cocaine. Patients sleep and eat better even when receiving the stimulants because their pain has been decreased. Such combinations may be effective, but their use has probably been overemphasized. One frequently used combination is methadone 1 mg/ml plus amphetamine 0.5 mg/ml in a liquid preparation.

5. **Parenteral narcotics.** Step 3 requires the use of parenteral strong narcotics or narcotic antagonist analgesics for the relief of serious pain. Its initiation usually necessitates hospitalization, where parenteral medication can be administered and dose adjustments made to achieve pain control without undue risk. Once a relatively stable dose or range has been established, a hospice or other chronic care facility can usually administer parenteral narcotics safely. Often family members can be taught to administer parenteral medications, or trained personnel can make scheduled visits so the patient can be kept comfortable and at home. Parenteral analgesia in the home is often facilitated if the patient has a semipermanent central catheter or implanted vascular access port (see Chap. 38). Parenteral meperidine or morphine—or if the patient has not already being on long-term narcotic treatment, the parenteral partial agonist-antagonists such as butorphenol, nalbuphine, pentazocine, or buprenorphine—may be prescribed.

Step 3A is the use of a parenteral nonnarcotic such as methotrimeprazine.

At each step nonsteroidal anti-inflammatory analgesics can be added if appropriate. In some patients normeperidine, the major metabolite of meperidine, may accumulate, resulting in paradoxical CNS stimulation and even seizures.

6. **Adjunctive therapy** should be considered at every pain level. Nondestructive techniques include the epidural–intrathecal use of opioids via an implanted catheter or local anesthetic block of nerves and sympathetic ganglia. Destructive neurosurgical procedures include injections of neurolytic agents (phenol or alcohol) and insertion of freezing probes into nerves and ganglia. Marked relief of pain was observed in 65.5% of a group of cancer patients treated with calcitonin. The investigators also showed a decrease in the quantity of other analgesics used. The underlying mechanism for calcitonin in analgesia is not well understood. However, inhibition of the synthesis of algogenous peptides can be involved.

Physicians can now choose from among many forms of treatment, including transepidermal neurostimulation (TENS), neurosurgical ablative procedures, nerve blocks, heat, cold, and braces. Neurosurgery may always be considered when the pain no longer responds to conservative treatment methods or responds only at the cost of undesirable side effects. Cordotomy, indicated for patients with unilateral pain, is currently the most effective and most durable treatment form.

7. **Behavioral approaches.** Marked advances have been made in the use of psychologic techniques, including teaching patients a variety of behavioral approaches to pain control. Behavioral techniques should be integrated into nearly all treatments for chronic pain patients, particularly for those who do not obtain pain relief from narcotics or other analgesics or who have side effects from analgesics.

V. New developments in pain control

A. **Patient-controlled analgesia.** The exciting development of patient-controlled analgesia in hospital settings remains of interest. Patients can administer analgesics to themselves, particularly medications given IV through reliable drug administration systems equipped with fail-safe controls. Such systems may be valuable in achieving pain-free periods. Patients in self-dosing, self-controlled analgesia studies requested lower total analgesic doses over a 3-day period after surgery than a comparison group. During the first 24 hours after abdominal surgery, however, they administered on the average 500 mg of parenteral meperidine, a dose that is much higher than physicians usually prescribe. In a study involving patient-controlled analgesia for severe cancer pain, morphine sulfate dosages ranged from 1 to 5 mg. The lockout intervals ranged from 15 to 90 minutes. The patients self-administered more doses during the first 4 hours than during the remaining time of treatment. Significant pain relief was produced in all patients without causing undue sedation. Patient acceptance of this mode of therapy was excellent. Most patients preferred this type of analgesia to other forms of pain treatment. Other methods, e.g., controlled IM analgesia and patient-controlled epidural injection of narcotic analgesics, may also offer important benefits.

B. **New agents.** Continued research on endorphins and enkephalins may result in the achievement of orally active derivatives of these fascinating materials. Further definition of the specific opioid receptors may result in the development of medications that selectively stimulate analgesic receptors with no or minimal euphoria, sedation, cardiovascular effects, and tolerance. The pharmaceutic industry is continually searching for more effective orally administered nonnarcotic analgesics. Physicians should follow the literature and use these drugs as soon as they become available, and their efficacy for cancer pain is apparent. Although we have neither the perfect drug nor agents that accomplish all of our goals, we certainly can do a better job in using the available drugs more effectively and more rationally.

Selected Reading

American College of Physicians. Drug therapy for severe chronic pain in terminal illness (review). *Ann. Intern. Med.* 99:870, 1983.

Breitbart, W. Psychiatric management of cancer pain. *Cancer* 63(suppl. 11):2336, 1989.

Breitbart, W. Psychotropic adjuvant analgesic drugs for cancer pain. *J. Pain Symptom Manag.* 4(suppl. 3):2, 1989.

Citron, M. L., et al. Patient-controlled analgesia for severe cancer pain. *Arch. Intern. Med.* 146:734, 1986.

Foley, K. M. The treatment of cancer pain. *N. Engl. J. Med.* 313:84, 1985.

Graves, D. A., et al. Patient controlled analgesia. *Ann. Intern. Med.* 99:360, 1983.

Hanks, G. W. Controlled release morphine (MST Contin) in advanced cancer: the European experience. *Cancer* 63:2378, 1989.

Hill, C. S. Pain management in a drug-oriented society. *Cancer* 63:2383, 1989.

Inturrisi, C. E. Management of cancer pain: pharmacology and principles of management. *Cancer* 63:2308, 1989.

Levy, M. H. Integration of pain management into comprehensive cancer care. *Cancer* 63(suppl. 11):2328, 1989.

Magni, G., Conlon, P., and Arsie, D. Tricyclic antidepressants in the treatment of cancer pain: a review. *Pharmacopsychiatry* 20:160, 1987.

Payne, R. Role of epidural and intrathecal narcotics and peptides in the management of cancer pain. *Med. Clin. North Am.* 71:313, 1987.

Siegfried, J. Electrostimulation and neurosurgical measures in cancer pain. *Recent Results Cancer Res.* 108:28, 1988.

Sundaresan, N., DiGiacinto, G. V., and Hugues, J. E. Neurosurgery in the treatment of cancer pain. *Cancer* 63(suppl. 11):2365, 1989.

Ventafridda, V., et al. Clinical observations on controlled-release morphine in cancer pain. *J. Pain Symptom Manag.* 4:124, 1989.

Walsh, T. D., and West, T. S. Controlling symptoms in advanced cancer. *Br. Med. J.* 296:477, 1988.

Principles of Oncology Nursing and Safe Handling of Chemotherapeutic Agents

Jane W. Ringlein

Since the early 1970s the specialty of cancer nursing has grown, and its members have become one of the largest groups of health professionals caring for persons with cancer. Nurses must offer skilled and sophisticated care to patients, understand disease mechanisms, and provide patient education and emotional support to continually meet the needs of persons with cancer.

The administration of chemotherapy is a skill that has fallen under the domain of the registered professional nurse. The purpose of this chapter is to discuss aspects of the administration of chemotherapeutic agents and review data on safe handling practices.

I. **General guidelines.** Antineoplastic agents are administered in a variety of settings, including outpatient clinics, physicians' offices, patients' homes, and inpatient hospital units. To ensure safe delivery of a drug to the patient, the Oncology Nursing Society has developed a list of qualifications the registered nurse must possess.

   A. The nurse must be designated as qualified to administer chemotherapy by a variety of routes after educational preparation, depending on individual institutional policies and procedures.

   B. The nurse must have current licensure as a registered nurse in his or her state of employment.

   C. Current cardiopulmonary resuscitation (CPR) certification is recommended for all nurses who administer chemotherapy.

   D. The nurse should demonstrate knowledge and skill in the following areas.

   1. Pharmacology of antineoplastic agents
   2. Handling and preparation of antineoplastics
   3. Principles of chemotherapy administration
   4. Venipuncture and IV therapy
   5. Resolution of common problems encountered by patients and families
   6. Side effects of chemotherapy and nursing interventions

   E. Evaluation of knowledge and skill in chemotherapy administration may be determined by the administrative authorities of the institution each year.

   F. Attendance at continuing educational offerings on chemotherapy and cancer care is recommended periodically to update the nurse's knowledge.

   It is necessary to check the Nurse Practice Act in any individual state to determine any further requirements for practice.

Prior to administration of any antineoplastic agent, **informed consent** must be obtained. A written consent is necessary when a patient is participating in a research study, but oral consent should be obtained and documented for all drugs. The physician is responsible for obtaining informed consent. The nurse shares in this responsibility by providing further explanation and discussion of the treatment and expected benefits and side effects. It is recommended that these explanations to patients be documented in the patient chart.

II. Routes and methods of chemotherapy administration

A. Oral route. Although this method is fairly simple and straightforward, care must still be taken to ensure proper dosing and scheduling, as oral chemotherapy is potentially toxic. Patients must be educated about side effects and taught to monitor themselves, as they may not view oral medications as having the serious implications of parenteral medications.

B. Subcutaneous and intramuscular routes are reserved for those agents that are not vesicants and do not cause irritation or damage to the tissues. The smallest-possible-gauge needle for the viscosity of the medication should be used. The subcutaneous route is also used for the injection of slow release pellets. Because of the large gauge needle required, the needle puncture site and track must first be anesthetized with a local anesthetic. Patients may complain of pain at the injection site due to alcohol or other irritating substances being present in the diluent of the medication, as well as to the medication itself. These routes are generally avoided when the patient is thrombocytopenic (platelets $< 50,000/\mu l$).

C. IV administration is the method most often used for the delivery of antineoplastic agents. IV administration can refer to IV push, IV sidearm, IV "piggyback," or IV continuous infusion method.

1. **IV push** is a method that is reserved for nonvesicants. It involves the use of two syringes: a medication syringe and a flush syringe. After a needle is inserted into the vein, the flush syringe is attached and a flush solution of normal saline is infused, using 2–3 ml to establish patency. The flush syringe then is detached, the medication syringe is attached, and medication is pushed into the vein at a rate appropriate for the type of medication; the medication syringe is next detached, the flush syringe reattached, and 3–5 ml of flush solution is infused to clear the line. IV push is a cost-effective method of administering agents that are not harmful to the vein wall.

2. **IV sidearm** is the preferred method for vesicant administration. A needle is placed in the vein, and IV tubing is attached with solution freely running. A medication syringe with needle is inserted into the Y site, the rubber arm of the tubing, and the chemotherapy is infused. The person administering the chemotherapy is then able to observe the site contin-

uously to monitor for potential extravasation. It is important to let the IV solution run at a wide open rate while administering the chemotherapy to dilute the agent, making the medication less caustic to the vein and to ensure continual free flow of medication to the vein. During the interval between the administration of each agent it is important to flush with the IV solution for 20–30 ml to ensure that the medication is completely infused before giving another drug.

3. **IV piggyback** is useful for medications that require a large volume of dilution and need to be given over a longer period than other IV methods allow. It is usually not employed for vesicants because the IV site is not in constant view of the nurse, and so extravasation can occur without notice. IV solution is run through a needle that has been put in the vein. Chemotherapeutic medication is placed in a smaller bag of solution, generally 50–250 ml. Piggyback IV tubing is inserted into the smaller bag, and a needle is placed at the end of the tubing. The needle is then inserted into the Y site of the main IV tubing. This piggyback medication is infused over a specified period of time. When completed, the IV solution that was first begun is used for the flush.

4. **Continuous infusion method** is usually used for medications that are to be infused over 24–96 hours. Medications are added to the infusing solution, then run at the appropriate rate for the medication. This method is not appropriate for vesicant therapy through peripheral veins. For vesicants, the IV line must be connected to a central venous access device. Continuous infusion therapy can be carried out successfully at home through the use of both portable ambulatory pumps and implantable pumps.

D. **Intraarterial therapy** is given by means of an arterial catheter. When the hepatic artery is selected, medication can be given by either an implanted or an external infusion pump. Other methods of delivering intraarterial chemotherapy involve use of the femoral artery or brachial artery.

E. **Intrathecal therapy** is given by injecting antineoplastic agents directly into the cerebrospinal fluid (CSF). A lumbar puncture is performed, and medication is given directly into the intrathecal space. This application is the responsibility of the physician. Specially trained nurses can administer intrathecal therapy with the use of an Ommaya reservoir, a device in which a catheter is inserted into the frontal horn of the lateral cerebral ventricles. The reservoir is implanted subcutaneously in the scalp or lumbar area. The skin is prepared with a iodine-povidone (Betadine) solution and wiped with alcohol. Sterility is critical throughout this procedure. The reservoir is accessed obliquely with a 25- or 23-gauge butterfly (or a butterfly Huber-point) needle to ensure the self-sealing capacity of the reservoir diaphragm. CSF 3 ml is withdrawn, and the medication is then administered slowly, over 5 minutes or more. The reservoir is then flushed with the 3 ml of CSF. Family members can be taught this procedure, especially if the reservoir is used for pain medication.

F. Intraperitoneal therapy is facilitated by inserting a catheter or an implantable port attached to a catheter into the peritoneum. The catheter is similar to that used for peritoneal dialysis, e.g., a Tenckhoff catheter. A "belly bath" is given with solution, followed by medication. It is left in place for a specified period of time and then removed. Although residual medication is often removed, systemic absorption has taken place, and nurses should be aware of side effects of the medication.

G. Intrapleural therapy is usually performed by inserting a chest tube. Any fluid accumulated in the pleura is drained for 24–48 hours. Medication is then instilled through the chest tube, and the tube is clamped for 1–2 hours. The patient is turned frequently during this time to help distribute the medication. The tube is then connected to suction or water seal. This procedure is the responsibility of the physician. However, nurses are responsible for the patients when they are turned and for monitoring the patients for side effects.

III. Vascular access

A. Insertion of intravenous needles. For many patients, insertion of an intravenous needle prior to the administration of chemotherapy can be the most anxiety-producing event of the treatment. Thus the skill of the nurse and the ease of insertion can have considerable impact on the comfort and emotional well-being of the person receiving chemotherapy.

  1. Site of venipuncture. Proper selection of veins for chemotherapy administration is important. Upper extremities are always chosen to decrease the risk of thrombophlebitis unless the physician specifies that the lower extremities be used. Limbs with compromised circulation (postmastectomy arms, fractured arms) and veins that are sclerosed or inflamed (phlebitis) are to be avoided.

  The best site for placing the needle is in an area of controversy. The antecubital fossa is generally avoided for the following reasons.

  a. Arm mobility is restricted.

  b. It is difficult to spot extravasation because of the presence of a large amount of subcutaneous tissue.

  c. If extravasation should occur, increased morbidity could follow because of the required extensive reconstruction of the area.

  d. If venous fibrosis should occur because of the caustic effects of the drugs, drawing blood from that vein would be difficult.

  Those who favor the use of the antecubital fossa do so because of the large vein size that allows rapid administration of the drugs, which enables the drugs to reach the circulation sooner and decrease the irritation to the vein. Distal veins, as in the dorsum of the hand, are preferred by some nurses because of their easy access and allowance for additional venipuncture when necessary.

2. **Needle size** is another controversial area. A 19- or 21-gauge needle allows rapid administration of the drugs, decreasing exposure of the vein to the drug. A small (22 or 23) gauge needle may be easier to insert, produce less scar tissue, be less painful, and cause less mechanical phlebitis. For short-term insertions, a 23-gauge butterfly needle is frequently used, as its ease of insertion and minimal vein irritation decreases the risk of infection. A Teflon catheter is frequently used for longer infusions or for the administration of cisplatin, as an aluminum needle can cause cisplatin to precipitate.

3. **Problem veins.** Many persons with cancer have had repeated needle sticks for diagnostic procedures as well as for chemotherapy administration that result in scarring, irritation, and sclerosing of veins. Thus a large vein with a firm wall may be difficult to find. Applying moist heat for 5–10 minutes helps to distend the veins, making them more visible and easier to palpate. An inexpensive heating pad may be used to warm the arm. Fragile veins that roll can be difficult to access successfully. Applying countertension on the vein may be helpful. Even those experienced at venipuncture can have an "off" day. A general rule of thumb is to limit venipuncture attempts to three when trying to start an intravenous infusion. It is then wise to call in a colleague for consultation. The goals of successful venipuncture are to avoid patient anxiety, discomfort, infection, and thrombosis and to deliver medication safely.

B. **Venous access devices.** The advent of venous access devices has made the administration of cancer chemotherapy easier, safer, and more comfortable for individuals with cancer. Peripheral veins can eventually become difficult to manage. It is wise to anticipate the need for a venous access device early during treatment to allow the patient full benefit of the treatment. Potential benefits of venous access devices include prevention of extravasation, increased patient comfort, promotion of self-care, and facilitation of continuous infusions.

1. **Semipermanent central catheters.** Of the Silastic right atrial catheters, the most frequently used are the Hickman, Broviac, and Groshong. These catheters can be used to draw blood and to administer blood products, antibiotics, chemotherapeutic agents, and total parenteral nutrition products. They are tunneled under the skin, inserted into a large vein, and threaded into the right atrium. The exit site is usually on the chest wall. Patient or family involvement is required for dressing changes and

flushing the catheter. The procedure for dressing change and flush solution is controversial, with additional research needed in the area. Dressing changes have been recommended anywhere from one to three times per week, usually by clean technique. The Groshong catheter does not require heparin for flush. It is recommended that the catheter be flushed with 5 ml of normal saline once every 7 days. After administration of viscous solutions the catheter should be flushed briskly with 20 ml of normal saline to prevent crystallization at the catheter tip.

Hickman and Broviac catheters do require a heparin flush, the amount of which varies in the literature. Amounts of flush solution can range from 2 to 5 ml, generally of normal saline with heparin 100 units/ml. It has been reported in the literature to flush anywhere from daily to once every 7 days.

    2. Implanted vascular access ports. The implanted port is another type of right atrial catheter that is attached to a port and implanted under the skin. Three brand names are Portacath, Infusaport, and Mediport. Each has a self- sealing septum and silicone catheter. The port itself is either metal or plastic. These devices can be used for blood sampling, IV bolus medications, IV infusions of medications, total parenteral nutrition, chemotherapy, and blood products. A special Huber point needle must be used to prevent damage to the port septum. Right-angled Huber needles and butterfly Huber needles are available for infusion therapy. Port maintenance is required after each use and every 4 weeks when not in use. A heparin flush of 5 ml of heparin (100 units/ml) followed by 10 ml of normal saline should be done briskly to prevent clotting of the port. Because of the cosmetic effect and ease of use, the ports are becoming increasingly favored. A blood return should be obtained prior to the administration of any medication to ensure proper catheter placement and prevent extravasation. Some physicians are reluctant to use implanted ports for vesicant chemotherapy because of the severity of slough that could occur in the event of extravasation.

    3. Temporary catheters. Small-gauge Silastic catheters may be used for patients requiring less than 2 months of IV therapy. They can be placed nonsurgically and can be used for infusions of chemotherapeutic agents or bolus injections. The catheters are generally too small for drawing blood. They are less convenient to use than other forms of venous access because they require daily irrigation and sterile dressing changes every other day.

IV. Safe handling of chemotherapeutic agents. The potential risk to the health care worker involved in handling cytotoxic agents is a complex issue. It was first discussed in the United States during the late 1970s. Ongoing controversy exists, complicated by the confusion and fear felt by the health care worker.

Anecdotal reports began appearing in the medical literature about health care workers who suffered headaches, alopecia, lightheadedness, dizziness, nasal mucosal sores, flulike symptoms, and various other symptoms when mixing chemotherapeutic agents. Many chemotherapeutic agents, such as the alkylating agents, are known to be carcinogenic in therapeutic doses. Studies were done using the Ames test to measure mutagens in the urine of health care personnel who handle antineoplastic drugs. These studies produced conflicting results. Some studies demonstrated a significant amount of sister chromatid exchanges and chromosomal breaks, whereas others did not. There are no data on the amount of absorption needed before these abnormalities become apparent. Studies have demonstrated that body fluids of persons who received cytotoxic agents contain active metabolites of the medications and should be a consideration when employing safe handling practices. Mutagenicity does not mean carcinogenicity, but there is a strong correlation between the two.

Because there are many unanswered questions on this topic and a lack of long-term worker follow-up, the Occupational Safety and Health Administration (OSHA) issued guidelines in 1986 for proper workplace practices. They do not constitute mandatory standards. They do assume that potential risk exists, and that these risks are minimized by compliance with the guidelines. Many health care workers still do not comply with the guidelines, and institutions are urged to set standards and policies to be followed. The following guidelines constitute the OSHA recommendations.

A. Personnel

1. Those individuals who work with chemotherapeutic agents must receive special training in safe working procedures with cytotoxic agents.
2. Individuals should document any acute exposure to antineoplastic agents.
3. Personnel should be provided with periodic health examinations. There are no clear guidelines on testing that should be done. It is recommended that a registry be established of all staff who routinely prepare or administer antineoplastic drugs.
4. Women of childbearing age should exercise caution when handling cytotoxic drugs. Those who are trying to conceive, are pregnant, or are breast feeding should be informed of potential risks of exposure.
5. All chemotherapeutic agents should be mixed in an approved Class II Biologic Safety Cabinet with a high efficiency particulate air (HEPA) filter and vertical laminar flow hood.
6. Syringes and IV sites should contain Luer-Lok fittings.
7. Use of latex surgical gloves and a low permeability gown with cuffed long sleeves is recommended when

compounding the drugs. Use of gloves when administering the drugs is also recommended.

8. Hand washing should occur prior to putting on gloves and when removing them, as all gloves have some permeability.

9. When no biologic safety cabinet is available, e.g., with home use, a hydrophobic filter is recommended to vent the drug vials.

10. IV tubing should be primed with a noncytotoxic agent.

11. Sterile gauze should be used to wrap around all chemotherapy needles and syringes when removing them from injection ports.

12. Syringes should not be recapped, as this action can cause an increase in needle sticks.

13. Double gloving and gowns, goggles, masks, and shoe covers are recommended to be worn when cleaning up a spill.

14. There should be no eating, drinking, smoking, or applying cosmetics in the drug preparation area.

15. All antineoplastic drugs should have a chemotherapy hazard label.

16. Gloves and gown should be worn when handling body fluids of persons who have received antineoplastic drugs.

B. Disposal procedures

1. All equipment used for the compounding and administration of chemotherapeutic agents should be placed in a closed, leakproof, puncture-proof container labeled hazardous waste.

2. Housekeeping personnel should receive instruction on safe handling procedures and should wear surgical latex gloves and gowns with cuffs and back closure when handling hazardous waste containers.

3. If chemotherapy is administered in the home, the leak-proof container should be taken to a designated area for disposal.

4. The two major methods of safely disposing of antineoplastic drugs are incineration at temperatures of 1000°C (1800°F) or landfill. Both methods should be done at places with Environmental Protection Agency approval.

These techniques constitute responsible practices for nurses working with antineoplastic agents. The nurse is urged to keep abreast of current research in this area to promote safety among all personnel exposed to antineoplastic drugs.

Selected Reading

Camp, L. D. Care of the Groshong catheter. *Oncol. Nurs. Forum* 15:745, 1988.

Falck, K., et al. Mutagenicity in urine of nurses handling cytostatic drugs. *Lancet* 1:1250, 1979.

Goodman, M. S., and Wickhane, R. Venous access devices: an overview. *Oncol. Nurs. Forum* 11:16, 1984.

Knobf, M. K. Intravenous guidelines for oncology practice. *Oncol. Nurs. Forum* 9:30, 1982.

Larson, D. L. What is the appropriate management of tissue extravasation by antitumor agents? *Plast. Reconstr. Surg.* 75:397, 1985.

McNally, J. C., et al. *Guidelines for Cancer Nursing Practice.* Orlando: Grune & Stratton, 1985.

Montrose, P. A. Extravasation management. *Semin. Oncol. Nurs.* 3:128, 1987.

OSHA Work Practice Guidelines for Personnel Dealing with Cytotoxic Drugs. OSHA Instructional Publication 8-1.1. Washington, DC: Office of Occupational Medicine, 1986.

Valanis, B., and Shortridge, L. Protective practices of nurses handling antineoplastic drugs. *Oncol. Nurs. Forum* 14:23, 1987.

Wainstock, J. M. Making a choice: the vein access method you prefer. *Oncol. Nurs. Forum* 14:79, 1987.

Management of Nausea and Vomiting and Other Acute Side Effects of Cancer Chemotherapy

Jane W. Ringlein

Chemotherapeutic agents for cancer are potent, with the potential for many side effects. Toxicities and side effects are frequently found as the result of damage to rapidly dividing cells. Cells that are most vulnerable by virtue of rapid cell division are those of the bone marrow, hair follicles, and lining of the gastrointestinal tract. Other toxicities are characteristic of the individual agents and may or may not be related to mechanism of action of the drug. Side effects may range from those that are a nuisance or of cosmetic importance to those that are life-threatening.

I. Acute reactions

A. Extravasation

refers to the leaking or infiltration of drug into subcutaneous tissues. If the drug is a *vesicant,* it is capable of producing tissue necrosis or sloughing. An *irritant* is a drug that causes inflammation or pain at the site of extravasation.

1. **Vesicant agents** that are commonly used include the following.

   Dactinomycin (actinomycin D, Cosmegen)
   Daunorubicin Cerubidine)
   Doxorubicin (Adriamycin)
   Estramustine (Estracyte, Emcyt)
   Mithramycin (Mithracin)
   Mitomycin (Mutamycin)
   Mechlorethamine (nitrogen mustard, Mustargen)
   Vinblastine (Velban)
   Vincristine (Oncovin)
   Vindesine

2. **Commercially available agents** generally considered to be irritants are as follows.

   Carmustine (BCNU, BiCNU)
   Dacarbazine (DTIC)
   Etoposide (VP-16, Vepesid)
   Streptozocin (Zanosar)

3. **Management of extravasation** is controversial, and there is a need for more research. Most data have been obtained from animal studies. Studies concerning humans have had a small sample size. It has been estimated that extravasation occurs in 1/1000 venipunctures, even when correct protocol is followed. Primary prevention of extravasation is obviously the best form of management.

   To prevent or lessen the serious complications of extravasation, only experienced registered nurses should administer cancer chemotherapy. All supplies necessary for dealing with potential extravasation should be assembled in a kit that can be taken to the area of drug administration when vesicants or irritants are being given.

a. General procedures. If extravasation or suspected extravasation occurs, the following steps should be taken. It is recommended that standing orders for these procedures be obtained to avoid delay.

  (1) Stop administration of the drug immediately.

  (2) Leave the needle in place.

  (3) Aspirate any residual drug in the tubing.

  (4) Remove the needle.

  (5) Avoid applying pressure to the site.

  (6) Photograph the suspected area of extravasation when possible.

  (7) Elevate the arm.

  (8) Apply warm compresses or cold packs as indicated by the specific drug used.

  (9) Consider consulting a plastic surgeon to review situation.

b. Recommended procedures for specific agents. The following antidotes and dosages are recommended based on current data. There are no clear data on antidotes for other chemotherapeutic agents. With regard to investigational agents, the nurse is encouraged to review all existing literature to determine if the agent in question is a vesicant and what antidote for extravasation is recommended.

  (1) **Mechlorethamine extravasation.** Isotonic sodium thiosulfate 2.6% or 1/6 M solution is the antidote. Administer liberal subcutaneous injections (5–6 ml total) into surrounding tissue of extravasated area. Sodium thiosulfate is thought to cause chemical neutralization of mechlorethamine.

  (2) **Plant alkaloid vinblastine, vincristine, etoposide, vindesine) extravasation.** Hyaluronidase (Wydase) 150 units/ml is the recommended antidote. Administer 1–6 ml SQ around the extravasation site. Hyaluronidase is an enzyme that breaks down hyaluronic acid in the interstitial fluid, allowing the vesicant to be dispersed and absorbed. It should be followed by warm compresses. Application of cold and corticosteroids has been found to increase skin toxicity and should not be used.

  (3) **Doxorubicin extravasation.** Doxorubicin is taken into cells in the extravasation area by the process of endocytosis; it binds to DNA in the cells and has been found in the tissues up to 5 months after extravasation. It has a slowly developing and prolonged tox-

icity. Ice should be applied immediately following suspected extravasation. The length of time for the ice to remain in place is controversial. Most studies have found that 30 minutes qid for the first 72 hours is the preferred schedule. Steroids have been found to worsen skin toxicity. Other IV, SQ, and topical antidotes have been studied with conflicting results. Local cooling is the preferred treatment.

(4) **Mitomycin extravasation.** Mitomycin is also a DNA binding agent, with a prolonged course for healing of an extravasation. These ulcers appear resistant to conservative treatments. Application of neither heat nor cold has had any proved benefit. Some reports in the literature have recommended a local injection of pyridoxine into the extravasation site. It is thought that pyridoxine converts in the tissues to pyridoxal and pyridoxal-5-phosphate, forming complexes with mitomycin. This proposal bears further investigation.

B. **Anaphylaxis.** Some chemotherapeutic agents can potentially cause an allergic response. Although an accurate allergy history should be obtained and documented, it is not likely to predict an allergic reaction to chemotherapy. When administering a chemotherapeutic agent associated with a high incidence of allergic response, a test dose may be given. Prophylactic administration of hydrocortisone or diphenhydramine may prevent some local reactions, such as the flare or urticaria that has been associated with doxorubicin administration. For a generalized allergic response, such as anaphylaxis, IV epinephrine is needed. The chemotherapy treatment area must be stocked with readily accessible epinephrine (10 ml of 1:10,000 solution is preferable to 1 ml of 1:1000 epinephrine because of easier titration when given IV) preferably already in a syringe, so appropriate therapy is immediately available. It is important that if an anaphylactic reaction occurs, the IV needle is not withdrawn but maintained with a nonmedicated IV solution to facilitate administration of an appropriate antidote. Usually 1–3 ml of epinephrine (1:10,000) is administered slowly with additional increments as needed to correct hypotension, bronchospasm, and laryngospasm. Diphenhydramine and hydrocortisone may be used as ordered by the physician. It is recommended that all supplies for management of an allergic response be assembled into a kit to be kept in the area of drug administration.

C. **Nausea and vomiting.** Much effort has gone into preventing or controlling the side effects of nausea and vomiting. Patients frequently think that all persons undergoing chemotherapy experience this reaction and so become fearful. Patients receiving cancer chemotherapy rank vomiting as the most distressing side effect, followed by nausea. The psychologic response as well as multiple physiologic factors can trigger anticipatory nausea and vomiting. A significant improvement in the quality of life of persons receiving chemotherapy can be made by controlling nausea and vomiting.

Nausea is a subjective feeling of stomach distress that may be accompanied by the feeling of wanting to vomit. Nausea can begin earlier and last longer than actual vomiting. Vomiting, also called emesis, is the expulsion of stomach contents. Certain chemotherapeutic agents are more likely to cause emesis than others (Table 37-1). The dose of the agent given also can increase the amount of nausea and vomiting.

1. Antiemetic drugs. Much of the research emphasis in controlling nausea and vomiting has been aimed at the use of antiemetic drugs. Some of the standard antiemetic regimens, as well as new drugs that appear promising, appear in Table 37-2. Combinations of drugs are frequently used. It is clear that prophylactic treatment with antiemetics is the most effective treatment for nausea and vomiting. It is preferable to prevent nausea and vomiting because once experienced they can become conditioned responses and may not respond to antiemetic therapy.

Table 37-1. Chemotherapeutic agents with known emetic actions

Nausea with low potential for emesis*	Nausea with moderate potential for emesis†	Nausea with high potential for severe emesis‡
L-Asparaginase	Azacytidine	Cisplatin
Bleomycin	Carboplatin	Cyclophosphamide
Chlorambucil	Cytarabine§	Dacarbazine
Hydroxyurea	Daunorubicin	Dactinomycin
L-Phenylalanine	Doxorubicin	Ifosfamide
Mercaptopurine	(Adriamycin)	Mitomycin
Methotrexate§	Etoposide (VP-16)	Mechlorethamine
Tamoxifen	Fluorouracil	(nitrogen
Thioguanine	Hexamethylmelamine	mustard)
Thiotepa	Mithramycin	Nitrosoureas
Vinblastine	Mitoxantrone	
Vincristine	Procarbazine	
Steroids (most)	Streptozocin	

*A drug that is associated with a 20% or lower incidence of eliciting nausea or vomiting, or both, has low potential for emesis.
†A drug that is associated with a 25–70% incidence of eliciting nausea or vomiting, or both, has moderate potential for emesis.
‡A drug that is associated with a 75% or greater incidence of nausea or vomiting, or both, has high potential for severe emesis.
§At low doses. Potential increased at higher doses.

Table 37-2. Antiemetics commonly used for prevention and treatment of chemotherapy-induced nausea and vomiting

Generic name	Trade name	Route	Dosage*
Prochlorperazine	Compazine	IM or IV†	10 mg
		PO	10 mg
		PR	10 or 30 mg
Thiethylperazine	Torecan	IM or PO	10 mg
Trimethobenzamide hydrochloride	Tigan	PO	250 mg
		IM, PR	200 mg
Metoclopramide	Reglan	PO	10 mg
		IV drip over 20 minutes	1–2 mg/kg
			Repeat at 2-hour intervals for 3–5 doses
Droperidol	Inapsine	Slow IV	1.25 mg
		IM	2.5 mg
Haloperidol	Haldol	IM or PO	2–4 mg
		IV	2 mg
Lorazepam	Ativan	IM or IV	1–2 mg
		PO or SL	0.5–1.0 mg

Hydroxyzine	Vistaril	IM, PO	25–100 mg qid
	Atarax	IM, PO	25–100 mg qid
Dexamethasone	Decadron	IV	10–20 mg‡ to start, then 4 mg PO q4h for 6 doses, then q6h for 4 doses, then q12h for 2 doses
		PO	
Scopolamine	Transderm Scōp	Patch (transdermal)	0.5 mg over 3 days
Diphenhydramine	Benadryl	PO	25–50 mg
		IV	25–50 mg
Ondansetron§	Zofran	IV	0.15 mg/kg over 15 minutes before and at 4 and 8 hours after chemotherapy, or 8 mg before, then 1 mg/hour as continuous infusion for 24 hours
Dronabinol	Marinol	PO	5–10 mg/m^2

*Unless otherwise indicated, doses may be repeated at 4- to 6-hour intervals for 24 hours or for as long as significant nausea and vomiting are present.
†With prochlorperazine and several of the other antiemetics, there is increased potential for severe postural hypotension when the agent is given IV. The patient must therefore be closely observed and assisted when attempting to sit up or get out of bed.
‡Single IV dose prior to chemotherapy usually followed by tapering oral doses.
§Investigational.

2. **Example of combination antiemetics.** For antiemetics with high emesis potential, combinations are often used, as in the following example.

Dexamethasone 10 mg IV 30 minutes prior to chemotherapy, followed by 4 mg IV or PO q4h × 6 doses, then q6h × 4 doses, *and*

Lorazepam 1–2 mg IV 30 minutes prior to chemotherapy followed by 0.5–1.0 mg IV q4h for 4 doses, *and*

Metoclopramide 1–2 mg/kg IV over 20 minutes. Repeat q2h × 3 doses, then q4h if nausea persists or returns, *and*

Benadryl 25–50 mg IV with first metoclopramide. Repeat with every other dose of metoclopramide, *and*

Compazine (begin 20 hours after the chemotherapy) 10 mg PO q4–6h for 24 hours or longer if nausea persists.

3. **Holistic interventions.** If anticipatory nausea and vomiting are the major problem, many patients receiving chemotherapy are helped by the use of relaxation techniques, with or without guided imagery. Music therapy has also been studied and found to be successful in the prevention of nausea and vomiting. Self-hypnosis has been tried with adults and children, with positive results; a skilled professional must spend 30–60 minutes with each patient until he or she can master these skills. A major part of the effectiveness of these interventions seems to be allowing patients a sense of control over their treatment effects.

Other nursing interventions include teaching patients to eat foods at room temperature and to take a clear liquid diet when nauseated. Carbonated beverages and dry crackers, as well as avoiding foods with offensive odors, may be helpful. Giving an antiemetic 30 minutes before eating and providing smaller meals may make food more tolerable. Frequently, sleeping during periods of nausea can alleviate much of the discomfort.

D. **Nonacute reactions**

1. **Hematologic reactions.** The major side effects and toxicities of the rapidly dividing cells of the bone marrow are anemia, thrombocytopenia, and leukopenia. Medical aspects of these three hematologic nonacute reactions are discussed in Chapters 32 and 33.

a. **Anemia.** Cancer treatment, the cancer itself, or both, can contribute to the patient becoming anemic. Disease-related causes include invasion of the bone marrow by cancer cells, loss of blood from the gastrointestinal tract or other sites, and hemolysis. If the anemia is treatment-related and not owing to hemolysis, it is generally not seen for 60–90 days after treatment is begun. Circulating red blood cells have an expected life of 120 days, and only newly proliferating cells of the bone marrow are affected.

The major problem from which anemic patients suffer is fatigue. They may also notice pallor and experience shortness of breath and tachycardia. Nursing interventions should be directed toward helping patients to conserve their strength. Such interventions may involve helping them to plan their activities with frequent rest periods, encouraging self-care but providing assistance as needed. The head of the bed can be elevated to facilitate easier breathing. Hemoglobin and hematocrit levels need to be monitored. Transfusions of packed red blood cells are usually given if the hemoglobin is less than 7–8 gm/dl or the patient has substantial anemia-related symptoms.

   b. **Thrombocytopenia** is an abnormal decrease in the number of circulating platelets, which may leave the patient at risk for bleeding or hemorrhage. Generally, a platelet count of less than 50,000/μl is associated with an increased risk for bleeding. Spontaneous bleeding usually does not occur with a platelet count of more than 20,000/μl. If the decreased platelet count is treatment-related, it may not manifest until 10–14 days after treatment or, in the case of drugs such as carmustine, until 3–4 weeks have elapsed.

   The nurse can perform many interventions to lessen the risk of bleeding in the thrombocytopenic patient. Avoidance of trauma to the skin by using only electric razors and no sharp instruments and avoidance of intramuscular or subcutaneous injections when possible can be part of the plan of care. Injection sites should have pressure applied for at least 5 minutes. Adequate hydration and bulk in the diet decrease the likelihood of straining with bowel movements and so may prevent tears in the rectal mucosa. Aspirin products and alcohol are contraindicated, as they increase the risk of bleeding. Soft toothettes are preferable to hard bristle toothbrushes in order to prevent bleeding gums. A water-based lubricant should be used prior to sexual intercourse in order to avoid damage to the mucous membranes. Gentle blowing of the nose and humidification of the air decrease the risk of epistaxis. Platelet counts should be monitored frequently and platelet transfusions administered in accordance with the physician's orders.

   c. **Leukopenia.** Infection is one of the major causes of morbidity and mortality in the patient with cancer. Significant leukopenia exists when the total white blood cell (WBC) count is less than 2000/μl or the total neutrophil count is less than

$1000/\mu l$. At that point the patient is at eminent risk for infection. If leukopenia is related to cancer treatment, it is important to know when the expected low point (nadir) of the WBC count is expected to occur for the drug regimen used.

Strategies the nurse uses to prevent infection in the patient at risk of leukopenia always include good hand washing. Proper hand washing can be the most important procedure for the nurse to perform. Leukopenic patients in their home environment should be instructed to monitor themselves for fever, cough, burning upon urination, sore throat, and anal or rectal pain. They should also be advised to avoid crowds and people with known contagious illness. Hospitalized leukopenic patients are frequently put in a private room. In some cases, protective isolation is used, primarily to remind the staff to keep up with hand washing. Patients must be assessed for signs and symptoms of infection in the groin, axilla, and rectal area and on any mucosal surface. Injections as well as rectal suppositories and rectal temperature-taking should be avoided. Cut flowers in the patient's room and ingestion of raw fruits and vegetables are to be avoided, as they are thought to carry pathogens. Temperatures are monitored frequently, and IV sites are changed every 48–72 hours. Sexual practices should include the use of a water-based lubricant and a condom to decrease infection risk. If a patient is neutropenic, there may be no inflammatory response to infection. Granulocyte transfusions may be administered in accordance with physician orders, generally when the neutrophil count is less than $500/\mu l$.

2. **Stomatitis** is an inflammation of the oral mucosa often caused by the effects of chemotherapy and radiation treatments. It can begin as dryness of the mouth and progress to erythema, difficulty in swallowing, and ulceration. Two grading systems—one anatomic and the other functional—have been developed to help evaluate the degree of toxicity.

   a. Grading—anatomic

Grade I	Erythema of oral mucosa
Grade II	Isolated small ulcerations
Grade III	Confluent ulceration covering more than 25% of the oral mucosa
Grade IV	Hemorrhagic ulceration

   b. Grading—functional

Grade 1	Soreness
Grade 2	Ulcers, can eat
Grade 3	Ulcers, cannot eat

   Stomatitis may involve the entire gastrointestinal tract, down to the anal mucosa. A daily oral assessment should be performed for all patients on chemotherapy, and the rectal area should be assessed as well. Intervention can minimize patient discomfort.

Oral care should be with a safe toothette and the mouth rinsed with a 1:4 hydrogen peroxide solution. Most commercial mouthwashes should be avoided, as they contain alcohol and are irritating to mucosal surfaces. An exception is Peridex, which appears clinically useful for cleansing the mouth and minimizing secondary infection. Lemon glycerin swabs should never be used, as they contribute to further dryness.

If oral pain occurs, a topical anesthetic such as lidocaine (Xylocaine 2% viscous solution) may be used. Vitamin E capsules broken open and swabbed in the mouth have been reported to promote healing. Dentures should be avoided until lesions have healed. Cold foods such as ice cream can be soothing, but extremes in temperature of foods should be avoided. Narcotics may be useful until severe pain subsides.

In the case of oral thrush, nystatin oral suspension or clotrimazole may be prescribed. It is also important to maintain hydration and nutritional status so healing may occur.

3. **Alopecia.** Chemotherapy-induced alopecia is one of the most painful psychologic blows that patients with cancer receive. This self-perceived negative change in body image is attributable to the importance placed on the hair as it contributes to the overall appearance of the individual.

Hair loss occurs either by total atrophy of the hair follicle or partial atrophy, causing the hair shaft to break off. It is usually temporary, and hair growth returns within 1–2 months after treatment stops. Hair may then grow back in a different texture or color than previously.

   a. **Chemotherapeutic agents** with the greatest potential for producing alopecia are doxorubicin, cyclophosphamide, ifosfamide, and vincristine. Alopecia occurs in almost 80% of patients receiving these drugs. Other drugs capable of causing alopecia are bleomycin, dactinomycin, daunorubicin, etoposide, fluorouracil, hydroxyurea, methotrexate, mitomycin, mitoxantrone, and vinblastine.

   b. **Nursing interventions** include informing persons with cancer of the possibility of alopecia and encouraging preparedness. Attractive wigs or scarves can be purchased before alopecia occurs to allow the patient to become used to wearing them. Encouraging verbalization of feelings in regard to the changes in body image can help patients deal with their fears of rejection or embarrassment.

   c. **Several methods of scalp hypothermia** are available that cause vasoconstriction of the scalp vessels and minimize the exposure of the hair follicles to the chemotherapeutic agent. A scalp tourniquet can also be used with or without hypothermia to aid in restricting the amount of drug to the hair follicles. These methods have been found to be most effective when doxorubicin is used because of the short plasma half-life of this drug. Unfortunately, many patients receive combinations of agents, and the effectiveness of scalp hypothermia diminishes. Scalp hypothermia is not recommended for tumors that have a high incidence of scalp metastases, e.g., leukemia and lymphomas. The cooling of the scalp can become uncomfortable as well.

Selected Reading

Baker, T. *Cancer Chemotherapy: A Manual for Nurses.* Boston: Little, Brown, 1981. Pp. 372–396.

Cotanch, P. M. and Strum, S. Progressive muscle relaxation for antiemetic therapy for cancer patients. *Oncol. Nurs. Forum* 14:33, 1987.

Cubeddu, L. X., et al. Efficacy of ondansetron (GR 38032 F) and the role of serotonin in cisplatin-induced nausea and vomiting. *N .Engl. J. Med.* 322:810, 1990.

Keller, J. F., and Blausey, L. A. Nursing issues and management in chemotherapy induced alopecia. *Oncol. Nurs. Forum* 15:603, 1988.

Marty, M., et al. Comparison of the 5-hydroxytryptamine (serotonin) antagonist ondansetron (GR 38032 F) with high dose metoclopramide in the control of cisplatin-induced emesis. *N. Engl. J. Med.* 322:816, 1990.

Wickhan, R. Managing chemotherapy related nausea and vomiting: the state of the art. *Oncol. Nurs. Forum* 16:563, 1989.

Yasko, J. *Guidelines for Cancer Care Symptom Management: A Self-Learning Module for the Nurse Caring for the Client with Cancer.* Reston, VA: Reston, 1983.

Venous Access, Infusion, and Perfusion

Hollis W. Merrick

The ability to gain reliable access to the vascular system is an important part of the management of patients with cancer. Progressive loss of peripheral veins makes subsequent treatments increasingly more difficult and dangerous; thus fear of needle sticks during intravenous therapy often becomes one of the most traumatic aspects for the patients undergoing chemotherapy. Fortunately, there have been significant advances in vascular access with the introduction of new devices, and increasing numbers of patients are gaining benefit from their use early in the treatment of cancer. These devices spare the patient discomfort, preserve the remaining peripheral venous sites, and prevent major problems such as extravasation of toxic chemicals and resultant tissue slough. Similar devices have been developed that permit administration of chemotherapeutic agents into arteries and the peritoneal cavity, facilitating these important routes of regional therapy.

I. **Venous access.** The use of Silastic right atrial catheters is simple and safe, even in leukopenic and thrombocytopenic patients. Complications associated with the insertion of these catheters are uncommon; and the incidence of problems associated with their use, e.g., phlebitis, thrombosis, and infection, is lower than that with peripheral venous access sites. Right atrial catheters are easy for the nursing staff to use, as they are essentially central lines with which the nurses have had much experience. Their use avoids the need for venipuncture, and the ensured access facilitates proper blood testing and adherence to chemotherapy scheduling.

Dual-lumen catheters are used particularly for patients who are hospitalized and who require uninterrupted administration of hyperalimentation in addition to their regular cancer therapy. Patients can resume normal activities, including showering and swimming, with the catheter in place.

A. **Types of devices**

1. **Percutaneous devices.** In 1971 Broviac described the use of a *permanent central venous catheter* for hyperalimentation, and during the late 1970s the catheter began to be used for chemotherapy. In 1979 Hickman described an improved version of this catheter that had a larger diameter to facilitate infusion of drugs and fluids as well as sampling of blood. Dual-lumen catheters have been developed that allow flexibility in administering fluids and drugs and in taking blood samples simultaneously. The first dual-lumen catheters were simply two Hickmans or a Hickman and a Broviac attached side to side. They required placement by a direct operative approach to

the internal jugular vein. More modern dual-lumen catheters are round with a septum in the lumen. They are small enough to be introduced to the subclavian approach using a "peel away" sheath introducer. Table 38-1 outlines the characteristics of percutaneous vascular access devices currently available.

2. **Implantable devices.** A subcutaneously implantable *right atrial catheter and injection port* have also been developed. These devices are introduced into the subclavian vein by a peel-away catheter, and the port is then placed in the same incision, as outlined in **I.B.** These devices are entirely under the skin and therefore more cosmetically appealing. They are usually irrigated monthly. The subcutaneous ports and catheters offer the same advantages as the percutaneous catheters but require a percutaneous needle stick with a special Huber needle for access into the port. Nurses must be trained to use them and recognize when the needle is not positioned properly. If the needle is not securely docked in the port, subcutaneous infusion of drugs occurs and with vesicants this occurrence can be hazardous. Currently, several types of implantable devices are available. They are listed in Table 38-2.

B. Technique of catheter placement. The catheters are usually placed by way of the subclavian or internal jugular vein. Placement via the subclavian vein is performed in the operating room under fully sterile conditions.

The patient is placed supine in the Trendelenburg position, and an incision is made inferior to the clavicle under local anesthesia. After infiltrating with local anesthesia under the clavicle, a needle on a syringe with

Table 38-1. Percutaneous central vascular access devices

Catheter	Description
Right atrial catheters	
Broviac*	Pediatric age group; 2.7–6.6 French
Hickman*	Adult patients; 9.6 French
Groshong*	Slit-valve end; requires less frequent irrigation; 3.5–9.5 French
Hemed†	4.0–14.0 French
Dual-lumen catheters	
Broviac*	
Hickman*	
Groshong*	
Quinton‡	Temporary hemodialysis catheter
Permacath‡	Permanent hemodialysis catheter

*Davol, Inc. (C.R. Bard, Inc.), Cranston, RI.
†Gish Biomedical, Inc., Santa Ana, CA.
‡Quinton Instrument Co., Seattle, WA.

Table 38-2. Implantable vascular access devices

Device name	Manufacturer
Infus-a-port	Infusaid Corp. (Norwood, MA)
Mediport	Cormed (Medina, NY)
Port-a-cath	Pharmacia (Piscataway, NJ)
Lifeport	Strato (Beverly, MA)
Hickman port	Davol (Cranston, RI)
Groshong port	Davol (Cranston, RI)

heparinized saline is introduced underneath and parallel to the clavicle. To best estimate the angle of approach, it is useful to place the index finger of the other hand in the suprasternal notch and aim at the tip of the finger. Placing the patient in the Trendelenburg position maximally dilates the subclavian vein and facilitates entry. Once blood can be freely aspirated, the syringe is removed and a guide wire is introduced through the needle into the right atrium. The needle can then be removed from the subclavian vein.

An additional incision is placed in the lower anterior midchest wall, and a tunneler is passed from this point up to the subclavicular incision. A Hickman catheter, placed on the lower end of the tunneler, is drawn up through the subclavicular incision. It is convenient at this point to estimate the length of catheter required by placing it on the anterior chest wall. The excess catheter can be removed where the tip would be in the right atrium. A peel-away sheath introducer and sheath can then be advanced over the guide wire into the subclavian vein. This step should be done slowly and carefully in order to not tear the subclavian vein on entry or lacerate the innominate vein or superior vena cava. The sheath introducer should advance easily after passing under the clavicle. Once in position, the wire and introducer should be withdrawn, leaving the sheath in place. Use of the Trendelenburg position allows blood to flow out through the introducer and prevents air from entering the central venous system. Finally, the catheter is threaded into the sheath, which is then peeled away. Proper placement of the catheter tip in the right atrium can be confirmed by fluoroscopy or chest film after the procedure.

The most frequent complications of the procedure are pneumothorax and hemothorax. A postoperative chest film can rule out the presence of either complication.

C. Management of access catheters varies considerably. Our practice has been to flush the catheters twice daily with 2 ml of heparinized saline solution (100 units/ml). The dressings are changed twice weekly, and a small amount of iodine-povidone (Betadine) ointment is placed around the catheter at the entry site. The patient and family are taught home care of the device by the nursing staff at the time of implantation. The subcutaneously implantable devices are flushed monthly.

D. Blocked catheters. Catheters that become blocked can usually be cleared by flushing with heparinized saline. If this step is not successful, infusion with streptokinase or urokinase has been found to be effective in unblocking the catheter.

Commonly, blocked catheters become difficult from which to draw blood despite the fact that substances can be infuse through them easily. This difficulty is due to either the position of the catheter tip against the vessel wall or the presence of a small thrombus or fibrin sheath at the catheter tip. Forceful flushing with heparinized saline, a change in patient position (including Trendelenburg), or infusion with urokinase may be successful in reopening the catheter. A chest film is helpful to verify satisfactory positioning of the catheter, as it may be accidentally moved from its original position. If these maneuvers are unsuccessful, the catheter can be surgically repositioned or replaced.

E. Catheter infection. Infection remains one of the most persistent problems and consists in two major components, subcutaneous infection and fever.

    1. Subcutaneous infection. The patient may show signs of infection with inflammation or drainage around the catheter at the skin entry site. The subclavian incision may break down, and the catheter or cuff may become visible. The wound should be sampled for cultures and treated with warm compresses and antiseptic dressing changes; the patient should be treated with appropriate antibiotics. The catheter is usually not removed unless the infection does not clear after an extended course of therapy.

    2. Fever. The patient may show no local signs of catheter infection and may demonstrate only a fever. Blood cultures are commonly positive when fever occurs during the nadir leukopenia due to chemotherapy. Culture samples should be taken from the catheter and a peripheral vein and appropriate antibiotics then administered. If the patient's condition deteriorates, the catheter should be removed. In most circumstances, however, catheter infection usually can be cleared with the catheter still in place (See chapter 32).

F. Catheter repair. Damaged catheters can easily be fixed with a repair kit from the particular manufacturer.

G. Catheter removal. A catheter is easily removed in the clinic or the patient's hospital room using a simple cutdown set. The position of the cuff of the catheter is established by gentle traction on the catheter, and a cutdown is made over this point. The cuff is mobilized; and after placing clamps over and below it, the cuff is removed from the catheter. The upper end of the catheter can then be withdrawn from the central track and the lower portion withdrawn through the catheter entry site. Simple pressure over the venous tract is all that is necessary to control bleeding. It is essential to culture the tip of the catheter (rather than the tunnel) at the time of removal to determine if potential bloodstream infection from the catheter exists. Culture of the tunnel does not suffice, as it is invariably contaminated.

II. **Arterial access.** Intraarterial chemotherapy has become increasingly popular for the treatment of localized malignant disease in the extremities, head and neck, abdomen, and liver.

A. **Hepatic artery infusion.** There is renewed interest in the treatment of hepatic tumors by infusion. Access to the hepatic artery has been gained with both percutaneous and implantable devices. Whichever technique is used, it is vitally important to obtain preoperative arteriograms to verify the vascular anatomy of the liver, as it is highly variable. Catheterization of the hepatic artery by way of the gastroduodenal artery provides full infusion coverage of the liver in only 60% of patients. The reason is that the major right hepatic artery arises from the superior mesenteric artery in 12% of patients, and the major left hepatic artery arising from the left gastric artery supplies the left lateral segment of the liver in 25% of patients. Catheterization of these additional arteries may be necessary to gain complete coverage of the arterial system of the liver. Complete coverage of the hepatic circulation is essential for successful infusion therapy. Infusion by implantable and percutaneous devices can be carried out by placing a Hickman or other similar catheter in the appropriate vessel(s). The percutaneous infusion can then be carried out with a portable external infusion pump, such as that manufactured by Cormed.

B. **Implantable devices.** The Infusaid pump is currently available for permanent implantation by placement in the subcutaneous tissue of the abdominal wall. The catheter is brought through the abdominal wall and placed in the appropriate vessel. This pump allows continuous infusion without the presence of external catheters. Its use has eliminated many of the technical problems associated with the use of external pumps and catheters. However, the response rate of tumors is similar to that achieved by percutaneous infusion, and no improvement in survival has been proved. Publications have reported a significant incidence of biliary sclerosis that was not found in previous studies using percutaneous infusion.

C. **Percutaneous devices.** Percutaneous catheters have been utilized for arterial or portal vein infusion. Catheters can be placed by the radiologist in the main hepatic artery by way of the femoral or brachial arteries. These catheters can then be used for continuous or intermittent percutaneous infusion.

III. Cavitary access intraperitoneal chemotherapy

A. Rationale. Direct instillation of chemotherapeutic agents into the peritoneal cavity offers the advantage of increasing drug levels at the site of disease compared to those that could be achieved by systemic therapy. Drugs with a low lipid solubility and high molecular weight have low peritoneal clearance and thus have a pharmacologic advantage with this route of administration. The rate of clearance from the peritoneal cavity is controlled by the peritoneal membrane permeability and by the size of the peritoneal surface area. After systemic absorption, the drug is cleared by the usual mechanisms. The ideal drug must have a slow peritoneal clearance, a steep dose-response relation and acceptable local peritoneal toxicity.

The initial clinical use of this method has been for cancers of the ovary and colon. When ovarian carcinoma is primarily confined to the abdominal cavity, combinations of IV chemotherapy give a 60–80% response rate, but complete remission is achieved in only 10–15%. Intraperitoneal (IP) chemotherapy may offer the means to improve these results. Intraperitoneal spread of colon cancer is a common feature of advanced disease. Ninety percent of IP fluorouracil can be extracted from the blood as it passes through the portal system; consequently, IP chemotherapy offers the potential for high drug levels in the peritoneal cavity as well as in the liver.

B. Technical considerations. IP chemotherapy has been administered by means of a temporary or a semipermanent peritoneal dialysis catheter such as the Tenckhoff catheter (Table 38-3). The optimal means of delivering IP chemotherapy has yet to be established. The use of a peritoneal dialysis catheter has been demonstrated to function well with an acceptable incidence of complications. It can be used for both drug administration and assessment of response by peritoneal cytology or computed tomography scans of the abdomen following instillation of contrast medium. A small number of peritoneal catheters become blocked with a fibrin sheath that prevents complete evacuation of the infusate. Patients may experience abdominal pain that is due to peritonitis secondary to chemotherapy instillation. The use of a totally implantable system for peritoneal dialysis has also been reported.

Table 38-3. Cavitary catheters

Device type	Manufacturer
Percutaneous peritoneal catheters	
Tenckhoff	Davol (Cranston, RI)
Trocath	McGaw (Puerto Rico, VI)
Implantable peritoneal catheter	
Port-a-cath	Pharmacia (Piscataway, NJ)

Selected Reading

Abraham, J. L., and Mullen, J. L. A prospective study of prolonged central venous access in leukemia. *J.A.M.A.* 248:2868, 1982.

Balch, C. M., et al. A prospective phase II clinical trial of continuous FUDR regional chemotherapy for colorectal metastases to the liver using a totally implantable drug infusion pump. *Ann. Surg.* 198:567, 1983.

Broviac, J. W., Cole, J. J., and Scribner, B. H. A silicone rubber atrial catheter for prolonged parenteral alimentation. *Surg. Gynecol. Obstet.* 136:602, 1973.

Cohen, A. M., and Wood, W. C. Simplified technique for placement of long term central venous silicone catheters. *Surg. Gynecol. Obstet.* 154:721, 1982.

Gyves, J., et al. Totally implanted system for intravenous chemotherapy in patients with cancer. *Am. J. Med.* 73:841, 1982.

Hickman, R. O., et al. A modified right atrial catheter for access to the venous system in marrow transplant recipients. *Surg. Gynecol. Obstet.* 148:871, 1979.

Hohn, D., et al. Biliary sclerosis in patients receiving hepatic artery infusion of floxuridine. *J. Clin. Oncol.* 3:98, 1985.

Hurtubise, M. R., et al. Restoring patency of occluded central venous catheters. *Arch. Surg.* 115:212, 1980.

Linos, D. A., and Mucha, P. A. A simplified technique for the placement of permanent central venous catheters. *Surg. Gynecol. Obstet.* 154:248, 1982.

Markman, M., et al. Intraperitoneal chemotherapy with high-dose cisplatin and cytosine arabinoside for refractory ovarian carcinoma and other malignancies principally involving the peritoneal cavity. *J. Clin. Oncol.* 3:925, 1985.

Myers, C. E. The use of intraperitoneal chemotherapy in the treatment of ovarian cancer. *Semin. Oncol.* 11:275, 1984.

Niederhuber, J. E., et al. Totally implanted venous and arterial access system to replace external catheters in cancer patients. *Surgery* 92:706, 1982.

Niederhuber, J., et al. Regional hepatic chemotherapy for colorectal cancer metastatic to the liver. *Cancer* 53:1336, 1984.

Ozols, R. F., Myers, C. E., and Young, R. C. Intraperitoneal chemotherapy. *Ann. Intern. Med.* 101:118, 1985.

Raaf, J. H. Two Broviac catheters for intensive long-term support of cancer patients. *Surg. Gynecol. Obstet.* 158:173, 1984.

Sugarbaker, P. H., et al. Prospective randomized trial of intravenous vs intraperitoneal 5-FU in patients with advanced primary colon or rectal cancer. *Surgery* 98:414, 1985.

Wade, J. C., et al. Two methods for improved venous access in acute leukemia patients. *J.A.M.A.* 246:140, 1981.

Appendix A

Nomogram for Determining Body Surface of Adults from Height and Mass*

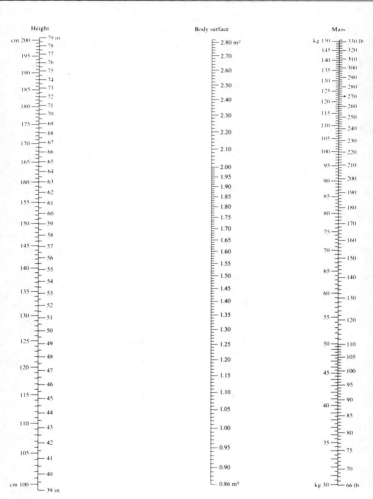

Height | Body surface | Mass

*From the formula of Du Bois and Du Bois. *Arch. Intern. Med.* 17:863, 1916 [$S = M^{0.425} \times H^{0.725} \times 71.84$, or $\log S = \log M \times 0.425 + \log H \times 0.725 + 1.8564$ (S = body surface in cm^2; M = mass in kg; H = height in cm)]. Source: C. Lentner (ed.), *Geigy Scientific Tables* (8th ed., vol. 1). Basel, Switzerland: Ciba-Geigy, 1981. P. 227.

Nomogram for Determining Body Surface of Children from Height and Mass*

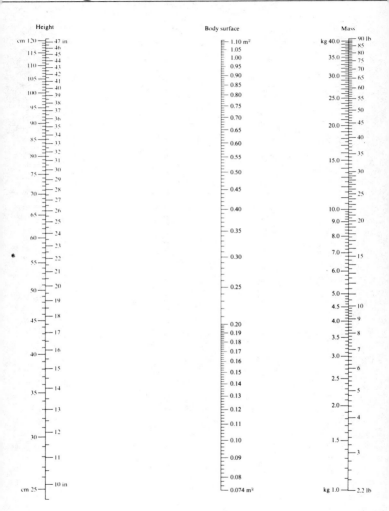

Height	Body surface	Mass

*From the formula of Du Bois and Du Bois. *Arch. Intern. Med.* 17:863, 1916 [$S = M^{0.425} \times H^{0.725} \times 71.84$, or $\log S = \log M \times 0.425 + \log H \times 0.725 + 1.8564$ (S = body surface in cm²; M = mass in kg; H = height in cm)]. Source: C. Lentner (ed.), *Geigy Scientific Tables* (8th ed., Vol. 1). Basel, Switzerland: Ciba-Geigy, 1981. P. 226.

Index

Index

of ever seeing him again. If he had said firmly: "Till next ye
have been perfectly content, or almost. I would have had to 1
"schizophrenic"—in the sense Sartre and I gave that word—to 1
ine that Algren would accommodate himself to that state of thing
often grieved to myself that he didn't make the effort to accept
but I also know perfectly well that he could never have done so.

Then should I have refused our affair and limited myself to enjoying the fellow feeling I had for Algren? That he had agreed with
me in despising such prudence would not suffice to excuse me; what I
said earlier about Sartre and M. is valid here. I possessed an in-
communicable knowledge of my bond with Sartre; from the very first
the dice were loaded; even the most truthful words still betrayed the
truth. But in this case as well, the great distance involved forced us
into an all-or-nothing situation: one doesn't cross the ocean, one
doesn't cut oneself off from one's life for weeks on end, just for fellow
feeling; it could only last by turning into a more violent experience.
I don't regret that it existed. It brought us more than it tore from us.

Sartre had kept me in touch with what was happening in France;
at the end of May he wrote to me: "Some ex-Resistance members
from La Charbonnière near Lyon kidnapped Sacha Guitry as he was
coming out of one of his eternal self-justification lectures (or as he
was going to it, I can't remember which) and forced him to take off
his hat in front of a monument to the Resistance members killed in
1944, and then made him clear out. *Paris-Presse* paid a million
francs[1] for a picture of Sacha (a bit blurred but still fairly striking),
head bare, eyes like a frightened rabbit, running a hand over his bald
pate. No one talks about anything else." It was just one episode in
the struggle between the ex-Resistance members and the ex-collaborators. The Vichyists won an important victory: on June 20th, at
Verdun, De Gaulle paid homage to the "victor of Verdun," and
almost went so far as to forgive Pétain for his politics on the grounds
that he was "swept along under the influence of his age, by the
wholesale desertions."

Sartre, like all the non-Communist Left, put great hope in the
break between Tito and the U.S.S.R. If Yugoslavia could refuse to
choose between the two blocs, the cause of neutralism would be
strengthened. For the moment, the chances of peace were very uncertain. The creation of the new *Deutsche Mark* by the Americans

[1] $2,000.

was obviously a prelude to the setting up of a government in West Germany; the Russians' countermove, the Berlin blockade, had brought international tension to fever pitch. In France and in Italy, this crisis aggravated existing dissensions. I had just gotten back to Paris, when on the 14th of July, at about eleven in the morning, a student called Ballante, the son of a Fascist volunteer killed on the Russian front, fired a revolver three times at Togliatti. The Italian proletariat reacted so violently that some thought there would be a revolution.

America Day by Day had just been published by Morihien and had a fair critical success. I resumed my study of the feminine condition. Sartre was reading a lot of political economy and history; he was still filling notebook after notebook with minuscule handwriting in his attempt to work out his system of morality. He had begun a study on Mallarmé.[1] And he was working on *Troubled Sleep*. We were expecting to take a vacation together toward the end of July; unexpectedly, M. telephoned him from New York. She couldn't bear being away from him any longer; she wanted to spend a month with him; she sobbed across the ocean; they were burdensome tears, but nonetheless genuine; he agreed to her request. But during the whole of the month they spent touring the South of France together, he held this piece of capricious coercion against her, he had exchanged his guilt for resentment; it was, for him, a good bargain.

I regretted having cut short my stay in the States. I sent a cable to Algren suggesting I return to Chicago. "No, too much work," was the answer. I was hurt—work was only an excuse; but I was also relieved: these meetings and partings, these rejections and impulsive offers were getting to be too much for me. For a month I stayed in Paris, working, reading and seeing friends.

At last I set out with Sartre for Algeria; we wanted sun, we loved the Mediterranean; it was a vacation, a pleasure trip; we would go touring, write, talk. One day Camus had said: "Happiness exists, and it's important; why refuse it? You don't make other people's unhappiness any worse by accepting it; it even helps you to fight for them. Yes," he had concluded, "I find it sad the way everyone seems to be ashamed of feeling happy nowadays." I agreed with him completely, and the first morning I looked out of my room in the Hôtel Saint-Georges at the blue sea with a light heart. But that afternoon we

[1] He wrote several hundred pages of it that he afterward lost.

walked around the Casbah, and I realized that tourism, as we had practiced it in the old days, was dead and buried; what had been picturesque before no longer seemed so: what we encountered now in those narrow streets was misery and bitterness.

We stayed in Algiers for two weeks, and the owner of the hotel confided to some journalists that he was astonished by Sartre's "simplicity": when we wanted to go into town on our first day there, we had taken a trolley bus! When Bernstein was working, he asked that all the clocks be stopped; the hotelkeeper seemed disappointed that Sartre hadn't come up with any such demands. I wrote sitting in front of my window; we ate dinner in the garden under the palm trees and drank a heavy wine from Mascara; we followed the roads along the coast in a taxi, we walked among the pines, over the hills. But Camus, now that I thought it over, had put the question badly; we weren't refusing to feel happy, we just couldn't.

No word came from Algren; I sent him a cable to which he didn't reply. I decided to forget him for the time being; I'd had enough of that particular sadness. One morning, I was walking along by the sea at Tipaza, crushing the mint leaves and inhaling the age-old odor of the Mediterranean scrub warmed by the sun, and suddenly I was twenty again: no regrets, no great expectations, simply the earth and the water, and my life. But in the cities I froze: how dismal Cherchell was! We went on with the trip simply out of curiosity; we no longer expected any pleasure from it.

"Don't go to Kabylia. I always carry a revolver when I can't avoid going," one of the people staying at the Saint-Georges had told us; other *colons* had agreed in chorus. We booked several days at the Hôtel Transatlantique in Michelet. We walked through some of the villages: huts of beaten earth, stuck one against the other, and sunken alleys so narrow that they gave us the impression of walking along hallways. No fountains. The men were working a long way off in the valley; outside the houses we saw only children and women with kohl-smeared eyes. It was impossible to tell what they were thinking. There was a fair at Michelet. Just men and animals; the air was full of the greasy smell of sheep's wool. I had a strange feeling that evening when I went back up to my room: a pack of cigarettes I had left on a table was missing; I discovered that some sweaters and money that had been inside a closed suitcase had been taken; and someone had vomited on my balcony. I was forced to tell the hotelkeeper that someone had been in my room. "Was anything stolen?" I said no, but had some difficulty convincing him. That night I locked myself in, and thank goodness I did, because someone turned the doorknob very noisily. In the morning they found a butcher from a nearby village dead drunk and asleep in an unoccupied room. The hotelkeeper hesitated for a while but finally decided against calling the police. There was something sinister about this pitiful and clumsy attempt at theft that made me sick at heart for a long while.

Bost joined us at Bougie. We spent several days together in a deserted palace, on the beach at Djidjelli; all around us there was nothing but sand and sea, and we swam day and night. I wanted to see Ghardaïa which I had missed two years before. I went down in a bus with Sartre as far as Bou Saâda; a taxi took us on to Djelfa, where the people were living not even in caves but in holes. The heat was still scarcely bearable, the buses ran only at night. Once more I was forced to give up the idea of seeing Ghardaïa.

CHAPTER IV

I'D HAD ENOUGH OF LIVING IN A hotel, where there was very little protection against journalists and inquisitive people generally. Mouloudji and Lola told me about a furnished room they had lived in in the Rue de la Bûcherie: the tenant who had taken it after them wanted to leave. I moved into it in October; I put red curtains up at the windows and bought some green bronze lamps designed by Giacometti and executed by his brother; I hung on the walls and from the big ceiling beam many of the objects I had brought back from my travels. One of my windows overlooked the Rue de l'Hôtel-Colbert which led down to the banks of the Seine. I could see the river, ivy, trees and Notre-Dame; opposite the other window was a hotel full of North Africans, with a café called Le Café des Amis on the first floor; they were always fighting inside. "You'll never be bored," Lola had told me. "All you have to do is go to the window and look out." She was right: in the morning, the rag pickers wheeled up perambulators piled high with old newspapers to sell to the junk merchant on the corner; bums of both sexes sat on the stepped sidewalk drinking their liters of red wine, sang, danced, talked to themselves and bickered. Hordes of cats wandered over the roofs. There were two veterinarians on my street; women brought their pets to them. The house, once a private mansion now beginning to come apart at the seams, was full of the sound of barking dogs, the ones in the clinic "under the patronage of the Duke of Windsor" and my concierge's big black one keeping up a constant exchange that echoed right up to my landing; the daughter of the impresario Betty Stern, who lived opposite me, had four dogs. Everyone knew each other. Mme D., the concierge, a slim, lively little woman who lived with her husband, her tall son and a tall nephew, helped me keep house. Betty, who had been very beautiful, who had known Marlene Dietrich intimately and Max Reinhart very well, often came and talked to me. She had spent a year hiding in the *maquis* during the Occupation. Below me lived a woman who worked as a film editor and who shortly after I moved in gave up her apartment to the Bosts. Finally, upstairs there was a dressmaker I occasionally patronized. Neither the façade nor the staircase were much to look at, but I was very pleased with my new home. We spent most of our evenings there because people were always bothering us in the cafés.

Every week I found in my mailbox an envelope with a Chicago postmark; I found out why I had received letters so rarely from Algren while I was in Algeria: he had written to me in Tunis instead of Ténès. The letter was returned to him; he sent it to me again. It was lucky it got lost, because I would have found it painful reading at the time. While speaking at rallies for Wallace, he had fallen in love with a young woman, he wrote; she was being divorced and he had thought of marrying her; she was in analysis and didn't want to get involved in a relationship of that sort until the analysis was finished; by the time the letter finally reached me in December they had almost stopped seeing each other. But he explained what he felt in detail: "I won't have an affair with this girl, she doesn't really mean anything to me. But that doesn't change the fact that I still want what she represented for me for two or three months: a place of my own to live in, with a woman of my own and perhaps a child of my own. There's nothing extraordinary about wanting such things, in fact it's rather common, it's just that I've never felt like it before. Perhaps it's because I'm getting close to forty. It's different for you. You've got Sartre and a settled way of life, people, and a vital interest in ideas. You live in the heart of the world of French culture, and every day you draw satisfaction from your work and your life. Whereas Chicago is almost as far away from everything as Uxmal. I lead a sterile existence centered exclusively on myself: and I'm not at all happy about it. I'm stuck here, as I told you and as you understood, because my job is to write about this city, and I can only do it here. It's pointless to go over all that again. But it leaves me almost no one to talk to. In other words, I'm caught in my own trap. Without consciously wanting to, I've chosen for myself the life best suited to the sort of writing I'm able to do. Politicians and intellectuals bore me, they seem to be unreal; the people I see a lot of these days are the ones who do seem real to me: whores, thieves, junkies, etc. However, my personal life was sacrificed in all this. This girl helped me to see the truth about us more clearly; last year I would have been afraid of spoiling something by not being faithful to you. Now I know that was foolish, because no arms are warm when they're on the other side of the ocean; I know that life is too short and too cold for me to reject all warmth for so many months."

In another letter, he returned to the same subject: "After that wretched Sunday when I began to spoil everything in that restaurant in Central Park, I had that feeling I told you about in my last letter—of wanting something *of my own*. To a great extent it was because of this woman who seemed so near and dear to me for several weeks (it's over now; but nothing has changed). If it hadn't been her it would have been someone else; it didn't mean I had stopped loving you, but you were so far away, it seemed so long before I would see you again. . . . I feel it's a little silly to talk about things we've gone past. But it's just as well, since you can't live in exile in Chicago nor I in Paris, since I'd always have to come back here, to my typewriter and my loneliness, and feel the need of someone close to me, because you're so far away. . . . "

There was nothing I could say in reply; he was absolutely right which didn't make it any easier to bear; I would always have felt a painful regret if our affair had ended then. The happiness of the nights in Chicago, on the Mississippi, in Guatemala, and the sudden botched-up ending would have turned it into no more than a dream. Happily, Algren's letters gradually grew warm again. He told me about his daily life. He sent me newspaper clippings, edifying tracts against alcohol and tobacco, books, chocolate, and two bottles of old whisky concealed in two enormous bags of flour. He also wrote that he would come to Paris in June and was booking his passage on a boat. I grew easy in my mind again, but every now and then I realized with anguish that our relationship was doomed to come to an end, and soon. Forty. Forty-one. Old age was growing inside me. It kept catching my eye from the depths of the mirror. I was paralyzed sometimes as I saw it making its way toward me so steadily when nothing inside me was ready for it.

Since the beginning of May, my study on *La Femme et les Mythes* had begun appearing in *Les Temps Modernes*. Leiris told me that Lévi-Strauss was criticizing me for certain inaccuracies in the sections on primitive societies. He was just finishing his thesis on *Les Structures de la Parenté*, and I asked him to let me read it. I went over to his place several mornings in succession; I sat down at a table and read a typescript of his book; it confirmed my notion of woman as *other*; it showed how the male remains the essential being, even within the matrilineal societies generally termed matriarchal. I continued to go to the Bibliothèque Nationale; it is pleasant and restful to fill one's eyes with words that already exist, instead of having to wrest sentences from the void. At other times I wrote, in my own room in the morning, and at Sartre's in the afternoon. From my table, I would glance over between erasures at the terrace of the Deux Magots and the Place Saint-Germain-des-Prés. The first volume was finished during the fall and I decided to hand it over to Gallimard right away. What should I call it? I thought about it for a long time, with Sartre's help. *Ariane, Mélusine:* that sort of title was no good because my work was a rejection of the myths. I thought of *The Other, the Second*: that had already been used. One evening, in my room, Sartre, Bost and I spent several hours trying out words. I suggested: *The Other Sex?* No. Bost changed it to *The Second Sex* and when we thought it over that was exactly right. Whereupon I set to work like a beaver on the second volume.

Twice a week I went to a gathering of all the regular contributors to *Les Temps Modernes* in Sartre's office: Merleau-Ponty, Colette Audry, Bost, Cau, Erval, Guyonnet, Jeanson, Lefort, Pontalis, Pouillon, J. H. Roy, Renée Saurel, Stéphane, Todd; a lot of people for such a small room, and it soon filled up with smoke; we drank brandy Sartre's family sent him from Alsace, passed the world in review, and made plans.

In October or November, Gaston Gallimard asked Sartre to have a talk with him. Malraux had been discussed in the July issue of *Les Temps Modernes* in a manner which had displeased him. Merleau-Ponty had quoted an article in *The New York Times* which congratulated Malraux on rallying to Gaullism and thereby remaining faithful to his old Trotskyist position; the indignant reaction of Trotsky's widow was then printed after the quotation. *"Malraux was never a sympathizer of Trotskyism, quite the contrary. . . . Malraux gives the appearance of having broken with Stalinism, but he is still serving his old masters by trying to establish a link between Trotskyism and the reactionaries."* The dossier was completed by a letter from an American revealing that Trotsky had twice asked Malraux to speak out on his behalf, and that on both occasions he had avoided doing so. Merleau-Ponty recalled that before 1939 Malraux had in fact supported Stalin against Trotsky; he reproached him for pretending the contrary now and for likening Gaullism to Trotsky-ism. Malraux had immediately gone to see Gallimard and threatened him with reprisals if we weren't dropped. Sartre took the matter lightly to the great relief of Gaston Gallimard, who announced in emotional tones to his collaborators: "Now *he* is a real democrat!" We were taken in by René Julliard. Malraux tried to intimidate his partner, Laffont, who was about to publish De Gaulle's memoirs: it would scarcely please the General to be published by the same house as *Les Temps Modernes,* and he might very well withdraw his manu-script. Nevertheless we moved over to the other side of the Rue de l'Université in December.

Sartre had another setback. The production of *Red Gloves* in New York was a flop. The script had been sabotaged. Boyer, playing Hoederer, had also balked at the line "He's vulgar." He had made Jessica say: "He looks like a king." They had stuck in a speech about the assassination of Lincoln and butchered the whole thing. The play came out like an incredible melodrama; Sartre tried to make them take it off and brought suit against Nagel, who had authorized the whole thing without his permission.

Things in general were still going as badly as ever. The R.P.F. had collapsed, for the good reason that the bourgeoisie no longer needed it; reunited and strong again, they had won an ominous vic-tory over the divided proletariat, which turned out to be the losers in the battle over wages. Despite Marshall Plan aid, despite increased production and an excellent harvest, prices had doubled between the summer of '47 and the fall of '48; the purchasing power of the work-ers had never been so low. On October 4th, 300,000 miners began a strike which lasted eight weeks. Jules Moch once more set the C.R.S. on them, and two men were killed, 2,000 put into prison, 6,000 fired. The stevedores and the railroad workers also stopped work. In vain. The Socialist dreams of 1944 were truly dead. Every issue on the C.N.R. program had petered out. The class in power was resolutely colonialist. The verdict on Tananarive was delivered on October 5th: six men condemned to death, including two deputies. In Indo-china, the leaders were putting the Bao Daï operation into effect against the Vietminh,[1] though its futility was obvious. *Les Temps Modernes* had been denouncing the imbecility and horror of this war

1 On March 8th, the Bao-Daï-Auriol agreements were signed.

since 1947. We often saw Van Chi, the cultural attaché to the Vietnam delegation—which still existed, paradoxically enough—and he introduced us to its president. Bourdet took part in these discussions.

The Berlin blockade was still going on. In China, Mao Tse-tung was winning a series of smashing victories. Nanking was collapsing; there was some doubt as to whether the United States would intervene. If so, it was thought, it would concentrate its forces in the Far East, and if it abandoned Europe even temporarily the Russians would invade; the two Great Powers would then confront each other in Germany and in France. One of the most ardent of the American warmongers, Forrestal, began to have such horrible visions of the Red Army flooding across the whole world and into New York, he let out such howls that they had to lock him up; he threw himself out of the sixteenth story of the hospital. In France, the Right was scientifically propagating panic; it used two themes which it thundered out either alternately or together: 1. The Soviet regime is cruel and terrible and inevitably entails poverty, famine, dictatorship and murder. 2. Without the help of America, we shall be defenseless; the Red Army will reach Brest in less than a week and we shall be subjected to all the horrors of Occupation. It was in this spirit of planned panic that *Carrefour*—in the same issue in which it triumphantly announced: *Thomas Dewey, the 33rd President of the United States, will enter the White House with a broom in his hand*—launched an inquiry: *"What would you do if the Red Army occupied France?"* The real danger was in fact the Atlantic Pact that Robert Schumann, a partisan of "Little Europe," was preparing to sign: it would cut the world in two for good and involve France in the war if America should ever launch it.

A great number of pacifist movements were born and developed at that time. The most publicized was that of Gary Davis. This "little man," as he was then called, took up a stand under the peristyle of the United Nations Building, which was considered international territory, and declared in interviews that he was giving up his American citizenship in order to become a "citizen of the world." On October 22nd a "council of solidarity" was constituted around him which included Breton, Camus, Mounier and Richard Wright, who had recently come to live in Paris; the day in November when Davis made a scene at the United Nations, Camus gave a press conference in a café during which he defended him; Bourdet reinforced Camus' support with an editorial, and from then on *Combat* devoted a page every month to the "World Government Movement." On December 3rd there was a rally in the Salle Pleyel during which Camus, Breton, Vercors and Paulhan defended this idea. Camus was hurt that Sartre refused to participate, and announced to us triumphantly that the rally on December 9th at the *Vel' d'Hiv'* had drawn twenty thousand people. Sartre was in complete agreement with the Communists that the Gary Davis affair was nothing but hot air. We couldn't help laughing when the Right accused Davis of being "in Moscow's pay." His idea wasn't new; there had once been a great deal of talk for a whole year about a "World Federation." Even his activities weren't particularly astonishing; America is swarming with inspired eccentrics solemnly proclaiming platitudinous slogans. The significant thing was that he should have been taken seriously by European "left-wing" intellectuals.

A few days after the meeting on December 9th at which Camus had spoken for peace, Van Chi presented him with a petition being circulated by Sartre and Bourdet against the war in Indochina. He didn't sign it: "I don't want to play the Communists' game." Camus rarely descended from lofty principles to particular cases. Sartre thought that it was by opposing wars one by one that we could work for world peace.

The R.D.R. wanted to unite all the Socialist forces in Europe behind a definite policy of neutralism. Sartre envisaged it as a group of moderate size, but dynamic enough to affect public opinion and influence events. Rousset wanted mass action. "There are fifty thousand of us now," he said in February (five thousand would have been nearer the truth). "There must be three hundred thousand of us by October, or we'll have lost." We felt much less sympathetic toward him than we had at first. He was possessed by an ambition that was all the more disquieting for being without any clear aim; his self-confidence covered abysses of uncertainty and ignorance; his admiration of himself was breathtaking. The sound of his own voice intoxicated him; all he had to do was talk in order to believe what he was saying. He conjured up images of the immense "audience" the movement had already reached, without giving a thought to the woeful deficiencies of its organizational aspects: often when people came to a district meeting they would find the door locked and no one would have a key. All Rousset liked were the rallies; at these he could declaim himself into a state of ecstasy. The R.D.R. organized one at the Salle Pleyel at the beginning of December; intellectuals from different countries were invited to talk about peace. Camus took part, as did Rousset, Sartre, Plievier, the author of *Stalingrad*, Carlo Levi, and Richard Wright, whose speech I translated. Many people attended, and there was much applause. Rousset delivered himself of a diatribe against the Communists. A split was beginning to appear within the R.D.R.; the majority wanted to align itself with the social action of the Communist Party; a minority—which included most of those responsible for its conception—on the pretext that the Communists were treating the movement with hostility, were slipping toward the Right.

Rousset announced that he had found a way of procuring the money the R.D.R. needed: he was going to the United States with Altmann in February; they would contact the C.I.O.[1] We were not aware to what extent the C.I.O. was supporting the government in its struggle against Communism, but we knew that it practiced class collaboration, and Sartre didn't approve of this step. The R.D.R. was a European movement; Americans were free, like Richard Wright, to sympathize with it but not to finance it.

The label "left-wing American" was in any case a very uncertain guarantee; we realized this the afternoon when Wright got together a group of French and American intellectuals in the public rooms of a big hotel. I made the acquaintance of Daniel Guérin and discussed with him the economic aspects of the American color problem; also that of Antonina Vallentin, the author of excellent biographies of Heine and Mirabeau. Sartre and some others said a few words. The American Louis Fischer, who for several years had been a journalist in Moscow and a Communist, stood up and delivered an attack on the U.S.S.R. He dragged Sartre over into a corner and treated him to an account of the horrors of the Soviet regime. He continued it while we were having dinner at Lipp with the Wrights. His eyes glittering with wild fanaticism, Fischer poured out an unending stream of stories of disappearances, betrayals and liquidations, of which, though they were probably all true, we could grasp neither the meaning nor the general significance. Then he sang the praises of America and its virtues.

Sartre conceived of the R.D.R. as a mediating influence between the advanced wing of the reformist *petite bourgeoisie* and the revolutionary proletariat: those were the circles from which the Com-

---

[1] The C.I.O. was the farthest to the left of the American trade union groups, and Rousset was playing on this misunderstanding.

munists recruited their members. More clearly than ever Sartre was now an adversary in their eyes. At the Wroclaw Congress, which was intended to seal an alliance between intellectuals throughout the world, Fadeev had referred to him as "a jackal with a fountain pen" and accused him of "dragging man down onto all fours." With the Lysenko affair, Stalinist dogmatism had penetrated even into the realm of science; Aragon, who knew nothing about it, demonstrated in *Europe* that Lysenko was right: Art was no longer free; all Communists were obliged to admire Fougeron's "The Fishmongers" exhibited at the Salon d'Automne. Luckács, passing through Paris in January, attacked "the decadent cogito of Existentialism." In an interview in *Combat,* Sartre replied that Luckács didn't understand the first thing about Marxism. Luckács' retort and Sartre's second reply were printed together in the next issue. Ehrenburg was in Paris in February and explained that Sartre had once inspired him with pity; since *Red Gloves* however, he felt nothing but contempt for him. Finally, Kanapa had been put in charge of *La Nouvelle Critique,* almost every number of which contained an article attacking Existentialism in general and Sartre in particular.

He was no less harshly treated by the magazine which began appearing in February under the editorship of Claude Mauriac called *Liberté de l'Esprit,* and which was dedicated to defending "Western values." Its writers included R.P.F. members and ex-collaborators. A newcomer, Roger Nimier, author of a poor little novel called *Les Epées,* called attention to himself in the first issue by writing apropos of the war: "We shall not wage it with M. Sartre's shoulders nor with M. Camus' lungs (and even less with the beautiful soul of M. Breton)." The allusion to "M. Camus' lungs" disgusted so many people that Nimier was forced to apologize. In the issues that followed, "Western values" were conspicuous by their absence, but the anti-Communist crusade was going great guns.

The anti-Soviet campaigners were leaving no stone unturned. In November a White Russian girl named Kosenkina jumped out of the window of the Soviet Consulate in New York. This melodramatic event was given enormous publicity.

In January, the Kravchenko trial opened; he was bringing suit against *Les Lettres Françaises* for defamation: the newspaper had revealed that his book *I Chose Freedom* had been fabricated by American government services. I went with Sartre to one of the hearings which was very unexciting; yet this affair, which filled the newspapers for weeks, was of the greatest interest: it was the trial of the U.S.S.R. The anti-Communists, supported by M. Queuille and by Washington, mobilized hordes of witnesses; the Russians on their side sent witnesses from Moscow. No one won. Kravchenko got damages, but they were very much smaller than he had claimed, and he emerged from the trial pretty well discredited. However, whatever lies he told, however great his venality, and despite the fact that most of the witnesses were as suspect as himself, one truth did emerge from their evidence as a whole: the existence of work camps. Logical, intelligent and confirmed in any case by numerous facts, the account given by Mme Beuber Newmann carried conviction. As soon as the Russo-German pact had been signed, the Russians handed over to Hitler deportees of German origin. They did not execute their prisoners in large numbers, but exploited them in such a way, and illtreated them to such an extent, that many died. The number of victims was not established, but we began to wonder whether the U.S.S.R. and the People's Democracies deserved to be termed socialist countries. Certainly Cardinal Mindszenty was guilty; how had he been persuaded to admit it? He confessed everything they wanted him to. What was happening in Bulgaria? What was the meaning of Dimitrov's "rustication"? The Communists were launching a peace offensive in countries all over the world; we began to think the reason must be that it was in their interest to prolong the truce to give themselves time to prepare for war.

Sartre continued to reflect on his split position and to search for a means of surmounting it; he read, and his notebooks were piling up. He was also writing the sequel to *Troubled Sleep,* which was to be called *The Last Chance.* In order to be able to work quietly, we went to the South of France. I picked out an isolated hotel on the Esterel coast; it was built in the shape of a ship, and stood directly over the water; at night, the sound of the waves came into my room, and I felt I was on the high seas. But the solemnity with which the meals were served in the vast, empty dining room took away our appetites. There were very few places to walk to because the mountains rose steeply just behind the hotel. We migrated to a less forbidding place: Le Cagnard, high up in Cagnes. We had pleasant rooms on the top floor; mine opened onto a terrace where we could sit and talk. An agreeable smell of woodsmoke came up from the tiled roofs below, and we could see the sea in the distance. We walked among the trees which were in bloom and visited Saint-

Paul-de-Vence, less mundane then than it is now; sometimes we went for an outing in a taxi. Sartre was very gay, but uneasy because M. was thinking of coming to France to live; he was trying to dissuade her.

The first volume of *The Second Sex* was about to appear; I was finishing the second and wanted to publish some extracts of it in *Les Temps Modernes*. Which ones? The final chapters were suitable, but they didn't exactly convey the basic point of the book. We settled for the chapters I had just finished, on female sexuality.

For some time I had been thinking about a novel. I often let it run through my mind as we drove through the pinewoods or walked through the lavender fields. I began to take notes.

When we got back to Paris after three weeks, the date set for the signing of the Atlantic Treaty—April 4th—was drawing near. Gilson, supported by Beuve-Méry, attacked it in *Le Monde*. In *Combat*, Bourdet suggested the creation of a "neutral bloc," fully armed, but pledged to the defense not of American bases but of an independent Europe. Also, the Peace Movement created by the Communists held a rally of its "partisans" in the Salle Pleyel on April 20th under the presidency of Joliot-Curie. The Congress, for which Picasso designed the emblem, his famous dove, ended with a mass demonstration.

Rousset had returned to France, bringing back with him from America a project for "study courses" devoted to peace which would go into operation ten days after the Pleyel rally. We realized at once that he intended his project as a rejoinder to the Peace Movement. In *Franc-Tireur*, Altmann ran a series of reports on America. An idyl! The regime was not socialist, of course, but it was not capitalist either; it was a trade-union culture. There was not complete equality either, of course; there were even slums—but what comfort! There was a series of anti-Communist trials going on, all right—but people could speak freely in the streets. Whites and blacks fraternized together. And, to sum up, it was the workers who governed the country.[1] As for Rousset, he gave me the most unpleasant impression. He told us what a triumph his tour had been, what banquets had been given for him, what an "audience" he had succeeded in winning. He came up with a defense for the American union leaders, for Mrs. Roosevelt and for American liberalism. He had garnered flattery and a few subsidies, and he had turned his coat. (Unless he was already wearing it that way around before. . . .) I questioned his view on

[1] "The dignity and defense of labor influence public affairs with all their weight."

the United States. He pointed an accusing finger at me and said in his most orotund voice: "It is easy, Simone de Beauvoir, in France today, to speak ill of America!" Among the people he expected to take part in the projected debates, he mentioned Sydney Hook. I had met him in New York; this ex-Marxist had become a frenzied anti-Communist. Sartre asked if, instead of holding public debates with foreigners, we might not convene an internal congress which would include as many active members from the provinces as possible; Rousset objected that we lacked funds for that. In which case who was financing the "Day of Resistance to Dictatorship and War"? And also what dictatorship in particular was to be resisted? Richard Wright was being pressed by the American Embassy to take part in the demonstration and told Sartre that he found their insistence suspicious. Sartre was wondering if he should attend in order to defend his own point of view against Rousset's or if he should abstain from attending; for once I gave him a piece of political advice: not to go. On April 30th, Merleau-Ponty, Wright and Sartre sent a collective message to the *Vel' d'Hiv'* directed against the policies of the State Department. Woolly messages from Gary Davis and Mrs. Roosevelt were read out. Sydney Hook and a Socialist member of the Dutch Parliament glorified the virtues of the Marshall Plan as opposed to Stalinist dictatorship; someone contributed a justification of the atomic bomb; there were disturbances on the floor, and the platform was taken over by Trotskyites. Sartre organized a meeting of the Congress of the R.D.R. at his own expense which pronounced its opposition to Rousset. The movement ceased to exist. At the time, we imagined that Sartre's only mistake had been to place his faith in Rousset and Altmann who, being more ambitious and more disturbed, had prevailed over more honest men; the group was still so limited in extent that small matters of this sort could still have important consequences, especially when they concerned the question of personality; the collapse of the association did not prove that it had been doomed to failure from the start. Soon, Sartre came to think the opposite: *"Splitting up of the R.D.R. Hard blow. Fresh and definitive apprenticeship to realism. One cannot create a movement."*[1] To attract the masses had not been his ambition; but to be satisfied with such a small movement was mere idealism: if four workers from the R.D.R. had participated in a Communist-organized strike, they would not have been able to modify its course or its

1 Unpublished notes.

intent. *"Circumstances merely appeared to be favorable to the association. It did answer to an abstract need, defined by the objective
situation, but not to any real need among the people. Consequently
they did not support it."*[1]

I enjoyed Queneau's *Saint-Glinglin* very much, his language, his
savage humor, his calmly horrific view of existence. I admired—
though slightly less than his earlier works—Genet's *Pompes Funèbres.*
Plievier's *Stalingrad* was a terrifying document. In America, Dr. Kin-
sey's report on *Sexual Behavior in the American Male* had just come
out: a great deal of noise over very little.

After having lived in Vienna and then in Belgrade, my sister and
Lionel had come back to Paris. They rented a pretty eighteenth-
century house at Louveciennes, a bit dilapidated and flanked by a big
garden that had run to seed. We saw a great deal of each other. One
evening I went with Olga to hear some jazz at the Rose Rouge in the
Rue de la Harpe, run by Mireille Trépel—who had once been at the
Flore—and Nico; they had moved to the Rue de Rennes and were
living opposite the building where I had spent my adolescence. I
heard the Frères Jacques there; they were becoming enormously successful, and deservedly so. At the Théâtre des Champs-Élysées, Boris
Kochno put on a new ballet called *La Rencontre;* Cocteau and
Bérard asked Sartre to write a text for the program; we went to a
rehearsal; we saw Leslie Caron, in black tights, lending the Sphinx
all the mystery of her fifteen years with grave and graceful diligence.
She completely conquered the glittering horde of first-nighters. We
found the ballets of Katherine Dunham of little interest, though they
were the rage of Paris. We abstained from Camus' *L'Etat de Siège,*
though not out of lack of friendship. We attended the production of
Les Fourberies de Scapin at the Marigny: Barrault had chosen to be
no more than a purveyor of entertainment.

Sartre was politically very close to Bourdet—who was to write the
political column in *Les Temps Modernes* shortly afterward—and
asked me one afternoon to go to a cocktail party Ida was giving. She
was a good hostess and there was an enormous number of people—too
enormous. All those people, separated by so many things and going
around slapping each other on the back, made me very uncomfortable. Altmann, who at the time I took to be a member of the
Left, fell into Louis Vallon's arms; and the hands I shook! Van Chi

[1] Unpublished notes.

wandered about in the crush, looking as unhappy as myself. To smile at opponents and friends alike is to debase one's commitments to the status of mere opinions, and all intellectuals, whether of the Right or Left, to their common bourgeois condition. It was that condition which was being imposed on me here as my truth, and that was why I was experiencing such a burning sensation of defeat.

At the beginning of June, I put on the white coat I had worn two years ago in Chicago and went to the Gare Saint-Lazare to meet Algren's boat train. How were we going to get on with each other now? We had parted badly; but he was coming. With my eyes I devoured the rails, the train, the flood of passengers. I couldn't find him; the last cars were emptying; they were empty; Algren wasn't there. I waited there a long while; by the time I turned and left there was no one left on the platform; I walked away slowly, glancing back over my shoulder several times—in vain. "I'll come and look for him when the next train comes in," I told myself and went home in a taxi. I sat down on my divan and lighted a cigarette, too upset to read. Suddenly I heard an American voice in the street; a man carrying a vast amount of luggage was going into the Café des Amis. He came out again and came over to the door. It was Algren. He had recognized my coat from the train window, but he had got into such a mess with his luggage that he didn't manage to get off the train until long after all the other passengers had left.

He brought me chocolate, whisky, books, photographs and a flowered housecoat. As a G.I. he had spent two days in Paris, at the Grand Hôtel de Chicago, out near Batignolles. He had seen almost nothing. It was odd reminding myself as I walked with him down the Rue Mouffetard: "This is really the first time he has ever looked at Paris; what do they look like to him, these houses, these shops?" I was anxious; I didn't want to see that sullen face he had sometimes turned on me in New York. He confided to me later that my excessive solicitude during those first days made him uncomfortable. But I soon grew more confident; his face was always radiant.

On foot, in cabs, once in a fiacre, I took him everywhere and he loved it all: the streets, the crowds, the markets. Occasionally little things shocked him. There were no fire escapes down the fronts of the houses, there was no railing along the Canal Saint-Martin: "So, if there's a fire, you just burn alive? I begin to understand the French. If you burn, you burn! If a child is drowned, it drowns—no interfering with fate!" He thought all the drivers were mad. French cooking and Beaujolais filled him with delight, even though he preferred sausage to foie gras. He particularly liked shopping in the stores nearby; the ceremonial exchange of conversation was a delight to him: *"Bonjour,* Monsieur, how are you today, thank you very much, very well and you, fine weather, nasty weather today, *au revoir,* Monsieur, thank you, Monsieur"; in Chicago, one shops in silence, he told me.

I took him to meet all my friends. With Sartre, conversation was a bit difficult because Sartre doesn't know English and I haven't enough patience to be an interpreter; but they got on well. We talked a bit about Tito and a lot about Mao Tse-tung. China was so little known that it provided matter for all sorts of extravagant notions. People were amazed that Mao Tse-tung should write verses, because they were unaware that every general in his country has a go at the pen. Because they were also literate, these revolutionaries were being endowed with an antique wisdom that combined with Marxism into some mysterious and seductive amalgam. Beautiful, and also true, stories were being told about education in the fields, theatrical performances in the army, and the liberation of women. It was thought that "the Chinese road to Communism" would be more flexible and more liberal than the Russian way, and that the entire face of the socialist world would be changed by it.

At the Rose Rouge, Bost and Algren swapped infantry reminiscences. Olga seduced Algren utterly by listening to all his stories with eyes wide in astonishment. He knew hundreds, and when he ran out he made them up. The four of us had dinner together in the restaurant on the Eiffel Tower—crammed with Americans. The food and drink were terrible, but the view very beautiful—and he talked for two hours straight about his friends the drug addicts and thieves, till I could no longer tell what was true and what wasn't. Bost didn't believe a word; Olga lapped up everything. I got up a little party at the Vians'; we invited Cazalis, Greco, and Scipion. I took Algren to a cocktail party given by Gallimard in honor of Caldwell. We often went for drinks at the Montana with various people. At first, the "leftists" of our group, Scipion among others, eyed this American with suspicion. Annoyed by this antagonism, he delighted in giving out with paradoxes and unseemly truths. But when they found out he had voted for Wallace and that his friends were all being forced out of work in radio and television because of their anti-American-ism, and above all when they got to know him better, he was in. He was very fond of Michelle Vian, whom he called Zazou and who very conscientiously interpreted everything for him, even when we all got carried away by the heat of our own conversation. On the 14th of July, after rushing about in a group to all the neighborhood street dances, one after the other, we all collapsed in one of the big cafés that didn't close till dawn. Queneau was in top form and from time to time I would turn to Algren and say: "He just said something very funny!" Algren would reply with a sketchy and rather forced smile, whereupon Michelle sat down beside him and translated everything that was said. He also liked Scipion very much because of his laugh, and thought he had the prettiest nose in the world. At the Library over the Club Saint-Germain, he met Guyonnet, who was trying to translate his latest novel and was having difficulty with all the Chicago slang. Guyonnet invited him one morning to go and box with him and Jean Cau. When he met me for lunch on the terrace of the Bouteille d'Or, down by the Seine, he collapsed into his chair exhausted. "These Frenchmen, they're all crazy!" he said. Following Guyonnet's instructions, he had gone up to a sixth-floor room, and was greeted by a shout of: "Here's the brave American!" He looked out the window and saw Cau and Guyonnet beckoning him to join them on a terrace to which the only means of access was the gutter leading to the roof. For Algren, who suffers from vertigo, it was a terrifying experience. The terrace was about as big as a pocket handkerchief and had no railing; they were boxing on the edge of a precipice. "All mad!" Algren repeated, still not quite recovered.

To show him a Parisian crowd, I took him to the celebration on June 18th: the Avenue d'Orléans was being rebaptized "Avenue du Général-Leclerc" in a ceremony presided over by the General's widow. As we were walking along in the crowd under the burning sun a man recognized me: "You have no right to be here!" He looked at me with murder in his Gaullist eyes. We went together to see the Van Goghs and the Toulouse-Lautrecs at the Jeu de Paume. I took him to the Musée Grévin as well; he was so filled with wonder at the "palace of mirages" with its endless forests and columns, its stars and lusters, its tricks of light—especially the "black light"—that he sent all his fellow Americans there whenever they came to Paris. One afternoon, Sartre hired a Slota; with Bost, Michelle and Scipion we went for a grand tour of the suburbs. We walked around the dog cemetery at Clichy, a little island in the middle of the Seine; at the entrance we were greeted by the statue of a Saint Bernard who saved, as I remember it, ninety-nine people. The inscriptions on the graves declare the superiority of animals over men; they are guarded by plaster spaniels, fox terriers and hounds. Suddenly Algren aimed an angry kick at a poodle, whose head fell off and rolled along the ground. "But why?" we asked him, laughing. "I didn't like the way it was looking at me," he answered. This cult of animals irritated him.

I thought he would enjoy a day at the races at Auteuil, but he couldn't make head or tail of the French betting system or understand the announcements of the results. On the other hand, he was very interested in the boxing matches at the Central. He filled me with confusion because I had managed to acquire a certain amount of respect for human beings since my childhood, whereas he didn't have a shred. He took photographs while the contestants were actually fighting, using flashbulbs and a reflector.

I went with him to the Club Saint-Germain, started a year earlier by Boubal. Vian and Cazalis had migrated there. The New Orleans style was still in vogue at the Tabou, but here it had yielded to bebop. The cellar was packed; a bearded lady smiled from a frame. At the Rose Rouge, I heard the Frères Jacques again in *Les Exercices de Style*. Algren liked them, but he liked Mouloudji even more, and also Montand, who was singing at the A.B.C. For the first time in my life I drank champagne at the Lido, because of an act there that Sartre had recommended: a ventriloquist called Winces who used his left hand as a dummy; two boot buttons for eyes, two fingers painted red for the lips; on top he popped a wig and arranged a body underneath; the doll moved its mouth, opened it wide enough to swallow a billiard ball, smoked and stuck out its tongue—a third finger. It was so alive that one really did believe it was talking, and when he took it to pieces it was as though some charming and impertinent little being had died.

Algren wanted to see the Old World. Spain was closed to us; there could be no question of setting foot in Franco's territory. We took a plane to Rome. It was amazing to me to be able to see the city, the sea and vast parched stretches of the Campagna all at the same time. And I was overcome by the strangeness of having been in Paris in the morning and then having lunch in the Piazza Navona! We walked a lot and saw a great deal. We went up to the Janiculum to have dinner and bowled with Carlo Levi in a little tavern there; we had lunch with Silone and his wife; we saw *Aïda* in the Baths of

Caracalla. I liked hearing a plane thrumming in the sky over one of Verdi's great arias. One night, a *fiacre* took us through a storm along dark streets streaming with water. But there were too many ruins and the city was too quiet for Algren's taste. We took a bus to Naples. We stopped at Cassino; the ruins scorching under the sun seemed as remote as those of Pompeii.

Algren loved Naples; he had known poverty and still brushed elbows with it everyday; he didn't feel the slightest bit uncomfortable walking through the overcrowded slum districts. When he began taking photographs I was even more embarrassed than I had been at the Central; actually the people all smiled at his flashes, and the children squabbled over the hot bulbs as they fell to the ground. They greeted him as a friend when he came back to hand around the prints.

He found the Italians charming. When we reached Porto d'Ischia where we wanted to spend a few days, we went into a restaurant; he asked for a glass of milk; there wasn't any; the waiter, who came up to Algren's waist, lectured him: "But you shouldn't drink milk! You should drink wine, Monsieur; that's the way to get big and strong!" The little port with its dusty oleanders and plumed horses didn't take our fancy. We pushed on as far as Forio; our little hotel, from which we looked straight down into the sea, was completely empty; there was a shady dining room and a terrace; the woman who ran it stuffed us with baked lasagna. Out in the square where we took our coffee, someone pointed out Mussolini's widow. We went for excursions in a carriage. We lounged on the beach for hours on end. In our memories, Ischia remains our paradise. But we were happy at Sorrento too, and at Amalfi and Ravello, and as it turned out Algren was deeply impressed by the ruins of Pompeii.

A plane took us from Rome to Tunis; the *souks* and the Mellah fascinated Algren. I can't remember now how we met Amour Hassine, a chauffeur who was driving his family to Djerba to celebrate the end of Ramadan; for a small sum he took us along with them. The island was in a state of frenzy the evening we arrived; among Moslems all over the world, lookouts were keeping a watch out for the moon; if it appeared during the course of the night, they would advise their fellow worshippers of it by telegram and the fast would be over; if not, it would go on for yet another day until the next evening; eating, drinking, dancing, smoking, scouring the sky with their eyes, everyone was killing time at a pitch of tension that did not seem to me to be justified by the prospect of one day's postponement. Sitting at a café table, surrounded by maniacal music and chanting, Algren smoked a narghile with Amour Hassine; the latter confessed to us that he sometimes drank wine during the year and often disobeyed the Koran, but during Ramadan he did not swallow as much as a crumb or smoke a single cigarette between dawn and dusk. "That, God would never forgive!" he said. The tension and the fatigue of these days of abstinence explained the crowd's impatient frenzy. The moon did not appear. The following night everything was calm because there was no longer any uncertainty: Ramadan was over.

We stayed on the island for three days. In the Jewish village Algren gazed with astonishment at the beautiful women with their dark eyes and their heads wrapped in the traditional black shawls. "I know women exactly like that in Chicago," he told me. We visited the synagogue to which Jews come on pilgrimage from all over the world. We spent quite a long time in a grotto that had been made into a tavern; the bottles of beer lay in the water of a little pool, in which the owner would dabble his feet to cool them off. He gave Algren some *kiff* to smoke: "You'll see; you'll fly away!" All the customers watched and waited. Algren felt a slight shudder that lifted him off the ground, but he came down again almost immediately.

At the house of some cousins of Amour Hassine, we ate vermilion-colored stew and drank violet syrup. We returned to Tunis with him by way of Médenine and Kairouan. In front of the *gorfa*, Algren stared wide-eyed: "I just don't know where I am!" Amour Hassine showed us a photograph of himself with a telephone against his ear. "I was calling Paris!" he told us with great pride. He was also proud to be driving an American, but found it difficult to understand why the American didn't have a car of his own. "Not everyone's rich over there," Algren told him. Hassine pondered over that; he noticed that we bought a lot of fritters and cakes and asked: "Are there eggs in America? And milk?" ". . ." "Then take me back with you; we'll set up at a crossroads somewhere, we'll make fritters and cakes and we'll be rich." There were two things he hated: France and Israel. He only expressed his opinions on the former in guarded allusions because of me; but on the subject of the Jews, since Algren didn't even flinch, he poured out his bitterness: "They've never even had a flag; and now they want a country of their own!"

After Tunis came Algiers, then Fez and Marrakesh; so much light, so many colors and sights, so many wounds; Algren's eyes opened wider and wider. He wanted to have another look at Marseilles where he had waited for his ship back to the States when the war was over. Afterward Olga and Bost welcomed us to their house at Cabris; the windows overlooked terraces of olive trees with the sea in the distance. The village had scarcely changed since 1941. One evening we hired a car to go and lose a little—a very little—money at the casino in Monte Carlo. In a loft in Antibes, to which the Club du Vieux-Colombier had migrated, we listened to Luter play; Greco sang "Si tu t'imagines" and "La rue des Blancs-Manteaux." Algren drank a lot; he danced with Olga and then, very gracefully, with a chair.

Back in Paris, the month of September was magnificent. We had never got on better together. Next year I would go to Chicago; I was certain when I said good-bye to him that I would see Algren again. And yet there was something terribly tight around my heart as I accompanied him to Orly. He went through the door to Customs; he disappeared; that in itself seemed so impossible that everything became possible, even or especially, that we would never meet again. I went back to Paris by taxi: the red lights on top of the pylons were all omens of some dreadful calamity.

I must have been mistaken. Algren's first letter was brimming over with high spirits. When they landed at Gander, he discovered from a magazine that he had been awarded the National Book Award. Cocktail parties, interviews, radio and television appearances: New York celebrated his return. A friend had driven him back to Chicago. He was very happy about his trip through Europe, very happy to be back home. He wrote: "We drove all Saturday and all Sunday, and it was marvelous to see American trees again, and the big American sky, the great rivers and the plains. It isn't as colorful a country as France; it doesn't captivate you in the same way as the little red roofs you see coming into Paris on the boat train or when you fly over them in the plane from Marseilles. Nor is it awesome like the gray-green light of Marrakesh. It's just huge, warm and friendly, confident and sleepy and taking its time. I was glad to think I belonged to it, and sort of relieved at the thought that wherever I go, this is the country I'll always be able to come back to."

He repeated that he was looking forward to seeing me over there, and my confidence returned.

The first volume of *The Second Sex* was published in June; in May, *Les Temps Modernes* had printed the chapter on "Woman's Sexual Initiation" and followed it up in the June and July issues with the chapters on "The Lesbian" and "Maternity." In November, Gallimard published the second volume.

I have described how this book was first conceived: almost by chance. Wanting to talk about myself, I became aware that to do so I should first have to describe the condition of woman in general; first I considered the myths that men have forged about her through all their cosmologies, religions, superstitions, ideologies and literature. I tried to establish some order in the picture which at first appeared to me completely incoherent; in every case, man put himself forward as the Subject and considered the woman as an object, as the Other. This assumption could of course be explained by historical circumstances, and Sartre told me I should also give some indication of the physiological groundwork. That was at Ramatuelle; we talked about it for a long time and I hesitated; I hadn't expected to become involved in writing such a vast work. But it was true that my study of the myths would be left hanging in midair if people didn't know the reality those myths were intended to mask. I therefore plunged into works of physiology and history. I didn't merely compile; even scientists, of both sexes, are imbued with prejudices in favor of man, so I had to try to dig for the exact truth beneath the surface of their interpretations. From my journey into history I returned with a few ideas that I had never seen expressed anywhere: I linked the history of woman to that of inheritance, because it seemed to me to be a byproduct of the economic evolution of the masculine world.

I began to look at women with new eyes and found surprise after surprise lying in wait for me. It is both strange and stimulating to discover suddenly, after forty, an aspect of the world that has been staring you in the face all the time which somehow you have never noticed. One of the misunderstandings created by my book is that people thought I was denying there was any difference between men and women. On the contrary, writing this book made me even more aware of those things that separate them; what I contended was that these dissimilarities are of a cultural and not of a natural order. I undertook to recount systematically, from childhood to old age, how they were created; I examined the possibilities this world offers women, those it denies them, their limits, their good and bad luck, their evasions and their achievements. That was what I put into the second volume: *L'Expérience Vécue*.

I spent only two years[1] on this work. I already knew some sociology and psychology. Thanks to my university training, I had the habit of efficient working methods; I knew how to sort books out and strip the meat off them quickly, how to reject those that were merely rehashes of others or pure fantasies; I made a pretty exhaustive inventory of everything that had appeared on the subject in both English and French; it was one that had given rise to an enormous literature but, as is usually the case, only a small number of these studies were important. When it came to the second volume, I also profited from the continual interest that Sartre and I had had for so many years in all sorts of people; my memory provided me with an abundance of material.

The first volume was well received: twenty-two thousand copies were sold in the first week. The second one also sold well, but it shocked people. I was completely taken aback by the fuss it provoked when the extracts from the book appeared in *Les Temps Modernes*. I had completely failed to take into account that "French bitchiness" Julien Gracq mentioned in an article in which—although he compared me to Poincaré making speeches in cemeteries—he congratulated me on my "courage." The word astonished me the first time it was used. "How courageous you are!" Claudine Chonez told me with an admiration full of pity. "Courageous?" "You're going to lose a lot of friends!" Well, I thought to myself, if I lose them they're not friends. In any case, I had written this book just the way I wanted to write it, but there had been no thought of heroism in my mind at any time. The men whom I knew well—Sartre, Bost, Merleau-Ponty, Leiris, Giacometti and the staff of *Les Temps Modernes*—were real democrats on this point as well as on any other; if I had been writing it for them I would have been in danger of breaking down an open door. In any case I was accused of doing just that; also of inventing, parodying, digressing and ranting. I was accused of so many things: everything! First of all, indecency. The June, July and August issues of *Les Temps Modernes* sold like hot cakes; but they were read, as it were, with averted eyes. One might almost have believed that Freud

[1] It was begun in October 1946 and finished in June 1949; but I spent four months of 1947 in America, and *America Day by Day* kept me busy for six months.

and psychoanalysis had never existed. What a festival of obscenity on the pretext of flogging me for mine! The good old *esprit gaulois* flowed in torrents. I received—some signed and some anonymous— epigrams, epistles, satires, admonitions, and exhortations addressed to me by, for example, "some very active members of the First Sex." Unsatisfied, frigid, priapic, nymphomaniac, lesbian, a hundred times aborted, I was everything, even an unmarried mother. People offered to cure me of my frigidity or to temper my labial appetites; I was promised revelations, in the coarsest terms but in the name of the true, the good and the beautiful, in the name of health and even of poetry, all unworthily trampled underfoot by me. Certainly it is monotonous writing inscriptions on lavatory walls; I could under-stand that many sexual maniacs might prefer to send their lucubra-tions to me for a change. But I was a bit surprised at Mauriac! He wrote to one of the contributors to *Les Temps Modernes:* "Your employer's vagina has no secrets from me," which shows that in private life he wasn't afraid of words. When he saw them printed, it upset him so much that he began a series in *Le Figaro Littéraire* urging the youth of France to condemn pornography in general and my articles in particular. Its success was slight. Although the replies of Pouillon and Cau, who had flown to my rescue, were suppressed— and probably those of many others as well—I had my defenders: among others, Domenach; the Christians were only gently indignant, and on the whole the youth of the nation did not seem excessively outraged by my verbal excesses. Mauriac lamented the fact bitterly. Exactly at the right moment to close his series, an angelic young lady sent him a letter so perfectly calculated to grant his every wish that a lot of us got a great deal of amusement out of what was obvi-ously a godsend for Mauriac! Nevertheless, in restaurants and cafés— which I frequented much more than usual because of Algren—peo-ple often snickered as they glanced toward me or even openly pointed. Once, during an entire dinner at Nos Provinces on the Boulevard Montparnasse, a table of people nearby stared at me and giggled; I didn't like dragging Algren into a scene, but as I left I gave them a piece of my mind.

The violence and level of these reactions left me perplexed. Among the Latin peoples, Catholicism has encouraged masculine tyranny and even inclined it toward sadism; Italian men have a tendency to combine it with coarseness, and the Spaniards with ar-rogance, but this sort of meanness was particularly French. Why?

Primarily because in France a man feels himself economically threatened by feminine competition; to maintain, or to assert the maintenance of a superiority no longer guaranteed by the customs of the country, the simplest method is to vilify women. A tradition of licentious talk provides a whole arsenal calculated to reduce women to their function as sexual objects: sayings, images, anecdotes and the vocabulary itself. Also, in the erotic field, the ancestral myth of French supremacy is being threatened; the ideal lover is now generally attributed to the Italian rather than the Frenchman; finally, the critical attitude of liberated women wounds or tires their partners; it makes them resentful. This meanness is simply the old French licentiousness taken over by vulnerable and spiteful men.[1]

In November, the swords were unsheathed once more. The critics went wild; there was no disagreement: women had always been the equal of men, they were forever doomed to be their inferiors, everything I said was common knowledge, there wasn't a word of truth in the whole book. In *Liberté de l'Esprit,* Boideffre and Nimier outdid each other in contempt. I was a poor neurotic girl, repressed, frustrated, and cheated by life, a virago, a woman who'd never been made love to properly, envious, embittered and bursting with inferiority complexes with regard to men, while with regard to women I was eaten to the bone by resentment.[2] Jean Guitton, with great Christian compassion, wrote that *The Second Sex* had affected him painfully because one could so clearly see running through it the thread of "my sad life." Armand Hoog outdid himself: "Humiliated by being a woman, agonizingly conscious of being imprisoned in her condition by the eyes of men, she rejects both their eyes and her condition."

This theme of my humiliation was taken up by a considerable number of critics who were so naïvely imbued with their own masculine superiority that they could not even imagine that my condition had never been a burden to me. The man whom I placed above all others did not consider me inferior to men. I had many male friends whose eyes, far from imprisoning me within set limits, recognized me as a human being in my own right. Such good fortune had protected

[1] There exists a hatred of women among American men. But even the most venomous writings such as Philip Wylie's *A Generation of Vipers,* do not descend to the level of obscenity; their sights are not on degrading women sexually.

[2] When Christiane Rochefort's *Warrior's Rest* appeared ten years later, there was less scandal, but there were still plenty of male critics ready to chant the old refrain: "She's an ugly and frustrated woman!"

me against all resentment and all bitterness; my readers will know too that I was never infected by such feelings during my childhood or my adolescence.[1] Subtler readers concluded that I was a misogynist and that, while pretending to take up the cudgels for women, I was damning them; this is untrue. I do not praise them to the skies and I have anatomized all those defects engendered by their condition, but I also showed their good qualities and their merits. I have given too many women too much affection and esteem to betray them now by considering myself as an "honorary male"; nor have I ever been wounded by their stares. In fact I was never treated as a target for sarcasm until after *The Second Sex;* before that, people were either indifferent or kind to me. Afterward, I was often attacked as a woman because my attackers thought it must be my Achilles' heel; but I knew perfectly well that this persistent petulance was really aimed at my moral and social convictions. No; far from suffering from my femininity, I have, on the contrary, from the age of twenty on, accumulated the advantages of both sexes; after *She Came to Stay,* those around me treated me both as a writer, their peer in the masculine world, and as a woman; this was particularly noticeable in America: at the parties I went to, the wives all got together and talked to each other while I talked to the men, who nevertheless behaved toward me with greater courtesy than they did toward the members of their own sex. I was encouraged to write *The Second Sex* precisely because of this privileged position. It allowed me to express myself in all serenity. And, contrary to what they suggest, it was precisely this placidity which exasperated so many of my masculine readers. A wild cry of rage, the revolt of a wounded soul—that they could have accepted with a moved and pitying condescension; since they could not pardon me my objectivity, they feigned a disbelief in it. For example I will take a phrase of Claude Mauriac's which perfectly illustrates the arrogance of the First Sex. "What has she got against me?" he wanted to know. Nothing; I had nothing against anything except the words I was quoting. It is strange that so many intellectuals should refuse to believe in intellectual passions.[2]

1 I by no means despise resentment and bitterness, or any other of those negative emotions; they are often justified by circumstances and one might consider that I have missed something in not having experienced them. If I reject their attribution to me here it is because I would like *The Second Sex* to be understood in the spirit in which I wrote it.

2 A novelist-pamphleteer of the Right, having been sharply attacked by Bost in *Les Temps Modernes,* exclaimed, very hurt: "But why so much hate? He doesn't even know me!"

I stirred up some storms even among my friends. One of them, a progressive academic, stopped reading my book and threw it across the room. Camus, in a few morose sentences, accused me of making the French male look ridiculous. A Mediterranean man, cultivating Spanish pride, he would allow woman equality only if she kept to her own, and different, realm; also, he was of course, as George Orwell would have said, the more equal of the two. He had blithely admitted to us once that he disliked the idea of being sized up and judged by a woman: she was the object, *he* was the eye and the consciousness. He laughed about it, but it is true that he did not accept reciprocity. Finally, with sudden warmth, he said: "There's one argument that you should have emphasized: man himself suffers from not being able to find a real companion in woman; he does aspire to equality." He too wanted a cry from the heart rather than solid reasoning; and what's more, a cry on behalf of men. Most men took as a personal insult the information I retailed about frigidity in women; they wanted to imagine that they could dispense pleasure whenever and to whomever they pleased; to doubt such powers on their part was to castrate them.

The Right could only detest my book, which Rome naturally put on the blacklist. I had hoped it would be well received by the extreme Left. Our relations with the Communists couldn't have been worse; all the same, my thesis owed so much to Marxism and showed it in such a favorable light that I did at least expect some impartiality from them! Marie-Louise Barron, in *Les Lettres Françaises,* confined herself to remarking that *The Second Sex* would at least give the factory girls at Billancourt a good giggle; which implies a very low estimate of the factory girls at Billancourt, replied Collette Audry in a "review of the critics" she did for *Combat. Action* devoted an anonymous and unintelligible article to me, delightfully decorated with the photograph of a woman held fast in the passionate embraces of an ape.

The non-Stalinist Marxists were scarcely more comforting. I gave a lecture at the *École Émancipée* and was told that once the Revolution had been achieved, the problem of woman would no longer exist. Fine, I said; but meanwhile? The present apparently held no interest for them.

My adversaries created and maintained numerous misunderstandings on the subject of my book. Above all I was attacked for the chapter on maternity. Many men declared I had no right to discuss women because I hadn't given birth; and they?[1] They nevertheless produced some very distinct opinions of their own in opposition to mine. It was said that I refused to grant any value to the maternal instinct and to love. This was not so. I simply asked that women should experience them truthfully and freely, whereas they often use them as excuses and take refuge in them, only to find themselves imprisoned in that refuge when those emotions have dried up in their hearts. I was accused of preaching sexual promiscuity; but at no point did I ever advise anyone to sleep with just anyone at just any time; my opinion on this subject is that all choices, agreements and refusals should be made independently of institutions, conventions and motives of self-aggrandizement; if the reasons for it are not of the same order as the act itself, then the only result can be lies, distortions and mutilations.

I devoted a chapter to the problem of abortion; Sartre had already written about it in *The Age of Reason,* and I myself in *The Blood of Others;* people were always rushing into the office of *Les Tempes Modernes* asking Mme Sorbets, the secretary, for addresses. She got so irritated that one day she designed a poster: WE DO IT ON THE PREMISES, OURSELVES. One morning, when I was still asleep, a young man knocked on my door. "My wife is pregnant," he said distractedly. "Give me an address . . ." "But I don't know any," I told him. He swore at me and left. "No one ever helps anyone!" I didn't know any addresses; and I should scarcely have been inclined to have any confidence in a stranger endowed with so little self-control. Women and couples are forced by society into secrecy; if I can help them I have no hesitation in doing so. But I did not find it very pleasant to discover that I was apparently thought of as a professional procuress.

There were people who defended *The Second Sex:* Francis Jeanson, Nadeau, Mounier. It provoked public controversy and lectures, it brought me a considerable amount of correspondence. Misread and misunderstood, it troubled people's minds. When all is said and done, it is possibly the book that has brought me the greatest satisfaction of all those I have written. If I am asked what I think of it today, I have no hesitation in replying: I'm all for it.

Oh! I admit that one can criticize the style and the composition. I could easily go back and cut it down to a much more elegant work. But at the time I was discovering my ideas as I was explaining them,

1 They went out and questioned mothers; but so did I.

and that was the best I could do. As for the content, I should take a more materialist position today in the first volume. I should base the notion of woman as *other* and the Manichaean argument it entails not on an idealistic and *a priori* struggle of consciences, but on the facts of supply and demand; that is how I treated the same problem in *The Long March* when I was writing about the subjugation of women in ancient China. This modification would not necessitate any changes in the subsequent developments of my argument. On the whole, I still agree with what I said. I never cherished any illusion of changing woman's condition; it depends on the future of labor in the world; it will change significantly only at the price of a revolution in production. That is why I avoided falling into the trap of "feminism." Nor did I offer remedies for each particular problem I described. But at least I helped the women of my time and generation to become aware of themselves and their situation.

Many of them, of course, disapproved of my book; I disturbed them or opposed them or exasperated them or frightened them. But there were others to whom I did some service, as I know from numberless testimonies to the fact, especially from the letters that I am still receiving and answering after twelve years. These women have found help in my work in their fight against images of themselves which revolted them, against myths by which they felt themselves crushed; they came to realize that their difficulties reflected not a disgrace peculiar to them, but a general condition. This discovery helped them to avoid the mistake of self-contempt, and many of them found in the book the strength to fight against that condition. Self-knowledge is no guarantee of happiness, but it is on the side of happiness and can supply the courage to fight for it. Psychiatrists have told me that they give *The Second Sex* to their women patients to read, and not merely to intellectual women but to lower-middle-class women, to office workers and women working in factories. "Your book was a great help to me. Your book saved me," are the words I have read in letters from women of all ages and all walks of life.

If my book has helped women, it is because it expressed them, and they in their turn gave it its truth. Thanks to them, it is no longer a matter for scandal and concern. During these last ten years the myths that men created have crumbled, and many women writers have gone beyond me and have been far more daring than I. Too many of them for my taste take sexuality as their only theme; but at least when they write about it they now present themselves as the eye-that-looks, as subject, consciousness, freedom.

I should have been surprised and even irritated if, when I was thirty, someone had told me that I would be concerning myself with feminine problems, and that my most serious public would be made up of women. I don't regret that it has been so. Divided, lacerated, in a world made to put them at a disadvantage, for women there are far more victories to be won, more prizes to be gained, more defeats to be suffered than there are for men. I have an interest in them; and I prefer having taken a limited but real hold upon the world through them to drifting in the universal.

It was still beautiful, warm weather when I returned to Cagnes with Sartre in the middle of October. I went back to my same room, to our little lunches on my balcony, to my glossy table under a little window with red curtains. The book Lévi-Strauss let me read had just come out, and I did a review of it for *Les Temps Modernes*. Then I made a start on the novel I had been thinking about for so long already; I wanted it to contain all of me—myself in relation to life, to death, to my times, to writing, to love, to friendship, to travel; I also wanted to depict other people, and above all to tell the feverish and disappointing story of what happened after the war. I dashed down a few words—the beginning of Anne's first monologue—but the blank paper made me feel giddy. I had no lack of things to say; but how to set about it? This was to be no potboiler, oh no! I was high with excitement, but frightened. How long would it take, this new adventure? Three years? Four? A long time anyway. And where would it land me?

To both calm and stimulate myself, I read *The Thief's Journal*, one of Genet's finest books. I took walks with Sartre. Pagniez, who was staying at Juan-les-Pins with Mme Lemaire, came over to see us with his children. His wife's death had brought us closer again. The doctors had not been mistaken. She had dragged on for two years. Confined to her bed, growing weaker and more emaciated all the time, it was heartbreaking to hear her making plans. She was convinced she was on the road to recovery when, during the winter, she died.

We went by taxi to Sospel and Peira-Cava, and took tea on the terrace. We were surprised several days later, on opening *France-Dimanche*, to find an account of our afternoon. The cartoonist Soro, who helped write the gossip column for the paper, was taking his holiday at the Cagnard; he found it ludicrous of us to be entertaining a father and his children. He took a sarcastic tone about my conversations with Sartre, without being able to make up his mind whether it was their hermetic quality he objected to or their simplicity. The contents of such articles were in themselves a matter of indifference to me; but I found it unpleasant to feel that I was being stalked even in my quietest retreats.

The third volume of *The Roads of Freedom,* called *Troubled Sleep,* appeared shortly after our return to Paris. I prefer it to the other two; in the transparency of each particular vision, the world still keeps its opacity; everything is outside, everything is inside; one grasps reality in both its aspects, the heavy weight of things and what we must after all call liberty. Yet the novel was less successful than its predecessors. "It's a sequel, yet it isn't the conclusion, so people hesitate to buy it," said Gaston Gallimard, who would have liked to put it out at the same time as the final volume. The readers were also influenced by the critics of course. Sartre shocked the Right by depicting officers deserting their troops. The Communists were indignant because the French people, civilians and soldiers alike, were shown as passive and apolitical.

Troubled Sleep left several questions unanswered: Was Mathieu dead or not?[1] Who was this Schneider whom Brunet found so interesting? What happened to the other characters? *The Last Chance* was to answer these questions. The first episode appeared at the end of 1949 in *Les Temps Modernes* under the title: *Drôle d'Amitié.* A newly arrived prisoner at the Stalag, Chalais, a Communist, recognized Schneider as the journalist Vicarios who had left the Party at the time of the Russo-German pact; the Communist Party had circulated a warning about him because they supposed him to be an informer. Chalais expressed his conviction that the U.S.S.R. would never enter the war and that *Humanité* was taking collaboration as the order of the day. Uneasy, indignant, distressed, when Brunet discovered from Vicarios that he was going to escape in order to confront his slanderers, he decided to go with him. This shared escape sealed the friendship which Brunet still felt for Vicarios despite the feelings of the others. Vicarios was killed, Brunet recaptured. The rest was still in a rough first draft. Having escaped, Mathieu,

1 Sartre had an insert printed so that readers would know he was in fact still alive, but you couldn't tell from the story itself.

tired of being free "for nothing" all his life, finally and happily decided in favor of action. Thanks to his help, Brunet escaped and reached Paris; there he discovered, with stupefaction, that—with a change of policy analogous to the one that forces Hugo to suicide at the end of *Red Gloves*—the U.S.S.R. had entered the war, and that the Communist Party had condemned collaboration. Having succeeded in rehabilitating Schneider, he resumed his role as a militant member of the Resistance; but the doubt, the scandal and the solitude he experienced had revealed his subjectivity to him: in the depths of his commitment he had rediscovered his freedom. At the same time Mathieu was moving in the opposite direction. Daniel, who was collaborating, had managed to have him recalled to Paris as the editor of a newspaper controlled by the Germans. Mathieu avoided the post and went into hiding. In the Stalag, his activities had still been those of an individualistic adventurer; now, by submitting himself to a collective discipline, he arrived at genuine commitment: starting in one case from alienation from the Cause and in the other from abstract liberty, Brunet and Mathieu were the embodiments of the authentic man of action as Sartre conceived him. Mathieu and Odette returned each other's love; she left Jacques and they experienced the fullness of a freely shared passion. Then Mathieu was arrested and died under torture, a hero not in essence, but because he had *made himself* a hero. Philippe too joined the Resistance, to prove to himself that he was not a coward, and also as a revenge against Daniel. He was shot down during a raid on a café in the Latin Quarter. Mad with grief and rage, Daniel hid in his briefcase one of the grenades Philippe used to keep hidden in the apartment; he attended a meeting of German officials and blew up both them and himself. Sarah, having fled to Marseilles, threw herself out of a window with her child when the Germans came to arrest her. Boris was parachuted into the *maquis*. Everyone, or almost everyone, being dead, there was no one left to become involved in the problems that arose after the war.

But they were precisely the problems that at this time interested Sartre; he had nothing to say about the Resistance because he conceived the novel as a form that poses questions, and under the Occupation one knew exactly what to do: there could be no perplexity, no ambiguity about how to behave. For his heroes at the end of *Drôle d'Amitié*, the die was cast; the critical moments of their stories are those when Daniel wildly rushes along the path to evil, when

Mathieu is finally no longer able to bear the vacuum of his liberty, when Brunet abandons his old ideas; all that remained for Sartre to do was to harvest the fruits so delicately ripened; but he prefers to clear the ground, to plow, to plant. Without having abandoned the idea of a fourth volume, he always found work that needed his attention more. To skip ten years and hurl his characters into the anxieties of the present would have been meaningless; the last volume would then have disappointed all the expectations roused by the one before it. The last volume was too imperiously predetermined for Sartre either to change his original intentions or to conquer the distaste which the idea of conforming to them aroused in him.

I was very pleased that Merle's *Weekend at Zuydcoote,* published in *Les Temps Modernes,* won the Prix Goncourt. I saw several films; I shared Cocteau's opinion of *Bicycle Thief:* it was Rome and a masterpiece. With *Festivals of Hell* Paris discovered Ghelderode. At Agnès Capri's theater, they were doing Queneau's *Les Limites de la Forêt,* in which the leading role was played by a dog; there were other acts. I singled out the delicious Barbara Laage who was later to be in the film of *The Respectful Prostitute.* The audience was largely composed of members of the fourth sex: diamond-covered ladies of about fifty next to the young girls they were manifestly keeping.

Camus came back from South America, he had done too much and looked very tired on the opening night of *Les Justes;* but the warmth of his greeting brought back the best days of our friendship. Perfectly acted, the play seemed to us academic. He accepted all the handshakes and compliments with a smiling and skeptical simplicity. Rosemonde Gérard, humpbacked, ravaged and extravagantly dressed, rushed up to him. "I like it better than *Red Gloves,*" she said, not having seen Sartre nearby. Camus turned to him with a smile of complicity and said: "Two birds with one stone!" for he disliked people treating him as a rival of Sartre's.

We visited Léger's studio; he gave Sartre a painting and me a very pretty watercolor. Since his stay in America his canvases had begun to have much more warmth and color than before. The Musée d'Art Moderne gave a huge exhibition of them; later, at the same place, I saw the sculptures of Henry Moore.

Since he no longer had a theater of his own, Dullin had been making exhausting tours of France and Europe. Camille didn't make his life any easier for him, since she was having difficulties of her own and drinking excessively. Crippled and exhausted, he was suddenly seized with such violent pains that they took him to the Saint-Antoine hospital; they opened his abdomen and closed it again hurriedly; he had cancer. As he lay dying, two journalists from *Samedi-Soir* passed themselves off as pupils of his and forced their way into his room. "Fuck off!" Dullin yelled; but they had already taken a picture. This way of behaving shocked people; *Samedi-Soir* whined and defended itself. After fighting for two or three days, Dullin died. I hadn't seen him for a long time; old and in pain, his end was not tragic in the way Bourla's was, but I am always moved when I recall my memories of him. A whole stretch of my past went with him, and I had the feeling that my own death was beginning.

During our traditional retreat at La Pouèze, Sartre worked at a preface for the works of Genet that Gallimard had asked him to do. I revised my translation of Algren's novel and went on with my own. Having heard on a radio program that I had described her as a courtesan in *The Second Sex,* Cléo de Mérode brought suit against me; there was some talk about it in the newspapers; I put the case in the hands of Suzanne Blum and didn't think about it.

In February, Dullin's friends and pupils organized a "Tribute to Dullin" at the Atelier. We called for Camille to take her there. The door was opened by the ravishing Ariane Borg in dismay. To enable her to face the evening, Camille had been drinking red wine; we carried her, in tears, her hair tumbling down and her clothes in disorder, from the taxi into a box where she hid herself and sobbed through the whole ceremony. Salacrou and Jules Romains made brief speeches; an actor read Sartre's. Olga did a scene from *The Flies* in costume, very well. We heard Dullin's recorded voice in the soliloquy from *The Miser.*

During March, I went to the Théâtre de Poche to attend a few rehearsals and then the opening of two little plays by Chauffard: *Le Dernier des Sioux* and *Un Collier d'une Reine.* Claude Martin directed. It was a young troupe who worked together very happily all the time without dissensions. I thought what a pity it was that things were always so different with Sartre's plays! Denner[1] played the king, Loleh Bellon was a charming queen and Olga, who was getting back to acting at last, struck sparks; the critics showered her with com-

[1] Whose performance as Landru had just made him famous.

pliments. Sartre was hoping to have *The Flies* revived when she was completely recovered.

Just next to my house was a little newspaper vendor and I often used to stop and chat with him. "I'm Martin Eden," he told me one day. He used to read a lot and also went to school. He had decided that he would help all the people who were trying to teach themselves in our district: "Because I found it so very hard myself." He had managed to organize a sort of club in a room in the Rue Mouffetard and he was asking intellectuals to come and give lectures. Sartre gave one on the theater, Clouzot one on the film. I spoke about the condition of women; it was the first time I had come into contact with a truly working-class public, and I discovered that, contrary to what Mme Barron had said, they felt very much concerned with the problems I spoke about.

The attempts of the neutralists had come to nothing. On the pretext of joining forces with a conscientious objector called Moreau, Gary Davis tore up his identity papers and started a publicity campaign on his own that disgusted his partisans. The R.D.R. had finally collapsed and disappeared. It was now certain beyond doubt that there could be no third course between adherence to one of the two blocs. And the choice between them remained impossible. The State Department continued to support Chiang Kai-shek, who had taken refuge on Formosa, against the Chinese People's Republic that had been proclaimed on November 1st. It had also given financial aid to Franco; it was, as the title of an article published in *Les Temps Modernes* expressed it, "The End of Man's Hope" for Spain. In Greece, with the connivance of the English, America had assured the triumph of the reactionaries: the Communists and all the others who had opposed that triumph were dying in Makronisos' camp. Yet it was not possible to decide without reservations in favor of the U.S.S.R. when so many half-public, half-concealed dramas still continued to succeed one another in all the Stalinist countries. Our ears were still numb from the admissions of Cardinal Mindszenty when Rajk started confessing in his turn—treason and plotting—before being hanged on October 15th in Budapest. Kostov admitted nothing and was hanged in Sofia in December. By the fate of these two "criminals," who were in fact paying for Tito, Stalin was denouncing "cosmopolitanism" and "cosmopolites."

Sartre had been a member of a committee formed to obtain a

retrial in Tananarive, but he had by now practically given up all political activity. He was busy with Merleau-Ponty on the magazine, which was going through a slack period: four years before we had been everyone's friends, now we were looked upon by everyone as enemies. He began two works that had no connection with our circumstances at that time. *La Reine Albemarle et le Dernier Touriste* was intended to be the *Nausea* of his maturity, as it were; in it he gave a capricious description of Italy, its present structure, its history and its countryside, and also meditated on what it means to be a tourist.[1] Also his preface to the works of Genet turned into a long book in which he attempted to give an account of one man that would go far deeper than his *Baudelaire*. He had moved closer to both psychoanalysis and Marxism, and it seemed to him at that time that the possibilities of any individual were strictly limited by his situation; the individual's liberty consisted in not accepting his situation passively but, through the very movement of his existence, interiorizing and transcending it in order to give it meaning. In certain cases the margin of choice left to him came very close to zero. In others, the choice continued over a period of many years; Sartre was telling the story of Genet's choice; he examined the values which his options brought into play—holiness, demonism, good and evil—in relation to their social context.

Sartre abandoned his work on morals proper that year because he was convinced that *"the moral attitude appears when technical and social conditions render positive forms of conduct impossible. Ethics is a collection of idealistic tricks intended to enable us to live the life imposed on us by the poverty of our resources and the insufficiency of our techniques.*[2] He worked mainly in the fields of history and economy. The young Marxist philosopher Tran Duc Thao suggested to him that they have a series of discussions that could afterward be collected to form a book; Sartre agreed.

In November, Roger Stéphane came to see Sartre; there had come into his hands a copy of the "Soviet Code of Corrective Labor" which had just been republished in England[3] and though still un-

---

[1] He wrote several hundred pages of it, but never had the inclination or the time to revise them and only published tiny fragments of them later.

[2] Unpublished notes.

[3] It had been published there as early as 1936; the existence of the camps was already known; but the French Communist Party was too small and the U.S.S.R. too far away for public opinion to pay much attention to them. We had both been so indifferent to politics then, Sartre and myself, that we had never given the matter a thought.

known in France had been the object of a discussion in the U.N. at the beginning of August. It confirmed the revelations made during the Kravchenko case about the existence of labor camps. Did Sartre want to publish it in *Les Temps Modernes?* Yes, he did. Sartre, as I have said, believed in socialism. He expressed his thoughts on the subject a few years later in *Le Fantôme de Staline:* taken as a whole, the Socialist movement *"is the absolute judge of all other movements because the exploited experience exploitation and the class struggle as their reality and as the fundamental truth of bourgeois societies . . . it is the movement of man in the process of creating himself; the other parties believe that man is already created. Socialism is the absolute standard of reference by which any political undertaking is to be judged."* Now the U.S.S.R., in spite of everything, had been, and still remained, the mother country of socialism: the revolutionary seizure of power had been accomplished. Even if its bureaucracy had become stratified, even if its police had arrogated enormous power to itself, even if crimes had been committed, the U.S.S.R. had never in any way questioned the original appropriation of the means of production; its political system differed radically from those which aimed at establishing or maintaining the domination of one class. Without denying the faults of its rulers, Sartre was of the opinion that if they presented so much ground for criticism it was partly because they refused the excuse provided for bourgeois politicians by the so-called "economic laws"; they assumed responsibility for everything that happened in and to their country.

It was being said that the Revolution had been betrayed and was now entirely unrecognizable. This was untrue, replied Sartre: it has been embodied; the universal, in other words, has been reduced to the particular. Made real in this way, it immediately encountered contradictions that kept it from attaining the purity of the original conception; yet over the dream of a socialism without defect, Russian socialism had the immense advantage of existing. On the subject of the Stalinian era, Sartre's thoughts were already those expressed recently in an as yet unpublished chapter of *La Critique de la Raison Dialectique: "The regime in the U.S.S.R. was really socialism, but socialism characterized by the practical necessity of disappearing from the world or of becoming what it is at the cost of a desperate and bloody effort. . . . In certain circumstances, this reconciliation of contradictions may be synonymous with hell."* In *Le Fantôme de Staline,* he also wrote: *"Must we call this bloody monster that tears at its own flesh by the name of Socialism? My answer is, quite frankly, yes."*

Nevertheless, despite this essential right to recognition that he allowed the U.S.S.R., he refused the *either—or* in which both Kanapa on one side and Aron on the other sought to imprison him; he offered the French people the choice of safeguarding their liberty. Such a course implies the necessity of looking truth in the face, no matter what the circumstances. He was determined never to place a mask on truth, not from any abstract principle but because he believed in the practical value of truth. Even if he had been closer to the U.S.S.R. than he was, he would still have chosen to tell this truth, for in his eyes the role of the intellectual is not the same as that of the politician; it is his duty, not by any means to judge an undertaking according to moral rules that are external to him, but to keep it from contradicting its principles and its goal in the process of its development. If the police methods of a socialist country were compromising socialism, then they should be denounced. Sartre came to an agreement with Stéphane that he would publish and comment on the Soviet Code in the December issue of *Les Temps Modernes*.

But on November 12th, the *Figaro Littéraire* blazoned across its pages in enormous capitals: APPEAL TO THOSE DEPORTED TO NAZI CAMPS. HELP THOSE BEING TAKEN TO SOVIET CAMPS. The cry came from Rousset. He quoted from the articles of the code which authorized "Administrative Internment," in other words, all the arbitrary arrests and deportations. With the collaboration of *Figaro,* he was assembling a splendid anti-Soviet machine. The following numbers of the *Littéraire* and the right-wing press in general exploited it to the full. An unbelievable chorus! Hundreds of stories, memoirs, eyewitness accounts suddenly appeared out of drawers and were printed anywhere and everywhere. There were also terrible photographs of armored trains and "musulmans" that matched the pictures of the Nazi trains and camps feature for feature. They seemed identical—and they were: old photographs had been unearthed and disguised. This hoax was exposed, but it got no one any nearer to the truth. Perfectly indifferent to the 40,000 people killed at Sétif, the 80,000 murdered Malgaches, the famine and poverty in Algeria, the burned-out villages of Indochina, the Greeks dying in their camps, the Spaniards shot by Franco, the hearts of the bourgeoisie suddenly burst when confronted by the misfortunes of the people imprisoned by the Russians. The truth was that they gave a great sigh of relief, as though all the crimes of colonialism and all the exploitations of capitalism had been annulled by the camps in Siberia. As for Rousset, he had found a job.

Nevertheless, the fact remained that the administration had discretionary powers, there was nothing to protect the individual against the arbitrariness of its decisions. In January, *Les Temps Modernes* published an account of the debates in the United Nations on the work camps and an editorial, written by Merleau-Ponty and signed by Sartre as well as himself, which put the affair in its proper perspective.[1] A serious appraisal and correlation of the information available from various sources placed the figure of those deported at ten million.[2] "There can be no socialism when one citizen out of twenty is in a concentration camp," some declared. They accused the Communists of bad faith. Successively and almost simultaneously, we read Wurmser's assertion in *Les Lettres Françaises:* There are no camps! and Daix's proclamation that the camps were the U.S.S.R.'s greatest claim to glory. Merleau-Ponty then took Rousset to task: Rousset's demand for the opening of a commission of inquiry was simply another maneuver in his anti-Communist crusade. He pointed out those parts of the Russian Delegate's reply to the United Nations in which he compared the Russian work camps and the millions of unemployed in the West; when he said: "The colonies are the labor camps of the democracies," the Russian was not cheating; the two systems—Russian socialism and Western capitalism—should be considered in their totality; it was not by accident that the Soviet spokesman implicated Western unemployment and colonialist overexploitation.

This article displeased everyone, or almost everyone. It did nothing to improve our relations with the Communist Party. In any case, the Communist intellectuals were heartily sick of us. Their attitude to *The Second Sex,* however, and the repeated attacks of Kanapa annoyed us less than the hatred with which Aragon was pursuing Nizan. In his novel, *Les Communistes,* he had depicted him as a

[1] *The Mandarins* presents an extremely fictional account of this incident, quite remote from the facts; I even went so far as to use the supposition that French intellectuals had discovered the extent of the concentration camp phenomenon in the U.S.S.R. as early as 1946. It was permissible since the evidence was available, but it was simply an imaginative gesture.

[2] The figure is doubtful; so is the number of years that the deported spent in the camps (it was often five years), and equally so the number of deaths and even the meaning and purpose of the phenomenon. Today the Russians consider it as one of Stalin's "bloody crimes" and do not minimize it; but their appraisals vary.

traitor. Orfilat in the novel was, like Nizan, in charge of the foreign-politics page of *Humanité;* like him he was a philosopher, like him he had demolished Brunschvicg and the bourgeois ideologists, like him he had written a study on a Greek philosopher (Heraclitus; Nizan's had been on Epicurus); the non-Communists said of him, as they did of Nizan: "He's the only intelligent Marxist of the lot, the only one you can talk to." Having thus made it clear whom the character represented, without possibility of mistake, Aragon showed Orfilat-Nizan sobbing with fright, after the German-Soviet pact, at the idea of going to the front, and then going off to plead for a post at the Ministry of Foreign Affairs, where an honest liberal made him feel ashamed of his betrayal. The literary vacuity of this portrait did not in the least attenuate its perfidy. Elsa Triolet did her bit by launching "the battle of the books"; in Marseilles, and then in the suburbs of Paris, the Communist writers gave lectures in which they praised their own merchandise to the skies and treated all "bourgeois" writing as horse shit: Breton, Camus, Sartre.

The scandal of the slogans which erupted at the beginning of 1950 unmasked the real nature of what Beuve-Méry called "The war of filth." This was an affair which brought a great deal of profit to a very few people, but the war continued nonetheless. The victory of Mao Tse-tung had changed the situation. Recognized by China and the U.S.S.R., Ho Chi-minh emerged from the semineutrality with regard to the two blocs behind which he had sheltered up till then. The war in Indochina was henceforth presented by the French propaganda services as an episode in "the anti-Communist crusade." The West was shaking with fear because on October 9, 1949, General Bradley had announced that the day of the "Red Atom" had arrived; the U.S.S.R. now possessed atomic bombs. There began to be talk of a new weapon much more powerful even than the atom bomb. In January 1950, on the orders of President Truman, the H-bomb went into production. Its effects were described everywhere at great length; *Match* complacently demonstrated on a photograph what would happen if one fell on Paris: 80 square kilometers reduced to nothing. The fear it engendered became cosmic: flying saucers were seen in America and in France, sometimes in the sky, sometimes on the ground; some people had even seen Martians. The newspapers helped to maintain this state of panic. The only one we read with sympathy was *Combat,* but Bourdet resigned from it because Smadja, who was financing it, was trying to interfere with the editorial policy.

After that, Rousset and Sérant were able to spread themselves out. Bourdet, supported by Stéphane, started *L' Observateur;* at that time it was only a tiny, boring weekly with very few readers.

I hadn't been away anywhere with Sartre the summer before, so we planned a trip for the spring. Leiris, an ethnographer whose specialty is Black Africa, suggested to Sartre that we go and see what was happening there for ourselves. The Europeans had tried, in vain, to repeal the Houphouet law voted by the Constituent Assembly in 1947 which suppressed forced labor. Having failed to achieve their ends by due process of law, they managed, on each payday, to provoke incidents that were disorganizing the system.[1] The R.D.A. was attempting, through the unions, to protect the small African producers; but the large trading companies were putting pressure on the administration to oppose it. There had been a reign of terror on the Ivory Coast since December of 1949. Many of the R.D.A. leaders had been arrested, tortured or shot down; members of the group, sympathizers and people suspected of sympathizing with it had been massacred or thrown into prison; in February, there were fresh outbreaks whose repression resulted in—officially—twelve people being killed and sixty wounded. To make contact with the R.D.A. and to find out and publish the facts would be a useful piece of work. This project was not favored—as Leiris discovered while he was trying to get it going—by the Communist Party, to which many of the R.D.A. leaders belonged; but we thought that these latter would be less intractable in the event than their French comrades. Because I wanted to see the Sahara, we devised a plan that would take us from Algiers to Hoggar, then to Gao, Timbuktu, Bobo-Dioulasso, and Bamako, where Sartre would be met by members of the R.D.A. and invited to the Ivory Coast. I rushed around the tourist agencies. The trucks going from Ghardaïa to Tamanrasset carried a few passengers in their cabs; I booked space for two.

This time—it was my third attempt—I managed to get from Algiers to Ghardaïa without a hitch. The town was worthy of my perseverance; it was a magnificently constructed Cubist painting; white and ochre rectangles, brushed with blue by the bright light, were piled on each other to form a pyramid; at the top of the hill was stuck, slightly awry, a piece of yellow earthenware that might that

[1] Colonel Lacheroy played a large role in the provocations and the "repressions" of January 1949.

moment have sprung—gigantic, extravagant and superb—from the hands of Picasso: the mosque. The streets were teeming with merchants and merchandise: carrots, leeks and cabbages with skins so shiny that they seemed more like fruit than vegetables. Plump, with a look of deep repose, the Mozabites seemed to be very well fed; most of the grocers in Algeria had come from the M'Zab, and returned there once their fortunes had been made. Up above, in the main square, tanned and wiry-looking men from the desert were busy among their kneeling camels.

We liked the hotel and stayed several days; there was a big patio with a gallery running around it giving access to all the rooms; I worked on the terrace in the mornings; toward eleven, the sky would begin to flame and I would retreat into the shade. In the afternoons we went to see some of the other Mozabite towns near Ghardaïa, more provincial but quite as beautiful: Bénis-Isguen, Melika. We wished we could paint; it would have been a good excuse to stay there for hours looking at them. Some officers asked Sartre to give a lecture and he accepted. We were opposed to the colonialist system, but we had no *a priori* prejudices against the men who administered native affairs or supervised the construction of the roads.

I was very excited when I climbed at dawn into the cab of our first truck; even when one is traveling, a real beginning is rare. I had never forgotten the great orange moon behind Aegina, at the moment when our little boat left the Piraeus for the Islands. That morning, when the truck had climbed above the cliff that dominates the valley, an enormous red currant rose out of the earth: a sun as simple as a childhood memory. Sartre watched it with the same jubilation as myself. In the sky shone, marvelously fresh and still untouched, all the joys·we were setting out to reap together. That sun too is inlaid in my memory like a blazon of bygone happiness.

Five miles farther on, we passed two young Germans wearing white caps and sitting on a great pile of luggage under a murderous sun; they were hitchhiking. "They're mad!" said the driver. The truck was loaded with goods and people, there wasn't room to squeeze in a hummingbird; the road was quite likely to remain deserted the whole day; if by some chance a car did pass, it would certainly be packed to the bursting point. In the Sahara the unforeseen is so strictly limited that there is no margin left for adventure; yet such madmen abound, the driver told us.

We ate lunch in a *bordj* and had two flat tires; they were both very pleasant stops. The Arabs jumped down from the truck, pulled up some of the thornbrush between the rocks and in the wink of an eye had a fire going and a kettle simmering over it; the water, which they got from a skin bottle hanging on the side of the truck, smelled a bit greasy, but the tea they offered us in painted glasses was excellent. As soon as the wheel had been changed they stamped the fire out and whisked all their apparatus out of sight as if by magic.

The day stretched on over two hundred miles. Three more days, exactly the same, brought us to Tamanrasset, with two stops of twenty-four hours each at El Goléa and In-Salah. To us, the time never seemed long; we were learning a whole new world. First of all there was the road. We discovered with surprise that it was really only an ideal axis around which the navigable track meandered; there were laborers working on it and steamrollers rolling it, but we never drove on it: either it had just been resurfaced for a stretch of several miles and we mustn't spoil it; or else—most of the time—it hadn't been resurfaced, in which case it was so full of crevices, so bumpy, patchy, wavy, lumpy and full of holes that the sturdiest vehicle would have been jolted to bits in five minutes. All of which did not prevent the military engineers from expending an enormous amount of energy and zeal on these six hundred miles, or the "road" from constituting an object of pride. "La route, c'est moi," we were told successively by the Commandant of El Goléa, who was director of the operation as a whole, by scattered officers who were in charge of particular sections, by engineers who had done the surveying and planning, by contractors and even by one or two foremen. Only the laborers had nothing to say; we came into close contact with one team—one of them having just been bitten by a snake—but they had no boasts to make.

Except when we crossed a *hammada* the color of anthracite, in which there was literally nothing to be seen—as we were coming out of El Goléa—the Sahara was a spectacle as alive as the sea. The tints of the dunes changed according to the time of day and the angle of the light: golden as apricots from far off, when we drove close to them they turned to freshly made butter; behind us they grew pink; from sand to rock, the materials of which the desert was made varied as much as its tints; sinuous or sharp-edged, their forms produced an infinity of modulations within the deceptive monotony of the *erg*. From time to time we would see a mirage shimmering with metallic lights, it would become still, then vanish into thin air; sand storms would arise, swirling wildly upon themselves, lonely vortices unable to shake the stillness of the world.

We passed two or three caravans. The desert was becoming huger around us, measured by the swinging steps of camels; at least the number of men and beasts and the amount of the loads was in keeping with its size. But where did he come from, where was he going, that man who suddenly appeared from nowhere, walking along with great strides? We followed him with our eyes until he was completely swallowed up again by the great absence that enveloped us.

During the last days of the journey we drove through gorges, beneath giant citadels with battlements and Cyclopean walls black as lava; we crossed plateaus of white sand stuck full of needles and bristling with black lace: the atmosphere had been blown away, and our Earth had changed into a moon. "Incredible!" we said to each other; and yet a painting or even a photograph of that landscape would have astonished us even more. We were in it, therefore it became natural; the fantastic can exist only in images: once embodied it is destroyed. That's why it is difficult to tell about one's journeys; the reader is taken either too far or not far enough.

Thirsty, dusty, stunned and slightly paralyzed, it was pleasant to arrive in the evening, no matter where it was we stopped. At El Goléa, when I went into the hotel with its profusion of patterned carpets, its brass lanterns and all its Sahara bric-a-brac, it seemed like a palace from the Arabian Nights. On the lawn, some Americans had organized a big *méchoui* in honor of Shell. I was jolted back to my own century. In the morning we walked through the town and saw the market and the old Slave Quarter where the Negroes still live. We had lunch with the head of the Engineers. His wife, who was one of our readers, had come to invite us herself; she gave us a French lunch with fresh spring vegetables, and her husband told us about "his road."

At In-Salah, Sartre shut himself in his room to work as soon as we got out of the truck; I walked across the dunes, which were fringed with reeds (or, perhaps frayed palms); evening was coming on; the sand I lay down on was as soft as flesh; I almost expected to feel it move beneath my cheek. Along a path I saw tall Negro women passing in single file, draped in blue with their faces uncovered; golden rings swung from their ears. They were coming back from the fields, they did not speak and their bare feet made no sound; in the still of the falling dark, there was something touching in that quiet cortege.

I was also moved when I leaned out of my window the following morning; it overlooked a vast square—or rather a stretch of waste-land—across which men and women were moving, quickly, slowly, each absorbed in his or her own progress; I had seen paintings which expressed the maleficent quality of space that separates even as it unites. But in that moment I seemed to surprise it at work in life itself. The houses of In-Salah were made of red earth with battle-ments; they had been half swallowed up by the sand, despite the barriers and obstacles put up across the streets. In the market I again saw beautiful black women swathed in blue.

Our last stop was only for one night, in the depths of the Arak gorges, at the foot of a black granite fortress; there was a travelers' hut where we found beds, but nothing to eat; two young men were camping out on the terrace and their radio was playing music from another world. They were traveling in a jeep, without an escort, though the rule is that no vehicle has the right to risk traveling alone along the desert tracks. "It's dangerous," our driver told us. He was our third, because we had made two stopovers during our journey, and more loquacious than his predecessors, though sharing their conviction that all tourists are mad. He pointed to the framework of an automobile lying by the side of the track. "Cross the Sahara in that! It caught fire from spontaneous combustion!" According to him, the heat of the sun had been sufficient to send it up in flames. He told us more stories while we ate lunch in the shade of a thorny bush, the only one we encountered on the whole journey; there wasn't enough shade to cover more than half our heads, but there was water nearby and grass growing as fresh and as green as a Nor-mandy meadow. "As soon as the rain comes everything is covered with grass and flowers," the driver told us; he added that the rain came very rarely, but that when it did it was usually torrential. One or two years before, a Dodge had been immobilized by one of these storms; the official period of delay having elapsed, he was sent in his truck to rescue it; at last he saw the car, lost like an Ark amid the waves; but then, before he reached it, he too was caught and held fast by the mud. At first no one was apprehensive when he did not re-turn; in this way he and the tourists spent, they a week and he five days, without food or water other than the muddied water of the flood. As he was talking, a soldier was throwing empty food cans into the air and shooting at them with a distracted air; he in his turn recounted somber dramas of the desert; our fellow travelers, the people we met by chance when we stopped, were all full of extraordinary and terrible stories, and they all discounted the ones we had already heard: "I know the man who told you that, he's crazy," they would say; and then they would assure us that their own stories were guaranteed to be one hundred percent true. There must have been some that were true out of so many; but which ones?

The evening came when we had finished this first lap of our journey. We arrived at Tamanrasset and the little hotel of the S.A.T.T. It was impossible to choose any other: the S.A.T.T. had a monopoly on the transport and lodging of tourists; moreover, on the pretext of guaranteeing their rescue, should the need arise, they demanded large sums from independent travelers as security. I had often heard protests against these privileges; at Tamanrasset, it was whispered that the lack of any competition encouraged the hotel-keeper to behave like a potentate. Always laughing, with bright snapping eyes, he did indeed seem very confident of his rights; but his hotel, though a terrible barracks of a place, was well run and kept well provisioned by truck and plane. "At Christmas we had oysters. One of the pilots brought them straight from the sea!" he told us proudly. Everything considered, it was an ideal holiday resort. Because it was more than 5,000 feet above sea level, the mornings were temperate enough for me to work in the garden, facing the black, deforested mass of the Hoggar; there were strips of camel meat hanging from the trees to dry and I was secretly grateful that they didn't serve it to their customers. We had no desire to go climbing up the mountain; it would have been a full-scale expedition, with guides and camels. We contented ourselves with a few automobile rides and the magnificent sunsets that bathed the inky mountains in their light.

The society of Tamanrasset was very closed; the wives of the officers and civil servants lived as though they were at Romorantin; they wore hats, kept tabs on each other and gossiped. We discovered that we were not viewed with favor. A captain bestowed a short visit on us and left it at that. But we were lucky enough to be taken in hand by the teachers, Monsieur and Madame B., and by the explorer Henri Lhote. Mme and M. B. had both French and Tuareg pupils; the latter, they told us, were intelligent but nervous and unstable, and their parents only sent them to class at irregular intervals. In certain villages, at a two or three days' walk in the mountains, the children received no instruction at all; a mobile classroom had been started: at that very moment there was a teacher camping out up in the highlands.

Henri Lhote was searching through the Hoggar for cave paintings and sculptures; he had already amassed a vast collection of photographs and sketches whose authenticity was being somewhat contested at the time. His stories also aroused a certain amount of skepticism. He had narrowly escaped death a hundred times in the course of the most dramatic and extravagant series of events; one day, for example, almost dead with thirst, he reached the edge of a well at the bottom of which he could see the light glinting on a bit of water: the rope tied to the bucket was too short! He twisted an extra length from his clothes and went on, his thirst assuaged, naked across the *erg;* one couldn't help wondering why he hadn't been burned to death by the sun. But it didn't particularly matter; his inventions had a lyric quality that enchanted us.

When we went to visit B. and his wife, we constantly met several tall boys wearing veils who were there playing cards, chatting or dozing: the sons of the Amenokal, their cousins and their friends; they came there as though it were a club; apart from one or two brothels where they found some amusement in the evenings, Tamanrasset had no other distractions to offer them. Now that their wars and raids were forbidden them and they were no longer allowed to exploit slave labor, this warrior people was simply dragging out an empty and almost poverty-stricken existence with all their former occupations gone. Their principal resources were raising sheep and, above all, the salt mines of Amadror, not far from Tamanrasset. From July to September, they came in great numbers from the villages and hewed out the salt with axes. From October to February, they rode in caravans up to the Sudan, where they exchanged their merchandise for millet and manufactured articles. But such trade was beneath the dignity of the great chiefs and their families. I bought some camels made of braided string from Mme B: "The eldest son of the Amenokal makes them," she told me. "It brings him in a bit of pocket money, but he couldn't bear anyone to know about it." In the old days the chiefs stuffed their wives with food to such an extent that they needed the help of several servants when they wanted to penetrate one of these lumps of fat. But those days were long past. "Take a pound of tea," B. told us when he and his wife drove us out to see the Amenokal; such visits represented for him a by no means negligible source of income. His tent stood among several others about eight miles outside the town; hung with carpets, furnished with coffers, it was luxurious enough, but too small to hold us all; we sat outside around a fire that didn't keep us very warm. Even with blankets thrown around our shoulders, we shivered as we drank our tea; but I enjoyed the strangeness of being there, under those new stars, in this encampment that was really so far away from me in space and time. Freed from the slavery of past opulence, thin, nervous, her face proud and hard, the wife of the Amenokal managed the reception with authority and courtesy; she was in fact, we were told, the real chief. As we left, Mme B. swept the infinitude of the desert with her hand. "You see what sort of life they have, those boys!" And indeed few people I have seen seemed to me less adapted to the world of today than those young princes, proud and stony broke. They were so impressive in their indigo robes, their somber eyes glittering above their veils. One afternoon, Mme B. asked one of the Amenokal's sons to uncover his face: "There's a good boy, take off your veil, just for a moment, Chéri." (Chéri was his real name, and it was strange to hear this woman quite calmly coaxing him: Chéri, Chéri . . .) He shrugged, laughed, drew away the cloth. His face was disfigured by a great nose like an eagle's beak; every time I caught a glimpse of a Tuareg's face I recognized this same nose, the same disappointing homeliness beneath the dark brilliance of the eyes. The women were luckier. Though it wasn't very easy to get to meet them; the only way Henri Lhote could think of in the end was to invite all the prostitutes of the neighborhood one evening; most of them were being treated for syphilis at the hospital; he got permission for them to be released for a few hours, and we all sat on a carpet in the school garden and drank tea together.

We spent more than a week at Tamanrassett; we were kept informed of all the gossip circulating between Laghouat and the Hoggar. The Europeans scattered along the more than six hundred miles of the road, surrounded by spaces of dizzying immensity, knew each other, spied on each other, loathed each other, slandered each other, and bickered with each other with all the enthusiasm and attention to detail one would have expected in a small provincial town. All this "long-distance" chatter was fascinating to us; the night before we left it kept me up very late. After dinner we went up on a roof to see the Southern Cross. Then Sartre went off to bed. I stayed up and stood at the bar drinking and joking with the hotel-keeper and two truck drivers, one of whom was as blond and handsome as Jean Marais at twenty. They talked about the people I had met along the road from Ghardaïa, and in particular about an ex-convict who gave truck drivers very good free bed and board as long as "the rest" was included; each one gaily accused the other of having profited from this generous offer. Then they began to tell the story of their lives. The stories were interesting and I wasn't bothered by the coarseness of their language; I am perfectly able to use their vocabulary myself when the need arises. We all bought several rounds, the hotelkeeper included, and at about three in the morning I went up to bed still laughing. I was stupefied to hear someone opening my door; it was our host, who came over and propositioned me in a whisper. I was all the more astonished in that his wife did not look at all like a woman with a tolerant disposition. The following morning, he rushed up to me with a wide smile and a basket of oranges. They were a fruit rarely seen in Tamanrasset, so I realized that he was trying to buy my silence. It was a deal; I'd had no intention of making a fuss anyway. He then talked, not about his attempts at seduction, but about my own alcoholic and verbal debauch: opening *Samedi-Soir* several days later, I came across an account of our drinking bout. I read that my trooper's vocabulary had made the truck drivers blush; then there were other kind words that have slipped my mind,[1] but that made me rather uneasy at the time. Since Sartre and I were so closely linked, any filth thrown on me was always intended for him as well; I blamed myself for having provided the opportunity. But did that mean that I must live perpetually on the defensive and calculate every word I spoke and every drink I took? "The advantage of our position," Sartre said to me, "is that we can do whatever we want: it will never be worse than what they say we do."

A three-hour flight; from above, the diversity of the Sahara was flattened out. It seemed monotonous, but uniformity, so insipid when it indicates the repetition of human effort, fascinates me when I see in it one of the original aspects of our planet; perpetual snows, a sky of flawless blue, a plain of clouds seen from the cockpit, a desert. During the whole journey I riveted my eyes on the redness of the sun. I was not blasé; flying over the Niger seemed to me like a miracle; it was a wide road of gray water, but as the plane wheeled and came down, I caught sight of an island the color of pale coral opposite a golden beach of sand; at that point the river was made of

---

[1] The article did not appear in the Paris edition. It exceeded in its vileness even the low standards *Samedi-Soir* set for itself.

blue enamel. "Oh how lucky," I thought to myself, "to be alive today and not at any other time, and see these things with my own eyes!" But I found the ground itself disappointing; it was no longer pure mineral; it was made messy by clumps of lank grass and sour-looking little bushes. As I stepped from the plane onto the asphalt, the sun hit me on the head like a mallet; we took refuge under a hangar. Yet the sky was as gray as the river. They had warned us: "Down there, it's never blue; it's like being under glass." A canopy of vapor filtered the sunlight without lessening the violence of its attack. As we got out of the bus at the hotel, our hostess exclaimed: "But you must have helmets, you'll be dead by this evening!" Despite our dislike of tourist gear, we walked off to the bazaar she pointed out to us; even crossing those few yards of street we felt as though we were going to collapse. In the shade, the temperature was 104 degrees. "It's bearable here because it's dry," people told us; it was certainly dry, but it didn't seem all that bearable. According to our original plans, we should have arrived at Gao three weeks earlier, but Sartre had been detained and we had thought: "What are three weeks more or less?" Actually, in this place those three weeks mattered: water traffic on the Niger had just stopped for several months.

Duly helmeted, we took a walk through the market on the main square just in front of the hotel. Suddenly, at long last, instead of the veiled phantoms that haunt the Arab towns, there were women. Beautiful Negro women, swathed in brilliant cotton stuffs, their hair piled up in complicated structures of twisted braids, displayed their faces, their shoulders, their breasts, their smiles and their laughter; the young ones, with tawny skins and glistening white teeth, stood resplendent; the textured, dry nudity of the old women had nothing offensive about it; they chattered among themselves and argued with the men. And there was such variety, so many different types, so many different ways of dressing! There were the Peuhls, both sexes so beautiful with their finely cut profiles, the graceful carriage of their heads and the slimness of their waists; the women wore ornaments around their necks, their wrists and in their hair, made of the little cowrie shells that also serve as money. Some of the Negroes wore lurid boubous, others were in shorts, with felt hats and sunshades. A few Tuaregs, draped and veiled in blue, wandered through the crowd. Gao was a meeting place of many tribes on market day, and the population was extremely mixed; such variety gave an impression of luxuriance. The impression faded however when we became aware of the poverty of the merchandise being exchanged: poor quality bread, pitiful stuffs, tinplate. In this district, as we were informed later, the natives have almost nothing; even grain has to be distributed to them, otherwise they would have nothing to eat.

The town was built of mud in the Sudanese style; cubelike houses stuck one against the other along narrow alleys. The big attraction was the Niger. We went to look at it at about five in the evening. Flat as a lake, wan, it was bathed in a false dusk that reminded me of the light in Abisko at midnight; we went along it in a pirogue; it might well have been a landscape in Scandinavia, except for that feeling of anguish you only find in hot countries. A whole nation of people was encamped along its banks; they were lighting fires, cooking, getting ready for the night. We went back early in the morning and saw them waking up. Tuaregs, holding mirrors, coquettishly scrutinized their unveiled faces; as we approached they hurriedly replaced their veils. How long were they going to stay here on these banks? How did they live?

The misery and the gaiety of Gao disconcerted us. Roaming through the streets in the afternoon, we heard a tom-tom; we searched to find where the sound was coming from; we came to a courtyard full of laughter and songs: a wedding. There was a group of Negroes watching the festivities through the doorway from the street, and for a long time we watched with them, captivated by the exuberance of the dances and the voices.

To get to know the country a bit we would have had to know people there. We saw almost no one. We were invited over by a young geologist bored by geology; he entertained us on his roof, and we took tea with the Moslems from whom he rented his room; as we talked, I contemplated the town below me, and the undefined country around it, no longer the desert but not yet the savanna. He asked Sartre to look at his pictures: his father was a well-known artist, and he too would have liked to paint. He showed us his canvases, still very immature, but Sartre did not hesitate a moment. "If you really want to paint, go ahead," he told him. The young man has since followed that advice.

We had dinner at the home of the Administrator; young and a bachelor, he had just lost a lioness he had lovingly raised from a cub. He had little to tell us about the natives, though he did say that their poverty was made even worse by their religion, which forbade those who lived on the banks of the river to eat fish; they were undernourished but did not fish. He placed an automobile at our disposal for the following day. We saw several wretched villages along the banks of the Niger. The countryside seemed to me decidedly unrewarding; its most interesting feature was the anthills bristling all over it; if you went to sleep in the shade of one, the driver assured us, you woke up without a stitch left on your body.

One of the places I had wanted to see most of all was Timbuktu, 250 miles from Gao. From Paris the distance had seemed trifling; even if there were no boats, there were sure to be trucks making the journey. I inquired about it and was simply laughed at for my pains: in the present heat, the track—rarely used at any season—was impassable. I resigned myself to this fact with an ease that surprised me. The same thing happened again several times later on; a place that had seemed to me, when we began our journey, the principal attraction of one of its stages, lost its importance when we got nearer to it. From afar, its name had symbolized a whole country; when we got there, the country had many other ways of showing itself to us. In the market at Gao, along the banks of the Niger, I had already seen embodied the images of Timbuktu that I had previously conjured up in my mind's eye.

Perhaps my regrets were also routed by fatigue: twelve hours in a truck under that sun—I hadn't the strength to want anything that much. The heat raged unchecked all day; at siesta time, the electric fan in our room merely stirred up the burning air, and we could not sleep a wink. The shower was a bucket that you tipped; the water fell all over you in one short-lived splash, and it was scarcely any cooler than the air. Toward evening, big birds that they called "gendarmes" began to preen themselves in the trees; they flew about and sang. But the heat scarcely subsided at all. Everyone slept outside; our beds, covered by mosquito netting, were installed in an isolated corner of the roof; I liked going to sleep under the stars, but the nights were so heavy we could scarcely bear the weight of a sheet on top of us. At about four in the morning, a light breeze would begin to catch the netting over us. "Fair stands the wind for France," I would think, mistily, and half in a dream I would float for a few minutes over the cool depths of a great lake; a gentle light made the sky opalescent, it was a delicious moment—the only one of the day; the sun soon became savage again. We would go down to our room; couples would be lying with closed eyes in the inner court, more united in sleep than in their daily lives. The last night at dinner, the Adjutant and his wife had quarreled bitterly; now her head was resting gently on her husband's naked shoulder.

Two days after our arrival, Sartre was suddenly prostrated by it all. I called the doctor: "He's got a temperature of 104." He prescribed quinine; whereupon Sartre stuffed himself so full of it that he lost his sense of balance and could neither see nor hear. He stayed in bed for two days. Our hostess shrugged. "A temperature of 104! I get a temperature of 104 every week; it doesn't keep me from polishing the floors!" I managed to keep going, but I was suffering from a complaint as unpleasant as its name suggests: prickly heat. In the hollows of one's knees and elbows, and between the toes, the sweat begins to produce a sort of reddish lichen; it itches a great deal, but the main thing is not to touch it on any account: a scratch, the slightest infection, is enough to produce "cro-cro," real wounds that can rapidly become running sores. I spent two pretty awful afternoons in a room with Sartre lying there more or less unconscious; at three o'clock, I sat down at my table and worked; what else was there to do? The shutters were closed; outside, a raging sirocco was thrashing among the trees; the darkness and the noise of the wind both suggested the idea of coolness, but the wind was made of flames, and the thermometer on the wall said 110 degrees.

As soon as Sartre could stand on his feet we would leave, we had decided. But at the Tourist Bureau I received an unpleasant shock. Planes only arrived and took off at very irregular intervals; it was impossible to give me a definite date of departure. I loathed the idea of being imprisoned in that furnace.

At last they told me that a plane was to leave the following day for Bobo-Dioulasso. Sartre's fever had abated, and we took it. I looked down nostalgically at the forest beneath us, and at the red roads we would never drive along. There was a short stop at Ouagadougou. In the airport concourse, a Negro was selling lead figurines—tom-toms, witch doctors, antelopes. I bought an assortment.

"Bobo's unhealthy, it's so humid," I had been told at Gao. However, when we left the plane I found the moisture in the air a relief. A man with a sallow, puffy face was waiting for us at the airport; in Gao, the people still had tanned, Sahara skins; here, all the faces looked like boiled fish—Bobo was a saucepan with the lid on, perpetually simmering. "I'll take you to the hotel," the man said, though we didn't know who he was, and he helped us into his car. He was an official who had come to meet us on behalf of the administration. We drove into the town. "Bobo-Dioulasso's just like Normandy," a friend had told me. And the countryside was, in fact, rolling and green, but it was a very suspicious-looking green, and the smell of rotting earth was not the same as the smell of meadows in France; long, low, and thatched with dark straw, the houses made it plain that we were in the tropics; a few flowers made bright splashes in the gardens. Our guide deposited us in front of a hotel. Our room was not ready yet, and we sat down in the shade of the veranda on comfortable armchairs, opposite a little open-air dance floor. The assistant administrator, B., found us sitting there and passed on an invitation to dinner with his superior. Then he took us to a fairground around which all the different native districts rose in tiers; he pointed at one of them and said: "That side's pretty bad; it's under the control of the R.D.A. Whatever you do, don't go walking there!" He didn't show us much. "Let's go and have a drink before lunch," he suggested. We went back to the airport, the bar of which was used by the European elite as a meeting place because it stood a few feet above the town and the heat was therefore supposedly less torrid. It seemed to me quite as overpowering as it was down below; the impression of relief I had felt for the first hour had now completely evaporated. Before lunch we took our suitcases up to our room: the same shower system as at Gao; it smelled of disinfectant and felt like a steam room. We left the door to the courtyard open and went to lunch. A man we didn't know, a friendly planter from Guinea, came up and offered us an apéritif; we had already had a drink, but he insisted: "You must drink a lot here!" and told us the story of a young woman, proud of her looks, who drank only very little so as to keep her figure; within a matter of weeks she was dead of dehydration; newborn children had to be watered from morning to night, or else they dried up and died. So we gulped down one or two glasses of black currant syrup and water. During lunch a storm broke, brief but violent. When we got back to our room for our siesta, the beds were soaked; there were cockroaches coming out of the waste pipe in the shower and crawling all over the floor and ceiling. We fled and wandered around the native town. Steep *marigots*, running almost dry, split the hillsides from top to bottom. The women were doing their washing in the pools of water at the bottom of them, their children playing among the yellow rocks. But apart from these clefts, each district formed a compact and apparently hostile block; the houses presented walls unbroken by any window, and we passed almost no one in the alleys between. It was impossible to penetrate in any way without knowing the inhabitants. Our arrival had been reported in the local press, and Sartre had hoped we would find a message from the R.D.A at the hotel; we didn't.

We ate dinner with the Administrator, B., and his wife, a Creole girl from Martinique who was lamenting that her husband wanted to take her that summer to Paris, which she had never seen. "It's so cold there!" she said in a frightened voice. "It's hot in August," I assured her. "But August, that's nearly September; in September I'll catch a chill on my chest and it will kill me." Sitting on the terrace after dinner, I searched the sky for the Southern Cross: "They showed it to me at Gao." "It couldn't have been the real one; it's never the real one they show you." B. told us about the last elections. "I got the votes I needed," he told us, with a wink that made it obvious he had no doubt of our complicity. We left them while it was still early and went for a drink with the planter at the illuminated dance hall; in front of the door, a dressed-up monkey was dancing about on the end of a chain. We were ready to drop with fatigue, but we had difficulty getting to sleep; Sartre barely closed his eyes all night: his bed was still wet, the jazz across the road deafened him, and above all he was frightened of the cockroaches that were trotting about on the ceiling. He spent the night reading a biography of Mme Roland.

In the morning, an automobile provided by the Administrator took us into the forest. We visited a village and saw their fetish underneath a tree: a great ball stuck full of very dirty feathers. The women, dressed in loincloths, wore little bits of carved ivory fixed in their jaws by way of ornament (they made me think of the tooth I had pulled out of my own jaw one day); tall and vigorous, their hair smeared with cocoa butter and giving off the most nauseating smell, two of them were pounding grain in a mortar; on a stairway (some of the huts, wretched as they were, had two stories) among a lot of other naked children, there was a little albino boy; his pale skin didn't look natural; it was as though the top layer had been scoured off with acid and what was left was insufficient to protect him. We were quite close to the town, and yet these people seemed lost in the depths of a forest where time had always stood still. As we left, we passed two young boys coming along the road on bicycles; they were dressed in European clothes, very smart-looking, and they too lived in the hamlet we had just left; in a few years those naked children would become adolescents adapted to this century. We would very much have liked to know how the young cyclists managed the business of belonging to those two worlds.

But to Sartre's great disappointment, we heard nothing from the R.D.A that day either and were forced to content ourselves with questioning the white people we met at a cocktail party that was given for us. Sartre talked to two future administrators who were making a great display of their good intentions; when pressed a bit, however, it became apparent that they were already preparing to cut their ideas according to their situation. Our trip was becoming farcical and unpleasant. We had set out to make contact with the Negroes who were fighting against the administration; we hadn't met any, and furthermore we were being very honorably entertained by the administrators themselves. Perhaps we would be luckier at Bamako? We took a plane there that evening.

Sartre was coming down with a high fever again; he was shivering when we landed quite late at night. The principal hotel was full; they sent us to the station hotel; a young fellow grabbed Sartre's baggage and dragged him off with an air of authority, while another led me away with equal imperiousness in the opposite direction. I found myself alone, in a sort of cage, furnished with a chair and a pallet, that overlooked the station platforms. Fortunately there were very few trains going by, but on the other side of the wire screen that covered my window the air under the glass roof that covered the railroad tracks was heavy with smoke and soot; I had no idea of the number of Sartre's room and the thought of him lying ill in a prison like the one I was in was nightmarish; I spent an appalling night.

The next day Sartre had somewhat recovered, and the other hotel had saved us a room; there too we suffocated, despite the enormous electric fans, but at least we could sleep out on the balcony: it was an astonishing spectacle in the morning, that balcony piled with half-naked bodies. The food was good; they even gave us strawberries. But what made the stay really pleasant for us was the cordiality of the Air Force Commandant C. He had belonged to the Normandie-Niémen Squadron and spent some time in Moscow, with the result that he was completely without prejudice against left-wing writers; nor did we inspire him with very much curiosity. "I was in Gao at the same time as you were," he told Sartre. "I was told: 'Simone de Beauvoir's just arrived with Pierre Dac; then I found out it was you afterwards. . . .'" He hadn't particularly wanted to see us. But he cared very much about a young woman who read a great deal and who had urged him to come and talk to us. He called her Juju. She was a beautiful girl with a lively mind, and he was completely lost in admiration of her intelligence, culture and courage. She was married to an Air Force officer who was away from Bamako at the time. C. had a wife and children who were spending the summer at the seaside in Guinea. But it soon became apparent to us that they were both resolved to divorce and marry each other—which they did in fact shortly afterward. When love enters into people whose hearts are not withered, it makes them want to love everyone. We reaped the benefits of this kindly predisposition in them and also of their astonishment, for they had expected, they later admitted to us, to encounter monsters and not human beings; they were censured for compromising themselves with us, but the reproaches they received simply created a further complicity between them.

Juju and C. both lived on the outskirts of the town in vast, almost identical houses, surrounded by verandas and equipped with absolutely the latest thing in bathrooms: the tiled floors and light furniture gave an impression of coolness. Juju had a tom-tom displayed on a table just like the one I had bought, only larger; she also had other, well-chosen pieces of native work. We took our apéritifs every evening on her terrace, and she showed us the site of the great ultramodern hotel that was soon to be built. One of their friends, V.—also a flier—often came and drank with us; his vitality quite revived us. "You get used to the climate quickly enough; when I get a high temperature, I hop into my jeep and go off and shoot a buffalo, that gets rid of the fever." He admitted that the prickly heat was unpleasant; "When you go to bed, you have to dive under the sheet right away," and he gave a demonstration of an intrepid swimmer hurling himself into icy water. Big-game hunting—for buffalo and even lion—played a large part in their lives; Juju could shoot as well as a man; she often accompanied her men friends in their planes or on their expeditions in jeeps.

The first morning, we went out on our own, in a carriage, through the European part of the town—pretty enough with its old-fashioned colonial houses—and then through the native districts which we didn't get to see much of because the driver refused to stop. But after that we were always with our new friends. They took us to the market; the population of the town was less varied than at Gao, but the goods seemed more abundant and much gayer to the eye; the stuffs the women wore could be bought in profusion: muslins, made in Alsace, but printed in bold patterns that were at that time exclusive to Africa; I bought several rolls. In the evening, Commandant C. drove us in a jeep out to the Niger dam through a dull, thinly wooded landscape; on the road of red laterite I realized the truth of what I had always heard without giving it much credence: that an automobile can only withstand the corrugated surface if it goes more than 50 miles an hour; if it does less, it gets shaken to pieces. There were some Negro prisoners working on the side of the road, under the surveillance of armed guards; two of the prisoners, who were pointed out to us, were serving sentences for cannibalism. All their faces seemed to have been molded into expressions of despair and hate.

Bamako and the surrounding district teems with frightful diseases. There are long worms that find their way through the skin on the soles of the feet and dig caves inside for themselves; to get them out, you have to get hold of one end and roll it tight around a matchstick; you give the matchstick a turn every day; it's no good trying to pull it out all at once because it would break and then you'd never get rid of it. We were also given descriptions of the horrors of elephantiasis and sleeping sickness. One of the most widespread scourges was leprosy, and there was a really enormous leper hospital at Bamako.

The doctor in charge of it received us very cordially. He talked to me about *The Second Sex,* which he approved of. We went with him through a big village: huts and markets where men with barrows were offering a variety of products for sale; this was where the lepers lived with their families, for the disease was no longer considered as fatally contagious; furthermore, if caught in its very early stage, it could easily be held in check. The doctor showed us the dispensary where the mild cases were treated; the only indication of the disease on a young Negro woman being given an injection by a male nurse was a slight discoloration on her right arm. "She may live to be eighty without the disease making any further advance," the doctor told us. To check the disease they also used chaulmoogra oil, an old Hindu remedy; but at that time *asiaticoside* had just been discovered, and it was hoped that it might prove to be a means of reversing the course of the disease and even curing it altogether. However, there was a certain number of men and women who had only been hospitalized in the later stages of the malady and were in an advanced state of deterioration; we were taken into the dormitory where they were lying and I thought I would pass out, first because of the smell and then because of the "lion" faces, the mouths that had become muzzles, the noses eaten away, the mutilated hands. "Even these won't die as a direct cause of leprosy," the doctor told us. "Its progress is extremely slow, it's just that it weakens the organism; all it takes is a bout of flu and a leper will succumb to it." There were enormous numbers of lepers in the bush, and quite a few walking about in Bamako; we had certainly walked past some in the market. But there was no risk of contamination unless one went out barefoot.

Commandant C. introduced us to one of his Negro friends: a very old doctor who gave Sartre a copy of a voluminous work on the native pharmacopoeia of the region. He didn't discuss politics with us. Every day Sartre waited impatiently for the R.D.A. to contact him; every day brought a fresh disappointment. This silence was obviously deliberate and consequently affected him all the more. After a last evening with Juju and C. in an open air dance hall, we left for Dakar.

Dakar was part of my private mythology; it was *the* colony: men in white helmets, with yellow faces in the intolerable heat, drank whisky all day long until both their livers and their reason were undermined. People in Bamako thought of it as a haven of cool relief. "In Dakar you can sleep under a sheet," they told me nostalgically. Before we landed the pilot of our plane invited us into his cockpit and wheeled over the city so he could show us the port and the sea and the island of Gorée. We touched down, and for the first time since Tamanrasset I felt comfortable inside my skin: 75 degrees. We abandoned our helmets in the hotel and went out for a walk in the streets.

We saw no Negroes on the café terraces, no Negroes in the air-conditioned luxury restaurant where we ate lunch; officially, segregation didn't exist; society was split up in such a way economically that there was no need for it; no Negro, or almost none, could afford to frequent the places the whites went to. The European town was uninteresting and the coastline, which we went along for several miles in a taxi, just shabby, despite the splendor of the ocean: frail palms, huts without gaiety, the earth a mess of decayed and decaying vegetable matter. We found the island of Gorée charming, with its tawny, crumbling Portuguese fortress. But our interest was not really caught until the evening, when we went for a walk through the residential area; it was our first contact with natives who had become a proletariat. The muddy streets lined with straw huts had a countrified, village look about them, but they were wide and long and all at right angles to one another; the Negroes living in them were all workers; it evoked—paradoxically, it seemed to us—both the bush and Aubervilliers. We could not begin to imagine what was going on behind those faces, mostly handsome and calm, but closed. Like the boys we saw cycling back to the fetishist hamlet, these men belonged to two civilizations: how did they reconcile them inside themselves? We left Dakar without even beginning to know the answer. Our brief trip through Black Africa had been a failure. Back in Paris we were confirmed in our suspicions that heavy injunctions had been laid upon all the members of the R.D.A. and they had deliberately avoided meeting Sartre.

To recover from our weariness, and to work in peace, we spent two weeks in Morocco. We stopped for a while at Meknès and for a long time at Fez. This time it was spring, the trees were in bloom, the sky was light, and the Djalnai palace had opened its doors. They put me in the sultana's room, decorated with carpets and mosaics and opening onto a beautiful patio; I left my door open while I worked, and often visitors would come in and walk around my table as if I were an exhibit in a museum. The dining room had glass walls and looked out over all the whiteness of the town; we met Rousset there and exchanged unenthusiastic greetings.

Since June, my sister and her husband had been living in Casablanca; I spent a few days with them; we toured by car through the Middle Atlas and as far as Marrakesh where, beyond the red ramparts, I could see the high peaks glistening with snow.

Boris Vian was fined 100,000 francs for having written *I Spit on Your Grave*. His books, and Sartre's as well, were being held responsible for a good many suicides, criminal offenses, murders and the "crime of the J3" in particular. When Michel Mourre got up into the pulpit of Notre-Dame, this "sacrilege" too was imputed to the effects of Existentialism.

Sartre's thought, as I have said, was gradually stripping itself of all idealism; but he did not reject the existential postulates and continued to demand, within the realm of *praxis*, a synthesis of the two points of view. In a preface to Stéphane's *Portrait de l'Aventurier*, he expressed the wish that the militant might inherit the virtues of those men whom Stéphane termed adventurers. "*An action has two aspects: there is the negative aspect that belongs to the adventurer and the constructive aspect that comes from discipline. Negativity, doubt and self-criticism must be re-established within the framework of discipline.*" A similar concern inspired the essay he wrote introducing Dalmas' book on Yugoslavia. Stalinist objectivism, he said, annuls the subjectivism of his opponents by presenting them to the world, often on their own admission, as objective traitors. The case of Tito was unique: he had succeeded and therefore made it impossible for Stalin to recoup his losses in this way. His opposition effectively replaced subjectivism as a force within the Revolution. A truly revolutionary ideology would have to take as its task, in opposition to Stalinism, the reinstatement of subjectivity in its proper place.

Tito was the *bête noire* of the Communists. They had insulted Bourdet, Mounier, Cassou and Domenach, who had spoken out on his behalf, and the last two had even been excluded from the Peace Movement. Sartre's preface provided the Communists with a new grievance. He really didn't have much luck with them. He thought his discussions with Thao so feeble that he opposed their publication; Thao, taking advantage of the bourgeois legal system without the slightest embarrassment, filed suit against him, and Domarchi, who had sat in on the conversations without opening his mouth except to agree with Thao, joined with the latter in demanding a million francs in damages. The recent trials, the work camps, had so set us against Stalinism that we refused—and we were in the wrong— to have anything to do with the Stockholm Appeal, for which eight million signatures were collected throughout France in the last weeks of June. Yet we were still sickened by "the West"; we learned with regret that Silone was participating, side by side with Koestler, in the congress "for the defense of culture" which had been convened in Berlin under the aegis of the *Liberté de l'Esprit* movement.

Sartre also had personal troubles. In 1949, he had taken a trip with M. to Mexico and Guatemala, and had also visited Cuba, Panama, Haiti and Curaçao. They were not getting on well any more. Despite Sartre's opposition she had come to live in Paris. They quarreled and eventually separated.

Algren and I had kept up our correspondence throughout the past year. He had changed his tune since his return to America; the country was changing, very fast. The witch-hunt was affecting a great number of his friends. In Hollywood, which he had visited as a result of winning the National Book Award, all the left-wing film makers were out—many were emigrating to Europe; John Garfield was unable to play the lead in *The Man with the Golden Arm*. On his return from California, Algren had bought a house on Lake Michigan; we were to spend two months there together. For me the idea of having a real life with him was a great happiness.

Just as I was about to catch my plane, the North Koreans penetrated South Korea; immediately, the American Air Force and then the American Army intervened. If China attacked Formosa, a world war would break out; the Stockholm Appeal collected three million additional signatures in just a few days. Everyone was talking about France being occupied by the Red Army. *Samedi-Soir* chose as its headline: SHOULD WE BE AFRAID? and concluded that we should. Despite my desire to see Algren and my repugnance at letting him down once again, I hesitated a great deal before leaving France. "Go," Sartre told me, "you can always come back. I don't believe there's going to be a war." He gave me the arguments that he then repeated in a letter I received during August; in Paris there was panic, gold had soared from 3,500 francs to 4,200, people were queuing outside all the grocers to lay in stocks of canned food and sugar, and everyone was expecting the Red Army to arrive any day, then the bombs. But Sartre still continued to reassure me. "In any case, here is my opinion: A *bloody* war is impossible. The Russians haven't got the atomic bombs and the Americans haven't got the soldiers. Thus it cannot take place, mathematically, until a few years from now. So that leaves us with the fact that both will now, also mathematically, prepare for it. So in the end it comes to the same thing. Either some clumsy move on one side or the other will cause war to be declared without its being a real war: in that case the Soviet troops will come as far as Brest and we get three to five years before we're up against it; or else everyone will wait and arm themselves while they do so: which will result in the mythological spirit of war pervading the whole world, in censorship, espionitis, Manichaeism and, if you like to put it that way, camouflaged occupation by the Americans. If it comes to choice, I believe in the second hypothesis. . . ."

I did leave, but with a heart so full of anxiety that it made the sadness of my arrival in America even harder to bear. My first days in Chicago were very much like those Anne spent with Lewis in *The Mandarins* when they meet for the last time. For a whole year Algren had been writing me gay and tender letters; now suddenly he was telling me that he didn't love me any more. "We'll have a nice summer together, all the same," he assured me with deliberate thoughtlessness. And the next day he took me to the races with a lot of people I didn't know. I wandered through the crowd of strangers gulping down one drink after another. I had no intention of going back to France, unless there were suddenly some immediate danger. First of all I had to understand with my heart and my body words that I had not yet succeeded in even getting through my head; what a dreary task ahead! It was already enough of an effort to stitch all the little bits of time together. In the little house on Wabansia Avenue, the combination of the stifling heat and Algren's presence suffocated me. I went out: the streets were hostile. At a little hairdresser's in the Polish neighborhood, the girl who washed my hair asked me in a severe tone: "Why are you all Communists in France?" A French-woman equaled someone suspect, ungrateful, almost an enemy. And then, outside, I felt I was melting like the tar on the roads; in American bars one can neither read nor weep. I literally didn't know what to do with myself.

Finally a friend drove us to Miller and gradually time began to resume its flow once more; my days had a routine, and that did me good. I slept in a room of my own, I worked there, beside the window protected by a wire screen; or else, having sprayed myself with "insect repellent" to keep the mosquitoes away, I lay down in the grass with Sandburg's *Lincoln;* I read a lot of books on American literature and history; and Fitzgerald's heartrending *The Crack-up;* and also science-fiction stories, often disappointing but sometimes casting disquieting lights on the world today. The garden sloped down to a lagoon, and tall hedges on either side protected me from prying eyes; big, gray squirrels ran and jumped around me, and birds sang. Toward noon, we would cross the lagoon in a boat and scramble up and down over the dunes which burned our feet; then we'd get to Lake Michigan, wide and full of movement as the sea. There would be no one else on the sandy, endless beach, only white birds perched high on tall legs and pecking at the sand. I bathed and sunned myself. In the water I took great care not to lose my footing because I could barely swim. But one day, after a few tentative breast strokes, I put my foot down to find the bottom and couldn't; I panicked and sank; I called to Algren, who just smiled at me from a long way off; I called out more explicitly: "Help!" He still smiled, but all the same my gurglings did worry him in the end; when he did get hold of me, my head was already under the water and my face was wearing, or so he told me, a completely idiotic grin; he added that he had been very frightened, because he was a very poor swimmer too. We returned home on the double, drank a few shots of whisky and, in the euphoria produced by this dramatic rescue, friendship flamed into life between us as vividly as if it had been scoured completely free from the scar tissue of our lost love.

It had its pleasant moments; at night we would walk along the beach; in the distance the tall furnaces of Gary spat out their flames; a great reddish moon hung reflected in the lake, and we talked idly about the beginning of the world or about its end; or else we would watch television: news reels of famous boxing matches that Algren would explain to me, old films and on Saturday nights an excellent variety show. But quite often, without apparent reason—perhaps because he feared that one of us might be deceived by this apparent harmony—Algren's face would close up; he would move away and fall silent. One day, we had been to the races again with a friend, I had been bored; on the way back the radio in the car announced noisily that war was imminent. To have cut myself off from France in order to live through this private disaster suddenly seemed odious and absurd; so much so that I began to sob. "It's just propaganda, it doesn't mean anything," said Algren, who didn't believe in the war. But I had fallen to the bottom of an abyss from which it took me several hours to escape. Another evening Algren went to Chicago: I loved and feared the implacable silence of those days spent on my own; since morning I had mulled over many desolate thoughts before I finally sat down in front of the television screen. They were showing *Brief Encounter*, and I soaked the cushions with my tears.

After a month, Lise came to Miller. I had seen her again in 1947; as in the old days, we had fought a lot but also got on very well together. We fell into each other's arms. She had kept all her beauty and baroque sharpness; in the conventional world in which she lived, her behavior, which she had refused to correct, got her into all sorts of scrapes that she recounted very amusingly; however, our meeting was darkened by several shadows. Algren had balked at the idea of having a strange woman in his house, and in any case it was too small; he had found Lise a room about five hundred yards away, and that irritated her. She decided to stay for two weeks; I was going back to France in a month, and because of the very difficulty in my relations with Algren I felt the need to be alone with him. Against Lise's frankness I had always had only one weapon—an equal frankness on my part; I used it, and she called me once again "a clock in a refrigerator." Despite her coaxing and exuberant manner, Algren found Lise cold; he said she always looked as though she expected him to walk upside down or something; and indeed Lise's natural attitude was one of ironic defiance; to win her over one had to distinguish oneself by some feat or other. Algren even went so far as to tell me one morning that he was leaving for Chicago. We decided finally that it should be Lise and myself who would go there for two or three days.

Her feelings for me were ambivalent; in her opinion I had devoted less time to her during the war years than I ought to have done; she still had a grudge against me for having sacrificed her to my work, and this slight feeling of bitterness was directed against my work; she kept saying, indirectly but with transparent intention: "It's such a sad thing to be a second-class writer!" This sullenness also reflected her own relation to writing; she wanted to write and she didn't want to write: "What's the use when we're about to get a bomb on top of us?" The truth was that she was torn between the fact that she had a gift and the fact that she had no vocation; her talent showed itself in the short stories she had had published in magazines, and above all in her letters; she had the gift of concision and also that of choosing the wrong word with the happiest results; but alone in front of a sheaf of blank paper, her heart would sink; I think she wasn't interested enough in other people to have the patience to keep on talking to them page after page.

Her life wasn't going too well. She had come to the States because she was in love with a man and so she could eat; love had grown threadbare, and she was about to be divorced; she had got used to eating. There had been a time when she had hoped that motherhood would compensate for the misfortune of her early years, but that very misfortune had made her ill-suited to the care of a little girl with whom she identified herself both too much and too little. She was grateful to America for having taken her in, but she missed the sort of human and intellectual relationships she had been accustomed to in Paris. She was taking a teachers' training course; she was brilliant at her work, but many of her professors were put off by her aggressiveness. She was both disdainful and easily fascinated, and being cut off from people by the frostiness in her character that Algren had noticed, she would fling herself into the most complicated or impossible adventures. At that time she was obsessed by a pair of male homosexuals and very attached to Willy, the elder one; she was trying to convince him, in the name of Existentialism, that one cannot *be* homosexual: it was rather a question of a choice still reversible at any time. He was very fond of her, but that did not satisfy her. I recall a painful walk we took together through Chicago. I showed her Algren's house, my heart full of heavy memories, while she reiterated with all the scholastic passion of a medieval theologian her proof that Willy could demonstrate his liberty by loving her; one in silence, one aloud, we soliloquized through the heavy city heat, the streets stretching endlessly beneath our feet and neither of us advancing one step.

She left Miller ahead of me to go to Chicago, where Willy and his friend Bernard, who were traveling by car, had arranged to meet her. The morning I was supposed to go to join them the bus that was to take me to the station in Gary didn't arrive. Algren stopped a car on the road and put me in charge of the driver. As soon as he found out I was French, he began attacking me: "Is it true that you're all Communists? Is it true that in France white women sleep with Negroes?" I pretended I didn't understand English. I rather liked Willy and Bernard but I found it difficult to accept the trio they made with Lise. They wanted to go to sleazy strip joints, and once there they would comment on all the details of the girls' nakedness with snickers that somehow betrayed a resentment against the whole of humanity.

I returned to Miller alone. Algren, who had seen his ex-wife a few months before in Hollywood, told me that he was thinking of remarrying her. So be it, I thought. By that time my despair had drained me of all feelings and I could no longer react to anything. It was Indian summer by then; I walked around the lagoon, blinded by the beauty of the foliage, red-gold, green-gold, yellow-gold, copper and flame, my heart numbed, believing neither in what was past nor in whatever lay ahead. At brief moments I would come to and throw myself down on the grass. "It's all over, oh why?" It was a childish distress, because, like a child, I was battering myself against the inexplicable.

We returned, briefly, to Chicago. To keep ourselves in countenance we spent the last afternoon at the races; Algren lost all his cash. So that we could eat dinner he telephoned a friend who came over and stayed with us until the moment we got into the cab taking us to the airport. Algren didn't seem to mind. Chicago glittered behind fine gray gauze, to me it had never seemed so beautiful. I walked like a somnambulist between the two men and thought: "I'll never see it again. Never. . . ." In the plane, I stuffed myself with sleeping tablets once more and sat there sleepless, my throat torn with the pain of the cry that I was holding back.

Sartre was still reaping a rich harvest of insults. A certain Robichon, in *Liberté de l'Esprit* announced that his pernicious influence must be forcibly prevented from making further inroads on our youth, which in any case—he told his readers in the same breath—paid no attention to Sartre whatever. "Should we burn Sartre?" was the heading of an ironic rejoinder in *Combat,* where we still had a few friends. Sartre had printed several long extracts from his work on Genet in *Les Temps Modernes;* they had aroused interest. But what a fuss at the same time! Although a year earlier, apropos of *Deathwatch,* Mauriac had recognized Genet's talent, he now wrote an article in *Figaro* frothing with indignation at what he called "Excrementialism." Also some of our friends were expressing astonishment that the magazine had so far not devoted a single article to the Korean War. *L'Observateur* deplored the fact that *Les Temps Modernes* was not coming to grips with the events of our time. Merleau-Ponty, who to all intents and purposes ran the magazine, had been converted to an apolitical attitude by the Korean War itself: "The cannons speak and silence now is all our part" was more or less the substance of his explanation to us.

Sartre's second hypothesis was now proving to be true: the Americans were secretly occupying France. They were helping de Lattre to stabilize the situation in Indochina after his serious setbacks there. In exchange, Pleven publicly endorsed the principle of rearming Germany and consented to the establishment of American bases in France; when Eisenhower came over to establish his headquarters in Paris during January, the Communists demonstrated in vain. France was accepting the idea of a Europe supported by the Americans and pledged to fight for them. When Beuve-Méry once again defended the idea of neutralism, he merely got called "emasculated" for his pains by Brisson. "Is it simply a matter of having balls or not, then?" Beuve-Méry asked. Their argument got a great deal of publicity, but to no good purpose. When it was discovered that Gilson had accepted a chair at the University of Toronto he was accused of abandoning his country to the Red invasion, and there was indignation at this "preventive departure."[1]

In fact there was a good deal of talk about a Russian occupation. After the crossing of the 36th parallel by the American troops, after the "volunteer" Chinese Army entered North Korea and the American Air Force pounded Pyongyang, the United States announced that mobilization was imminent. MacArthur wanted to bomb China; in that case the Russians would intervene; in America 50 million radiation-resistant identity discs were distributed for the purpose of identifying victims after an atomic attack. Truman declared a state of emergency. If war were to break out, the Red Army would invade Europe as far as Brest in next to no time; what then? "The day the Russians march into Paris," said Francine Camus—as we were coming out of a communist-organized concert, during which we had heard some Bartók Dances based on folk tunes—"I shall kill myself and my two children." In one lycée class, some teen-agers, terrified by their parents' prophecies, made a collective suicide pact that would be effective in the event of a Russian occupation.

It didn't occur to me to wonder what I should do until the conversation we had with Camus at the Balzar: "Have you thought about what will happen to you when the Russians get here?" he asked Sartre; and then added with a great deal of emotion: "You mustn't stay!" "And do you expect to leave?" asked Sartre. "Oh, I'll do what I did during the German occupation." It was Loustaunau-Lacau, always one for secret societies, who started the idea of "armed and clandestine resistance"; but we no longer argued freely with Camus. He was too quickly carried away by anger, or at least by vehemence. Sartre's only objection was that he would never accept having to fight against the proletariat. "You mustn't let the proletariat become a mystique," Camus answered sharply; and he complained of the French workers' indifference to the Soviet labor camps. "They've got trouble enough without worrying about what's going on in Siberia," was Sartre's reply. "All right," said Camus, "but all the same, they haven't exactly earned the Legion of Honor!" Strange words: Camus, like Sartre, had refused the Legion of Honor which their friends in power had wanted to give them in 1945. We felt a great distance between us. Yet it was with real warmth that he urged Sartre: "You must leave. If you stay it won't

1 Gabriel Marcel wrote a play about it!

be only your life they'll take, but your honor as well. They'll cart
you off to a camp and you'll die. Then they'll say you're still alive,
and they'll use your name to preach resignation and submission and
treason; and people will believe them." I was shaken by these words
and in the days that followed I remembered Camus' arguments and
used them myself. Perhaps they would leave Sartre alone, on condition that he keep quiet; but things would happen—that we could no
longer doubt—about which he would not remain silent, and the way
Stalin dealt with intractable intellectuals was common knowledge.
During lunch one day at Lipp, I asked Merleau-Ponty what he
thought he would do; he had no intention of leaving. Suzou turned
to Sartre. "A lot of people will feel disappointed if you leave," she
said with a mixture of innocence and deliberate provocation. "Everyone's expecting you to commit suicide." Another day, Stéphane
begged Sartre: "In any case, Sartre, promise me you'll never give in
to them!" These heroic tableaux did not appeal to me at all, and I
returned to the attack. An alliance with the Fascists against the
French workers was out of the question; accepting everything equally
impossible; and open opposition would be the equivalent of suicide.
Sartre listened to me with a mulish look on his face; he rejected the
idea of exile to the very marrow of his bones. Algren, now convinced
that some headstrong action on the part of MacArthur might unleash
a world war at any moment, invited us both to Miller. But we had
never detested America more violently than we did at that moment.
In August, Sartre had been disturbed—less so than Merleau-Ponty,
but a little all the same—by the fact that the North Koreans had been
the first to cross the border and that the Communist press had denied
it. We now knew that they had walked into a trap; MacArthur had
wanted this conflict, hoping to profit by it in order to hand China
back to the Chinese lobby; and we also knew that the feudal leaders
of South Korea had their eyes on the industrial power of the North.
Manhunts, wholesale bombings, mopping-up operations—the American troops were waging a war as ferociously racist as that being
carried on by our own troops in Indochina. If we were to leave, it
would have to be for a neutral country. "Just imagine what it
would be like," Sartre said, "ending up in Brazil like Stefan Zweig!"
He was convinced that by going into exile, no matter how good the
reasons for doing so, one lost one's place in the world, and that one
could never quite recover it again. And we were considering flight
from a regime which was, in spite of everything, the embodiment of

socialism! We were finding ourselves in the same boat as the people on the Right; and they weren't just wasting words on the subject, they were using their wealth and their connections to make sure the necessary boats and planes would be ready for them. We had lunch with Clouzot and his wife Vera; she was dressed with studied casualness: black pants and top, a golden chain around her ankle, her magnificent hair cascading over her shoulders. André Gillois and his wife were there too; during the meal the conversation turned to the practical possibilities of leaving the country. Sartre could not accept being grouped with that camp. "Between American ignominy and Communist fanaticism, we really don't know whether there's room left for us on earth any more," I wrote my sister. Sartre was unable either to elude or to accept the now manifest fact that the Communists, by treating him as an enemy, were forcing him to act as though he actually was one. He never put much faith in the likelihood of a Russian occupation;[1] but envisaging it was enough to make him feel very sharply the paradoxical quality of our situation; the shock it inflicted on him played a great role in his subsequent development.

[1] *"These preparations did not cause me much alarm because I didn't believe in the invasion: to me they seemed no more than party games in which things were pushed as far as they would go and thus revealed to everyone the necessity of choosing and the consequent results of the choice so made. . . . Surrounded by these gloomy hallucinations, I felt cornered."—Merleau-Ponty Vivant.*

CHAPTER V

MY WAY OF LIFE HAD CHANGED. I
stayed at home a lot. The phrase itself had taken on a new meaning
for me. For a long time I had had no possessions, neither furniture,
nor wardrobe. Now in my closet there hung jackets and skirts from
Guatemala, blouses from Mexico, a suit and more than one topcoat
from the United States. My room was decorated with objects that
were without value but precious to me: ostrich eggs from the Sahara,
lead tom-toms, some drums that Sartre had brought back from Haiti,
glass swords and Venetian mirrors that he had bought in the Rue
Bonaparte, a plaster cast of his hands, Giacometti's lamps. I liked to
work facing the window: the blue sky framed in the red curtains
looked like one of Bérard's sets. I spent many evenings there with
Sartre; I kept a stock of fruit juice for him, since he'd given up
alcohol for the time being. And we listened to music. Since 1945, I
had listened to Schönberg's *Ode to Napoleon* conducted by Leibo-
witz, and several other concerts, but really only very few and quite
haphazardly. That winter Sartre and I heard *The Messiah,* and at his
home we listened with his mother to a broadcast of Berg's *Wozzeck.* I
wanted a phonograph; I asked Vian's advice about what machine to
buy and Sartre helped me assemble a little record library. He was
interested in Schönberg, Berg and Webern; he had explained the
principles of their music to me, but in France no recordings of their
works were to be had. I bought some classics, some early music,
Vivaldi's *Four Seasons* which all Paris was suddenly crazy about, a lot
of Franck, Debussy, Ravel, Stravinsky and Bartók. The latter we had
both discovered separately in America, where he was enjoying a great
wave of popularity and at that time—especially his last quartets and

the sonata for solo violin—he was the composer who moved us both the most. Also, on Vian's advice, I bought a lot of jazz: Charlie Parker, Ellington, Gillespie. Changing the record every five minutes, and the needle quite often too, what patience it took! And canned music at that time was a long way from being as fresh as the real thing. But it was pleasant to be able to organize my own concerts at home, with my own choice of program and whenever it suited me.

On Christmas Eve, which brought Olga, Wanda, Bost, Michelle, Scipion and Sartre all together in my room, there was another attraction: a tape recorder that M. had left with Sartre. I recorded several conversations without telling anyone. Words are by nature birds of passage; everyone is dismayed to hear over again, fixed, defined and promoted as it were to the undeserved dignity of a poem, the disparate phrases he or she has unthinkingly thrown out. Scipion had delivered himself of certain impassioned expressions when discussing the charms of Colette Darfeuil (whom he did not know) which it gave him no little stupefaction to hear himself repeat.

I went to the movies now and then. I liked the starkness of Bresson's *Diary of a Country Priest*, and also, despite the abuse of certain surrealist reminiscences, the cruelty of Buñuel's *Los Olvidados*. And *Casque d'Or* at last did justice to the beauty of Simone Signoret and revealed her talent to the world.

A new restaurant had recently opened where the old Procope used to be and had taken over the name—marble tables and leather banquettes; I liked it there. Upstairs there was a club where society people dined by candlelight. Below, one came across old inhabitants of the district, among others Louis Vallon, soused. He mumbled insults at me across the room; but then when he was finished he staggered over to talk to me, his eyes streaming with tears, about Colette Audry, whom he had loved before the war in the days when he was a Socialist. It was also at the Procope that I used to meet Antonina Vallentin for lunch every now and again, at least on those occasions when I didn't go over to her place during the afternoon. Badly dressed, in grotesque hats or draped in awful robes, I was amazed to see a photograph of her when she was young and beautiful; but her talent as a biographer was apparent in her conversation: she could talk extremely well about people. A friend of Stresemann's, she had known many politicians well and Einstein, about whom she was writing a book, intimately. She was also the author of works on Goya and Da Vinci which had both been great successes. She was on the staff of *Les Temps Modernes,* primarily as its art critic. We continued to see each other until August 1957, when she died of a heart attack.

Ever since he had taken over *Les Temps Modernes* from Gallimard, Julliard would occasionally invite us to lunch. His wife, the elegant Gisèle d'Assailly, enjoyed bringing together a group of well-known people who didn't always have much to say to each other; in this way we met Poulenc, Brianchon, Lucie and Edgar Faure, Maurice Chevalier and Jean Massin, a bearded priest who was still a believer but had left the Church; he used to say Mass in his bedroom; he explained his reasons for this and his problems. From time to time, Merleau-Ponty would stop him and say: "You should write this down for *Les Temps Modernes.*" And each time he would reply gently: "I couldn't care less about *Les Temps Modernes.*" Later he did cease to be a believer, married and collaborated with his wife in writing books of Marxist inspiration, some of which—on Mozart, Beethoven, Robespierre, Marat—are excellent.

Simone Berriau took me up to see Colette, whom she knew very well. When I was a young girl Colette had fascinated me. Like everyone else, I took great pleasure in her style and liked three or four of her books very much. "It's a pity she doesn't like animals," Cocteau had said to us one day; it is true that when she wrote about dogs or cats she was only writing about herself, and I preferred it when she did so openly; love, the wings of the music hall, Provence, these subjects suited her better than animals. Her self-satisfaction, her contempt for other women, her respect for a fixed set of values, none of these appealed to me. But she had lived, she had worked, and something in her face attracted me. I had been warned that she was not generally pleasant to women of my age, and she received me coldly. "Do you like animals?" "No," I replied. She stared me up and down with an Olympian gaze. I didn't mind; I hadn't expected any contact between us. It was enough for me to look at her. Crippled, her hair in a wild fuzz, startlingly made up, age gave her sharp face and her blue eyes the brilliance of lightning; surrounded by her collection of paperweights, silhouetted against the gardens framed by her windows, she appeared to me, paralyzed and regal, like some awful Mother Goddess. When we had dinner with her and Cocteau at Simone Berriau's, Sartre too had the impression of approaching a *"monstre sacré."* She had made the effort to leave her apartment mainly out of curiosity, because she wanted to see him, and knowing that she was the attraction of the evening for him; she assumed this role with an imperial good humor. She told anecdotes about her life and the people she had known; the vigorous Burgundy tones of her voice did nothing to blunt the pointedness of her wit. Colette's words flowed unimpeded from their source and, compared to this example of one of nature's great talkers, Cocteau's brilliance seemed dim and labored.

We had dinner with Genet at Léonore Fini's; she had done a portrait of him; together they would go visiting millionaires whom they would urge, with more or less success, to become patrons of the arts. I found her drawings very interesting, her collection of cats less so; and even less still her stuffed mice that enacted a little scene beneath a glass dome.

A person I ran into quite often in Saint-Germain-des-Prés was the painter Wols. He had done illustrations for a text by Sartre, *Visages;* Paulhan would buy a drawing or a watercolor from him from time to time; we liked his work very much. Wols was a German who had been exiled in France for a very long time, he drank a liter of *marc* a day and looked quite old, despite the fact that he was only thirty-six and had blond hair and a rosy complexion; his eyes were always bloodshot and I don't think I saw him cold sober once. A few friends used to help him; Sartre got him a room at the Hôtel des Saints-Pères; the man who ran it complained that they would find him asleep in the halls during the night and that he would bring friends home at five in the morning. One day I was having a drink with him on the terrace of the Rhumerie Martiniquaise; he was shabby, unshaven and looked like a tramp. A very well-dressed gentleman, very severe-looking and evidently wealthy, came over and spoke one or two words to him. When he had gone Wols turned to me. "I am sorry; that fellow is my brother: a banker!" he said in the apologetic tones of a banker admitting that the bum he has just spoken to is his brother.

Barrault had once told Sartre the story of Cervantes' *Il Rufio Dichoso* in which a bandit decides to reform on a throw of the dice. At La Pouèze, Sartre began to write a play inspired by this episode, though not without altering it: in his version the hero cheated in order to lose. Influenced by his study of Genet and by the reading he had been doing on the French Revolution, he wanted first of all to present an exhaustive picture of society: the nobility was embodied in a certain Dosia who gave him a great deal of trouble and was done away with to make room for Catherine and Hilda. He had finished the first act by the time we got back to Paris. Simone Berriau asked him to read it to Jouvet, whom she wanted to direct it. First of all we had the usual admirable dinner; Brandel told us that often, during Barrault's plays, he went to sleep in his box, hidden behind a pillar. When we had finished eating, Sartre began to read and Brandel to snore; his wife kept pinching him to keep him awake; Mirande too kept dozing off; Jouvet's face was like a death mask. When Sartre had finished there was a leaden silence; Jouvet did not so much as open his lips; Mirande, searching his old memory for some word of praise fashionable in his youth, exclaimed heartily: "Some of your lines are like vitriol!" But the vitriol didn't seem to have affected anybody that night. They discussed casting. For Goetz, Brasseur could be the only choice. For Heinrich, Sartre had thought of Vitold, but he wasn't free; Vilar, whom we had thought sensational in Pirandello's *Henry IV*, was suggested and accepted. The two women's roles were entrusted to Casarès and Marie Olivier. But first the play had to be finished, and Sartre got down to writing the second act.

Olga was pretty well cured, she had appeared on the stage again several times with success; despite her doctor's advice, she wanted to take on the role of Electra again as soon as possible. Hermantier, who had put on *The Flies* at Nîmes, wanted to do it again at the Vieux-Colombier; it seemed as though things were working out very nicely. As it happened, they were not. Hermantier thought of himself as another Dullin, but he didn't know how to direct the actors, he had no feeling for the text and he chose appalling sets and costumes. Olga still hadn't regained complete control of her powers; her voice, her breath, let her down. Sartre, preoccupied with *Lucifer and the Lord*, went to the rehearsals far too infrequently. I was very worried on opening night, and with good reason: the audience found the performance execrable. The supper at Lipp afterward, with Olga and a few friends, lacked gaiety. After that Hermantier hacked up the text until he was left with no more than a skeleton that was swiftly buried. It would have been a matter of small importance, if that particular failure had not made Olga decide to give up the theater, when her only mistake had in fact been to return to it too quickly.

To finish the new play, Sartre needed peace and quiet. I wanted to go skiing again, and Bost went with us to Auron. Stretched out in a deck chair, eyes dazzled with whiteness, skin burned by the sun, I rediscovered the taste of a happiness recalled from many years before. The instructors were more tolerant than they had been in 1946 and allowed stems; I had a lot of fun. Sartre was busy disposing of Dosia and also, since it was a long time since he had skied, he would have been an easy target for unpleasant remarks, so he didn't even put his nose out of the door; everyone at the resort assumed he was mad. At Montroc we tumbled headlong together down the trails, nobody knew us, and what a holiday that was! When I went into his room at five o'clock, light-headed from the air and the mountain smell, he would be writing away, rolled up in a cocoon of smoke. It was with the greatest difficulty that he would tear himself away even for dinner in the vast dining room, where a solitary young lady sat reading *Caroline Chérie*.

We had asked Michelle Vian, who had a house in Saint-Tropez, to find us an apartment there; it overlooked a narrow street, it was icy cold, and the chimney wouldn't draw. We moved to the Aïoli; red tiles on the floors, old cretonne on the walls: the rooms, furnished by a homosexual antique dealer who owned the hotel, had great charm and grace. I bought some more skirts from Mme Vachon, still almost unknown then. We visited Ramatuelle again, and Gassin; I worked and read. But Sartre stayed buried in sixteenth-century Germany; I could scarcely drag him out into the streets and along the paths.

Pierre Brasseur, wanting to talk to Sartre about his part, came and stayed nearby for a few days; he no longer resembled the young man who had taken those slaps on the face with so much talent in *Port of Shadows;* bearded now, he had the body and bearing of a hardened campaigner, and Goetz's comic quality. His eyes, glittering with uneasy mischief, he would tell stories about the famous people he had met; his imitations of them were a delight. Out on Sennequier's terrace, in the garden of the Auberge des Maures where the bees buzzed around a *gratin dauphinois* spiced with fennel and thyme, while the sun gilded the carafes of vin rosé, he gave us several unforgettable recitals. I had often seen his wife, Lina, in the bar of the Pont-Royal in the days when she had been a pianist, sitting alone with her black hair streaming down over her shoulders; she had given up the piano and cut her hair, but she was still as beautiful as ever. They stayed at Mauvannes, and we went over and spent two days with them. Henri Jeanson was there too, with his wife, very friendly but not particularly gay company, I thought; also the director of *Tire au Flanc* whom people called Rivers *cadet,* and who wanted to film *Red Gloves*. He had the reputation of never shooting a scene twice. Since she was expecting *Lucifer and the Lord* to open in May, Simone Berriau was wild with anxiety: "What's the matter with him? Can't he write any more?" Her stage whisper implied that Sartre was suffering from some shameful disease; she imagined that writing was some sort of natural secretion; if the writer dried up, then his case was more or less the same as that of a cow which stops giving milk: something was wrong organically. But she had every right to be worried. When Sartre got back to Paris the play was put into rehearsal without a line of the last few scenes having been written.

Even without them, the play already lasted longer than any normal theatrical production. Simone Berriau, daily growing more frantic, begged Sartre to finish it with another twenty lines and then demanded enormous cuts; Sartre claimed that her fingers, as she wandered through the theater, automatically imitated the action of a pair of scissors. She asked everyone who knew Sartre well to try to persuade him; Cau was the only one who yielded; his intervention was very badly received. Brasseur was on her side because his role was already too big for him to memorize. So that every time Sartre wrote a word he did so with the knowledge that the first thought of the producer and the leading actor would be to make him cut it again. The tenth scene gave him a great deal of trouble, even though it had been the first, or almost the first, to come into his mind; however violent Heinrich's indictment of Goetz, the scene still seemed didactic; it suddenly came to life only when Goetz, before a speechless Heinrich, began to arraign himself. Sartre took the manuscript to the theater. "I'll have it typed straightaway," said Simone Berriau. Cau, who happened to be passing her room, saw her hand over the text to Henri Jeanson, whom she had been hiding there; she distrusted Sartre and her own judgment. Jeanson reassured her.

Jouvet took no part in these debates. For all practical purposes he was already dead; his heart was bad, he knew he was more or less doomed, and on Ash Wednesday he'd had himself photographed receiving the Ashes. He loathed Sartre's blasphemies. His right thumb riveted to his left pulse, his eye on his watch, he pretended to be timing the scenes but in fact let them run through without making a single observation. Once I had dinner with him and Sartre at Lapérouse. He came to life slightly. It is perfectly possible, he told us, to replace one out of every four of Racine's alexandrines by any rhythmic gibberish you like, or even by obscenities, and the audience will never tell the difference. This contempt for a text made us uneasy.

The actors restored our spirits. Brasseur's version of Goetz in the first act was dazzling; unfortunately he played the second part as though Goetz were a hypocrite, when in fact the character, in the folly of his pride, is detaching himself with utter sincerity from a lying virtue; I thought it a pity, too, that he refused to learn the soliloquy Sartre had written under the inspiration of St. John of the Cross. In the last scenes he regained his full powers. Vilar *was* Heinrich; we saw him stop a taxi once and stand aside to let his devil get in first. Casarès, Marie Olivier, Chauffard, almost all the actors were excellent. I found the sets Labisse had designed a bit too naturalistic. And Sartre couldn't persuade them to slash and muddy Schiaparelli's beautiful costumes.

We went on seeing quite a lot of people during the rehearsal period. We got together quite often with Brasseur and Lina. We had dinner with Lazareff, who was helping Simone Berriau finance the production; despite all the things that separated him from Sartre, we had a very pleasant meal together. Camus would often come to pick up Casarès and they would have a drink with Sartre; there was a brief revival of their friendship.

Finally the play was ready; but the cost in intrigues and arguments had been so high that by the time opening night arrived we had quarreled with both Simone Berriau and the Brasseurs; Jouvet had left for the country. I waited for the curtain to go up standing at the back of the house beside Lina dressed in a sumptuous evening coat; both our hearts were gripped in the same iron hand, but we didn't speak a single word to each other. I knew what those three opening cue thuds meant: the sudden apparition, instead of a familiar script, of a public work; it was what I longed for, yet I waited for the moment more anxiously than I had ever done before. I was soon reassured; there was a whistle from somewhere in the house, a few moments of restlessness, but the audience was rapt. I wandered through the corridors feeling more relaxed, I sat down now and then in Simone Berriau's box, though without speaking to her.

Neither the author nor his friends were invited to the supper that she was giving at Maxim's; in any case we wouldn't have gone. We had supper with Camus, Casarès, Wanda, Olga, and Bost in a night-

club run by a woman from the Antilles called Moune. It was a pretty
dismal meal; the old warmth between Camus and ourselves seemed
beyond recall. We had spent a much gayer evening—after a preview—
with a group of friends, Merleau-Ponty and Scipion among others, at
the Plantation, run by Mireille Trépel on the Boulevard Edgar-
Quinet; there were Negro musicians playing very good jazz.

For or against, the play's reception was an impassioned one. The
Christians were annoyed. Daniel Rops, who wanted to set the tone,
had persuaded Simone Berriau to let him see it from the back of one
of the boxes four days before the opening; his review in *L'Aurore*
tore it to shreds. Mauriac and some of the others claimed that to
attack God so violently Sartre must really believe in Him. They took
him to task for blasphemies which had in fact been taken from sixteenth-century texts. But the play also had its champions. On the
whole, the critics preferred the first act to the others,[1] and the play's
meaning escaped them. Kemp was the only one to point out its relation to the study of Genet; the same themes are to be found in
both—Good, Evil, holiness, alienation, the demonic—and Goetz, like
Genet, is a bastard, bastardy being a symbol of the vital contradiction
Sartre had experienced between his bourgeois birth and his intellectual choice. They all made the enormous error of supposing that
Goetz, by committing the murder at the end of the last scene, was re-
turning to Evil. In fact, Sartre was once more confronting the vanity
of morality with the efficacy of *praxis*. This confrontation goes much
further than it had in his previous plays; *Lucifer and the Lord* is the
mirror of Sartre's entire ideological evolution. The contrast between
Orestes' departure at the end of *The Flies* and Goetz's final stance
illustrates the distance Sartre had covered between his original an-
archistic attitude and his present commitment. He himself has made
the following note: *"The Sentence:* We have never been freer than
we were during the Occupation, *is in opposition to the character of
Heinrich, an objective traitor who becomes a subjective traitor, then
a madman. Between the two, seven years and the divorce of the
Resistance."*[2] In 1944, Sartre thought that any situation could be
transcended by subjective effort; in 1951, he knew that circumstances
can sometimes steal our transcendence from us; in that case, no individual salvation is possible, only a collective struggle. However, this

---

[1] Ten years later, when Messemer played the second part better than the first, the
critics reversed this judgment.
[2] Unpublished notes.

play differed from its predecessors in that the militant, Nasty, did not triumph over the adventurer; it is the latter who produces the synthesis Sartre had projected in his preface to Stéphane's book: he accepts the discipline of the Peasant War without denying his own subjectivity, within the enterprise he preserves the negative moment; he is the perfect embodiment of the man of action as Sartre conceived him.

"I made Goetz do what I was unable to do."[1] Goetz transcended a contradiction Sartre had been feeling very sharply since the failure of the R.D.R. and even more so since the war in Korea, without managing to surmount it: *"The contradiction was not one of ideas. It was in my own being. For my liberty implied also the liberty of all men. And all men were not free. I could not submit to the discipline of solidarity with all men without breaking beneath the strain. And I could not be free alone."*[2] This situation was particularly painful for Sartre in the realm closest to his heart: that of communication. *"To talk to the being it is not possible to convince (the Hindu dying of hunger) otherwise all communication is compromised. That is certainly the meaning of my development and of my contradiction."*[3] To have afforded an esthetic solution to his problem was not enough for him. He was seeking the means of doing what Goetz had done.

By June I had finished a first version of my novel; contrary to my usual habit, I had so far shown none of it to Sartre; I found it painful to wrench it out of myself, and I could not have endured any other eyes, even his, to see those pages that were still warm. He was to read it during our vacation. Meanwhile, circumstances and my own pleasure led me to write about Sade. Two or three years earlier, the publisher Pauvert had asked me to do a preface for *Justine.* I didn't know much about Sade. I had found *The Philosopher in the Boudoir* ridiculous, the style of *The Misfortunes of Virtue* boring, and *The 121 Days of Sodom* too abstract and schematic. *Justine*'s epic extravagance was a revelation. Sade posed the problem of the *other* in its extremest terms; in his excesses, man-as-transcendence and man-as-object achieve a dramatic confrontation. But I needed time to study the subject; I sent the proofs back to the publisher. In 1951, Que-

1 Unpublished notes.
2 Unpublished notes.
3 Unpublished notes.

neau suggested me as a contributor to a series of books in preparation called *Les Ecrivains Célèbres*. I chose Sade. Even for a short review I wanted to read everything, and I began an essay intended for *Les Temps Modernes*. In the Enfer[1] of the Bibliothèque Nationale I was duly issued a charming eighteenth-century edition illustrated with engravings in which personages in wigs and court dress abandoned themselves with an air of indifference to the most complicated maneuvers. Often Sade's narratives were as lifeless as the engravings; then suddenly a cry, a light would spring from the page and redeem everything.

For years I had been having my work typed by Lucienne Baudin, a very pleasant woman my own age; she had a little daughter, about ten years old. Despite several affairs with men, her tastes were more inclined toward liaisons with other women; she lived with a woman in her fifties; they brought the child up together. She used to tell me about her problems, her financial difficulties, her friendships, her love affairs, and the whole lesbian world, so much less well known than the world of the male homosexual. I didn't see her often, but I always got on well with her when I did. After a certain length of time she began to do her work very badly and unpunctually; she became nervous. "I think I've got something wrong with one of my breasts," she told me. I urged her to see a doctor. "I can't stop working." A year later, she told me: "I've got a cancer; it's already the size of a nut." She was sent to the Cancer Institute at Villejuif; I went to visit her, and when I walked in she burst into tears; she was sharing a room with three other patients; one of them, who had just had a breast removed, kept shrieking with pain between her morphine injections; one of the others had had her right breast removed a few years earlier, and now the left one was infected. Lucienne was reduced to a state of terror. It was too late to operate and they were treating her with radiation. The treatment was not successful. They sent her home and injected her with male hormones. When I went to see her again I could scarcely recognize her: her face was swollen, an incipient moustache darkened her upper lip and she spoke in a man's voice; the only thing that was still the same was the shining whiteness of her teeth. Every now and then she would put her hand to her bandaged breast and groan. I sensed how fragile and painful that bundle of decaying glands was, and felt like running away. She

---

[1] Collection of proscribed books, so-called from the original rubric *Enfermé*, restricted.—Tr.

cried. She had written to faith healers, had tried miracle drugs, and dreamed of getting to America to consult specialists. And she cried. They took her to the hospital. In the beds on either side, old women were dying of cancer. They went on with the hormone injections. Puffed up like a balloon, bearded, grotesquely hideous, she went on suffering, unresigned to death. When I came back from Saint-Tropez, her friend told me that she was dying; the next day she was dead, after fighting for twenty-four hours. "She looks like a woman of eighty," her friend told me. I hadn't the courage to go and see her corpse.

Lucienne's end made even sadder a year which, despite my work and the pleasure and excitement I got from Sartre's play, was a melancholy one for me. Everyone seemed gloomy. Though MacArthur had been replaced, the fighting went on in Korea all the same, and the French economy suffered in consequence. The Vichyists and ex-collaborators turned Pétain's funeral into what looked like a triumphant demonstration of their return to power, and the June elections, thanks to the system of party alliances, was a victory for bourgeois democracy. Sartre viewed both the year's events and his own situation grimly, and that saddened me too. Olga's failure hurt me as well. And it was hard to write off my relationship with Algren. He hadn't remarried, but that made no difference. It was futile to wonder what his feelings were; even if he found it painful to cut himself off from me, he would still do it if he thought it necessary. The affair was over. I was less devastated by this knowledge than I would have been two years earlier; it was impossible now to change my memories into dead leaves, they had become worth their weight in freshly minted gold. And also, during those two months at Miller, I had shifted from stupefied unbelief to resignation. It didn't hurt any more. But every once in a while a void would open up inside of me, it was as though my life were coming to a stop. I would look at Saint-Germain-des-Prés: there would be nothing behind it. Once my heart had beat in other places at the same time; now, I was where I was, there and nowhere else. What austerity!

We wrote each other only rarely, and even then had little to say. In a letter that reached me in Saint-Tropez, he suggested I spend October with him at Miller. He was offering, in all honesty, the friendship it is always so easy to maintain when a rupture has been made without bitterness and the two people concerned are living in the same city. I consulted Sartre. "Why not?" he said. I accepted.

At the end of June, Lise come over to Paris with Willy and

Bernard. Her friends were overjoyed to see her, and when she arrived she was radiant; the subsequent disappointment was bitter on both sides: she no longer understood us, and seemed far away. She reduced Scipion to a state of stupefaction by scolding him for not working out a budget for himself every month. The United States had become her country; she admired and accepted almost everything about it. On the 14th of July, I went with her and a whole band of others to all the street balls of the neighborhood; we stayed for quite a while at the *bal des timides* opposite the Closerie des Lilas. But when I said good-bye to her I knew she had no desire to come back, even just to visit us again. We wrote each other for several years after that; little by little, the animosity in her mixed feelings for me gained ground. I ended the correspondence; as things are, we send each other Christmas cards. She has remarried, has more children, and is doing well, apparently despite serious physical troubles and some disappointments.

In the middle of July, we took a plane to Oslo and I left my melancholy behind me. Sartre's Norwegian publisher put a car and a chauffeur at our disposal so that we could drive across the Telemark; pines, lakes, old wooden churches standing alone in the middle of fields; then Bergen, its abandoned warehouses, its ancient houses of multicolored wood surrounding the quiet harbor, the animation of the fish market. In the evening we embarked on a boat; at each stop, buses took us on a tour. Sartre had seen all these places long before, with his parents. In the wooden towns to the north, there were gardens where rockeries took the place of lawns and flower beds. During the day, I would sit on deck and read Boswell's *Journal* and his *Life of Dr. Johnson*. In the evening I stared for hours at the sun hanging motionless near the horizon, and at the furious activity of the sky above. A ball of fire amid shadows: that was how a little girl in Sartre's first short story had imagined the midnight sun. The reality had disappointed her: it simply stayed light at midnight. I wasn't disappointed; the unaccustomed brightness of the night kept me there on the deck until an hour which elsewhere would have been the dawn. We sailed around snow-covered cliffs plummeting down into the sea. From Kirkenes, a bus took us to the Russian border; through the bushes and barbed wire, we made out sentinels with red stars on their uniforms. I was moved at seeing with my own eyes that forbidden country which meant so much to us. We sailed back, dropping anchor in other ports. The Bergesbne, which is one of Norway's prides, took us back to Oslo; it is the only railroad in the world that goes over glaciers; it never goes above an altitude of 4,000 feet, yet we traveled for hours through perpetual snows.

Sartre, like myself, had once landed in a plane on Iceland, and we had promised ourselves that we would see it. We spent ten days of astonishment there. This young volcano, inhabited only since the tenth century, had no prehistory, not so much as a fossil; the streams smoked, the central heating used water from under the ground; the most difficult thing in the hotel rooms was to get cold water; in the middle of the fields stood cabins that were "steam baths." Almost no trees—what we would call brushwood they called a forest; but deserts of lava, mountains the color of rotten eggs, spitting out sulphurous vapors and riddled with "devil's cookpots" full of boiling mud; weather-worn rocks that in the distance looked like fantastic towns. These volcanoes were capped with snow fields and glaciers that broke off into the sea. There was no railroad and very few roads; not only was one jostled in the airplanes by peasants carrying cages of chickens, but even the sheep of the island effected their seasonal changes of pasture by air. The peasants looked much more like American cowboys than like the traditional European peasant: well-dressed, well-shod, they lived in houses provided with every modern comfort and traveled on horseback.

But though the landscapes had a strange planetary beauty, the towns, their wooden houses roofed with corrugated iron, were dismal. A tremendous wind roared ceaselessly along the streets that made up the gridiron of Reykjavik. While there, we stayed, like all foreigners, at the Hotel Borg. Little flags on the dining room tables indicated the nationalities of the guests. We were greeted in a friendly manner by the French contingent there, among whom was Paul-Émile Victor. Several times a week he flew out to parachute food, medicaments and tools to the settlements in Greenland. In the evening, he would say: "I've been to Greenland," as though he'd been just outside Paris visiting in Meudon for the day. He told us about the Eskimos, about his expeditions, his experiences as a parachutist. There were also two film makers—one of them I had met in Hollywood, and the other was an habitué of the Flore—who were there making a documentary. They took us by car to the lake of Thingvellir, which is very blue and full of little volcanoes and a lot of "atolls," made of lava clinkers that looked just like gigantic molehills. We also met the son of the explorer Scott, who was capturing wild animals, and an Icelandic geologist who was hunting pebbles; he took us for a ride in his jeep through a landscape of rocks more brightly colored than any flower bed. We went by plane to sinister Akureyri, and from there I took a hydroplane along the wonderful northern coast as far as the little harbor situated at the extreme north of the island. My only companions were two bearded boys. "We're hitchhiking around Iceland," they told me.

The Icelanders are hard drinkers; they were capable of making alcohol out of shoe polish. The principal task of the police was to pick the drunks out of the gutters at night. Every Saturday evening there was a dance at the Hotel Borg, and on that night it would be men in tuxedoes with muddy shirt fronts that the cops were loading into their Black Marias.

There was a reception at the French Embassy; it was one of the only places in the world at the time where Russian and American officials could be seen drinking together. I spoke, in English, to the wife of a Soviet diplomat, who was wearing a whole jardiniere of flowers on her blond hair. "I should love to see Paris," she told me. "And I should love to see Moscow." We left it at that.

After Iceland, we went to Edinburgh. Though less extraordinary than Iceland, Scotland as we went through it by boat, from lake to lake, from island to island, was beautiful. We saw the pale, flat island of Iona with its Celtic remains, and the cliffs of Fingal though not its cave, which was made inaccessible that day by enormous waves; as we went through the Hebrides I read Boswell's account of the journey he and Johnson made there. We crossed a vast region of heath and hills; on the maps the famous sites were marked with two crossed swords for a battle and just one sword for a massacre. We passed through the landscapes described by Sir Walter Scott, we visited Melrose Abbey. But Scottish austerity was too much for us. It was very difficult to find rooms, and impossible to work in them: no table and no desk lamp. "If you want to write, go into the writing room," they told Sartre. He would put his papers on his bed table or just use his knees. Their meal hours were no less strict; once when we were waiting for a boat at ten in the morning in driving rain, not one hotel would serve us so much as a cup of coffee or a piece of bread: it was too late for breakfast and too early for lunch. Our hearts sank at the grimness of the towns.

We stopped in London for two weeks. By chance we happened to

run into Mamaine Koestler in a restaurant; she was divorced, as graceful as ever and even more delicate-looking than she had been before.
She took us, with her friend Sonia, George Orwell's widow, to one of
the private clubs that are the sole refuge of "night people" in London: the Gargoyle, up on a sixth floor somewhere. We met a few
people there—among others, Freud's nephew Lucian, a painter—and
drank. In the morning, when we were about to get on the plane back
to Paris, I suddenly felt very queasy. "That one's going to be sick
before we start," I heard a steward murmur, to my great shame.

During our cruise in Norway, I showed Sartre the first version of
my novel. It was going to be my best book, he told me, but I still had
a lot of work ahead of me. Well-made plots always irritated me by
their artificiality; I wanted to imitate the disorder, the indecision,
the contingency of life; I had let my characters and the events in the
book sprawl in every direction; I left out all the "necessary scenes";
all the important things happened offstage. I should have adopted an
entirely different technique, Sartre told me, or else, having decided
that this one suited my subject, I should have pursued it with much
greater rigor; as it stood, the book was badly constructed and discouraged the reader. He convinced me that I should link the episodes
more tightly, that I should make it clearer what things were at stake
for the characters, and that I should introduce some suspense. I had
understood the difficulty of the book's dialogue without overcoming
it; the intellectuals occasionally talk about their ideas, debate and
ratiocinate: even if cut and more skillfully inserted, such conversations are likely to be boring; mine decidedly were. Another thing
worried Sartre; to believe completely in my characters, the reader
would have had to know their work; I couldn't write their books for
them; thus their objective reality escaped; their work, which was the
essential element in their lives, was only suggested indirectly, in the
margin. This last defect was inherent in the undertaking itself. But
for the rest, I decided to rework the whole thing. In such cases, the
gossip columnists tell how the writer "tore it all up and started
over." Nobody does that. One uses the work already done as a foun-
dation.

I spent October with Algren. Plane, train, taxi: I was quite calm
when I arrived at the house on Forest Avenue; I had nothing to gain
and nothing to lose. Once again there was the splendor of an Indian
summer. Once again I bathed in the lake, read in the sun, watched
television; I finished my essay on Sade. I scarcely set foot in Chicago.

One evening I drank martinis with Algren at the Tip-Top-Tap, some twenty stories above the lights of the city; then we saw Renoir's *The River*: an indecent lie that put Algren to sleep. Another time, Algren gave a lecture to a Jewish club; since anti-Semitism was very pronounced in Chicago, I imagined that those who suffered from it would be inclined to protest against the established order of things. But when Algren took up the defense of the drug addicts, attacking the society that forced its youth into such somber avenues of escape, I saw nothing but frowns in the audience. "He doesn't speak as well as he writes," they murmured. He also denounced police corruption.[1] A judge answered him with a panegyric on the virtues of the "boys in blue" which received wild applause.

Algren was going to remarry his ex-wife. As I walked along the beach during the last days of October, between the dunes dusted with gold and the changing blue of the water, I thought to myself that I would never see him again, nor the house, nor the lake, nor the sand being pecked at by the little white waders; and I didn't know which I would miss most: a man, a landscape, or myself. We both wanted to keep our good-byes to a minimum; Algren would put me on a train at Gary toward noon; I would go to the airport alone. The last morning, the hours seemed to drag for both of us; we refused to talk to each other and were embarrassed by our silence. At last I said that I had had a very nice time there and that at least we still had a real friendship for each other. "It's not friendship," he replied brutally. "I can never offer you less than love." These words, suddenly, after those four peaceful weeks, brought all the old uncertainty back: if our love still existed, why these final, these definitive good-byes? All the past flooded back into my heart, all my work was undone, life was unbearable; in the taxi, in the train, in the plane, in a cinema in New York that evening, watching a Walt Disney film in which animals endlessly devoured each other, I wept without stopping. In my room in the Lincoln Hotel, my eyes brimming with tears, I wrote Algren a short letter asking if everything was all over or not. I got back to Paris on All Saints' Day. Everywhere there were chrysanthemums and people wearing black. And I knew the answer to my question.

"One can still have the same feelings for someone," Algren wrote

---

[1] Ten years later, it was acknowledged officially; a great many members of the police force were indicted for burglary, blackmail, complicity, etc. It had taken all that time for the scandal to break out into the open, but things were already going on in 1951 just as they did in 1960, and many people knew it.

to me, "and still not allow them to rule and disturb one's life. To love a woman who does not belong to you, who puts other things and other people before you, without there ever being any question of your taking first place, is something that just isn't acceptable. I don't regret a single one of the moments we have had together. But now I want a different kind of life, with a woman and a house of my own. . . . The disappointment I felt three years ago, when I began to realize that your life belonged to Paris and to Sartre, is an old one now, and it's become blunted by time. What I've tried to do since is to take my life back from you. My life means a lot to me, I don't like its belonging to someone so far off, someone I see only a few weeks every year. . . ."

There remained only to write the words "the end." And so I did.

During the Occupation, when Sartre and I were toiling up hills on our bicycles, we used to dream of having a motorcycle. By 1951 it had become easy to realize an even more ambitious project I had been nursing since before the war: buying a car. On Genet's advice, I chose a new model Simca, an Aronde. I took lessons with an instructor in the Place Montparnasse with the predestined name of M. Voiturin. Bost, who had just got his own license, would take me out on Sunday mornings to practice just outside Paris. What agonies! Going through a village, luckily at less than three miles an hour, I hopped the sidewalk, giving both other people and myself a terrible scare. All the same, having never operated the smallest machine of any kind, it was a miracle that this one obeyed me even approximately. Once I had my license, our excursions, on which Olga was often included, grew longer; they would last a whole day or even two. I loved the roads through the forests when their reddish pelt was edged with white fur in winter; I loved the spring in Normandy, the tarns of the Sologne, the villages of Touraine; I discovered churches, abbeys, châteaux. I went to Auvers; I saw Van Gogh's café, the church, the plateau and in the cemetery the twin gravestones hidden under the ivy.

To celebrate the hundredth performance of *Lucifer and the Lord,* Simone Berriau summoned *"le Tout-Paris"* to the Carlton; neither the author nor his friends made an appearance. We went back to the Plantation, where there was a female-impersonation act at the time. Cau dashed over to the Champs-Élysées and came back to tell us how the official celebration was progressing. On Christmas Eve, I gave an all-night party at my place, as I had the year before.

The contributors to *Les Temps Modernes* were still meeting regularly at Sartre's every Sunday afternoon, to the sound of the hornpipe: men in the next building were always doing the dances of their native Brittany while musicians in costume stood in the doorway playing for them. There were a few newcomers—Péju, Claude Lanzmann, Chambure; we'd bought some folding chairs so that everyone would have somewhere to sit. Lanzmann and Péju worked as rewrite men for various newspapers, a job that allowed them to earn a comfortable living and still left them time to do other things. They both had a sound basic training in philosophy, though politics came first for both of them. They helped Sartre "repolitize" the magazine, and it was they more than anyone else who oriented it toward that "critical fellow traveling"[1] which Merleau-Ponty had abandoned. Lanzmann I liked very much. Many women found him attractive; so did I. He would say the most extreme things in a completely offhand tone, and the way his mind worked reminded me of Sartre. His mock-simple humor greatly enlivened these sessions. We drank framboise and debated hotly; we made suggestions, digressed, and swapped the pearls we had culled from *Aspects de la France* or *Rivarol*. In November Sartre asked for a volunteer to review Camus' *The Rebel*. He wouldn't let anyone say anything bad about it because of their friendship; unfortunately none of us could think of anything good. We wondered how we were going to get out of the dilemma.

These meetings account for most of the red-letter moments in a period which was one of the darkest of my life. Both in France and abroad, things were going from bad to worse. In France "the most backward collection of employers in the world" stubbornly buried its head in the sand of Malthusianism; production just managed to reach the same level as it had in 1929, the price inflation continued while wages had scarcely budged. The bourgeoisie remained indifferent to this state of decline and pursued its savage war against Communism. The big financiers and the government paid Jean-Paul David to intensify his propaganda against "the Fifth Column"; he had a radio program and inundated Paris with posters and tracts. The Left was divided and unable either to stop the war in Indochina

----

[1] *Merleau-Ponty Vivant.*

or make any dents in the current colonialist policy,[1] despite the trouble brewing throughout Black Africa; except for a few *graffiti—* U.S. go home—they had no way of fighting the ichneumon-like invasion Sartre had predicted a year before. In the States, MacArthur had gone so far as to attack General Marshall during June, and then Dean Acheson as well; investigations were instituted into the lives of American officials working for the United Nations. These persecutions were presented undisguised as the preliminaries of a preventive war Eisenhower himself announced in an interview he gave to *Paris-Match* in October: the armies of the West were to prepare for imminent battle in the suburbs of Leningrad. An issue of *Collier's* printed a report on the state of the world five years after the end of the atomic war in 1960. My imagination balked at envisaging such catastrophes; but I didn't believe we were going to have peace either. As in 1940, the future lost all perceptible shape, and I vegetated without living; the subjection of France was almost as painful to me as it had been then. One evening, at the end of a long day's outing in my car, I had dinner with Olga and Bost in a hotel in Chinon; the dining room was pleasant, we were drinking a good wine and we were gay; two American soldiers came in and I felt a sudden tightening around my heart that I recognized. Bost said out loud, "They give me exactly the same feeling as the Chleuhs." Seven years before we had loved them, these tall soldiers in khaki who had looked so peaceful; they were our liberty. Now they were defending a country which was supporting dictatorship and corruption from one end of the world to the other: Synghman Rhee, Chiang Kai-shek, Franco, Salazar, Batista. . . . What their uniforms meant to us now was our dependence and a mortal threat.

Time grows shorter as we grow old: seven years means yesterday. That beautiful summer when everything had begun again still remained the true reality of my life, so much so that I wanted to call the novel I was working on *The Survivors*. But truth and reality had been made into a mockery and though my disillusionment had begun in 1948, I had not yet reached its depths. My feelings of revolt only aggravated the discouragement I was now sharing with most of my fellow countrymen.

The young men of 1945 had certainly changed their tune. The French cinema was drooping; except for the Communist newspapers

---

[1] In December occurred the trial of the 460 Ivory Coast Negroes, arrested in the circumstances I have already described.

the left-wing press no longer existed; budding film makers and journalists, where were the fruits by which we were to know them? As for
literature, their doubts about the age they were living in, and consequently their doubts about themselves as well, were too deep for
them to devote themselves to it with any fervor. Vian, once the most
ambitious, had virtually given it up; he composed songs and sang
them, he wrote a column on jazz in a newspaper. They were interested enough in politics to argue in the bars of Saint-Germain-des-
Prés, but not interested enough to find a way of life or a reason for
living. It wasn't their fault. What could they do? What could anyone
do just then in France? Once, hope had united us; now we scarcely
saw them any more. We were still bound to our older friends by the
past but—except for Genet, Giacometti, Leiris—we were not entirely
in agreement with any of them about the present and the future.
Those who had filled our lives before the war had all—except Olga
and Bost—more or less vanished. Mme Lemaire lived in the country,
Herbaud abroad. Pagniez had turned against Sartre once again, and
they had more or less quarreled. Since Dullin's death, Camille had
become a recluse.

I had buried my memories of Chicago a second time, and they no
longer caused me pain—but what sadness to feel the pain subside!
"Well, that's that," I said to myself; and I no longer even thought
about my happiness with Algren. Less inclined than ever to what are
called adventures, my age and the circumstances of my life left little
room, it seemed to me, for a new love. My body, perhaps as the result
of a deeply ingrained pride, adapts easily; it made no demands. But
there was something in me that would not submit to such indifference. "I'll never sleep again warmed by another's body." Never:
what a knell! When the realization of these facts penetrated me, I felt
myself sinking into death. The void had always frightened me, but
till now I had been dying day by day without paying attention to it;
suddenly, at one blow, a whole piece of myself was being engulfed
before my eyes; it was like some brutal but inexplicable amputation,
for nothing had happened to me. In the glass my face still looked the
same; behind me a burning past was still not far away, but, in the
long years stretching ahead of me, it would not flame up again; it
would never flame again. I suddenly found myself on the other side
of a line, though there was no one moment when I had crossed it. I
stood there, bewildered by astonishment and regret.

The future was barred to me by History—both personal and pub-

lic—and even my work was of no help to me in finding my way into
it. I was by no means certain I could remedy the weaknesses that
Sartre had pointed out; and in any case it would be another year or
two before I finished the attempt. The horizon was so black that it
took almost as much courage to keep going as it had to continue with
She Came to Stay in 1941. This book meant a great deal to me. In
1943 and 1945, my successes had satisfied me; they did so much less
now. *She Came to Stay* was a long way away; *The Blood of Others*
had faded; *All Men Are Mortal* had never been a success. *The Second Sex* was still going strong, but in France it had earned me only a
very equivocal reputation. I wanted something more. Unfortunately,
this book was not going to make much of a stir, of that I was convinced. I wrote, I crossed out, I began again, I tormented myself, I
wore myself out, without hope. History was no longer on my side,
far from it. There was no place left for those who refused to become
part of either of the two blocs. Sartre agreed with me that the novel
would offend both Right and Left; if I managed to get three thousand readers I should be doing well! This failure, which seemed to
both of us a foregone conclusion, saddened us not only in itself but
also because it was a sign of our exile. All political action had become
impossible for us and even our writing was going to trickle away into
the sand.

As always, Sartre was a great help to me. Yet he seemed further
away from me than ever before. His successes had not changed him,
but he had created a situation which in cutting him off from the
world also broke some of our ties; he no longer even set foot in the
cafés we had so loved before; he had not followed me down the ski
trails at Auron; the unknown partner of our life together had become, by the pressure of circumstances, a public figure. I had the
feeling that he had been stolen from me. "Oh, why aren't you an
obscure poet!" I used to say to him. Overhauling his political position, he was pursuing at the same time an exhausting inner development and studies which devoured his days. I missed his old insouci-
ance and the golden age when we always had so much time: our
walks, our strolls through Paris, our evenings at the cinema we never
seemed to go to any more. He invited me to follow him along his
path. "You should read this!" he would tell me, pointing to the
books piled up on his desk; he would insist: "It's fascinating." I
couldn't; I had to finish my novel. And then, although I too wanted
to know more about the world I was living in, it wasn't a necessity

for me as it was for him. The year before, he had been forced into
the position of making a hypothetical choice, in the event of a Russian
occupation, between two solutions, one impracticable—to stay, without submitting—the other odious—to leave; this had led him to the
conclusion that it was impossible to be what he was, and it was impossible for him to go on living without finding a way of surmounting that situation; thus, the urgency he felt now was forcing him
back into the project which he had never abandoned: the construction of an ideology which, while enlightening man as to his situation,
would also offer him a practical approach to life. Such an ambition
was foreign to me; my objective importance was too slight for a
putative Russian occupation to pose any personal problem for me; I
could not expect, and at the same time I did not desire, to play even
the smallest political role. So that for me to read the same books as
Sartre, and to meditate upon the same themes, would have been a
gratuitious activity; what he had undertaken concerned him too intimately for anyone, even myself, to help him with it. I knew all this;
yet it seemed to me that his solitude was isolating me from him. "It's
not like it used to be," I said to myself; loyal to my past, these words
were enough to upset me. I put into my heroine's mouth in *The
Mandarins* the words I was saying then to myself: "It makes me unhappy not to feel happy." I also told myself: "There are people
more unhappy than I am," but it was a truth from which I drew
little consolation—on the contrary; the delicate sadness inside me
was like a resonator that captured the vibrations of a whole concert
of laments from the outside world; a universal despair crept into
my heart until I began to long for the world to end.

All these circumstances explain the panic to which I fell a victim
toward the beginning of spring. Until then, I had never been under
any threat from my body: in 1935 I had been unaware of the seriousness of my state. Now, for the first time, I believed myself to be in
danger.

"It's nothing," I told myself at first; then I wondered: "But is it
something?" I kept getting a stab of pain in my right breast, and in
one particular spot there was a swelling. "It's nothing," I told myself
more and more often; and more and more often I fingered the unaccustomed little swelling. I remembered the hairy face of Lucienne
Baudin, and her agony; for an instant, fear gripped me: "What if it's
cancer?" I thrust the thought aside; I was feeling well enough. Then
the stabs of pain returned and with them my anxiety. My body no

longer seemed invulnerable; from year to year it was deteriorating insidiously; why should it not have begun to decay quite suddenly? With a show of offhandedness I mentioned it to Sartre. "Then you must go and see a doctor, so he can put your mind at rest," he told me. I was given the name of a specialist. I went to see him on one of those April days when summer suddenly falls prematurely out of the sky; I had put on the fur coat I had been wearing the day before, and I was almost dying of the heat as I walked up one of the gloomy avenues that branch off the Place de l'Alma. The surgeon was reassuring at first: in view of my age, it would be wise to perform an exploratory operation and have a biopsy immediately; but I didn't look like a cancer patient and the suspicious swelling moved about when he rolled it between his fingers, which meant that it was benign. However, to lend the consultation a gravity worthy of the price he was charging, he left a certain amount of doubt hovering in my mind; he asked me if I would agree to the removal of the breast if it should turn out to be a malignant tumor. "Yes of course," I replied. And I left, shaken. This time I would get off with an amputation at most; but I recalled the old women in the room with Lucienne: ten years later the other breast becomes infected,[1] one dies in appalling agony. Sweltering in my fur coat, sweating, my mouth thick with anxiety, I looked up at the blue sky and thought: If I really did have cancer, it would happen just like this, there would be no portents . . . I repeated to Sartre, in a strangled voice, what the doctor had said. His way of consoling me shows what clouds were lowering on our horizon: if the worst came to the worst, I could count on twelve or so more years of life; twelve years from then the atomic bomb would have disposed of us all.

I was to be operated on the following Monday; on Sunday I went out in the car with Bost to see the beautiful Abbey of Larchant; I drove badly and kept stalling the motor the whole time. Bost grew impatient. Instead of learning, I was regressing; he couldn't see the connection between my nervousness and what he took to be a very minor operation. "You know," I said to him as we came back into Paris, "I may have cancer!" He looked at me with stupefaction. "Don't be silly! How could that happen to *you!*" I marveled at the way he kept intact my old optimism. I went into the clinic that evening. I had dinner, I read, I went to bed early. A sister shaved my armpit. "In case they have to take everything off," she said with a

[1] This isn't always true, far from it; but it is what I believed.

smile. They gave me an injection and I went to sleep. I was resigned to what was to come—not out of curiosity, as I had been when the threat of the sanatorium had been hanging over me, but out of a kind of bitter indifference. Next morning, after another injection, they wheeled me out on a trolley, covered with just a sheet. At the door of the operating theater they put little white boots on my feet, which intrigued me a great deal; then a needle went into a vein in my left arm. I said: "I can taste garlic" and then all sensations stopped. When I came to, I heard a voice: "There's absolutely nothing wrong with you," and I closed my eyes again; angels came and rocked me to sleep. I came out after two days, my breast covered with bandages, but full of wonder at finding myself still whole and delivered from my fear.

Now the gaiety of springtime won me. We drove to the South of France, Sartre, Bost, Michelle and I. Michelle had separated from Boris, and Sartre, who had always found her very attractive, had become intimately involved with her. I liked her very much, everyone always liked her because she never put herself first. Gay and rather mysterious, very discreet and yet very much there, she was a charming companion. We had a pleasant journey down, visiting the Abbey of Saint-Philibert at Tournus and the house of the Factor Cheval at Hauterive. Bost and I fought fiercely about who was to drive; we both loved driving for long distances. Bost didn't stay long at Saint-Tropez; I took him one evening to the station at Saint-Raphaël and on the way back I was suddenly moved at the thought that I was driving alone for the first time. I became bolder. I left the Hôtel de l'Aïoli at dawn, and as I drove through the town with all its shutters closed I felt once more the way I used to feel on those holidays long ago. I would hitchhike in those days. What a marvelous feeling, when a car stopped and carried me off down the road! To me it was miraculous to be taken in ten minutes a distance it would have taken me two hours to walk. Now, driver and passenger at the same time, I kept wanting to say thank you to myself. Walking had brought me a different kind of pleasure; but the new pleasure I got from my car made me almost forget the old one. I saw Provence once more as I had loved it twenty years ago, and yet I saw it in a different light as well: past and present made an alliance in my heart. I became so bold that I even drove out along the little byways of Les Maures with Merleau-Ponty and his wife, both new arrivals in Saint-Tropez. They displayed great courage; it's true that they had driven down from Paris with a couple without a license between them; on the dangerous bits of road, the husband and wife had come to blows over who was to drive. A great many of the people I knew were learning to drive; after the postwar shortage, it was beginning to be possible to obtain cars again.

I worked a little; Sartre was writing on Mallarmé; on Senne-quier's terrace, in the bar of La Ponche, he told me about what he was doing and explained some of the poems. He had meetings to attend and went back to Paris by train. I drove on alone to Avignon, proud of my powers, but with the fear that I might break down and not know what to do always in the back of my mind. At Avignon, I met Bost at the early morning train, and he helped me drive back to Paris as we had arranged.

I left again soon afterward; Sartre was spending three weeks in Italy with Michelle, so Olga, Bost and I took a motor tour there, exploring side roads and finding places it was difficult to get to without a car: Volterra for example. It was very pleasant to be able to go where we wanted when we wanted, just as the fancy took us. I got back to Paris in time to see the magnificent Mexican Exhibition.

Two things marked the beginning of that summer: Sartre quarreled with Camus and effected a reconciliation with the Communists.

I saw Camus, for the last time, with Sartre in a little café on the Place Saint-Sulpice in April. He made fun of a lot of the criticisms of his book; he just took it for granted that we liked it, and Sartre had great difficulty in knowing what to say to him. A little later, Sartre met him in the Pont-Royal and warned him that the review in *Les Temps Modernes* would be fairly cool, if not harsh. Camus seemed disagreeably surprised. In the end, Francis Jeanson had accepted the task of doing the piece on *The Rebel;* he had promised to do it circumspectly; as it turned out, he got carried away. Sartre persuaded him to soften some of his strictures, but there was no censorship on the magazine. Camus, affecting to ignore Jeanson's existence, sent Sartre an open letter in which he addressed him as "Monsieur le directeur." Sartre replied in the next issue. And everything was over between them.

As a matter of fact, if this friendship exploded so violently, it was because for a long time not much of it had remained. The political and ideological differences which already existed between Sartre and Camus in 1945, had intensified from year to year. Camus was an idealist, a moralist and an anti-Communist; at one moment forced to yield to History, he attempted as soon as possible to secede from it; sensitive to men's suffering, he imputed it to Nature; Sartre had labored since 1940 to repudiate idealism, to wrench himself away from his original individualism, to live in History; his position was close to Marxism, and he desired an alliance with the Communists. Camus was fighting for great principles, and that was how he came to be taken in by the hot air of Gary Davis; usually, he refused to participate in the particular and detailed political actions to which Sartre committed himself. While Sartre believed in the truth of socialism, Camus became a more and more resolute champion of bourgeois values; *The Rebel* was a statement of his solidarity with them. A neutralist position between the two blocs had become finally impossible; Sartre therefore drew nearer to the U.S.S.R.; Camus hated the Russians, and although he did not like the United States, he went over, practically speaking, to the American side. I told him about our experience at Chinon. "I really felt I was back in the Occupation," I told him. He looked at me with an astonishment that was both sincere and feigned. "Really?" He smiled. "Wait a little while. You'll see a real Occupation soon—a different sort altogether."

These differences of opinion were too radical for the friendship between the two men not to be shaken. Also, compromise was not easy for a man of Camus' character. I suppose he felt how vulnerable his position was in some way; he would not brook challenge, and as soon as he saw one coming he would fly into one of his abstract rages, which seemed to be his way of taking refuge. There had been a sort of reconciliation between him and Sartre at the time of *Lucifer and the Lord,* and we had published his article on Nietzsche in *Les Temps Modernes,* although we weren't at all satisfied with it. But this tentative attempt had not lasted. Camus was ready, at the slightest opportunity, to criticize Sartre for his permissiveness with regard to "authoritarian socialism." Sartre had long believed that Camus was wrong all along the line and that furthermore he had become, as he told him in his letter, "utterly insufferable." Personally, this break in their relations did not affect me. The Camus who had been dear to me had ceased to exist a long while before.

During that year, some Communists had asked Sartre to be a member of the Committee for the Liberation of Henri Martin, and to collaborate on a book making the facts of the matter public; he was happy that the first step toward a reconciliation had been made. Circumstances had convinced him that the only path still open to the Left was to find a way back to unity of action with the Communist Party. And the contradiction that was tearing him apart had by then become intolerable. *"I was a victim of and an accomplice in the class struggle: A victim because I was hated by an entire class. An accomplice because I felt both responsible and powerless . . . I discovered the class struggle in that slow dismemberment that tore us away from them (the workers) more and more each day . . . I believed in it, but I did not imagine that it was total . . . I discovered it against myself."*[1] Sartre told me one day: "I've always thought against myself." But he had never done so as savagely as he did in the years from 1950 to 1952. The work he had begun in 1945 with his article on the writer's commitment was finished; he had utterly demolished all his illusions about the possibility of personal salvation. He had reached the same point as Goetz: he was ready to accept a collective discipline without denying his own liberty. *"After ten years of rumination, I had reached breaking point: one light tap was all that was required."*[2] It was a book that struck him first: Guillemin's *Le Coup du 2 Decembre*. In his youth, in opposition to Politzer, for whom the bourgeois were defined exclusively by their situation as exploiters, he had supported the view that they could, in their relations with each other, display certain virtues; he had a respect for his stepfather, an engineer, severe both with others and with himself and a hard worker who lived a life of austerity. The Collaboration[3] had first aroused Sartre's suspicion that all bourgeois virtues are inevitably perverted by alienation. *Le Coup du 2 Decembre* showed him what men just as upright as his mother's husband were capable of thinking and writing. All capitalists must speak with the voice of Capital; yet the bourgeois are nonetheless individuals of flesh and blood who, to defend their interests, employ means whose violence is scarcely masked. It was Guillemin who tore away the veils hiding this process. From that moment, Sartre saw the class struggle in all its clarity—men against men; from that moment too, friendships and rejections became a matter of passion. He was overwhelmed with anger when he learned in Italy of the arrest of Duclos, on the evening of the demonstration against Ridgeway,[4] then during

1 Unpublished notes.
2 Unpublished notes.
3 Most of his stepfather's friends collaborated, though his stepfather himself was a Gaullist.
4 Ridgeway was coming to take over from Eisenhower as the head of SHAPE. Three days earlier, André Stil had been arrested for having referred to him in *Humanité* as the "General of the bacteriological war."

the strike that failed on June 4th, at the triumphant reaction of the
Right, the arrests, the appropriations, the lies, including the most
grotesque of them all, the story of the carrier pigeons. *"In the name
of the principles it had inculcated in me, in the name of its human-
ism and its 'humanities,' in the name of Liberty, Equality and Fra-
ternity, I swore a hatred for the bourgeoisie that would die only with
my own death. When I returned abruptly to Paris, I had to write or
choke."*[1] He wrote the first part of *Les Communistes et la Paix* with
a fury that frightened me. "In two weeks, he's spent five nights without sleep, and the other nights he only sleeps four or five hours," I
wrote my sister.

The article appeared in *Les Temps Modernes* a month before his
"Réponse à Camus." These two pieces of writing had the same
meaning: the postwar period was over. No more postponements, no
more conciliations were possible. We had been forced into making
clear-cut choices. Despite the difficulty of his position, Sartre still
knew he had been right to adopt it. His mistake up to that point had
been, he thought, to try to resolve the conflict without *transcending*
his situation. *"I had to take some step that would make me 'other.' I
had to accept the point of view of the U.S.S.R. in its totality and
count on myself alone to maintain my own. Finally, I was alone
because I did not wish to be alone enough."*[2]

This epoch we had just lived through was what I had tried to
evoke in *The Mandarins*. The book was to take me several more
months of work to finish. But everything about it had already been
decided. This is the moment for me to explain my intentions in
writing it.

From 1943 onward, my happiness had been carried along by the
stream of events; I felt myself so joyfully at one with the times I lived
in that I had nothing to say about them. *All Men Are Mortal* reflects
my new awareness of History, but diffused in a moral fable that took
me away from my own century; when I asked myself in 1946: "What
shall I write now?" I thought of writing about myself and not about
the world and time I lived in; I took that for granted. And then,
while I was working on *The Second Sex*, things around me changed.
The triumph of Good over Evil ceased to be a matter of tacit assumption; it even seemed gravely threatened. From our collective

[1] *Merleau-Ponty Vivant.*
[2] Unpublished notes.

halcyon, I had fallen, like so many others, to the dusty earth below: the ground was littered with smashed illusions. As in the past, failure, disturbing my private life, had brought forth *She Came to Stay,* so once again it made me step back from my recent experiences to see them better, and filled me with a desire to redeem that failure with words. It became possible and necessary for me to embody it in a book.

An experience is not a series of facts, and I had no intention of composing a chronicle.[1] I have already explained what is for me one of the essential purposes of literature: to make manifest the equivocal, separate, contradictory truths that no one moment represents in their totality, either inside or outside myself; in certain cases one can only succeed in grouping them all together by inscribing them within the unity of an imaginary object. Only a novel, it seemed to me, could reveal the multiple and intricately spun meanings of that changed world to which I awoke in August 1944; a changing world that had not come to rest since then.

It swept me into its flux, and with me all those things in which I had believed: happiness, literature. What good is happiness if it not only does not bring me truth, but even hides it from me? Why does one write if one no longer feels oneself charged with a mission? Not only was I not weaving my life, but its shape, the shape of the time I lived in, the shape of all I loved, depended on the future. If I thought that humanity was on the road to peace, justice and plenty, my life would be colored very differently than if I thought it was rushing toward war or wading through seas of pain. The practical side of politics—committees, meetings, manifestoes, discussions—bored me as they had always done; but I was interested in all the things that made our world. I had felt what was then called "the failure of the Resistance" as a personal defeat: the triumphant return of bourgeois domination. My private existence had been deeply affected by it. In stormy quarrels, or else in silence, the friendships that had glowed around me after the Occupation had all more or less died down; their death had become inseparable from the death of the hopes we shared, and that death was the center around which I organized my book. To talk about myself I had to talk about *us,* in the sense in which we used that word in 1944.

1 Today I am telling the story of my past in an historical mode, but I am doing so as a result of a project—on which I shall interrogate myself later on—entirely different from the one I formed in 1949, in the light of a disappointment which I had neither overcome nor even understood at the time, and which was still painful.

The danger of the enterprise was only too plain: we were intellectuals, a race apart with whom novelists are advised to have nothing to do; merely to describe a collection of peculiar animals whose adventures would have been interesting as a series of anecdotes but nothing more—that was a project that could never have held my interest; but, after all, we were human beings, just a little more concerned than most people with giving our lives an integument of words. If the desire to write a novel became imperative for me, it was because I felt situated at a point in space and time at which each of the sounds that I could draw from myself had a chance to awaken echoes in a great many other hearts.

To represent us, I wrought a great number of characters and singled out two of them as "subjects." Although the central plot was the breaking and subsequent mending of a friendship between two men, I assigned one of these privileged roles to a woman, since a great many of the things I wanted to say were directly linked to my condition as a woman. There were many reasons that persuaded me to put a masculine hero beside Anne. First of all, to convey the density of the world it is convenient to employ more than one point of view; then, I wanted the relationship between Henri and Dubreuilh to be lived internally by one of the pair; above all, if I entrusted to Anne the burden of expressing the totality of my experience my book would have been, contrary to my intention, the study of one particular individual. Depicting, as I was, a writer, I wanted the reader to envisage him as a fellow being and not as an exotic animal; but a woman with a literary vocation is even more of an exceptional being than a man with that vocation. (By exceptional being, I mean not a monster or a natural marvel, but a rare statistical entity.) I entrusted my pen, therefore, not to Anne but to Henri; to Anne I gave a profession that she pursues with discretion; the axis of her life is the lives of others—her husband, her daughter; this dependency, which relates her to the majority of women, interested me in itself and also afforded one great advantage: while being profoundly involved in the conflicts I was recounting yet remaining outside them, Anne envisaged them from an entirely different point of view than either Dubreuilh or Henri. I wanted to present images of my postwar period that would be at once decipherable and confused, clear but never fixed; Anne provided me with the negative of the objects that were shown through Henri's eyes in their positive aspect. My attitude with regard to literature was ambiguous. There was no longer any question of didacticism or salvation-seeking; in the face of the H-bomb and the hunger of millions, words seemed futile; and yet I worked at *The Mandarins* with a furious doggedness. Anne did not write, but it was necessary to her that Dubreuilh should continue to do so; Henri sometimes wanted to stop writing, sometimes not; by combining all their contradictions, I could throw light on these things from different angles. The same thing was true when I tackled the characters' actions and the scandals aroused by them; and similarly with the misfortunes of the others, their death, my death, the passage of time. Again I used the basic opposition on which I had built *All Men Are Mortal*, giving Anne the sense of death and its concomitant taste for the absolute—which suited her passivity—while Henri contented himself with existing. Thus the two accounts of life that alternate throughout the book are not symmetrical; rather, I attempted to establish between them a sort of counterpoint, each reinforcing, diversifying, destroying the other.

Describing Henri as he experienced himself, in his familiarity with himself, I also wanted to show a writer in his excess, his mania; famous, already aging, much more fanatically devoted than Henri to politics and literature, Dubreuilh occupies a key position in the book, since it is in their relation to him that his wife, Anne, and Henri define themselves. While approaching him fairly closely, thanks to Anne's intimate knowledge of him, I retained his opacity; the acuity of his experience and the strength of his mind place him above the other two; and yet, because his soliloquy always remains secret, I conveyed much less of it through him than through them.

I took particular pains with two portraits: Nadine and Paule. When I began, I intended to avenge myself on Nadine for certain traits that had offended me in Lise and some of my other younger women friends—a sexual coarseness that revealed rather nastily their underlying frigidity, an aggressiveness that was a poor compensation for their feeling of inferiority; demanding their independence without having the courage to pay the price of it, they converted the anxiety to which they were condemning themselves into bitterness. I had also observed, in other contexts, that the children of famous parents often have difficulty achieving maturity; the character I was drawing seemed to me suitable, by her very ingratitude, for the role of Dubreuilh's daughter. Little by little, the circumstances which explained her unpleasant qualities began to appear to me as full of valid excuses; Nadine began to seem to me more to be pitied as a victim than to be blamed; her egoism flaked off; she became, beneath her touchy uncouthness, generous and capable of attachment. Without deciding whether she would take the opportunity, at the end of the book I offered her a chance of happiness.

Of all my characters, the one that had most trouble taking shape was Paule, because I approached her by so many paths that did not intersect. In Anne's case, dependence was palliated by a direct and warmhearted interest in people and events; I conceived Paule as a woman radically alienated from herself by an exclusive attachment to one man, and tyrannizing him in the name of her slavery: a woman in love. Even more than at the time of *The Blood of Others*, in which I had given a sketch of one of these unfortunate creatures under the name of Denise, I now knew how dangerous it is for a woman to commit all of herself in a liaison with a writer or an artist dedicated to his work; giving up her own predilections, her own occupations, she exhausts herself in an attempt to imitate him without ever being able to reach him, and if he should turn from her, she finds herself stripped of everything. I had seen many examples of such a bankruptcy, and it was a subject about which I felt I had something to say. I was thinking, too, of certain women, beautiful and extravagantly brilliant in their youth, and then exhausting themselves later in their attempts to make time stand still; many such faces haunted my memory. And I still remembered the ravings of Louise Perron. It took me some time to compose from these specific intentions, these tattered images, these burning memories, a character and a story that I could fit into the book as a whole.

I have sometimes been criticized for not having chosen, to represent my sex, a woman who assumed an equal role with men in the realm of professional and political responsibilities; in this novel I was avoiding exceptions; I depicted women as, for the most part, I saw them, and as I still see them today: divided. Paule clings to traditional feminine values, they are not enough, she is torn to the point of madness; Nadine manages neither to accept her femininity nor to transcend it; Anne comes nearer than the others to true freedom, but all the same she does not succeed in finding fulfillment in her own undertakings. None of them can be considered, from a feminist point of view, as a "positive heroine." I agree, but unrepentantly.

I have said that at first I only wanted to establish the loosest of links between all these characters; "well-made" novels always bored me. This was one of the criticisms Sartre made on reading the first version; given the form I had chosen, the vagueness of the plot was a weakness and not a clever device; I tightened it up. But it did not worry me that one long and important episode should remain marginal: the love affair between Anne and Lewis. I wrote it because it gave me pleasure to transpose into a fictional world a real occurrence that meant so much to me; and also, imprisoned in her role as a witness, Anne would have lacked reality. I wanted to give her a life of her own; also, in the years just after 1945, it was one of the things I found most wonderful, the way space had suddenly been opened up to us; I expressed this feeling of liberation by involving my heroine in a transatlantic affair. The extent to which I have made my account of it convincing is a direct function of its adventitious character; for when she meets Lewis, Anne has already existed a long time for the reader, he knows the world she moves in, he has had time to become attached to her. I was able to make her a familiar figure even before anything exciting happened to her, because the novel had other centers of interest. That is what people didn't understand when they said they liked the love story itself, but that they would have pre-ferred it if, for the sake of unity, I had given it a separate treatment; by detaching it from the whole I should have emptied it of its content since, whether imaginary or real, what is called a character's richness is the interiorization of his or her environment. Lewis, it is true, does not benefit from any context; but he is seen through Anne's eyes; it suited my purpose that he should not exist until the moment he exists for her, and that one should be able to get inside his skin only insofar as Anne herself is able to do so; if one believes in her, one is inclined to believe in him. Of all my characters, Lewis is the one who approaches closest to a living model; external to the plot, he was exempt from its necessities, I was completely free to depict him as I wished; it so happened—a rare coincidence—that Algren, in his reality, was very representative of what I wanted to represent; but I did not content myself with a mere anecdotal fidelity: I used Algren to invent a character who would exist without reference to the world of real people.

For, contrary to what has been said, it is untrue that *The Mandarins* is a *roman à clé;* I loathe *romans à clé* as much as I loathe fictionalized biographies: it is impossible to sleep and dream if my senses remain awake; it is equally impossible to move into the world of fiction while still remaining anchored to the real world. If he tries to encompass both real and imaginary worlds at the same time, the reader becomes confused; and one would have to be a very cruel author indeed to inflict such a palimpsest on him. The extent and the manner of the fiction's dependence upon real life is of small importance; the fiction is built only by pulverizing all these sources and then allowing a new existence to be reborn from them.[1] The gossips who poke about among the ashes let the work that is offered them escape, and the shards they rout out are worth nothing; no fact has any truth unless it is placed in its true context.

Then Anne is not me? She was made from me, true, but I have explained for what reasons I made her into a woman in whom I do not recognize myself. I lent her tastes, feelings, reactions and memories that were mine; often I speak through her mouth. Yet she has neither my appetites, nor my insistences, nor, above all, has she the autonomy that has been bestowed on me by a profession which means so much to me. Her relations with a man almost twenty years older than herself are almost like those of a daughter and, despite the couple's deep understanding, leave her solitary; she has only tentatively committed herself to her profession. Because she does not have aims and projects of her own, she lives the "relative" life of a "secondary" being. It was mainly the negative aspects of my experience that I expressed through her: the fear of dying and the panic of nothingness, the vanity of earthly diversions, the shame of forgetting, the scandal of living. The joy of existence, the gaiety of activity, the pleasure of writing, all those I bestowed on Henri. He resembles me at least as much as Anne does, perhaps more.

For Henri, whatever people have said, is not Camus; not at all. He is young, he has dark hair, he runs a newspaper; the resemblance stops there. Certainly Camus, like Henri, was a writer, enjoyed being alive and concerned himself with politics; but they both shared these traits with a great many other people, with Sartre, with myself. Henri's language, his attitudes, his character, his relations with others, his vision of the world, the details of his private life, his ideas—all these things differ completely from those of his pseudo model; Camus' profound hostility to Communism would alone be sufficient—both in itself and in its implications—to set a deep gulf between them; my hero, in his relations with the Communist Party and in his attitude to Socialism, resembles Sartre and Merleau-Ponty,

---

[1] A successful historical novel satisfies this demand. Alexandre Dumas projects history into an imaginary dimension; his Richelieu is unequivocally an imaginary character.

and not Camus in the slightest; and in fact, most of the time they are my own emotions, my own thoughts that inhabit him.

The identification of Sartre with Dubreuilh is no less aberrant; the only similarities between them are their common curiosity, concern with the world and fanaticism in work; but Dubreuilh is twenty years older than Sartre, he is marked by his past and fearful of the future, between politics and literature it is politics to which he gives his preference: authoritarian, tenacious, closed, unemotional and unsociable, somber even in his moments of gaiety, he could scarcely be more different from Sartre. Nor do their stories intersect; while Dubreuilh's creation of the S.R.L. is almost an act of fanaticism, Sartre simply linked himself, without any show of frenzy, to certain groups that asked for his support; at no time did he ever give up writing; he published the "Soviet Work Code" without hesitation as soon as he became aware of its existence. The plot that I elaborated also differs deliberately from the facts. First by a transposition in time; I described as happening between 1945 and 1947 events, problems and crises that actually took place later. The R.D.R. came into being at the time of the struggle for neutralism; the scandal of the Russian camps did not break out until 1949, etc. The intimacy which exists between Henri and Dubreuilh is much more like that which in fact existed between Bost and ourselves than like the distant friendship that linked us to Camus. I have described the way in which the final quarrel between Camus and Sartre was simply the final moment of a long disagreement; the rupture between Henri and Dubreuilh is so entirely unlike theirs that I had written a first version of it in 1950, and it is followed by a reconciliation, which did not happen between Sartre and Camus. As soon as we had been liberated, their political attitudes were already beginning to diverge. Camus belonged neither to the *Temps Modernes* group nor to the R.D.R.; there was never any collusion between the R.D.R. and *Combat,* which *L'Espoir,* incidentally, resembles far less than it does *Franc-Tireur;* Camus left his newspaper for reasons that had nothing to do with Sartre. He no longer had anything to do with it at the time of the "soviet camps" affair, and he was never faced with the question of whether or not to make their existence public. The same things hold true of the secondary characters and events: all the material I drew from memory was refracted, diluted, hammered thin, blown up, mixed, transposed, twisted, sometimes completely reversed, and in every case re-created. I would have liked people to take this book for what it is; neither autobiography, nor reportage: an evocation.

Nor is *The Mandarins,* in my opinion, a novel with a message. Such thesis-novels always impose a certain truth that eclipses all others and calls a halt to the perpetual dance of conflicting points of view; whereas I described certain ways of living after the war, without offering any solution to the problems that were troubling my main characters. One of the principal themes that emerges from my story is that of *repetition* in the sense in which Kierkegaard uses that word: truly to possess something, one must have lost it and found it again. At the end of the novel, Henri and Dubreuilh once more take up the threads of their friendship, their literary work and their political activities; they return to the point they started from; but in between there was a time when all their hopes had died. From that moment on, instead of being content with a facile optimism, they take upon themselves all the difficulties, the failures, the scandal implied in any undertaking. Their old enthusiastic adherences are replaced by austere preferences. I described their apprenticeship; but I offered no proofs. The final decision of these two men does not have the value of a lesson; given what they are and the circumstances in which they find themselves, the reader can understand that they should make that choice; but he can also predict that in the future their hesitations may return. More radically, their point of view— that of action, of the finite, of life—is implicitly questioned by Anne, in whom I embodied the point of view of being, of the absolute, of death. Her past inclined her to this contestation and in the novel's present it is imposed on her by the horror into which the world is plunged. That is another important theme of the book, which it has in common with *The Blood of Others;* but when I wrote *The Blood of Others* I had just discovered that horror. I tried to protect myself against it, and I asserted, through my hero, the necessity of taking it upon oneself; that is how the book became didactic. By 1950, the horror had become a familiar dimension of the world. I no longer sought to elude it. Dubreuilh does attempt to transcend it, but Anne allows herself to remain immersed in it, and contemplates the idea of affirming its intolerable truth by her own suicide; between these two attitudes I made no choice. In the end, Anne does not kill herself; this is because I did not want to repeat the error I made in *She Came to Stay* of attributing to my heroine an act motivated by purely metaphysical reasons. Anne is not made of the stuff of suicides; but her return to an acceptance of the everyday world seems more like a defeat than a triumph. In a short story I wrote at the age of eighteen, the heroine, on the last page, came down the stairs leading from her room to the living room: she was going to mingle with the others, she was going to submit to their conventions and their lies, betraying the "real life" she had glimpsed in her solitude. It is no mere coincidence that Anne, leaving her room to go and join Dubreuilh, walks down a staircase: she too is betraying something. And then, tomorrow, for her as well as for Henri, is uncertain. The basic confrontation of being and nothingness that I sketched at the age of twenty in my private diary, pursued through all my books and never resolved, is even here given no certain reply. I showed some people, at grips with doubts and hopes, groping in the dark to find their way; I cannot think I proved anything.

In *The Mandarins*, I remained faithful to the technique of *She Came to Stay*, though using it more flexibly; underlying Anne's narrative is a monologue occurring in the present, which allowed me to break up the narrative, elide it and comment on it freely. I know the drawbacks of this form, even though I kept to it; but if I had eluded the conventions it imposed on me, I should only have been obliged to adopt others that satisfied me even less. Just after the publication of *The Mandarins*, Nathalie Sarraute wrote an article condemning this traditional approach. But in my eyes her critique is null and void because it is based on a metaphysic that does not hold water. According to her, reality "today" has been forced to take refuge in "scarcely perceptible impulses"; a novelist who is not fascinated by the "dark places of psychology" can be nothing more than a *trompe-l'oeil* artificer. This is because she confuses exteriority with appearances. But the exterior world does exist. It is not impossible to write good books based on an outmoded psychologism, but one certainly cannot deduce from it a valid esthetic system. Nathalie Sarraute allows that there exist, outside herself, "great sufferings, great and simple joys, powerful needs" and that one might think of "evoking the sufferings and struggles of men in a plausible enough manner"; but these are tasks below the dignity of a maker of literature; with amazing unconcern, she abandons them to the journalists. At that rate, one could divert one's readers with clinical studies, psychoanalytic memoranda, the verbatim ravings of schizophrenics and paranoiacs. So scrupulous when it is a question of anatomizing an ambition or a grudge, does she think that the life of a factory or an

H.L.M. can be accounted for by reports and statistics? Collective enterprises, public events, crowds, the relations of men to each other and to things, all these very real phenomena, that cannot be reduced to the terms of our subterranean palpitations, deserve and demand to be explored in terms of art. That dialogue is a problem for a novelist I quite agree; but I certainly don't think speech is "the extension of subterranean movements"; it has a great many uses; most often, it is an act, demanded by a situation, which explodes into daylight, breaking with the silence, and we denature it by encysting it within the continuity of an interior monologue. Means must be invented which will aid the novelist to unmask more efficiently the truth of the world, but not to turn him aside from it to imprison himself in a maniacal and untruthful subjectivism.

As for the style of *The Mandarins*, it either pleases or fails to please, but it has often been criticized in an academic manner, as though there existed a standard "good style" from which I diverged. I deliberately kept close to the spoken word. These memoirs are written differently. A certain rigor is suitable for a narrative dealing with a past already fixed. But in my novel I was attempting to evoke existence at the moment it springs into being, and I wanted my sentences to correspond to that movement.

INTERLUDE

WHY THIS PAUSE, SUDDENLY? I know perfectly well that an existence cannot be analyzed into clear-cut periods, and 1952 did not represent a milestone in mine. But the country and the map are different things. My narrative demands a kind of summing-up before I can continue it.

One defect of diaries and autobiographies is that usually "What goes without saying" goes without being said, and thus one misses the essential. I too am falling into this trap. In *The Mandarins*, I failed to make clear how important their work was to the characters in the book; I was hoping to do better for myself this time. I was deceiving myself. There is scarcely any way of describing work; you do it, and that's all. And so it is that in this book it takes up very little space, whereas in my life it takes up so much; my whole life is organized around it. I am insisting on this point because the public is more or less aware of the time and trouble it takes to write an essay; but, on the whole, they imagine that a novel or a book of memoirs can just be dashed off in no time at all. "There's not so much to that. I could've done as much myself," a lot of young women said after reading *The Memoirs of a Dutiful Daughter*; it is no coincidence that they did not in fact do as much. With one or two exceptions, all the writers I know work enormously hard; I am like them. And contrary to popular belief, novels and autobiographies absorb me much more than an essay; they also give me more pleasure. I think about them for a long time in advance. I thought about the characters in *The Mandarins* until I believed they really existed. For my memoirs, I familiarized myself with my past by rereading letters, old books, diaries, newspapers. When I feel ready, I write three or four hundred pages straight off. This is arduous work: it requires intense concentration, and the rubbish that I accumulate appalls me. At the end of a month or two, I am so sickened I can't go on. I begin again from scratch. Despite all the material I have at my disposal the paper is blank once more, and I hesitate before taking the plunge. Usually I begin badly, out of impatience; I want to say everything at once; my narrative is lumpy, chaotic and lifeless. Gradually I become resigned to taking my time. Then comes the moment when I find the distance, the tone and the rhythm I feel are right; then I really get under way. With the help of my rough draft, I sketch the broad outlines of a chapter. I begin again at page one, read it through and rewrite it sentence by sentence; then I correct each sentence so that it will fit into the page as a whole, then each page so that it has its place in the whole chapter; later on, each chapter, each page, each sentence, is revised in relation to the work as a whole. Painters, Baudelaire says, progress from first sketch to finished work by painting the complete picture at each stage; that is what I try to do. So that each of my books requires two to three years' work—four for *The Mandarins*—during which I spend six or seven hours a day at my writing table.

People often have a much more romantic idea of literature. But it imposes this discipline precisely because it is more than just a profession: it is a passion or, let us say, a madness. When I wake up, an appetite or an anxiety obliges me to pick up my pen straightaway; it is only in the dark periods when I doubt everything that I observe an abstract schedule; and in the dark times even the schedule may be of no avail. But, except when I am traveling or when extraordinary events are occurring, a day when I do not write tastes of ashes.

And of course inspiration comes into it: without it, mere diligence would be no use at all. The desire to express certain things in a certain way is born, reborn, enriched and transformed in capricious ways. I do not decide the resonances an incident, a sudden understanding, or a flash of memory awaken in me, nor what image or what word may spring into my mind. I keep to my plan, but I leave room for my moods; if I suddenly want to write a certain scene, treat a particular theme, I do so, without holding myself rigidly to a pre-established sequence. Once the main body of the book exists, I willingly trust myself to chance. I let my thoughts wander, I digress, not only sitting at my work, but all day long, all night even. It often happens that a sentence suddenly runs through my head before I go to bed, or when I am unable to sleep, and I get up again and note it

down. Many passages in *The Mandarins* and my memoirs were written in one fell swoop under the influence of a sudden emotion;
sometimes I retouch them the next day, sometimes not.

When finally, after six months, a year, or even two, I submit the
results to Sartre, I am not yet satisfied, but I feel I'm at the end of my
tether; I need his severity and his encouragement to revive my en-
ergies. First of all he reassures me: "You've done it . . . It will be a
good book." And then little things begin to annoy him: it's too long,
too short, that's not right, that's badly expressed, it's a mess, it's
hopeless. If I weren't accustomed to his harsh way of putting things—
mine is no softer when I'm criticizing him—I would be utterly
crushed. As a matter of fact, the only time he really made me feel
uneasy was when I was finishing *The Mandarins;* ordinarily his criticisms stimulate me because they show me how I can improve the
defects I am already more or less aware of, and which often jump out
and hit me in the face as soon as he begins reading a book. He
suggests cuts and changes; but most of all he urges me to go further,
to go deeper, to face up to obstacles instead of trying to get around
them. His advice is always directed the way I myself want to go, and
then I need only a few weeks, or a few months at most, to give the
book its final shape. I stop when I have the impression, not of course
that the book is perfect, but that I can't do any more with it.

In the years I am describing, I took a great many vacations; that
means, generally speaking, that I went and worked somewhere else.
However, I did go on long journeys during which I did not write.
That is because my desire to know the world is closely linked with
my desire to express it. My curiosity is less barbaric than it was when
I was young, but it is still almost as demanding: one never stops
learning because there is never any end to ignorance. I do not mean
to imply that no moment is ever gratuitous for me; no instant has
ever seemed wasted if it brought me a pleasure. But through the
dispersion of my occupations, my diversions and my wanderings,
there is a constant desire to add to my store of knowledge.

The further I go, the more the world fills my life to the bursting
point. To tell it, I need a dozen registers and a pedal to sustain the
feelings—melancholy, joy, disgust—that have colored whole periods of
it, through the heart's intermittences. Every moment reflects my
past, my body, my relations with others, the tasks I have undertaken,
the society I live in, the whole of this earth; linked together, and
independent, these realities sometimes reinforce each other and

descant together, sometimes they interfere with, contradict, or neutralize each other. If their totality does not remain always present, I
shall say nothing exact. Even if I surmount this difficulty, I stumble
over others. A life is such a strange object, at one moment trans-
lucent, at another utterly opaque, an object I make with my own
hands, an object imposed on me, an object for which the world provides the raw material and then steals it from me again, pulverized by
events, scattered, broken, scored yet retaining its unity; how heavy it
is and how inconsistent: this contradiction breeds many misunderstandings. I was not as shaken by the war as I claim, some have said,
since in 1941 I was enjoying going for walks; some will say, no doubt,
that I was little affected by the war in Algeria because Rome, because
music, because certain books still held their attraction for me. But,
and everyone must have experienced this, it is possible to be amused
even as the heart mourns. The most violent, the most sincere emotion does not last; sometimes it instigates action, engenders obses-
sions, but it disappears. On the other hand an anxiety, temporarily
laid aside, does not cease to exist: it is present in the very care I take
to avoid it. Words are often no more than silence, and silence has its
voices. During the time Sartre was a prisoner, was I unhappy, or still
happy? I was as I have described myself, with my moments of gaiety,
my anxieties, my discouragements, my hopes. I have tried to capture
reality in its diversity and its fluidity; to summarize my story in final
words is as aberrant as to translate a good poem into prose.

The background, tragic or serene, against which my experiences
are drawn gives them their true meaning and constitutes their unity;
I have avoided linking them by transitions that would be unequivocal, hence artificial. Yet if this ever-present totality seems so necessary
to me, why have I subjected myself to chronological order instead of
choosing some other construction? I have pondered this matter, and
I have hesitated. But what counts above all in my life is that time
goes by; I grow older, the world changes, my relation with it varies;
to show the transformations, the ripenings, the irreversible deteriora-
tions of others and of myself—nothing is more important to me than
that. And that obliges me to follow obediently the thread the years
have unwound.

So that after this interlude I take up my story at the point where
I had left it.